PRAISE FOR THE
Insider's Guide to
Graduate Programs in Clinical and
Counseling Psychology

"The process of applying for admission to graduate programs in clinical and counseling psychology can be daunting. This valuable resource guides individuals through the process.... Recommended."
—*Choice*

"The authors have created a valuable guide for applicants. The wealth of practical information and insights gleaned from their research and personal experiences should help applicants make the strongest possible application to the schools of their choice. This well-written, encouraging book will be a great asset for anyone applying to clinical or counseling psychology programs."   —Barry A. Hong, Ph.D., **Washington University School of Medicine**

"Anyone considering applying to a graduate program in clinical or counseling psychology would be advised to consult this book, even if the application is a few years away."
—*American Reference Books Annual*

"Students need to realize that the *Insider's Guide* is much more than a shopping list of statistics about programs to be picked up before sending off the first wave of applications. In fact, this is a resource that all students seriously considering careers in professional psychology will find valuable as soon as they declare their major."
—Bryan D. Fantie, Ph.D., **Director of Behavioral Neuroscience, American University**

"*Insider's Guide to Graduate Programs in Clinical and Counseling Psychology* is a significant reference and an excellent comprehensive guide that will be useful to students, trainees, psychologists, libraries, and department offices in psychology, education, and other related areas of career mentorship."   —*APA PsycCRITIQUES*

"Your book is simply a godsend! I found it to be instructive, informative, and a great comfort."
—Emily M. Douglas, psychology undergraduate

INSIDER'S GUIDE TO
GRADUATE PROGRAMS
IN CLINICAL AND
COUNSELING PSYCHOLOGY

INSIDER'S GUIDE to

Graduate Programs in Clinical and Counseling Psychology

2008/2009 Edition

John C. Norcross
Michael A. Sayette
Tracy J. Mayne

THE GUILFORD PRESS
New York   London

© 2008 The Guilford Press
A Division of Guilford Publications, Inc.
72 Spring Street, New York, NY 10012
www.guilford.com

Printed in the United States of America

Last digit is print number: 9 8 7 6 5 4 3 2 1

ISBN-10: 1-59385-637-7
ISBN-13: 978-1-59385-637-3

ISSN 1086-2099

CONTENTS

CONTENTS

TABLES AND FIGURES

ABOUT THE AUTHORS

John C. Norcross received his baccalaureate *summa cum laude* from Rutgers University. He earned his master's and doctorate in clinical psychology from the University of Rhode Island and completed his internship at the Brown University School of Medicine. He is Professor of Psychology and Distinguished University Fellow at the University of Scranton, a clinical psychologist in independent practice, and editor of the *Journal of Clinical Psychology: In Session.* He is president-elect of the American Psychological Association's Society of Clinical Psychology and past-president of the APA Division of Psychotherapy. Dr. Norcross has published more than 250 articles and has authored or edited 16 books, the most recent being *Leaving It at the Office: A Guide to Psychotherapist Self-Care, Clinician's Guide to Evidence-Based Practice in Mental Health, Authoritative Guide to Self-Help Resources in Mental Health,* and *Psychotherapy Relationships That Work.* Among his awards are the Pennsylvania Professor of the Year from the Carnegie Foundation, Distinguished Practitioner from the National Academies of Practice, and the Distinguished Career Contribution to Education and Training Award from the American Psychological Association. Dr. Norcross has conducted workshops and research on graduate study in psychology for many years.

Michael A. Sayette received his baccalaureate *cum laude* from Dartmouth College. He earned his master's and doctorate in clinical psychology from Rutgers University and completed his internship at the Brown University School of Medicine. He is Professor of Psychology at the University of Pittsburgh, with a secondary appointment as Professor of Psychiatry at the Western Psychiatric Institute and Clinic, University of Pittsburgh School of Medicine. Dr. Sayette has published primarily in the area of substance abuse. His research, supported by the National Institute on Alcohol Abuse and Alcoholism and by the National Institute on Drug Abuse, concerns the development of psychological theories of alcohol and tobacco use. He has served on National Institutes of Health grant review study sections and is on the editorial boards of several journals. He also is an associate editor of *Journal of Abnormal Psychology* and a former associate editor of *Psychology of Addictive Behaviors.* Dr. Sayette has directed graduate admissions for the clinical psychology program at the University of Pittsburgh, and has presented seminars on applying to graduate school at several universities in North America and Europe.

Tracy J. Mayne received his baccalaureate from the State University of New York at Buffalo, where he graduated *magna cum laude* and *Phi Beta Kappa.* He received his Ph.D. as an Honors Fellow from Rutgers University and completed his internship and postdoctoral fellowship at the University of California at San Francisco Medical School and the Center for AIDS Prevention Studies. He spent two years as an international scholar at the Institut Nationale de la Santé et de la Recherche Médicale in France and three years as the Director of HIV Epidemiology and Surveillance at the New York City Department of Health, where he received the Commissioner's Award for Outstanding Community Research. Dr. Mayne spent five years conducting research in cardiovascular medicine at Pfizer Pharmaceuticals and currently works in Global Health Economics at Amgen Inc., conducting research in cancer-supportive therapies. Dr. Mayne has published numerous articles and chapters in the area of health psychology, health economics, and emotion, and is the coeditor of the book *Emotions: Current Issues and Future Directions.*

ACKNOWLEDGMENTS

To paraphrase John Donne, no book is an island, entire of itself. This sentiment is particularly true of a collaborative venture such as ours: a coauthored volume in its tenth edition comprising the contributions of hundreds of psychologists and of reports on doctoral programs provided by training directors throughout North America. We are grateful to them all.

We are also indebted to the many friends, colleagues, and workshop participants for their assistance in improving this book over the years. Special thanks to Jeannette Ellis, who collected and organized data on individual program reports, as well as Krystle Evans for conducting data analysis for this edition. William Burke, Director of Financial Aid at the University of Scranton, updates our sections on financial aid and loan options every two years. Seymour Weingarten and his associates at The Guilford Press have continued to provide interpersonal support and technical assistance on all aspects of the project. Special thanks to our families for their unflagging support and patience with late night work!

Finally, our efforts have been aided immeasurably by our students, graduate and undergraduate alike, who courageously shared their experiences with us about the application and admission process.

PREFACE

One of the benefits of applying to clinical and counseling psychology programs is that you earn the right to commiserate about it afterwards. It was a night of anecdotes and complaints (while doing laundry) that led us to review our travails and compare notes on the difficulties we each experienced during the admission process. We emerged from three diverse backgrounds: one of us (T. J. M.) graduated from a large state university, took time off, and then entered a doctoral program; one of us (M. A. S.) graduated from a private liberal arts college and immediately pursued a doctorate; and another one of us (J. C. N.) graduated from a liberal arts college within a major state university after 5 years and then pursued doctoral studies.

Although we approached graduate school in different ways, the process was much the same. We each attempted to locate specific information on clinical and counseling psychology admissions, looked to people around us for advice, took that which seemed to be sound, and worked with it. Not all the advice was good (one professor went so far as to suggest a career in the theater instead!), and it was difficult to decide what was best when advice conflicted.

All in all, there was too little factual information available and too much unnecessary anxiety involved. No clearly defined or organized system was available to guide us through this process. So we decided to write an *Insider's Guide to Graduate Programs in Clinical and Counseling Psychology*. That was 10 editions, 20 years, and 100,000 copies ago.

The last dozen years have seen the entire process of choosing schools and applying become progressively more difficult. Approximately 76,000 bachelor's degrees are awarded every year in psychology, and about 20% of the recipients go on to earn a master's or doctoral degree in psychology. Clinical and counseling psychology programs continue to grow in number and to diversify in mission: 232 APA-accredited doctoral programs in clinical psychology, 67 APA-accredited doctoral programs in counseling psychology, 10 APA-accredited programs in combined psychology, dozens of non-APA-accredited doctoral programs, and hundreds of master's programs.

How should you prepare for admission into these graduate programs? Which should you apply to? And which type of program is best for you—counseling or clinical, practice-oriented Psy.D. or research-oriented Ph.D.? We will take you step by step through this confusing morass and help you make informed decisions suited to your needs and interests.

In clear and concise language, we assist *you* through this process, from the initial decision to apply through your final acceptance. In Chapter 1, we describe the predominant training models in clinical and counseling psychology and alternatives to these disciplines. In the next chapter, we discuss the essential preparation for graduate school—the course work, faculty mentoring, clinical experiences, research skills, entrance examinations, and extracurricular activities. From there, in Chapter 3, we get you started on the application process and assist you in understanding admission requirements. In Chapter 4, we show you how to systematically select schools on the basis of multiple considerations, especially research interests, clinical opportunities, theoretical orientations, financial assistance, and quality of life. Then, in Chapter 5, we take you through the application procedure itself—forms, curricula vitae, personal statements, letters of recommendation, academic transcripts, and the like. In Chapter 6, we review the perils and promises of the interview, required by three-quarters of clinical and counseling psychology programs. Last, in Chapter 7, we walk you through the complexities of the final decisions. With multiple worksheets and concrete examples, we will help you feel less overwhelmed, better informed, and, in the end, more aware that *you* are the consumer of a program that best suits *your* needs.

In this new edition, we provide:

- Listings of each program's concentrations and speciality tracks (Appendix G)
- Updates on financial assistance and government-sponsored loans
- Discussion of APA's decision to discontinue its accreditation of Canadian programs
- Enhanced coverage of acceptance rates
- Data on each program's attrition (dropout) rate
- A section for applicants with disabilities

In addition, we describe how you can capitalize on the Internet revolution to ease the graduate school admissions process—locating compatible programs, communicating with potential faculty mentors, submitting application forms, and helping faculty send letters of recommendation electronically. We also provide specific advice for racial/ethnic minority and lesbian, gay, bisexual, and transgendered (LGBT) applicants. Throughout the book, we provide Web sites to access for additional information and direction.

We have conducted original studies on graduate psychology programs for this book in an effort to inform your decision making. These results provide information on the differences between clinical and counseling psychology (Chapter 1), the distinctions between Ph.D. and Psy.D. programs (Chapter 1), the importance of various graduate school selection criteria (Chapter 2), acceptance rates (Chapter 3), the probability of financial assistance (Chapter 4), interview policies (Chapter 6), research areas (Appendix E), clinical and practica sites (Appendix F), and more. Indeed, we have extensively surveyed all APA-accredited programs in clinical, counseling, and combined psychology for 20 years now and present detailed information on each in the Reports on Individual Programs. A detailed Time Line (Appendix A) and multiple worksheets (Appendices B, C, and D) also provide assistance on the heretofore treacherous journey of applying to graduate programs in clinical and counseling psychology.

This volume will assist anyone seeking admission to graduate school in clinical and counseling psychology, both master's and doctoral degrees. However, the primary focus is on Ph.D. and Psy.D. applicants, as the doctorate is the entry-level qualification for professional psychology. Just as a master's degree in biology does not make one a physician, a master's in psychology does not, by state licensure and APA regulation, typically qualify one as a psychologist. Forty-eight states require the doctorate for licensure or certification as a psychologist; almost half the states grant legal recognition of psychological associates, assistants, or examiners with a master's degree (APA Practice Directorate, 1999). But the material presented here is relevant for master's (M.A. or M.S.) applicants as well.

With this practical manual, we wish you an application process less hectic and confusing than ours, but equally rewarding in the end result. Good luck!

CHAPTER 1

INTRODUCING CLINICAL AND COUNSELING PSYCHOLOGY

If you are reading this book for the first time, we assume you are either considering applying to graduate programs in clinical and counseling psychology or are in the process of doing so. For even the best-prepared applicant, this can precipitate a great deal of stress and confusion. The mythology surrounding this process is foreboding, and you may have heard some "horror" stories similar to these: "It's the hardest graduate program to get into in the country"; "You need a 3.7 grade point average and 650s on your GREs or they won't even look at you"; "If you haven't taken time off after your bachelor's degree and worked in a clinic, you don't have enough experience to apply."

Having endured the application process ourselves, we know how overwhelming the task appears at first glance. However, we have found that much of the anxiety is unwarranted. It does not take astronomical test scores or years of practical experience to get into clinical and counseling psychology programs. Although these qualifications certainly help, they are not sufficient. Equally important are a knowledge of how the system works and a willingness to put in extra effort during the application process. In other words, in this book, we will help you to work smarter and work harder in getting into graduate school.

Clinical and Counseling Psychology

Before dealing with the question of "how to apply," we would like to address "why" to apply and what clinical and counseling psychology entail. Reading through the next section may be useful by making you aware of other programs of study that may better suit your needs.

Let us begin with clinical psychology, the largest specialty and the fastest growing sector in psychology. Two-thirds of the doctoral-level health service providers in the American Psychological Association (APA) identify with the specialty area of clinical psychology (VandenBos, Stapp, & Kilburg, 1981). A census of all psychological personnel residing in the United States likewise revealed that the majority reported clinical psychology as their major field (Stapp, Tucker, & Vanden-Bos, 1985).

A definition of clinical psychology was adopted jointly by the APA Division of Clinical Psychology and the Council of University Directors of Clinical Psychology (Resnick, 1991). That definition states that the field of clinical psychology involves research, teaching, and services relevant to understanding, predicting, and alleviating intellectual, emotional, biological, psychological, social, and behavioral maladjustment, applied to a wide range of client populations. The major skill areas essential to clinical psychology are assessment, intervention, consultation, program development and evaluation, supervision, administration, conduct of research, and application of ethical standards. Perhaps the safest observation about clinical psychology is that both the field and its practitioners continue to outgrow the classic definitions.

Indeed, the discipline has experienced a veritable explosion since World War II in numbers, activities, and knowledge. Since 1949, the year of the Boulder Conference (see below), there has been a large and significant increase in psychology doctoral graduates. Approximately 2,400 doctoral degrees are now awarded annually in clinical psychology—1,400 Ph.D. degrees and 1,000 Psy.D. degrees. All told, doctoral

TABLE 1-1. Popularity and Doctorate Production of Psychology Subfields

Subfield	% of doctoral-level psychologists	Number of Ph.D.s awarded		
		1976	1994	2002
Clinical	44%	883	1329	1312
Cognitive	1%	—	76	121
Counseling	11%	267	464	536
Developmental	4%	190	158	173
Educational	6%	124	98	54
Experimental & physiological	3%	357	143	201
Industrial/organizational	6%	73	124	154
Quantitative	2%	27	23	22
School	5%	143	81	89
Social and personality	4%	271	165	197
Other or general	12%	387	560	438
Total	100%	2,883	3,287	3,199[a]

Note. Data from Stapp, Tucker, & VandenBos (1985) and National Research Council (selected years).

[a]Plus 1,000 Psy.D. degrees awarded annually.

degrees in clinical psychology account for about 48% of all psychology doctorates (Norcross et al., 2005). Table 1-1 demonstrates the continuing popularity of clinical psychology and the growing number of clinical doctorates awarded annually.

These trends should continue well into the future. After a drop in the early 1980s, the percentage of psychology majors among college freshmen has continued to increase nationally to over 3%. In fact, the proportion of college freshmen who explicitly express an intention of becoming clinical psychologists has risen to 1.3% (Astin, Green, & Korn, 1987). A nationwide survey of almost 2 million high school juniors, reported in the *Occupational Outlook Quarterly,* found that psychology was the sixth most frequent career choice. Indeed, according to data from the U.S. Department of Education, interest in psychology as a major has never been higher (Murray, 1996). So, if you are seriously considering clinical or counseling psychology for a career, you belong to a large, vibrant, and growing population.

Counseling psychology is the second largest specialty in psychology and another rapidly growing sector. As also shown in Table 1-1, counseling psychology has experienced sustained growth over the past three decades. We are referring here to counseling *psychology,* the doctoral-level specialization in psychology, not to the master's-level profession of counseling. This is a critical distinction: our book and research studies pertain specifically and solely to counseling psychology programs, not counseling programs.

The distinctions between clinical psychology and counseling psychology have steadily faded. Graduates of counseling psychology programs are eligible for the same professional benefits as clinical psychology graduates, such as psychology licensure, independent practice, and insurance reimbursement. The APA ceased distinguishing many years ago between clinical and counseling psychology internships: there is one list of accredited internships for both clinical and counseling psychology students. Both types of programs prepare doctoral-level psychologists who provide health care services.

At the same time, five robust differences between clinical psychology and counseling psychology are still visible (Morgan & Cohen, 2003; Norcross et al., 1998). First, clinical psychology is larger than counseling psychology: in 2007, there were 232 active APA-accredited doctoral programs in clinical psychology and 67 active APA-accredited doctoral programs in counseling psychology (APA, 2006) currently accepting students. Table 1-1 reveals that these counseling psychology programs—in addition to some unaccredited programs —produce about 500 doctoral degrees per year. By contrast, clinical psychology programs produce approximately 2,400 doctoral degrees (1,400 Ph.D. and 1,000 Psy.D.) per year. Second, clinical psychology graduate programs are almost exclusively housed in departments or schools of psychology, whereas counseling psychology graduate programs are located in a variety of departments and divisions. Our research (Turkson & Norcross, 1996) shows that, in rough figures, one-quarter of doctoral programs in counseling psychology are located in psychology departments, one-quarter in departments of counseling psychology, one-quarter in departments or colleges of education, and one-quarter in assorted other departments. The historical placement of counseling psychology programs in education departments explains the occasional awarding of the Ed.D. (doctor of education) by counseling psychology programs.

A third difference is that clinical psychology graduates tend to work with more seriously disturbed patients and are more likely trained in projective assessment, whereas counseling graduates work with healthier, less pathological patients and conduct more career and vocational assessment. Fourth, counseling psychologists more frequently endorse a client-centered/Rogerian approach to psychotherapy, whereas clinical psychologists are more likely to embrace behavioral or psychodynamic orientations. And fifth, both APA figures (APA Research Office, 1997) and our research (Bechtoldt, Norcross, Wyckoff, Pokrywa, & Campbell, 2001) consistently reveal that 15% more clinical psychologists are employed in full-time private practice than are counseling psychologists, whereas 10% more counseling psychologists are employed in college counseling centers than are clinical psychologists. Studies on the roles and functions of clinical and counseling psychologists substantiate these differences, but the similarities are far more numerous (Brems & Johnson, 1997; Fitzgerald & Osipow, 1986; Watkins, Lopez, Campbell, & Himmel, 1986a, 1986b).

In order to extend this previous research, we conducted a study of APA-accredited doctoral programs in counseling psychology (95% response rate) and clinical psychology (99% response rate) regarding their number of applications, characteristics of incoming students, and research areas of the faculty (Norcross, Sayette, Mayne, Karg, & Turkson, 1998). We found:

- The average acceptance rates of Ph.D. clinical (6%) and Ph.D. counseling (8%) psychology programs were quite similar despite the higher number of applications to clinical programs (270 vs. 130).
- The average grade point averages (GPAs) and GRE scores for incoming doctoral students were nearly identical in Ph.D. clinical and Ph.D. counseling psychology programs (3.5 for both).
- The counseling psychology programs accepted more ethnic minority students (25% vs. 18%) and

master's students (67% vs. 21%) than the clinical psychology programs.
- The counseling psychology faculty were far more interested than clinical psychology faculty in research pertaining to minority/cross-cultural issues (69% vs. 32% of programs) and vocational/career testing (62% vs. 1% of programs).
- The clinical psychology faculty, in turn, were far more interested than the counseling psychology faculty in research pertaining to psychopathological populations (e.g., attention deficit disorders, depression, personality disorders) and activities traditionally associated with medical settings (e.g., neuropsychology, pain management, pediatric psychology).

Please bear in mind that these systematic comparisons reflect broad differences in the APA-accredited Ph.D. programs; they say nothing about Psy.D. programs (which we discuss later in this chapter) or nonaccredited programs. Also bear in mind that these data can be used as a rough guide in matching your interests to clinical or counseling psychology programs. The notion of discovering the best match between you and a graduate program is a recurrent theme of this *Insider's Guide*.

As shown in Table 1-2, clinical and counseling psychologists devote similar percentages of their day to the same professional activities. About one-half of their time is dedicated to psychotherapy and assessment and a quarter of their time to research and administration. A stunning finding was that over half of clinical and counseling psychologists were routinely involved in all seven activities—psychotherapy, assessment, teaching, research, supervision, consultation, and administration. Flexible career indeed!

The scope of clinical and counseling psychology is continually widening, as are the employment settings. Many people mistakenly view psychologists solely as practitioners who spend most of their time seeing patients. But in truth, clinical and counseling psychology are wonderfully diverse and pluralistic professions. Consider the employment settings of American clinical psychologists: 40% in private practices, 19% in universities or colleges, 5% in psychiatric hospitals, 9% in medical schools, 4% in general hospitals, another 5% in community mental health centers, 4% in outpatient clinics, and 11% in "other" placements (Norcross, Karg, & Prochaska, 1997a, 1997b). This last category included, just to name a few, child and family services, correctional facilities, rehabilitation centers, school systems, health maintenance organizations, psychoanalytic institutes, and the federal government.

TABLE 1-2. Professional Activities of Clinical and Counseling Psychologists

Activity	Clinical psychologists		Counseling psychologists	
	% involved in	Average % of time	% involved in	Average % of time
Psychotherapy	80	34	74	28
Diagnosis/assessment	64	15	62	12
Teaching	50	10	60	18
Clinical supervision	50	6	54	6
Research/writing	51	14	50	8
Consultation	47	7	61	7
Administration	53	13	56	15

Note. Data from Norcross, Karpiak, & Santoro (2005) and Watkins, Campbell, & Himmell (1986a).

Although many psychologists choose careers as clinicians in private practice, hospitals, and clinics, a large number also pursue careers in research. For some, this translates into an academic position. Uncertainties in the health care system increase the allure of academic positions, where salaries are less tied to client fees. Academics teach courses and conduct research, usually with a clinical population. They hope to find a "tenure-track" position, which means they start out as an assistant professor. After a certain amount of time (typically 5 or 6 years), a university committee reviews their research, teaching, and service, and decides whether they will be hired as a permanent faculty member and promoted to associate professor. Even though the tenure process can be pressured, the atmosphere surrounding assistant professors is very conducive to research activity. They are often given "seed" money to set up facilities and attract graduate students eager to share in the publication process. (For additional information on the career paths of psychology faculty, consult *The Psychologist's Guide to an Academic Career,* Rheingold, 1994, or *Career Paths in Psychology,* Sternberg, 2006.)

In addition, research-focused industries (like pharmaceutical and biomedical), as well as community-based organizations, are increasingly employing psychologists to design and conduct outcomes research. The field of outcomes research combines the use of assessment, testing, program design, and cost-effectiveness analyses within contexts as varied as clinical trials and community interventions. Although lacking the job security of tenure, industry can offer greater monetary compensation and is a viable option for research-oriented PhDs.

But even this range of primary employment settings does not accurately capture the opportunities in the field. About half of all clinical and counseling psychologists hold more than one professional position (Norcross et al., 1997a; Watkins et al., 1986a). By and large, psychologists incorporate several pursuits into their work, often simultaneously. They combine activities in ways that can change over time to accommodate their evolving interests. Of those psychologists not in full-time private practice, over half engage in some part-time independent work (Norcross et al., 1997b). Without question, this flexibility is an asset.

As a university professor, for example, you might run a research group studying aspects of alcoholism, treat alcoholics and their families in private practice, and teach a course on alcohol abuse. Or, you could work for a company supervising marketing research, do private testing for a school system, and provide monthly seminars on relaxation. The possibilities are almost limitless.

This flexibility is also evident in clinical and counseling psychologists' "self-views." About 60% respond that they are primarily clinical practitioners, 20% are academicians, 7% administrators, 5% researchers, 5% consultants, and 2% supervisors (Norcross et al., 1997b; Watkins et al., 1986a).

Also comforting is the consistent finding of relatively high and stable satisfaction with graduate training and career choice. Over two-thirds of graduate students in clinical and counseling psychology express satisfaction with their post-baccalaureate preparation. Moreover, 87 to 91% are satisfied with their career choice (Norcross et al., 2005; Tibbits-Kleber & Howell, 1987). The conclusion we draw is that clinical and counseling psychologists appreciate the diverse pursuits and revel in their professional flexibility, which figure prominently in their high level of career satisfaction.

According to *Money* magazine and Salary.com, psychologist is one of the 10 best jobs in America. And so, too, is college professor.

Combined Programs

APA accredits doctoral programs in four areas: clinical psychology, counseling psychology, school psychology, and combined psychology. The last category is for those programs that afford doctoral training in two or more of the specialties of clinical, counseling, and school psychology.

The "combined" doctoral programs represent a relatively new development in graduate psychology training, and thus are relatively small in number, about 3% of APA-accredited programs. In emphasizing the core research and practice competencies among the specialties, combined programs try to enlist their respective strengths and to capitalize on their overarching competencies. In doing so, the hope is that a combined program will be "greater than the sum of its parts" (Salzinger, 1998). For students undecided about a particular specialty in professional psychology and seeking broad clinical training, these accredited combined programs warrant a close look.

The chief reasons that students select combined doctoral programs are for greater breadth and flexibility of training and for more opportunity of integrative training across specializations. The emphasis on breadth of psychological knowledge ensures that combined training will address the multiplicity of interests that many students have and that many psychologists will need in practice (Beutler & Fisher, 1994). The chief disadvantages of combined programs are, first, their lack of depth and specialization and, second, the fact that other mental health professionals may not understand the combined degree. Our research on combined training programs (Castle & Norcross, 2002; Cobb, Reeve, Shealy, Norcross, et al., 2004) does, in fact, substantiate the broader training and more varied employment of their graduates. Consult the Reports of Combined Programs at the end of this book for details on these innovative programs. Also consult two special issues of the *Journal of Clinical Psychology* (Shealy, 2004) on the combined-integrative model of doctoral training in professional psychology.

The Boulder Model (Ph.D.)

The diversity in professional activities has produced a diversity of training models in professional psychology. Without a firm understanding of the differences in these training models, many applicants will waste valuable time and needlessly experience disappointment. Let us now distinguish between the two prevalent training models in clinical psychology—the Boulder model and the Vail model. Combined programs and counseling psychology have parallel differences in training emphases, however, they do not typically employ the same terms as clinical psychology and offer only a handful of Psy.D. degrees.

The first national training conference on clinical psychology was held during 1949 in Boulder, Colorado (hence, the "Boulder model"). At this conference, equal weight was accorded to the development of research competencies and clinical skills. This dual emphasis resulted in the notion of the clinical psychologist as a *scientist–practitioner*. Clinical psychologists were considered first and foremost as scientists and were to have a rigorous, broad-based education in psychology. Their training would encompass statistics, history and systems, and research, with core courses in development, biopsychology, learning, and the like. The emphasis was on psychology; clinical was the adjective.

The Boulder conference was a milestone for several reasons. First, it established the Ph.D. as the required degree, as in other academic research fields. To this day, all Boulder model, scientist–practitioner programs in clinical psychology award the Ph.D. degree. Second, the conference reinforced the idea that the appropriate location for training was within university departments, not separate schools or institutes as in medicine and law. And third, clinical psychologists were trained for simultaneous existence in two worlds: academic/scientific and clinical/professional.

The important implication for you, as an applicant, is to know that Boulder-model programs provide rigorous education as a researcher along with training as a clinician. Consider this dual thrust carefully before applying to Boulder-model programs. Some first-year graduate students undergo undue misery because they dislike research-oriented courses and the research projects that are part of the degree requirements. These, in turn, lead to the formal dissertation required by Boulder-model programs. Many applicants are specifically seeking this sort of training.

A recent movement toward a "bolder" Boulder model was crystallized by the 1995 creation of the Academy of Psychological Clinical Science (APCS). According to its Web site, APCS is "an alliance of leading, scientifically oriented, doctoral training programs in clinical and health psychology, committed to empirical approaches to advancing knowledge." "The Academy seeks as members those programs that are strongly

TABLE 1-3. APA-Accredited Clinical Psychology Programs That Are Members of the Academy of Psychological Clinical Science (APCS)

University of Arizona	University of Nevada–Reno
Arizona State University	Ohio State University
Boston University	University of Oregon
University of California–Berkeley	University of Pennsylvania
University of California–Los Angeles	Pennsylvania State University
University of California–San Diego	University of Pittsburgh
University of Delaware	Purdue University
University of Denver	Rutgers University
Duke University	San Diego State University
Emory University	University of Southern California
Florida State University	University of South Florida
University of Hawaii	State University of New York–Binghamton
University of Illinois at Urbana Champaign	State University of New York–Stony Brook
Indiana University	University of Texas
University of Iowa	University of Toronto
University of Kentucky	Vanderbilt University
University of Maryland	Virginia Tech
McGill University	University of Virginia
University of Memphis	University of Washington
University of Miami	Washington University–St. Louis
University of Minnesota	University of Wisconsin
University of Missouri	Yale University

committed to research training and to the integration of such training with clinical training." APCS includes 44 clinical psychology Ph.D. programs. These programs are listed in Table 1-3. More information on APCS can be found on their Web site: w3.arizona.edu/~psych/apcs/apcs.html.

Based on the data from our previous editions of the *Insider's Guide* we found that, compared to non-member programs, APCS programs admit a slightly lower percentage of applicants (who had higher GRE scores) and were more likely to provide full financial support. APCS programs also subscribe more frequently to a cognitive-behavioral orientation, report a stronger research emphasis, and engage more frequently in research supported by funding agencies than non-APCS programs (Sayette, Mayne, Norcross, & Giuffre, 1999). Students interested in a Boulder-model clinical Ph.D program may find these programs to be especially attractive in that they represent evidence-based, research-focused training.

Other applicants are seeking training focused on clinical practice. For these applicants, there is an alter-native to the Boulder model: the Vail model of training psychologists.

The Vail Model (Psy.D.)

Some dissension with the recommendations of the Boulder conference emerged at later meetings; however, there was a strong consensus that the scientist–practitioner model, Ph.D. degree, and university training should be retained. But in the late 1960s and early 1970s, change was in the wind. Training alternatives were entertained, and diversification was encouraged. This sentiment culminated in a 1973 national training conference held in Vail, Colorado (hence, the "Vail model").

The Vail conferees endorsed different principles than the Boulder model, leading to a diversity of training programs (Peterson, 1976, 1982). Psychological knowledge, it was argued, had matured enough to warrant creation of explicitly professional programs along the lines of professional programs in medicine, dentistry, and law. These "professional programs" were to be added to, not replace, Boulder-model programs. Further, it was proposed that different degrees should be used to designate the scientist role (Ph.D.—Doctor of Philosophy) from the practitioner role (Psy.D.—Doctor of Psychology). Graduates of Vail-model professional programs would be *scholar–professionals:* the focus would be primarily on practice and less on research.

This revolutionary conference led to the emergence of two distinct training models typically housed in different settings. Boulder-model, Ph.D. programs are almost universally located in graduate departments of large universities. However, Vail-model programs can be housed in three organizational settings: within a psychology department; within a university-affiliated psychology school (for instance, Rutgers and Adelphi universities); and within an independent, "freestanding" university (e.g., Alliant University, Argosy University). These latter programs are part of independent institutions, some of which are run as for-profit companies. Although they are titled "universities," they are frequently not comprehensive universities offering degrees in dozens of subjects. Rather, they only offer degrees in a handful of subjects and thus not "universities" in the traditional sense of comprehensive universities.

Table 1-4 lists APA-accredited clinical Psy.D. programs. (For a listing of non-accredited Psy.D. programs, see www.apadiv2.org/otrp/resources/brynolf07psyd .pdf)

Clinical psychology now has two established and complementary training models. The Ph.D. programs together produce approximately 1.2 times as many doctoral-level psychologists per year as Psy.D. programs collectively. Although Boulder-model programs still outnumber Vail-model programs, Vail-model programs enroll, as a rule, three to four times the number of incoming doctoral candidates. This creates almost a numerical parity in terms of psychologists produced.

Several studies have demonstrated that initial worries about stigmatization, employment difficulties, licensure uncertainty, and second-class citizenship for Psy.D.s have *not* materialized (see Hershey, Kopplin, & Cornell, 1991; Peterson, Eaton, Levine, & Snepp, 1982). There do not appear to be strong disparities in the pre-internship clinical skills of Ph.D. and Psy.D. students as evaluated by internship supervisors (Snepp & Peterson, 1988). Nor are there discernible differences in employment except, of course, that the more research-oriented, Boulder-model graduates are far more likely to be employed in academic positions and medical schools (Gaddy, et al., 1995). While Vail-

model graduates may be seen as second-class citizens by some Boulder-model traditionalists, this is not the case among health care organizations or individual patients.

Which training model do clinical psychologists themselves prefer? In one of our studies (Norcross, Gallagher, & Prochaska, 1989), we found that 50% favored the Boulder model, 14% the Vail model, and the remaining 36% both models equally. However, preferences varied as a function of the psychologist's own doctoral program: 93% of the psychologists trained in a strong Boulder tradition preferred the Boulder model or both equally. Likewise, 90% of the psychologists trained in a strong Vail tradition preferred the Vail model or both equally. In short, psychologists preferred the training model to which they applied and in which they completed their training.

Differences between Boulder and Vail Programs

The differences between Boulder-model and Vail-model programs are quantitative, not qualitative. The primary disparity lies in the relative emphasis on research: Boulder programs aspire to train producers of research; Vail programs train consumers of research. Even Vail programs require research and statistics courses; you simply cannot avoid research sophistication in any accredited psychology program. The practice opportunities are very similar for students in both types of programs.

At the same time, as we discuss in subsequent chapters, there are important trade-offs between Vail-model and Boulder-model programs. Here are 7 differences to bear in mind as you read through our book and as you become an informed consumer.

1. *Research skills.* Vail-model, Psy.D. programs provide slightly more clinical experience and courses but less research experience and courses than do Boulder-model programs (Tibbits-Kleber & Howell, 1987). Psy.D. programs typically require a clinical dissertation, substantially less than an original research dissertation required by Ph.D. programs. An important caveat: if you desire to teach full time at a 4-year college or university, we strongly advise you *not* to seek the Psy.D. degree. The Psy.D. is an explicitly professional or practitioner degree; your training and expertise will be as a practitioner, not as a professor, researcher, or academician.

2. *Length of training,* The additional research training and the large dissertation required in Boulder-

TABLE 1-4. APA-Accredited Psy.D. Programs in Clinical Psychology

Adler School of Professional Psychology	Indiana State University
Alliant International University–Fresno[a]	Indiana University of Pennsylvania
Alliant International University–Los Angeles[a]	University of Indianapolis
Alliant International University–San Diego[a]	John F. Kennedy University
Alliant International University–San Francisco Bay[a]	La Salle University
Antioch University New England	University of La Verne
Argosy University, Atlanta Campus	Loma Linda University[a]
Argosy University, Chicago Campus	Long Island University/C.W. Post Campus
Argosy University, Honolulu Campus	Loyola College in Maryland
Argosy University, Phoenix Campus	Marshall University
Argosy University, San Francisco Campus	Marywood University
Argosy University, Schaumberg Campus	Massachusetts School of Professional Psychology
Argosy University, Tampa Campus	Nova Southeastern University[a]
Argosy University, Twin Cities Campus	Pacific Graduate School of Psychology/Stanford
Argosy University, Washington, DC Campus	University Consortium
Azusa Pacific University	Pacific University
Baylor University	Pepperdine University
Biola University[a]	Philadelphia College of Osteopathic Medicine
California Institute of Integral Studies	Ponce School of Medicine
Carlos Albizu University–Miami Campus	Regent University
Carlos Albizu University–San Juan Campus[a]	Roosevelt University
Chestnut Hill College	Rutgers University[a]
Chicago School of Professional Psychology	Spalding University
University of Denver[a]	Virginia Consortium in Clinical Psychology
Florida Institute of Technology	Wheaton College
Forest Institute of Professional Psychology	Widener University
Fuller Theological Seminary[a]	The Wright Institute
George Fox University	Wright State University
George Washington University[a]	Xavier University
University of Hartford	Yeshiva University[a]
Immaculata University	

[a]These institutions also have APA-accredited Ph.D. programs in clinical psychology.

model Ph.D. programs translate into an additional year of training, on average. Students in Ph.D. programs take significantly longer, 1 to 1.5 years longer, to complete their degrees than do Psy.D. students (Gaddy et al., 1995; Norcross, Castle, Sayette, & Mayne, 2004). Various interpretations are given to this robust difference, from "Psy.D. training is more focused and efficient" on one pole, to "Ph.D. training is more comprehensive and rigorous" on the other.

3. *Acceptance rates.* Both Vail and Boulder programs have similar admission criteria, which favor grade point average, entrance examination scores, letters of recommendation, and so on. (All these topics are covered in detail in later chapters.) But Vail-model programs afford easier admission than Boulder-model programs. On average, clinical Ph.D. programs accept 6 to 10% of applicants, whereas clinical Psy.D. programs accept 41 to 50% of applicants (see Table 3-1 for details).

4. *Financial assistance.* Admission rates are higher in Psy.D. programs, but financial assistance is lower. These numbers are plainly visible in the Reports on Individual Programs. As a rule, only 3 to 10% of Psy.D. students will receive full financial assistance (tuition waiver plus a paid assistantship), whereas 61 to 81% of clinical Ph.D. students will. (See Table 4-3 for details.).

5. *Loan debt.* The paucity of financial assistance to Psy.D. students translates into increased personal debt. If the program does not provide funding, then students are forced to rely on personal funds or loans. The median debt for Psy.D. recipients is now $90,000 (Wicherski & Kohout, 2005). The median debt for clinical Ph.D. recipients is $50,000, lower but still substantial. (For comparison, the median debt for psychology Ph.D.s in non-clinical fields is $21,500; Wicherski & Kohout, 2005).

6. *Accredited internships.* All doctoral students in clinical and counseling psychology will complete the equivalent of a year-long, full-time internship before receiving their degrees. Students desire an internship accredited by APA or APPIC (Association of Psychology Postdoctoral and Internship Centers). The competition for an APA or APPIC-accredited internship can be keen, and in recent years, only 75% of intern applicants matched with an accredited internship. The research consistently demonstrates that students enrolled in large, freestanding Psy.D. programs match at a lower rate than students enrolled in smaller, Ph.D. programs (APPIC, 2006).

7. *Licensure exam scores.* One disconcerting trend is that Vail-model, Psy.D. graduates do not perform as well as Ph.D. graduates on the national licensing examination for psychologists (Kupfersmid & Fiola, 1991; Maher, 1999). That is, doctoral students who graduate with a professional degree (the Psy.D.) score lower, on average, than doctoral students who graduate from a traditional clinical psychology Ph.D. program on the Examination for Professional Practice in Psychology (EPPP), the national licensing test. Higher EPPP scores have been reliably associated with smaller-sized clinical programs and larger faculty-to-student ratios, in addition to traditional Ph.D. curricula.

These 7 differences between Boulder-model, Ph.D. programs and Vail-model, Psy.D. programs do not reliably favor one training model over the other. As a potential applicant, you will probably prefer the shorter training and higher admission rates among Psy.D. programs, on the one hand. You will prefer the greater probability of financial assistance, accredited internships, and higher licensure scores among Ph.D. programs, on the other hand. These truly represent choice points for an informed student.

Moreover, these broad differences must be interpreted carefully. Psy.D. programs, in particular, constitute a heterogeneous bunch—some are small, university-based programs accepting 10 students a year and others are huge, for-profit campuses accepting hundreds per year.

In order to become an informed applicant, know these broad differences. But more importantly, know the specific data on programs to which you will apply. The Reports on Individual Programs later in this book present these data—length of training, acceptance rates, financial assistance, students securing accredited internships, and more—for each APA-accredited program.

The key task for you as a potential applicant is to recognize the diversity in training emphases. We describe this as the practice–research continuum. On one end of the continuum are the practice-oriented Psy.D. programs. These account for roughly one-third of APA-accredited doctoral programs. In the middle of the continuum are the equal-emphasis Ph.D. programs that, as the name implies, emphasize both research and practice. These programs account for another one-third of APA-accredited clinical, counseling, and combined programs. On the other end of the continuum are the research-oriented Ph.D. programs that account for the final one-third of the accredited programs.

The bottom line for applicants to psychology doctoral programs is one of choice, matching, and parity. You have the choice of two training models (and all the programs in between the two extremes). The choice should be matched to your strengths and interests. Parity has been achieved in that almost half of all doctorates in clinical psychology are awarded by Vail-model programs. The choices are yours, but make informed decisions.

A Word on Accreditation

Accreditation comes in many guises, but the two primary types are institutional accreditation and program accreditation. Institutional applies to an entire institution. Seven regional accreditation bodies, such as the Commission on Higher Education of the Middle States Association of Colleges and Schools, oversee accreditation for the university or college itself. A school receives accreditation when it has been judged to have met minimum standards of quality for postsecondary education.

Beware of any institution that is not accredited by its regional accreditation body. A degree from this institution will probably not be recognized by licensing boards, certifying organizations, or insurance companies (Dattilio, 1992). It is necessary to be particularly careful about nontraditional or external degree programs that offer the option of obtaining a degree based on independent study, typically away from the institution itself. Some of these are reputable programs, but many are "diploma mills" (Stewart & Spille, 1988). Many diploma mills have names similar to legitimate universities, so you must be vigilant. Here are several diploma mills with potentially misleading titles: Columbia State University (Louisiana), La Salle University (Louisiana), Chadwick University (Alabama), American State University (Hawaii), American International University (Alabama). (For additional information about diploma mills, consult the fact sheets at the Council for Higher Education Accreditation at www.CHEA.org, www.degreefinders.com/distance_learning/diploma .php and www.web-miner.com/deun accredited.htm).

If you have any doubt, inquire thoroughly into whether the institution as a whole is recognized by professional associations. This can be accomplished by referring to the document, *Doctoral Psychology Programs Meeting Designation Criteria,* jointly published by the Association of State and Provincial Psychology Boards (ASPPB) and the National Register of Health Service Providers in Psychology (2005). You can access an updated list at www.nationalregister.org/ designate.htm.

The second type of accreditation pertains to the clinical or counseling psychology program itself. Specialized accreditation of the discipline is performed by the American Psychological Association (APA). This accreditation is a voluntary procedure for the doctoral program itself, not the entire institution. Most programs capable of meeting the requirements of APA accreditation will choose to apply for accreditation. Accreditation of a clinical or counseling psychology program by the APA presumes regional accreditation of the entire institution.

As of 2007, APA had accredited 232 active clinical psychology programs (60 of these awarding the Psy.D. degree), 67 active counseling psychology programs (3 of these awarding the Psy.D. degree), and 10 active combined professional–scientific psychology programs (Accredited, 2006). The Reports on Individual Programs in this book provide detailed descriptions of these 300 clinical psychology, counseling psychology, and combined programs, respectively.

Take note that APA does *not* accredit master's programs. Accordingly, references to "accredited" master's psychology programs are to regional or state, not APA, accreditation.

The program accreditation criteria can be obtained from the APA Office of Accreditation (www.apa.org/ ed/accreditation/). The general areas assessed include institutional support, sensitivity to cultural and individual differences, training models and curricula, faculty, students, facilities, and practicum and internship training. These criteria are designed to insure at least a minimal level of quality assurance.

The APA (Accredited, 2005) recognizes three categories of accreditation. Accreditation is granted to programs that meet the criteria in a satisfactory manner. "Accredited, inactive" is the designation for programs that have not accepted students for 2 years. This indicates that the program is taking a hiatus as part of a restructuring process, or is phasing out the program (for example, New York University's Clinical Psychology program). "Accredited, probation" is the designation for programs that were previously accredited but are not currently in satisfactory compliance with the criteria.

For more than 30 years, doctoral psychology programs in Canada have enjoyed the option of simultaneous accreditation by the Canadian Psychological Association (CPA) and the American Psychological Association (APA). This dual accreditation enabled United States citizens to travel north to attend APA-accredited Canadian programs and facilitated internship placement and licensure in the United States for both American and Canadian students. Graduates of APA-accredited programs, whether located in Canada or the United States, were eligible for same privileges.

In 2007, the American Psychological Association decided to phase out accrediting Canadian psychology programs. The phase out will occur gradually over a 7-year period. Mutual recognition agreements will continue, but formal APA accreditation of Canadian programs will not. Most jurisdictions in the United States recognize CPA-accredited or National Register-designated programs for the purposes of licensure. But a few do not. Thus, be aware of this transition and the potential consequences on internship and licensure in selected USA states. We do *not* want to discourage anyone from attending excellent Canadian doctoral programs in psychology; we *do* want you to be informed consumers.

Our Reports on Individual Programs provide crucial descriptive and application information on each APA-accredited doctoral program in clinical, counseling, and combined psychology. The APA Education Directorate updates the listing of accredited programs annually in the December issue of the *American Psychologist* and bimonthly on their Web site, www.apa.org/ed.

How important is it to attend an APA-accredited program? The consensus ranges from slightly important to absolutely essential. APA accreditation ensures a modicum of program stability, quality assurance, and professional accountability. Graduates of APA-accredited programs are practically guaranteed to meet the educational requirements for state licensure. Students are in a more advantageous and competitive position coming from an APA-approved program in terms of their internship choices (Drummond, Rodolfa, & Smith, 1981) and their eventual employment prospects (Walfish & Sumprer, 1984). The federal government, the Veterans Administration, and most universities now insist on a doctorate and internship from APA-accredited programs. Graduates of APA programs also score significantly higher, on average, than do students of non-APA-accredited programs on the licensure exam (Kupfersmid & Fiola, 1991). Licensure and employment as a psychologist are not precluded by attending a non-APA-accredited program, but the situation is tightening. Five states now license only graduates from APA-accredited programs. All other things being equal, an accredited clinical or counseling psychology program gives you a definite advantage over a non-accredited program.

Online Graduate Programs

Practically every institution of higher education now offers some online courses and distance education. Some institutions have gone further to create graduate programs that are almost entirely online, with all discussions being conducted electronically on bulletin boards and all assignments being submitted by computer. The only on-campus contact might be a couple of weeks or several weekends per year.

Several of these online or distance learning institutions offer doctoral programs in clinical and counseling psychology, including Walden, Capella, and Fielding. Fielding Graduate University requires several weeks of in-person residency per year, making it the only distance program that is APA accredited. Capella and Walden are both regionally accredited.

We are frequently approached by students intrigued with these and other distance learning doctoral programs and asked whether we think they are credible programs. Our answer is that they are credible but definitely not preferred for several reasons. First, we recommend that students favor APA-accredited programs, and only one of these programs has met the minimum educational criteria set forth by APA. Second, many psychology licensing boards will not issue licenses to graduates of distance learning programs (Hall, Wexelbaum, & Boucher, 2007). Third, online programs lack quality control over their clinical supervisors, who are scattered around the country. Fourth, much of the learning in doctoral programs occurs in close, interpersonal relationships with faculty on a daily basis. Frequent computer contact is useful, but in our opinion, not equivalent. And fifth, without sounding too stodgy, we believe online programs are still too new and alternative to have developed a track record of producing quality psychologists. Most internship directors and potential employers feel likewise; graduates of non–APA-accredited distance programs have experienced difficulty in securing employment as psychologists.

Of course, each online program needs to be evaluated on its own merits, and each graduate student must be considered for his or her individual abilities. In the end, graduate students will get out of a program what they put in—whether through a traditional, bricks-and-mortar institution or an innovative, online program. The early research on distance and online education indicates that it produces comparable outcomes to traditional education, at least in acquiring knowledge and academic skills. Unfortunately, there is insufficient research on the online preparation of professional psychologists to render any conclusions.

Should you decide to apply to online doctoral programs in psychology, we would advise you to:

- complete your master's degree in a conventional program to secure one in-person degree and to meet the admission prerequisites of most online doctoral programs.
- obtain information on the program's track record of producing graduates who secure APA-accredited internships and eventually licensure as psychologists.
- determine the residency requirement (how much time per year is expected on campus).
- expect no financial assistance from the online institution itself (but loans are available).
- become very comfortable and savvy with computers, as most of your contact and assignments will be conducted online.
- be an organized, self-motivated individual who can meet deadlines without supervision.
- realize that the vast majority of interaction with fellow students and professors will occur online, not in a conventional classroom.
- be prepared for intensive research and writing on your own.

Practice Alternatives

In addition to doctoral programs in clinical and counseling psychology, we would like to describe several alternative programs of study that should be considered. We have classified these programs along the practice–research continuum. The practice-oriented programs are outlined first. Portions are abstracted from APA's (1986) *Careers in Psychology,* which can be found online at www.apa.org/students/brochure/index.html. Additional details on helping professions can also be accessed online at www.teachpsych.org/otrp/resources/resources.php. *A Student Guide to Careers in the Helping Professions* by Melissa Himelein provides information on typical job duties, potential earnings, required degrees, and the like.

You are restricted neither to clinical/counseling psychology nor even to psychology in selecting a career in mental health. School psychology, as discussed below, is a viable alternative. Also note that psychology is only one of five nationally recognized mental health disciplines, the others being psychiatry (medicine), clinical social work, psychiatric nursing, and counseling.

We do not wish to dissuade you from considering clinical or counseling psychology, but a mature career choice should be predicated on sound information and contemplation of the alternatives. A primary consideration is what you want to do—your desired activities. Conducting psychotherapy is possible in any of the following fields. Prescribing medication is currently restricted to physicians and some nurses, although psychologists are steadily securing prescription privileges around the country. Psychological testing and empirical research are conducted by psychologists. As discussed previously, psychologists also enjoy a wide range and pleasurable integration of professional activities. Following is a sampling of alternatives to a doctorate in clinical and counseling psychology.

1. School Psychology. Some undergraduates have a particular interest in working with children, adolescents, and their families. Admission into the Boulder-model programs with a child clinical track is particularly competitive. A doctorate in school psychology is much more accessible, with two or three times the acceptance rate of clinical psychology programs. The APA (Accredited, 2006) has accredited 56 of these programs, which provide doctoral-level training in clinical work with children in school settings.

One disadvantage of pursuing a career as a master's-level school psychologist lies in the fact that, unlike the other alternatives, one's professional work may be limited to the school. If this limitation is not a concern, then training as a school psychologist can be an excellent option for those interested in working with children and families (Halgin, 1986).

At the doctoral level, school psychologists are credentialed to function in both school and nonschool settings. Research finds substantial overlap in the coursework of child clinical programs and school psychology programs (Minke & Brown, 1996). Some differences remain, of course—such as more courses in consultation and education in school programs and more courses in psychopathology in child clinical programs—but the core curricula are quite similar. School psychology training at the doctoral level is broadening to include experience outside of the school setting and with adolescents and families as well (Tryon, 2000).

For further information, check out the following Web sites:

- www.indiana.edu/~div16/
  (APA's Division of School Psychology)
- www.naspweb.org
  (National Association of School Psychologists)
- www.ispaweb.org/
  (International School Psychology Association)
- www.schoolpsychology.net
  (comprehensive links to the field and graduate schools)

2. Community Psychology. This field shares with clinical and counseling psychology a concern with individual well-being and healthy psychological development. However, community psychology places considerable emphasis on preventing behavioral problems (as opposed to only treating existing problems), adopting a broader ecological or community perspective, and changing social policies.

Graduate training in community psychology occurs within clinical-community psychology programs or within explicitly community psychology programs. The former are clinical psychology programs with an emphasis on or a specialization in community; these doctoral programs are listed in Appendix E (Research Areas) and Appendix G (Program Concentrations) under "community psychology." Ten universities in the United States offer a doctorate in community psychology, and an additional 12 offer a doctorate in community-clinical psychology. If your interests lean toward prevention and community-based interventions, then by all means check out community psychology. The Web sites at www.scra27.org and www.communitypsychology.net provide further information about the field and training programs.

3. Clinical Social Work. A master's degree in social work (M.S.W.) is a popular practice alternative these days. One big advantage of this option is a much higher rate of admission to M.S.W. programs, with about 65% of applicants being accepted to any given program, on average (O'Neill, 2001). Other advantages are GREs less often required for admission, fewer research requirements, an emphasis on professional training, and completion of the M.S.W. in less than half the time necessary to obtain a psychology doctorate. With legal regulation in all 50 states and third-party vendor status (insurance reimbursement) in 49 states, social workers are increasingly achieving autonomy and respect, including more opportunities for independent practice.

The major disadvantages lie in the less comprehensive nature of the training, which is reflected in a lower pay scale as compared to psychologists. Not becoming a "doctor" and not being able to conduct psychological testing also prove troublesome for some.

Students interested in clinical social work as a career should peruse an introductory text on the profession, consult career publications (for example, Wittenberg, 2003), and contact the National Association of Social Workers (NASW). This organization provides detailed information on the emerging field, student membership, and accredited programs in clinical social work. NASW resources can be accessed via the Web (www.naswdc.org) or the telephone (1-800-742-4089). Three other Web sites on social work programs also prove handy: www.petersons.com/graduate_home.asp?path=gr.home; www.socialworksearch.com; and www.gradschools.com.

4. Psychiatry (Medicine). Students often dismiss the possibility of applying to medical schools, believing that medical school admission is so difficult that it is out of the question (Halgin, 1986). However, the student interested in neuroscience and the more severe forms of psychopathology may find this an attractive choice. Although the application process necessitates more rigorous training in the "hard" sciences than most psychology programs, the admission rate may also be higher than the most competitive doctoral programs in clinical and counseling psychology. Of the 40,000 people applying to medical school annually, about 45% are admitted, and half of them are women. The average GPA of applicants accepted to medical school is between 3.5 and 3.6 (see aamc.org for details).

Medical school thus remains an attractive option for many students headed toward a career in mental health. For further information and demystification of this subject, refer to the data-driven *Medical School Admission Requirements 2008-2009: The Most Authoritative Guide to U.S. and Canadian Medical Schools* (Chanatry, 2007) and *Medical School Admissions: The Insider's Guide* (Zebala, Jones, & Jones, 1999). Prime Web sites include www.premedonline.com and www.aamc.org, the official Web site of the Association of American Medical Colleges.

The advantages of a medical degree should be recognized. First, an M.D. (allopath) or D.O. (osteopath) allows one to prescribe medication. Second, the average income for psychiatrists is higher than for psychologists. Third, a medical degree permits more work in inpatient (hospital) facilities. Applicants should not dismiss this possibility out of hand, and should explore medicine as a career, especially if their interests lie on a physiological level.

5. Psychiatric Nursing. Although sometimes regarded as the handmaiden of psychiatry, master's-level psychiatric nursing is an autonomous profession. The employment opportunities for nursing are excellent at this time, especially for psychiatric nurses who have the flexibility of working in hospitals, clinics, health centers, or private practice. Of course, psychiatric nurses are nurses first and are required to obtain a bachelor's degree (B.S.N.) and to become registered (R.N.) prior to obtaining their Master of Science in Nursing (M.S.N.). They do not conduct psychological testing and rarely perform research, but psychiatric nurses practice psychotherapy in both inpatient and outpatient settings. Further, certified nurse practitioners now have the authority to write medication prescriptions in 47 states. Consult a textbook on mental health nursing and visit the Web site of the American Psychiatric Nurses Association at www.apna.org/ to learn more about psychiatric/mental health nursing and its graduate programs.

6. Counseling. A master's degree in counseling, as distinct from a doctorate in counseling psychology, prepares one for state licensure as a professional counselor. The high acceptance rates of counseling programs, their two years of practical training, and eligibility for state licensure in 49 states represent definite assets. Master's-level clinicians, such as social workers and counselors, have become the front-line providers of most mental health services in community clinics and public agencies. For those students committed to practice and untroubled by the lack of training in conducting research and psychological testing, the profession of counseling deserves consideration. Visit the webpage of the American Counseling Association (www.counseling.org/) for more information on careers and the webpage of accredited counseling programs (www.cacrep.org/directory.html) to locate counseling programs of interest to you.

7. Psychology and the Law. There is a great deal of interest in the burgeoning amalgam of psychology and law, as evidenced by an APA division, two energetic professional societies, and many scholarly journals (Bersoff et al., 1997; Otto & Heilbrun, 2002). Doctoral students must be trained in both fields, of course, increasing the length of graduate training. At least five programs now award law degrees and psychology doctorates together—joint J.D. and Ph.D./Psy.D. programs (Arizona, Drexel, Nebraska, Pacific, and Widener Universities). Graduates pursue both practice and research careers—practicing law in mental health arenas, specializing in forensic psychology, working in public policy, and pursuing scholarship on the interface of law and psychology, for example. This is an exciting career, albeit one requiring extra commitment in terms of effort and knowledge during doctoral studies.

Another two dozen clinical programs offer Ph.D.s or Psy.D.s with specializations in forensic psychology or clinical forensic psychology. (Consult Appendix G and the following Web sites for a list of the programs.) These clinical psychologists specialize in the practice of forensic psychology. It's a growing and exciting specialization in psychology, but one that rarely involves the criminal profiling featured in television shows and *Silence of the Lambs!* Instead, forensic psychologists are far more likely to conduct child custody evaluations, assess a patient's psychological damage, evaluate a person's competence to stand trial, consult with lawyers on jury selection, and conduct disability evaluations. For tips on undergraduate preparation and graduate training in forensic psychology, consult these Web links:

- www.teachpsych.org/otrp/resources/resources
  .php?category=Advising
  (Undergraduate Preparation for Graduate Training in Forensic Psychology)
- www.ap-ls.org/ (APA's American Law–Psychology Society)
- www.abfp.com/ (American Board of Forensic Psychology)

8. Other. Marital and family therapy, student guidance, art therapy, occupational therapy, and a plethora of other human service programs present attractive alternatives to clinical and counseling psychology. They are typically less competitive master's-level programs

in which admission rates are quite high and in which the training is quite practical. Relative disadvantages of these programs, in addition to lack of a doctorate, include less prestige, lower salaries, diminished probability of an independent practice, and variable licensure status across the United States.

If one or more of these options seem suited to your needs, discuss it with a psychology advisor, interview a professional in that field, peruse the Web sites, or write to the respective organizations for additional information.

Research Alternatives

Some graduate students enter clinical or counseling psychology to become researchers. They are less interested in working with patients than researching clinical phenomena. If you are most interested in research, here are some nonpractice alternatives that might appeal to you.

1. Social Psychology. Social psychology is concerned with the influence of social and environmental factors on behavior. Personality, attitude change, group processes, interpersonal attraction, and self-constructs are some of the research interests. Social psychologists are found in a wide variety of academic settings and, increasingly, in many nonacademic settings. These include positions in advertising agencies, personnel offices, corporations, and other business settings. Check out the official Web sites of the Society for Personality and Social Psychology (www.spsp.org) and the Social Psychology Network (www.socialpsychology.org) for additional resources.

2. Industrial/Organizational Psychology. This branch of psychology focuses on the individual in the workplace. Industrial/organizational psychologists frequently select and place employees, design jobs, train people, and help groups of workers to function more effectively. Master's programs generally prepare students for jobs in human resources and personnel departments, whereas doctoral programs are geared to preparing students for academic positions and for management and consulting work on larger-scale projects. Industrial/organizational psychologists earn among the highest median salaries compared to other areas of psychology (Kohout & Wicherski, 1992). Academics find positions in both psychology departments and business schools.

The Society for Industrial and Organizational Psychology (2006) produces a useful list of *Graduate Training Programs in Industrial/Organizational Psy-*

chology and Related Fields, which describes 200 plus graduate programs in "I/O" psychology and how to contact each. It is available free from the society's Web site (www.siop.org). Students interested in pursuing a career in I/O psychology should obtain, beyond psychology classes, courses in management, marketing, and organizational behavior as well as research experience.

3. Behavioral Neuroscience. For the student interested in biological research, the workings of the brain, and the influence of the brain on behavior, programs in neuroscience may be a better match. By employing animal subjects, researchers can control the conditions of their studies to a rigor often elusive when using human participants. Research areas include learning, psychopharmacology, memory, and motivation. For example, recent investigations on memory have provided valuable insight into the etiology and course of Alzheimer's disease. Go to www.andp.org/programs/gradgeo.htm for a splendid list of graduate programs in neuroscience.

Research demonstrates that neuroscience graduate programs expect entering students to possess course work and lab work beyond the standard psychology curriculum (Boitano, 1999). Essential courses would include biology, chemistry, calculus, and introduction to neuroscience. Desirable courses would sample from cell biology, biochemistry, and anatomy and physiology. These are all possible, with adequate planning, to incorporate into the psychology major, should you decide on this path relatively early in your undergraduate career. The Web site (www.undergraduateneuroscience .org/) of Faculty for Undergraduate Neuroscience (FUN) provides a bounty of useful information on preparing for a career in neuroscience.

4. Developmental Psychology. The developmental psychologist studies behavior change beginning at the prenatal stages and extending through the lifespan. Areas such as aging, identity, and development of problem-solving abilities are popular areas within developmental psychology. The characteristics of individuals at different age ranges, such as the work of Piaget on child cognition, are of particular interest to developmental psychologists.

Geropsychology, or the psychology of aging, has become a popular specialty as the elderly population in this country presents special needs that are insufficiently addressed. Employment opportunities in geropsychology are sure to grow over the next several decades. Visit the Web sites of APA's Division of Adult Development and Aging (apadiv20.phhp.ufl.edu/) and the friendly Geropsychology Central (www.premier.net/ ~gero/geropsyc.html) for more.

5. Cognitive Psychology. Cognitive psychology presents an attractive option for students whose interests lie in the exploration of human thought processes. Major areas include language structure, memory, perception, attention, and problem solving. Research in cognitive psychology has gained insight into what in the past was considered inexplicable behavior. For example, research into how moods affect the interpretation of ambiguous events has implications for the study of depression. Much research on the accuracy of eyewitness testimony has been conducted by cognitive psychologists. Cognitive programs emphasize artificial intelligence, cognitive neuroscience, and affective neuroscience. Indeed, interest in cognitive neuroscience and affective neuroscience has increased of late.

6. Experimental Psychology. Often a student is interested in research but has not yet defined an area of interest. Or a student is fascinated with a certain psychopathology but does not desire to practice. In both cases, a graduate program in experimental psychology might be the ticket. These programs allow a student to explore several research areas, such as learning, measurement, and memory. Other programs focus on experimental psychopathology, which is geared more specifically for the researcher interested in clinical populations.

Experimental programs offer excellent training in research methods, statistical analysis, and a great deal of hands-on research experience. In fact, some experimental programs now classify themselves as quantitative or measurement programs. If interested in these programs, consult www.apa.org/divisions/div5/ programs.html for a list of graduate psychology programs with a measurement and quantitative focus.

7. Sport Psychology. This emerging specialization typically entails both research and applied activities. Research focuses on all aspects of sports, whereas application involves psychological assessment, individual skills training, and group consultation. Research and training encompass stress management, self-confidence, mental rehearsal, competitive strategies, and sensory-kinetic awareness. Consult the *Directory of Graduate Programs in Applied Sport Psychology* (Sachs, Burke, & Loughren, 2006) for information on specific psychology programs. Consult, too, the Web site of APA's Division of Exercise and Sport Psychology at www.apa.org/about/division/div47.html for information on career possibilities in this area.

8. Medicine. A medical degree (M.D., D.O.) earned concurrently or sequentially with a psychology doctorate (Ph.D.) may allow the greatest flexibility of all the aforementioned programs of study. This option allows one to practice medicine and psychology while also affording a basic education in research and statistics. For an extremely bright and motivated student, this can be a real possibility, but it is certainly the most challenging of all the alternatives. Earning two doctoral degrees will take longer than earning either alone. This choice is for someone interested in the biological aspects of behavior in addition to gaining a rigorous education in the scientific study of human behavior.

Once again, if your interest lies in research, there are many options available besides clinical and counseling psychology. Talking to a professional in the relevant discipline and consulting textbooks about the discipline will help you to explore that option more fully. An increasing number of Web sites also offer valuable career advice. Five of our favorites are:

- www.psychwww.com/careers/index.htm
- www.lemoyne.edu/career_services/resources/index.htm
- www.apa.org/students/
- www.socialpsychology.org/career.htm
- www.gradschools.com

On "Backdoor" Clinicians

The APA ethical guidelines outline two pathways to becoming a clinical or counseling psychologist. The first is to complete a doctoral program and formal internship in clinical or counseling psychology. The second is to obtain a nonclinical psychology doctorate and then to complete a formal respecialization program in clinical or counseling psychology, which includes the internship. Formal training and supervised experience, not simply the desire to become a clinical or counseling psychologist, are required according to the APA ethical code.

In the past, some psychologists obtained doctorates in developmental, experimental, social, or educational psychology or in a psychology-related discipline and managed to practice as "clinical psychologists" or "counseling psychologists." This was possible because of the paucity of clinical and counseling psychology doctoral programs and because of generic state licensure laws, which recognize only one broad (generic) type of psychologist. However, this educational and licensure process circumvents the established pathway, increases the prospects of inadequate training, and in some cases results in unethical representation. Hence the term "backdoor"—unable to enter through the front door, they sneak in through the back entrance. Major universities, the federal government, the Veterans Administration, and practically all universities now insist on the doctorate (or respecialization) in clinical or counseling psychology for employment as a clinical or counseling psychologist. Although individuals with nonclinical psychology doctorates may be eligible for state licensure, they will be increasingly unable to identify themselves as clinical or counseling psychologists.

Circuitous routes to becoming a clinical or counseling psychologist may still exist, but they have become far less common and ethical. We emphatically recommend against these "backdoor" practices on both clinical and ethical grounds.

To Reiterate Our Purpose

The purpose of this book is to help you navigate the heretofore unknown and frightening process of applying to clinical and counseling psychology graduate programs. But nothing can eradicate the fact that gaining admission to such competitive programs requires a good deal of time and energy. There are the matters of taking the appropriate undergraduate courses, gaining clinical experience, acquiring research competencies, requesting letters of recommendation, locating the appropriate schools to which to apply, succeeding on entrance examinations, completing the application, creating personal statements, traveling to interviews, and deciding which program actually to attend. We have known people who have quit jobs or taken months off just to invest all their time to the application process. However, with this book and a fair degree of organization, you can make such extremes unnecessary.

Emotional strain is an inherent part of the application process. This is unlike many job interviews, where you are marketing yourself merely as a provider of services. Here you are marketing yourself as a human being. This is a personal process. The application forms and interviews require self-exploration and even a certain amount of justification. Why do you like clinical work? What do you enjoy about spending time with people who are disturbed? Do you really like research? You may end up questioning your answers and may feel compelled to examine the beliefs that have led you to this point in your life.

With the help of this book, you ultimately become the consumer for a program best fitted to you. And 86% of students say that their sense of fit with a program is the single most important factor in choosing a graduate program (Kyle, 2000). By negotiating this process in a systematic manner, you can become an informed consumer of psychology graduate programs. Many interviewers recommend that the final interview should be approached by the applicant in this way. With this approach to the admission process, much of the stress can be allayed.

Although the application process itself can appear intimidating, or the prospect of being rejected upsetting, we urge you *not* to allow fear to cause you to abandon the process altogether or to dismiss the option prematurely. Do not allow yourself to be one of the students who gets rejected unnecessarily. If you apply to the appropriate programs and present yourself with a certain savvy, your chances of getting in are vastly improved.

Our Approach

Having now counseled thousands of clinical and counseling psychology aspirants and conducted scores of workshops on applying to graduate school, the three of us have gravitated toward a particular approach to the topic. It might be called *realistically encouraging*.

It is realistic in that we present the hard facts about the competition for entrance into doctoral psychology programs. We will not resort to the disservice of feeding you illusions ("Anyone can become a psychologist!"), even though the reality may leave you feeling discouraged at times.

Still, our approach is unabashedly encouraging in that we support people seeking their goals. With knowledge and perseverance, most of our students have made it. Consider the real-life story of Justin, a success story in the quest for a doctorate in clinical psychology.

Justin almost flunked out of college during his first 2 years, before discovering his abiding interest in psychology. He took his GREs late in his senior year without adequate preparation but obtained combined verbal and quantitative scores of 1100. His applications to doctoral programs that year were hastily and poorly prepared. Justin was, to complicate matters, grossly unaware of typical admission requirements, acceptance rates, and application guidelines. He had no clinical experience whatsoever and had never engaged in research beyond course requirements. Not surprisingly, letters of recommendation about him were mildly positive but without detail or conviction (the deadly, two-paragraph "He/she's nice, but we haven't had much contact" letters). He received dismal rejections, not even a hint of a possible interview or finalist pool.

Well, as people are apt to do, Justin was about to give up and throw in the towel. But he then attended one of our workshops and began to understand that he had neglected virtually every guideline for sophisticated application to graduate school. The next year was devoted to preparing himself for the hunt: he took extra courses after receiving his degree in order to increase his GPA and to improve his GRE psychology score; he volunteered 10 hours a week at two supervised placements; he worked 20 hours a week for a small stipend as a research assistant; and he copublished three articles. Not surprisingly, his letters of recommendation were now enthusiastic and detailed. That year, Justin obtained six acceptances into clinical doctoral programs with full financial support at three of them.

There *are* concrete steps you can take to improve your application. It is as much knowing how to apply as it is your actual credentials. And if you do get rejected once, many steps can enhance the probability of acceptance the next time around, as in Justin's case. Knowledge of the process can make a tremendous difference. The following chapters provide suggestions and strategies that will increase your attractiveness as an applicant.

C H A P T E R 2

PREPARING FOR GRADUATE SCHOOL

People begin the graduate school application process at different stages in their lives. You may be a junior or a senior in college. Maybe you have a bachelor's degree in psychology and have worked for a year or two. Perhaps you are a master's-level counselor or social worker who has decided to return for a doctorate. Or maybe you were not a psychology major but have decided you want to make a career change. Depending on your situation, your needs will be somewhat different. Therefore, each situation is addressed separately throughout this chapter.

But whatever your current status, recognize this about becoming a clinical or counseling psychologist: *Do not wait until the year of your application to begin the preparation.* Securing admission into competitive doctoral programs necessitates preparation throughout your undergraduate career and any intervening years. Good grades, adequate test scores, clinical work, and research experience cannot be instantaneously acquired simply because you have made a decision to pursue psychology as your career.

Plan ahead of time using the knowledge and strategies presented in this chapter. Preparing for graduate study is *not* for seniors only (Fretz & Stang, 1980). Timeliness is everything, or, in the vernacular, "you snooze you lose" (Mitchell, 1996).

Much of the "advice" bandied about by fellow students and even some faculty is hopelessly general. Their well-intentioned comments are meant to be universal —one size fits all. However, this advice is akin to the bed of the legendary Greek innkeeper, Procrustes, who insisted on one size bed and who stretched or shortened his unfortunate guests to fit that bed! Do not fall prey to these Procrustean maneuvers; different applicants have different needs. Understanding your particular circumstances and needs will produce an individualized plan for applying to graduate school.

Different Situations, Different Needs

Underclassmen

Some of you will be undergraduates, not yet in your senior year. By getting a head start, you can take the appropriate courses and attain the optimal clinical and research training possible at your institution. The more time invested in preparation, the better able you will be to meet the requirements of the application process with confidence, which puts you in a very desirable position. This book will provide you with information that can help guide your undergraduate experiences, academic as well as practical. The "Time Line" presented in Appendix A outlines important steps to be taken during your freshman, sophomore, and junior years.

Seniors

Some of you are seniors, deciding whether to go directly on to graduate school. This is a difficult time, and you are likely to be given advice ranging from "everyone *must* take time off" to "if you take a year, you'll lose the momentum and study skills and never go back." Obviously, this decision is based on the needs and experiences of each individual. There are two guidelines, however, that can help you muddle through these decisions.

1. Are you primarily interested in becoming a practitioner and wish to have only a minimal amount of

research training? If so, a practice-oriented psychology program will probably best suit your needs. These programs tend to put the emphasis on clinical experience (Piotrowski & Keller, 1996). They favor applicants who have a master's degree or have been involved in a clinical setting and who will come into a program with some practice skills already in their repertoire. The average age of students admitted into these programs is slightly older than that in research-oriented programs, reflecting time spent out of school in a work environment. Consequently, if you are interested in a practice-oriented program, you could take time off to gain relevant experience in clinical work and research.

2. Are you interested in a program that is primarily research oriented? If you have a solid grounding in research as an undergraduate, such a program is less likely to emphasize the need for postgraduation clinical experience. The necessary and sufficient research experience can certainly be attained during an undergraduate education without taking time off. Adding work experiences and clinical skills to an application, however, can only improve your chances of acceptance into a research-oriented program.

The decision to postpone graduate school for a year or more can be influenced by the time constraints of the application process. Applications for doctoral programs in clinical and counseling psychology are typically due between mid-December and mid-February of the year before you plan to attend school. First-semester seniors just beginning an honors or research project may not be in a position to showcase their talents by application time. The additional preparation for the Graduate Record Examination (GRE) (see Entrance Examinations) may lead a potential applicant to wait a year before applying.

For all these reasons, first-semester seniors may not easily meet the requirements of the recommended Time Line presented in Appendix A. This is a frequent predicament, the solution to which is to wait another year to apply or to do what you can in the remaining time available. In either case, do not give up! Rather, review the Time Line carefully and check off what you have and have not accomplished before making the momentous decision to go for it this year, or to wait until next year. Some shortcuts may well be necessary to apply this year; the ideal time line will need to be modified to fit your reality (Keith-Spiegel, 1991). Some of the items will have to be sacrificed, some accomplished later or more hastily, and others with great energy.

Should you elect to wait a year after receiving your baccalaureate degree, you will begin the application process almost immediately after graduation. In addition to gaining research and clinical experience, the year away from school is spent applying to graduate school. This is not a year to relax or "goof off"; rather, it should be an intense year of preparation for graduate admission.

Our research on the admission statistics of APA-accredited clinical psychology programs demonstrates that, on average, approximately three-quarters of incoming doctoral students held bachelor's degrees only and one-quarter possessed a master's degree (Norcross et al., 2004; Oliver et al, 2005). However, this generalization is limited by significant differences among the types of programs: research-oriented Ph.D. programs enrolled a significantly higher percentage of baccalaureate-level students (85% on average; 15% master's), while Psy.D. programs enrolled more master's-level students (35% on average).

In summary, the advantages of taking time off depend on the type of psychology program you desire and the strength of your current credentials. If you desire to focus exclusively on clinical practice and a Psy.D. degree, it may be advisable to take time off to gain some practical experience and to save some money. If you are more research oriented and already possess skills in this area, you may be in a position to apply at present. If your current credentials—grades, GRE scores, research—are marginal, then another year may also be required.

In using this book, you will be introduced to the admission criteria for graduate school. And by using the worksheets, you can determine how well prepared you are to apply to schools at this point. Following the steps in this book will help you assess how prepared you are to apply to graduate school successfully and whether some time out in the "real world" would be advised.

Previous College Graduates

Some of you are college graduates and have already taken time off, or you are a member of the working world contemplating a career change. A solid work record and a mature perspective on psychology are certainly advantageous.

Those of you who have been out of school and in the real world for several years may feel at a disadvantage in terms of taking the GREs, finding academic letters of recommendation, and locating research opportunities. But by faithfully following the strategies in this book, you can master these steps—as have thousands of returning students before you. And by reviewing the admissions criteria for graduate programs and using the worksheets provided, you will be able to evaluate the degree of your preparation in order to decide whether it is prudent to begin the application process immediately or to bolster your credentials before beginning. Pay particular attention to the steps listed under "application year" in the Time Line (Appendix A).

Returning Master's-Level Clinicians

Some of you will be master's-level clinicians interested in obtaining the doctorate in clinical or counseling psychology. Although your wealth of clinical experience gives you an immediate edge over undergraduates in the admissions race to Psy.D. programs, you cannot ignore the importance assigned to entrance examinations and research experience.

Psy.D. programs and practice-oriented Ph.D. programs tend to accept proportionally more incoming students with master's degrees than with baccalaureate degrees only. Interestingly, counseling psychology programs also seem to prefer master's-level students: Two-thirds of incoming students in APA-accredited counseling psychology programs already held their master's. Of course, these are merely averages that mask the huge differences between, for example, the one-third of counseling psychology programs which *only* accept master's recipients and the one-tenth of programs which primarily accept baccalaureate recipients (Turkson & Norcross, 1996).

Hines (1985) conducted a survey of clinical psychology doctoral programs regarding their policies and experiences in accepting students with master's degrees in psychology. Following are several of the salient findings.

The first question was "What effect (if any) will having a master's degree have on an applicant's chances for admission to your program?" Most responses indicated that having a master's per se made little or no difference, with some respondents suggesting that it was the student's performance in the master's program that was more important. However, 10% answered that having a master's degree had a definite positive effect. Only 3% indicated that having a master's would have a definite negative bias.

The second question requested that respondents rate the importance of seven criteria for admission to their programs. Each criterion was rated on a 5-point, Likert-type scale ranging from least important to most important. The three highest ratings were for GRE scores, letters of recommendation, and research experience. The rest, in descending order of importance, were undergraduate grades, graduate grades, quality of the master's program, and practicum experience.

As you can see, GRE scores and research experience definitely count in admissions decisions for master's-level applicants. The lower ratings given to graduate grades and to undergraduate grades reflect a difference among schools in whether graduate or undergraduate grades are considered more important. The standard deviation for graduate grades was particularly high, indicating wide variability in the importance placed on graduate grades among different programs. Comments suggested that some schools tended to downplay graduate grades "because they are universally high"; another suggested that "high grades don't help, but poor grades hurt."

Having a master's degree in and of itself, then, neither helps nor hinders your chances in most doctoral admission decisions. It is not possessing the master's degree itself that matters, but the quality of performance in academic courses, clinical practica, and research experiences during master's training and thereafter that give a definite edge in the admission process.

Master's degree recipients with combined Verbal and Quantitative GRE scores below 1,000 can take hope from a study of similar students admitted to Ph.D. programs (Holmes & Beishline, 1996). Ten such applicants were admitted by virtue of "compensatory virtues," such as presentations or publications that helped mitigate the effect of low GRE scores. If you find yourself in this position, emphasize the other, positive elements of your application and, again, seriously consider Psy.D. clinical and Ph.D. counseling psychology programs that enroll a higher percentage of master's-level students (Norcross et al., 1998). Assuming other parts of your credentials are acceptable, master's recipients should not be discouraged from applying to doctoral programs on the basis of GRE scores alone.

While clinical experience is valued, for most doctoral programs this factor is a secondary consideration to research. The vast majority of clinical and counseling doctoral programs prefer a thesis or a journal article over a graduate internship or post-master's clinical experience (Keller, Beam, Maier, & Pietrowski, 1995). All programs value conducting empirical research: Ph.D. programs favor it over clinical experience and Psy.D. programs weigh it equally with clinical experience.

A Master's Degree First?

A common question during our graduate school workshops is whether students should secure a master's degree before seeking the doctorate. Fortunately, our workshop participants and you realize that no simple answer is possible to such a complex question. Nonetheless, the following are some broad reasons for seeking a master's degree first.

- *Low grade-point average.* The vast majority of doctoral programs will not consider applicants with a GPA below 3.0.
- *Weak GRE scores.* Similarly, doctoral programs rarely accept bachelor's-level applicants whose combined Verbal and Quantitative scores fall below 1,000.
- *Scarce research or clinical experiences.* Doctoral admission committees understandably desire that you have had some direct experience with those activities you intend to pursue for a lifetime.
- *Uncertain career goal.* Indecision about your subfield in psychology, or outside of psychology, is a strong indicator for a master's program initially.
- *Late application.* Doctoral programs hold to earlier deadlines than do master's programs, so those students waiting too late to apply will be redirected to master's programs.
- *Terse letters of recommendation.* By virtue of late transfer into a university or into psychology, some students lack sufficient contact with faculty for them to write positive and detailed letters of recommendation expected by doctoral programs.
- *Inadequate coursework in psychology.* Doctoral programs require a minimum level of education in the discipline prior to acceptance, typically at least 15 to 18 credits of psychology course work.

Completing a rigorous master's program in psychology can correct many of the foregoing impediments to acceptance into a doctoral program. As we describe in Chapter 7, students typically strengthen their grade point average, acquire clinical and research experience, sharpen their career goals, and establish close relationships with faculty during the 2 years of a master's program. For these and other reasons, many students opt for a master's degree at one institution before seeking the doctorate at another.

Doctoral psychology faculty were surveyed in detail regarding the value of a clinical master's degree for gaining admission to their programs (Bonifzi, Crespy, & Rieker, 1997). Assuming a *good* undergraduate GPA and *good* GREs, the effect of having a master's degree on the applicant's chances for admission was negative for 7% of the programs, neutral for 48% of the programs, and positive for 45% of programs. However, assuming *mediocre* GPA and *mediocre* GREs, the effect

of having a master's was more neutral than positive overall. Put another way, it is clearly the applicant's overall credentials—rather than possession of a master's degree—that carries the day.

This same study (Bonifzi et al., 1997) and our own research (Mayne et al., 1994; Norcross et al., 2004) consistently demonstrate that Ph.D. clinical programs hold a positive bias toward baccalaureate-level applicants. By contrast, Psy.D. clinical, Ph.D. counseling, and Ph.D. school psychology programs view master's degree recipients more favorably and accept higher proportions of master's-level applicants. Keep these biases in mind as you consider the selection criteria of graduate schools.

Graduate School Selection Criteria

As an applicant, your perceptions of graduate admissions criteria probably differ from those of the admissions committee. Some of the things you may think are important are actually not so important (Collins, 2001). For two examples, your GRE Psychology Subject score is less important than your GRE Verbal and Quantitative scores, and your extracurricular accomplishments do not count as much as you might like (Cashin & Landrum, 1991). On the other hand, you probably underestimate the importance of other admissions criteria; two examples are letters of recommendation and research experience, which students routinely underestimate compared to admissions committees (Nauta, 2000).

In this section we acquaint you with the evidence-based practices of graduate admissions committees. Learn what they value in graduate applicants and then tailor your application to those criteria in order to maximize your success.

A number of studies have been conducted to determine the relative importance of selection criteria in psychology graduate programs. The findings of our most recent and largest study (Norcross, Kohout, & Wicherski, 2005) are summarized in Table 2-1. This table presents the average ratings of various criteria for admission into 410 doctoral programs and 179 master's programs in psychology. A rating of 3 denotes high importance; 2, medium importance; and 1, low importance.

The top-rated variables for doctoral programs were letters of recommendation, personal statements, GPA, interview, research experience, and GRE scores. All received ratings of 2.50 and higher on the 3-point scale, indicative of high importance. Extracurricular activity and work experience were valued significantly lower.

TABLE 2-1. Importance of Various Criteria in Psychology Admissions Decisions

Criteria	Master's programs		Doctoral programs	
	Mean[a]	SD	Mean[a]	SD
Letters of recommendation	2.74	.49	2.82	.42
Personal statement/goals	2.63	.55	2.81	.41
GPA	2.75	.43	2.74	.45
Interview	2.30	.76	2.62	.60
Research experience	2.04	.74	2.54	.65
GRE scores	2.36	.66	2.50	.55
Clinically related public service	1.94	.70	1.91	.69
Work experience	1.91	.65	1.87	.68
Extracurricular activity	1.46	.54	1.41	.55

Note. Data from Norcross, Kohout, & Wicherski (2005).

[a]Means are calculated on ratings where 1 = low importance, 2 = medium importance, 3 = high importance.

The implications for enhancing your application are thus clear and embedded throughout this *Insider's Guide:* secure positive letters of recommendation, write compelling personal statements, maintain your GPA, ace the preadmission interview, secure research experience, and prepare thoroughly for the GREs. At the same time, being heavily involved in student organizations and campus activities does not carry nearly as much weight as these other criteria.

Another study (Eddy, Lloyd, & Lubin, 1987) investigated the selection criteria of only APA-accredited doctoral programs in clinical psychology. Program directors rated the importance of each type of undergraduate preparation on a scale ranging from very low importance, 1, to very high importance, 5. Table 2-2 presents the mean ratings and standard deviations for clinical psychology programs.

Research experience emerged as the top-rated variable. The authors of the study concluded that there is simply no better way to increase one's chances for graduate school acceptance than research. A personal visit to a department on an invited interview, computer proficiency, and paid clinical experience were also highly valued. However, as in the previous study, extracurricular activities, such as Psi Chi membership, were rated relatively unimportant.

Not all research experiences count equally in graduate admissions. The most important are published articles in referred journals and paper/poster presentations at national conferences. Of course, serving as

TABLE 2-2. Importance Assigned by Clinical Psychology Doctoral Programs to Various Types of Undergraduate Preparation

Preparation	Mean	SD
Research methods	4.28	0.91
Personal visit to department	3.14	1.41
Computer knowledge and skills	3.00	0.85
Paid human service experience	2.90	1.07
Volunteer human service	2.85	1.13
Double major with basic science	2.78	1.10
Master's degree	2.16	0.99
Double major with social science	2.08	0.84
Psi Chi membership	2.00	0.94

Note. From Eddy, Lloyd, & Lubin (1987). © 1987 Lawrence Erlbaum Associates. Reprinted by permission.

first author counts more than second or third author. Paper/poster presentations at regional conferences follow in importance, then state conferences. Publishing in nonrefeered or undergraduate journals bring less credit in graduate admissions decisions, but still credit (Kaiser et al., 2007; Keith-Spiegel et al., 1994).

To sum up, the results of these and other studies (e.g., Briihl & Wasielski, 2004; Mayne et al., 1994; Munoz-Dunbar & Stanton, 1999; Purdy, Reinehr, & Swartz, 1989) consistently indicate that the ideal applicant has high GRE scores, strong letters of recommendation, research experience, clinical experience, and high GPA. The results also consistently demonstrate that the admission requirements for doctoral programs are more stringent than for master's programs.

The remainder of this chapter highlights these pivotal criteria used by graduate admissions committees in selecting their students. We consider, in order, course work, faculty mentoring, clinical experience, research skills, entrance examinations, and extracurricular activities.

Course Work

Although graduate programs differ in the courses they prefer you to have taken prior to admission, there are some "core" courses that nearly all require (Smith, 1985). These include Introduction to Psychology, Statistics, Research Methods, Abnormal Psychology, Physiological Psychology/Biopsychology, and Learning/Cognition.

Our research on clinical doctoral programs in the United States and Canada reveals that both Vail- and Boulder-model programs hold similar expectations on desirable undergraduate courses (Mayne et al., 1994; Oliver et al., 2005). Approximately 60% of the programs require or recommend specific undergraduate courses, 15% require an undergraduate psychology major, 10% specify a minimum number of psychology credits (but not specific courses), and the remainder have no set policy on the matter.

Table 2-3 presents the percentage of psychology courses required (first column), recommended (second column), and either required or recommended (third column) for entry into APA-accredited clinical programs. Bear in mind that these figures systematically *underestimate* the actual percentage of programs requiring these courses as they do not include those graduate programs requiring a psychology major as a prerequisite and thus probably requiring most of the courses listed in Table 2-3. Introduction to Psychology was presumed to be a prerequisite for these advanced

TABLE 2-3. Undergraduate Courses Required or Recommended by APA-Accredited Clinical Psychology Programs

Psychology course	Percentage of programs		
	Required	Recommended	Either
Statistics	65	29	94
Research methods	48	19	68
Abnormal/psychopathology	29	22	51
Physiological/biopsychology	10	23	33
Learning/cognition	10	19	30
Personality	15	13	28
Child/developmental	11	13	24
Social psychology	7	16	23
History and systems	6	9	16
Psych testing/assessment	6	8	15
Laboratory course	6	5	11
Sensation and perception	3	2	5
Clinical/psychotherapy	1	1	2
Comparative psychology	1	1	2
Motivation and emotion	1	1	2
Neuropsychology	1	0	1

Note. Adapted from Mayne, Norcross, & Sayette (1994).

psychology courses and was therefore omitted from the table. Courses you should complete, according to these results, are Statistics, Research Methods, Abnormal Psychology, Physiological Psychology, Learning/Cognition, Personality, and Developmental Psychology.

Doctoral programs require more courses on average than do master's programs (Smith, 1985). Accordingly, both to meet admissions criteria and to improve your GRE Psychology Subject Test score, we heartily recommend that you complete Social Psychology, History and Systems, Psychological Testing, and at least one laboratory course. The safest plan, of course, is to complete a rigorous undergraduate major in psychology to satisfy all these courses, but a well-planned minor in psychology may suffice. The rule of thumb: the more competitive the graduate program, the more stringent the required undergraduate course work.

If you were not a psychology major, it is still important that you take the minimum of six core courses mentioned. In addition, you may have to invest additional time studying for the Psychology Subject Test of the Graduate Record Examination (more about this later).

If you have been out of college for several years and feel deficient in this course work, you might consider taking a course or two as a part-time student at a local university. This will shore up your record and prepare you more fully for admission and the GRE. Those of you who are not psychology majors but have studied extensively for this test and have done well will often be considered favorably by admissions committees.

Beyond these classes, we recommend an introductory computer science course, particularly if you are interested in research-oriented programs. Not only will it accustom you to the workings of computers, which are standard research tools, but it will also serve as a springboard for learning the statistical software used for data analysis. Recall that computer proficiency is rated a moderately important admission variable by doctoral programs.

Graduate selection committees prefer a broad undergraduate background in a variety of arts and sciences (Fretz & Stang, 1980). Exposure to biological sciences, math competency, and verbal skills are generally valued. If you are anxious or phobic regarding oral presentations, then by all means complete a public speaking course. Composition and writing courses are also vital; you may well face three or four major papers each semester in graduate school.

At this point, you may want to glance at the Reports on Individual Programs following Chapter 7 to get a better idea of which courses particular doctoral programs recommend or require of applicants. You will find the specific courses that each accredited clinical, counseling, and combined psychology program recommends or requires applicants to have taken.

For students who have gotten an early start or who are seniors, we would like to suggest considering advanced course work. To allay any anxieties, we would emphasize that the vast majority of applicants do *not* take these courses as undergraduates. Your application can be very strong without taking the courses we are about to mention. However, those fortunate enough to be in a position to add these to their academic transcripts should seriously consider taking advantage of the opportunity.

Consider an advanced or graduate statistics course. Statistical acumen is highly regarded, especially in research-oriented programs, and advanced knowledge may pave the way for funding as a graduate assistant or research assistant. Another suggestion would be to take a course specifically focused on one of the data analysis programs. Learning one of the major statistical packages—Statistical Analysis System (SAS) or Statistical Package for the Social Sciences (SPSS)—is a definite advantage. Such knowledge increases your employability and may catch the eye of a professor in need of a data analyst. Lastly, we suggest an advanced course in physiological psychology, biopsychology, or neuroscience. This is certainly helpful in increasing your understanding of the biological aspects of behavior, an increasingly important focus in psychology today. If you have the time and abilities, these courses can help distinguish a very good application from an outstanding one.

As mentioned earlier, your GPA is a very important criterion for admission. Three types of GPA may be considered by graduate programs: overall GPA, psychology GPA, and GPA during your junior and senior years. Most programs focus only on your overall or cumulative GPA. Determine which GPAs programs evaluate and also how much importance they place on them. For example, if you have an overall GPA of 3.2 (on a 4-point scale where $A = 4$, $B = 3$, $C = 2$, and $D = 1$), a psychology GPA of 3.6, and a junior/senior GPA of 3.5, you might concentrate on schools that emphasize the latter two averages.

Our research has shed light on the average GPAs among incoming doctoral and master's students in psychology (Norcross et al., 2005). For doctoral programs, the mean GPA is 3.54 for all undergraduate courses, 3.66 for psychology courses, and 3.67 for the last 2 years of course work. For master's programs, the mean GPA is 3.37 for all undergraduate courses, 3.48 for psychology courses, and 3.44 for the last 2 years of course work. Please employ your statistical sagacity in interpreting these figures: half of the incoming students will possess GPAs above these scores, and half of the students will possess GPAs below them.

Although we do not want to discourage anyone, a GPA below 3.0 is considered unsatisfactory by most APA-accredited programs. Regardless of the prestige of the institution, admissions committees view a GPA under 3.0 as below the acceptable limits of course performance. If your GPA is below 3.0, then consider the following steps:

- Take additional courses to bolster your GPA.
- Retake courses to improve it.
- Wait another year to apply in order for all of your senior-year grades to be factored into your GPA.
- Complete a master's program first to show doctoral admissions committees you can perform academically at a higher level.

Try to speak with an academic advisor about how best to improve your standing within the workings of your own institution. Academic performance in your junior and senior psychology courses is particularly vital. Your grades in these courses affect your overall, final 2 years, and psychology GPAs.

Your "academic" performance is not limited to exam grades in the classroom. Faculty members—several of whom may submit a letter of recommendation on your behalf—also assess your interpersonal skills, verbal ability, and professional commitment in the classroom, outside formal course work, and in everyday interactions. The direct implication is to avoid undesirable interpersonal behaviors—for instance, silliness, arrogance, and hostility—in any interactions with your professors (Keith-Spiegel, 1991). Although the wisdom of avoiding such undesirable behaviors may be obvious, students are frequently unaware of the importance faculty attach to good questions, genuine attentiveness, respectful disagreements, office visits, mature disposition, interpersonal responsibility, and so forth. These are the characteristics a student heading for graduate studies should manifest in and outside of the classroom.

Finally, there is a corpus of general knowledge regarding clinical and counseling psychology that may not have been covered in your courses. This body of information includes at least a cursory understanding of diagnosis, for example, the *Diagnostic and Statistical Manual*, 4th ed. (DSM-IV); various assessment devices, such as the Minnesota Multiphasic Personality Inventory-2 (MMPI-2) and the Wechsler Intelligence Scales (WAIS-IV, WISC-IV); and ordinary therapy practices, such as individual, group, and family therapy. You must have a passing familiarity with theoretical orientations, for example, cognitive-behavioral, psychodynamic, family systems, and integrative/eclectic, in order to understand program materials. If you are not already familiar with these concepts, it would be wise to review an introductory textbook in clinical psychology.

You should also be gaining knowledge specifically about psychology as a field and about the current issues within this field. Toward this end, we suggest you begin reading the *Monitor on Psychology,* a publication sent to all APA members and student affiliates, or the *APS Observer,* the newsletter distributed to all members of the American Psychological Society (APS). Both publications feature articles dealing with psychology in general and clinical/counseling psychology in particular. You can become an APA or APS affiliate and receive a subscription, peruse your library's copy, or ask to borrow a professor's old issues.

Faculty Mentoring

Learning about psychology and achieving good grades are important components of academic work. But classes are also important in that they provide you with the opportunity to become acquainted and form relationships with faculty. It is natural to feel shy around faculty, especially if you are part of a 300-person lecture class. Substantial courage is required to muster the nerve to ask a question or to stay after class and introduce yourself. Equally anxiety provoking is a visit alone to a professor's office during office hours. In the one case, you expose yourself in front of your peers; in the other, you are individually vulnerable and do not have a crowd of faces to blend into. *But find a way to become comfortable in approaching faculty members.*

The irony of student reticence to approach faculty is that professors generally would like more students to approach them. Many faculty sit alone during office hours wondering why students never come to see them. They love to have students come after class or during office hours with questions. Ideas for questions can include something mentioned in the lecture or something you encountered in the readings. You do not have to be a star pupil or ask brilliant questions to begin a conversation with a professor. If you want to develop a relationship, ask professors about their research or other courses they are teaching.

What is the importance of meeting faculty? Three compelling reasons spring to mind. First, having a mentor to advise you in your growth as a future psychologist is invaluable. There is no better way to learn about psychology than in a one-on-one, mentoring relationship. When you apply to graduate school, having a professor to guide you through the process is a huge advantage. Second, eventually you will need faculty to write letters of recommendation on your behalf. Whether you are applying to graduate school or for employment, everyone wants a few references regarding your performance and responsibility. Occasionally faculty members are asked to write a letter for a pupil who has taken a lecture course with 100 or more students—the professor may not even know the student until he or she requests a letter! It makes a huge difference if you have spent some office hours or time after class with a faculty member, and he or she knows you more personally.

And third, once you get to know professors, you may have the opportunity to work with them on a research project or as part of their clinical activities. You will be working closely with your major professor in graduate school, and you might as well begin as soon as possible as a colleague-in-training. Though more will be said about this later, we cannot overemphasize the need to cultivate such a relationship and obtain the rewards that can ensue.

To put it bluntly, the single largest contributor to preparedness for graduate school is students' interaction with faculty members at their undergraduate institution. That's what the research concludes and what graduate students report (Huss et al., 2002). Psychology students who had a mentor and who had high-quality interactions with faculty felt more prepared for graduate school. And the second largest contributor to graduate school preparedness is research activity—a point to which we shall return in a few pages.

Beyond meeting professors, read your textbooks with an eye toward graduate school. If you come across an interesting study, note the author and check in the back of the text for the reference. When you have time, go to the library or online and read the original article. If it is recent, note the author's university. You will be surprised at how much you can learn about the field just by doing your typical class work.

Clinical Experience

What is clinical experience? In its loosest sense, it involves spending time working in human service or mental health agencies. Graduate programs in clinical and counseling psychology expect that you will have some experience working with emotionally, intellectually, or behaviorally disadvantaged people. Many students volunteer or intern during their undergraduate years, whereas other people get paid as part of a summer job or during their time off. In research-oriented Ph.D. programs, you will be expected to have some clinical experience as a prelude to your clinical training and as an aid to researching clinically relevant problems. Experience of this nature will be considered essential.

What kinds of clinical experience count? Largely two types—paid and volunteer—under individual supervision. Paid part-time work in a clinical setting may be available in your community (but your involvement should not be at the expense of your academic performance). Returning master's-level clinicians will obviously have a multitude of employment possibilities, whereas undergraduates will have to search vigilantly for part-time employment.

For college students, a prime opportunity is to complete an undergraduate internship (or field experience) for academic credit. This is a great way to "kill two birds with one stone." One study (VandeCreek & Fleisher, 1984) found that over two-thirds of colleges and universities provided undergraduate internships in psychology. Further, students consistently rate field-work as one of the most rewarding experiences and relevant courses in their college career. Internships "pay" in multiple ways: clinical experience, academic credit, familiarity with human service agencies, professional supervision, potential sources for letters of recommendation, and a shot at a full-time job.

Check with your undergraduate advisor and the college catalogue to determine whether such an opportunity exists for you. To learn more about the specific placements, you should consult the Psychology Department or the faculty member responsible for internship placements.

In selecting a place to work or volunteer, please consider several factors. Although it may be difficult to accomplish, it is ideal to gain clinical experience in a setting that complements a research interest. For example, if your research is in the area of alcohol abuse, you might seek experience in a college counseling center or a substance abuse prevention program. Find out exactly what your responsibilities will entail.

The optimal program is one that will train you in clinical skills (such as crisis counseling on a hot line), will allow you to deal directly with clients, and will provide regular supervision by an experienced clinician.

Supervision is probably the most important consideration in choosing a clinical setting. It is important that you be supervised by a professional, one with at least a master's degree. Determine the qualifications of the person who will be supervising your work. Aside from the valuable insight supervisors can offer, they may also be familiar with faculty at different graduate programs and assist you in selecting schools. In addition, you may eventually decide to request letters of recommendation from them. Letters from a clinical supervisor are particularly important for practice-oriented graduate programs. In a later section we offer suggestions regarding approaching professors for letters of recommendation. The same strategies apply here.

If you are volunteering, you should insist on receiving supervision. Learn not only who will supervise you, but also how often and for what length of time. You will need to be assertive when searching out and interviewing possible agencies. If this seems difficult for you, try to remember that you are a volunteer—giving your time and energy, without financial compensation, to an agency that is in need of people like yourself. You seek only experience and supervision. You are a valuable commodity, so do not sell yourself short!

Numerous settings are available to people seeking clinical experience. Here are several excellent sources of hands-on experience that can be found in most communities:

- *Crisis hot lines.* These typically provide training in counseling skills, suicide prevention, and outreach services. The clientele range from sexual assault victims to suicidal teens to lonely elderly who need to talk with someone. Volunteers usually provide telephone counseling, although opportunities to work with an emergency outreach team may also be available. This can be a great way to gain exposure to a multitude of psychopathologies and to acquire fundamental helping skills. One word of caution: new members of most crisis hot lines are expected to take a large share of the midnight to 8 A.M. shifts. Be prepared to pay your dues.
- *Centers for homeless or runaway adolescents.* Much of what is done in these settings is similar to case management, in that these teenagers need to be put in contact with social service agencies. However, in-house counseling may also be provided to these youths, who frequently come from disadvantaged families. Be particularly careful about specifying the supervision arrangement before starting. The facilities are often understaffed and financially strapped, meaning you may have to be assertive to get the training you desire.
- *Schools for emotionally disturbed children and adolescents.* These placements offer exposure to both educational and clinical services. Educational activities might include tutoring, classroom management, and one-on-one homework supervision. Clinical activities typically involve recreational

supervision, art therapy, and perhaps individual, group, and family therapy.
- *Supervised homes for the developmentally disabled or chronically mentally ill.* These are unlocked transitional facilities where clients live and work in a therapeutic milieu (an environment consisting of peers). Depending on your prior experience, you might be expected to conduct skills training, recreational counseling, and work/school supervision. The programs are often behavioral, affording you experience with reinforcement schedules, shaping techniques, and token economies. Often the goal is to graduate clients to the outside world.
- *Summer camps for the physically challenged, developmentally disabled, or emotionally disturbed.* These can be either day or overnight camps, where counselors are expected to supervise recreation and train campers in skills and vocational activities. The positions are usually paid, ideal for college students who want to gain field experience while working for the summer. They also tend to be full-time positions, while they last. They offer short-term but intensive training.
- *Community mental health centers.* These provide experience with patients suffering from serious mental disorders, such as schizophrenia, bipolar disorders, substance abuse, and anxiety disorders. The programs vary but are likely to include an outpatient department, partial (day) hospitalization, and an education/outreach wing. Duties may include helping out during recreational activities or assisting with individual and group therapy. Though supervising recreational activities allows contact with patients, you might not be observing any clinical methods. Do not be shy about asking for greater responsibilities!
- *College peer programs.* These provide students with peer education and assistance on specific disorders, such as bulimia or substance abuse. Less common but still available is peer counseling on more general concerns, for example, "Need to Talk? Call Us." Both peer education and peer counseling programs are typically flexible in the number of hours you must work and usually provide training in listening and counseling skills. They may also provide an opportunity to begin learning about a specific clinical problem.
- *Women's resource centers.* These are multiservice centers that offer or coordinate a plethora of human services for women—rape crisis counseling, domestic violence education, "safe homes" for victims of abuse, and so on. Possible activities likewise vary, but the training and *esprit de corps*

are highly regarded. Students with abiding interest in women's issues and feminist therapy will find these placements particularly satisfying.

- *Drug and alcohol treatment facilities.* These offer a variety of detoxification and rehabilitation interventions designed to help patients cope with addiction. Although not all "D & A" programs will afford undergraduate placements, substance abuse is one of the most popular research areas in clinical and counseling psychology (see Appendix E). Students can gain exposure to several models of addiction, interact with a multidisciplinary treatment team, and observe clinical services with substance abusers across gender, racial, and socioeconomic lines.
- *Psychiatric hospitals.* These offer comprehensive behavioral care in an inpatient setting and typically feature individual psychotherapy, group counseling, psychoactive medication, psychological assessment, occupational therapy, and recreational therapy. Students are likely to observe patients with severe disorders receiving many treatments provided by multidisciplinary staff. In addition, large state hospitals depend upon the kindness of volunteers to staff social events, community outings, and recreational opportunities for patients.
- *Legal and probation offices.* These offer ideal experiences for students interested in forensic applications. Students frequently volunteer or intern with District Attorney's offices, probation officers, criminal lawyers, state police, and other criminal justice professionals. In these settings, ask to be exposed to the psychological or psychiatric side of criminal justice.

A word of caution about initial clinical encounters. Be careful not to generalize from one experience. One of the authors worked with runaways at a crisis center for adolescents in the Times Square area of New York City. The rate of employee turnover at this facility was exceptionally high. The "success" rate for clients was low, and the population was difficult indeed. Although it was a rich experience, some of the volunteers became disillusioned with psychology as a result of working there. Settings vary considerably, depending on the populations they serve and the resources available. An unpleasant experience may only mean that the specific population you were working with was not ideally suited to you. Try something else, and you may feel quite differently.

Though clinical work is important (and often rewarding), remember it is only one of several experi-

ences you must acquire for admission to graduate school. Some Ph.D. applicants make the mistake of accumulating a wealth of clinical experiences at the expense of gaining research training. By doing so, you may be inadvertently presenting yourself as being uninterested in research or perhaps better suited to a Psy.D. than a Ph.D. program. Clinical experience must be balanced with research competencies. This balance will be weighted toward clinical work or research depending on your desire to gain either a Psy.D. or Ph.D. or whether the Ph.D. program is practice or research oriented.

Research Skills

Research experience, as discussed earlier in this chapter, consistently emerges as a top admission criteria to nearly all Ph.D. programs in clinical and counseling psychology. To a lesser but still significant degree, Psy.D. programs also value your research experience for what it communicates about your intellectual ability and professional commitment. Recall the conclusion of one study on graduate school admission: there is simply no single better way to enhance an application than by obtaining research experience (Eddy et al., 1987). The desired skills—to critique the literature, to apply methodological reasoning, to write in scientific language, among others—are essential. Even though all psychologists need not produce original research, all must intelligently consume and apply research.

The benefits of student research, according to recent research (Landrum & Nelsen, 2002), boil down to two dimensions. The first might be labeled specific skills and abilities. These skills include developing clear research ideas, conducting literature searches, choosing appropriate measures, analyzing data, using statistical procedures, preparing conference presentations, and improving writing ability. The second dimension might be called interpersonal goals. These tend to be overshadowed by the specific technical skills listed above, but they are critical benefits in preparing and mentoring psychologists-in-training. These entail influencing decisions about graduate school, meeting other students involved in research, getting to know faculty members better, improving teamwork, forming relationships for the basis of letters of recommendation, developing leadership, and improving interpersonal communication. You seek *both* types of benefits in securing a research experience or assistantship.

Gaining research experience is largely dependent on your own initiative. It can be an intimidating process, and a knowledge of the potential opportunities can help you to maximize your gains during the course of your research.

Common Paths

Let us begin by outlining six common avenues for students engaging in scholarly research. The first is probably the most frequent—volunteering to work with a faculty member on one of his or her research projects. A second avenue is to complete a student research program for a notation on your transcript but not academic credit. Students identify potential professors to work with from a faculty directory of research interests, jointly complete a learning contract, and then devote a minimum number of hours (say, 75) throughout a semester working directly with the faculty sponsor. A third option is to enroll in independent psychology research for academic credit. This entails individual study and research under the supervision of a faculty member and is ordinarily limited to junior and senior psychology majors.

A fourth and increasingly common approach is to work or volunteer for a researcher outside of your university—in a hospital, medical center, research institute, industry, or community-based organization, for example. Especially in large cities, researchers with major grants depend upon individuals (both pre- and post-baccalaureate) for many elements of study management, data collection, and statistical analyses. Many industries, especially biomedical and pharmaceutical research, offer summer research internships. These positions can provide valuable experience, in randomized controlled trial research. Conversely, community-based organizations commonly conduct outcomes research around clinical or community interventions and accept interns throughout the year. If you have taken a statistics or research methods course that included SPSS or SAS, you may have sufficient skills for an entry-level position on an active research team outside of a university.

A fifth alternative, restricted to matriculated undergraduates, is to complete an honors thesis in either a departmental or a university-wide honors program. As with additional courses and post college work, an honors thesis is a "feather in your cap." For students desiring to move straight into a Ph.D. program, it is one means of presenting evidence to graduate admissions committees that you are capable of performing graduate-level work. Many schools allow motivated students to complete an honors thesis, an original study that the student conceptualizes, conducts, analyzes, and has some hope of presenting at a regional conference or even publishing. An honors thesis shows a genuine commitment to psychology and is a palpable sign of ability in the applicant.

A sixth and final avenue toward acquiring research competencies is restricted to master's students. A comprehensive paper or a formal master's thesis, requiring original research, practically guarantees additional experience with research. For this reason, undergraduates denied admission directly into doctoral programs frequently enter master's programs to gain valuable research (and clinical) competencies. And remember: the majority of clinical psychology doctoral programs prefer master's-level applicants to have completed a thesis (Piotrowski & Keller, 1996).

Whatever avenue you eventually pursue, the procedures are quite similar. Following is a step-by-step guide to help you make the most of your research experience.

Determining Your Interests

The first step is finding a research area that interests you. If you are not interested in the work, it will diminish your energy and enthusiasm and probably your decision to apply to graduate school. A good place to begin is to read through your department brochure or Web site describing faculty interests and current research. If you are out of school, check with a local university. Look for professors who have a proven track record of scholarly publications. If the program has a graduate psychology faculty, so much the better —look to those professors first.

Once you have a list of faculty interests, you may find someone interesting but not be sure exactly what the research is all about ("I've heard about autism and think I'd like to study it, but I don't really know much about it. . . ."). If specific publications are not provided in the Web site or brochure, or if reprints are not posted in the department, then you can go to *PsycLIT* or *PsycINFO* (found in most university libraries; ask at the reference desk) and read what that professor has published in the area over the last 5 to 7 years. This should make it easier to decide which professor you would like to approach to volunteer to do research with. *Do not narrow your choices too quickly!* Find at least two or three professors whose work initially interests you.

Selecting Professors

Next, find out more about that professor as a person. Do you know people who have taken a class with him or her? What did they think? Are there other undergraduate or graduate students working with this professor now? What do they do, and what is it like working under this person? Is the professor easy to get along with? Is the professor helpful to students? Do not be afraid to approach people and ask questions.

Having narrowed the choice to two or three professors whose work interests you and with whom you think you might get along, consider the rank of the professor. There are tenured faculty (a *full* or *associate* professor) and untenured (an *assistant* professor), both with respective advantages and disadvantages.

Full or associate professors have been in the field longer and will probably have colleagues at other universities. If the professor is well known, it gives your letter of recommendation that much more weight. If your professor's reputation in the field is strong, with a long list of publications, you are also likely to learn more and increase your own attractiveness as a candidate. However, once a faculty member becomes tenured, he or she is no longer under the same pressure to produce research as when he or she was pursuing tenure. Certainly if these faculty members are still conducting grant-funded research, they are likely to be committed to maintaining their productivity. Regardless, you should establish that tenured faculty are actively engaged in research and are currently publishing their work.

Assistant professors are newer to the field, probably 1 to 6 years post doctorate. They are often in more need of undergraduate help and will likely involve you to your full potential. The possibility of being included on a presentation or publication as a coauthor may also be increased. What they lack in terms of a reputation built on years of publications may be balanced by their energy and their motivation to produce.

One word of caution: some professors maintain large research facilities and employ vast numbers of undergraduates to help them with their data management. If there are 10 or 15 undergraduates working in a lab, the attention given to each individual tends to decrease, as well as the value of the research experience. On the other hand, some large laboratories provide unique research opportunities unavailable elsewhere. The key is to talk to students who have worked there to learn about their experiences and to determine if former students have had success applying to graduate school.

An optimal research context, then, is one in which there is a faculty member or research mentor who has an established reputation in his or her field of inquiry, a record of producing publishable research, similar interests to your own, a history of working successfully with students, a propensity to share authorship credit with students, and the ability to construct discrete research projects. Be guided by these general principles

in selecting professors to approach, but do not expect all these qualities to be available to you.

Making Initial Contact

Having chosen a professor you would like to work with, it is now time to make yourself known to him or her. You need to schedule an appointment or approach the professor during posted office hours. It is natural for you to be nervous! However, the more familiar with his or her work you are, the more secure you are likely to feel. Once again, read what the professor has written. Additionally, it helps to remember that you are coming to the professor to offer your services.

A good opening line might be, "Hello, Dr. Jones, my name is Chris Smith. I've been doing some reading on autism and came across several articles you've written. I'm pretty interested and was wondering if I could help with your research project." As the conversation progresses, let the professor know your long-term goals as well as your immediate desire both to contribute as a member of the research team and to acquire research skills. Let him or her know you are seriously considering graduate study in clinical or counseling psychology—it will increase your appeal.

Negotiating Research Responsibilities

"Well Mr./Ms. Smith, I'd be very interested in speaking with you about helping out with my research. . . ." You have made the contact. If the professor does not need help, you have lost nothing and gained the experience. Ask if he or she knows of someone with similar interests who is looking for help, or simply approach the next person on your list.

After the initial contact, your next move is dictated by your professor's needs and your abilities. Regardless of all your wonderful qualities, be prepared to run some of the grunt work! Photocopying needs to be done, literature searches need to be conducted, and at times you might well be expected to do some lab cleanup. You are "low person on the totem pole," so approach this with humility. But if you have experience with test administration or statistical analysis, let the professor know, being aware that ultimately your activities will be dictated first by his or her needs. However, if grunt work is the full extent of your duties, your needs are not being addressed properly. Spending a year doing nothing but photocopying would be a waste of time.

Research experience is, above all, an opportunity to learn. Volunteer to be trained to be of more use. For example, learn the computer skills to input data and conduct statistical analyses. Learn to score and, more importantly, to *understand* a Minnesota Multiphasic

Personality Inventory-2 (MMPI-2) or a Beck Depression Inventory (BDI-II). Learn how to calibrate and run psychophysiological equipment. Whatever equipment or tests, find out about them and their use. And always ask questions about what you do not understand. When it comes time to put your research on your curriculum vitae, these are the responsibilities you will want to list.

Some researchers have a weekly lab group or research meeting with graduate students, undergraduates, or both. These might entail a discussion of the project at hand, or a presentation on another area within the field, or a training session for new people. In any of these cases, it is an opportunity to learn more about your area of interest. If you have not been invited to these meetings, go ahead and ask about them. Optimize your contact with your professor! Convey your willingness and enthusiasm. Give your professor reason to write an outstanding letter of recommendation.

Finally, there are some instances where undergraduates are solely supervised by graduate students and have little contact with the professor in charge of the project. This can happen if faculty members have a large number of students working with them or if they are well known and are continually approached by masses of students. Being supervised exclusively by a graduate student is an undesirable situation for a potential applicant. Although there is much to be learned from graduate students—and they are fresh from the application process themselves—a letter of recommendation from a graduate student does not carry the same weight as one from a professor. Moreover, a lack of interaction with the professor means that he or she must depend solely on graduate students for feedback on your work, thus detracting from the value of his or her assessment.

This is *not* to say that you must avoid research opportunities that are primarily supervised by graduate students. Personal access to the faculty member is, however, one of several important factors to be considered in your decision on where to volunteer for research experience.

Arranging Credit and Semesters

Most colleges allow students to complete a certain amount of research experience for academic credit. If the opportunity is available, take advantage of it. Some professors may even demand that you sign up for credit, because it institutes a contract between them and you as to the number of hours per week required and how long they can count on you to work with them. Generally speaking, multiply the number of course credits by 3, and this will give you the number of weekly hours that you should spend doing research.

Expect to spend two semesters on a project. This demonstrates your commitment and allows ample contact between you and your professor. Thus, it is a good idea to work with someone at least 1 year before you plan to apply to graduate school. For instance, begin research in fall 2007 if you are applying in fall 2008 for a fall 2009 entrance to graduate school.

In consultation with your faculty advisor, consider applying for a university or national grant to fund your research project. These grant monies may be used to purchase equipment, pay postage for surveys, reimburse research participants for their time, and send you to a convention to present your findings. In most colleges and universities, these small grants are called undergraduate research grants, summer research fellowships, or something similar. At the University of Scranton, for example, the summer grants allow students to live on campus free for the summer, provide a tidy stipend, contribute up to $500 for research supplies, and fund travel to a conference in order to present the research. At the national level, Psi Chi and several publishers provide small awards and grants for research. Go to www.psichi.org/awards to access the list.

In terms of research, there is no such thing as too much for a Ph.D. applicant. The longer you have worked on a project and the greater your responsibilities, the more attractive you are as an applicant. Ideally, you would work with two professors over the course of your undergraduate education. This is not necessary, but when schools expect three letters of recommendation, having two letters summarizing two different research experiences is particularly strong. Although they will allocate less attention to research than Ph.D. applicants, Psy.D. applicants are reminded that research is still an important admission criterion.

One word of caution: do not overextend yourself. Be realistic about the amount of time you can commit. Some students juggle two or three research projects at once and end up performing poorly on them all. It is far more important to concentrate your energies and perform solidly on one project than it is to spread yourself too thin. Do as much research as your academic studies and other commitments allow.

An ideal time to begin research is during the summer, when you can balance it with a part- or full-time job. Since most undergraduates and some graduate students leave during the summer, professors may be short-staffed during this period. It is a prime opportunity to optimize your usefulness at the outset and increase your chances of picking up desirable skills.

The net result of your research experiences will be skill enhancement and professional identification. Depending on the nature of your project, you will probably have engaged in a literature search, hypothesis generation, experimental design, data collection, statistical analyses, and the write-up.

Presenting and Publishing Research

Presenting or publishing your research is a definite asset. Opportunities for presentation are numerous: a department or university colloquium, a local or regional undergraduate psychology conference, a state or national psychology convention. Participation in research conferences is viewed favorably as an index of your professional identification and commitment. Check with your advisor about these opportunities and other possibilities for your work to be seen by colleagues.

Publication of your research in a scholarly journal is held in very high regard by graduate admissions committees. As we discuss in Chapter 6, research experience leading to a coauthored publication is the most highly rated final selection criterion for Ph.D. (though not necessarily Psy.D.) admission decisions following the interview. The peer-review process by which journals accept papers for publication gives a seal of collegial affirmation that the research contributes to the scientific understanding of behavior. Although not common, undergraduate publication is slowly becoming more frequent.

If your research project is not quite up to the standards of a competitive, peer-reviewed journal, then consider sending the paper to a journal publishing student research in psychology. One such publication is the *Psi Chi Journal of Undergraduate Research,* which has the twofold purpose of fostering the scholarly efforts of undergraduate psychology students and of providing them with a valuable learning experience. Other publications for student research in psychology are *Modern Psychological Studies, Journal of Psychology and Behavioral Sciences,* and *Journal of Psychological Inquiry.* All these journals publish research in psychology conducted and written by students. Look for their instructions to authors on the Web (puffin.creighton .edu/psy/journal/studentjournals.asp), on departmental bulletin boards, or in *Eye on Psi Chi* (the national newsletter of Psi Chi).

Of course, though submission to these journals can be instructive, publishing in them does not carry as much weight as publication in established peer-reviewed journals. In fact, recent research suggests that a student publication in an undergraduate journal may be judged neutral or even unfavorably by research-oriented professors in a doctoral programs (Ferrari & Hemovich, 2004). So, always aim to publish your research in peer-reviewed, scholarly journals.

Still impressive is a paper/poster presentation at a state, regional, or national meeting. Only between 10% and 20% of undergraduate psychology majors present their research at some type of research conference, whether local, regional, or national (Terry, 1996; Titus & Buxman, 1999).

Most regional and national meetings are listed in each issue of the *American Psychologist, APS Observer,* and *Eye on Psi Chi.* These meetings are also listed on the Psi Chi Web site. Psi Chi members who present papers can receive a certificate recognizing their excellence in research. This award should be duly noted on your curriculum vitae and application. Refer to *Eye on Psi Chi,* ask your local Psi Chi moderator or consult their Web site at www.psichi.org/pdf/postcert.pdf to receive the form entitled "Certificate Recognition Program for Paper Presentations by Psi Chi Members."

Different graduate programs will assess your research experience in different ways, of course. Nonetheless, as an aid to applicants, we reproduce below (with permission) two rating scales employed at different times by one clinical program (University of Rhode Island) over the past 10 years. The first rating scale emphasizes research activity. Examples of relevant activities might include producing honors theses, serving as a research assistant, conducting independent research, coauthoring scientific publications, and developing research skills, such as data analysis and interviewing.

Rating	Criteria
5	Senior author of one or more articles in significant journals in addition to experience that provided a basis for extensive mastery of one or more directly related research skills.
4	Coauthor of one or more articles in significant journals in addition to experiences providing considerable familiarity with one or more directly relevant research skills.
3	Project leadership or significant participation in research activity (beyond activities connected with course work) serving to provide for considerable development of mastery of one or more relevant research skills.
2	Experience that provides a basis for some familiarity with relevant research skills.
1	Little if any experience according to these criteria.

The second rating scale, now in use at the University of Rhode Island, favors four criteria in evaluating research experience.

1. *Demonstrated research productivity:* sole or co-authorship of research publications, presentation of papers at scientific meetings, other tangible indications of research achievement.
2. *Breadth and quality of experience:* development of one or more research skills, data collection with different populations, work on more than one project.
3. *Research interest:* the strength of interest in research can be inferred from research activity over a sustained period of time and recommendations from research supervisors documenting skills, motivation, participation, and accomplishments.
4. *Individual autonomy:* responsibility for planning, implementing and carrying out research tasks as a member of a research team or evidence of independent work.

Rankings are based on the aforementioned criteria and assigned as follows:

Rating	Criteria
5	Satisfies all four criteria
4	Satisfies three criteria
3	Satisfies two criteria
2	Satisfies one criterion
1	Evidence of some prior research involvement or interest

Balance is the key. On the one hand, an absence of research experience is usually seen as a drawback to an application. On the other hand, over committing yourself to multiple projects at one time can lead to poor performance and a neglect of clinical experience and GRE preparation. And do not forget, research also provides you with the opportunity to make professional contacts. The professors or graduate students with whom you collaborate are excellent sources of information about the field and about applying to graduate schools.

Entrance Examinations

About 90% of doctoral clinical psychology programs (Mayne et al., 1994; Steinpreis, Queen, & Tennen, 1992) and 80% of doctoral counseling psychology programs (Turkson & Norcross, 1996) require you to complete two exams: the Graduate Record Examination (GRE) General Test and the GRE Psychology Subject Test.

The two GRE tests are often used to complement each other in admission decisions because the General Test is a measure of broad abilities and the Subject Test is an index of achievement in a specific field of study. The Miller Analogies Test (MAT) is required by fewer programs, about 3% of doctoral programs and 9% of master's programs in psychology (Murray & Williams, 1999; Norcross et al., 2005).

Blanket statements about entrance exams are difficult because not all schools require all tests, and some schools require additional testing (e.g., in the past the University of Minnesota required clinical psychology applicants to take the MMPI—a personality inventory!). Moreover, not all schools weight these tests equally among the application criteria. Some schools clearly state a minimum score that all applicants must obtain, whereas others state that they have no such criteria. Interestingly, a study at Boston University (Rem, Oren, & Childrey, 1987) showed that even without an imposed cutoff, applicants admitted into its Ph.D. program had GRE scores of 600 or better. This suggests that even if a program does not emphasize entrance exams, (1) scores can still play a major role in the selection of candidates, or (2) applicants with high exam scores are also the applicants considered most desirable on the other admissions criteria.

Consequently, the best assistance that can be offered is a brief description of each test, an overview of minimum and actual GRE scores of incoming graduate students, guidelines for deciding how much preparation will be needed, and some suggestions as to the available study aids for each test.

GRE General Test

Use of GRE scores for admission to clinical and counseling psychology programs continues to be the norm and continues to be controversial (Dollinger, 1989; Ingram, 1983; Sternberg, 1997). The traditional rationale—buttressed by some evidence—is that the GRE is ordinarily more valid than undergraduate GPA in predicting graduate school success (Boudreau et al., 1983; Goldberg & Alliger, 1992). Another rationale is that GRE performance is an "equalizer" among the diverse curriculum requirements and grading practices in thousands of undergraduate institutions. The entrance exam is probably the only standardized measure of all applicants that an admissions committee has. Does a 3.7 GPA and stellar letters of recommendation from Backwater College reflect more, the same, or less knowledge than a 3.3 GPA and strong letters of recommendation from Ivy League University? Since all students take the identical GRE test, the playing field is leveled.

The empirical research indicates that the GRE General Test has modest predictive validity for graduate school performance. A meta-analysis of studies conducted in psychology and counseling departments found that GRE scores predicted about 8% of the variance in graduate school GPA (Goldberg & Alliger, 1992). A later meta-analysis of two dozen studies encompassing more than 5,000 test takers similarly reported that 6% of the variance in graduate-level academic achievement was accounted for by GRE scores (Morrison & Morrison, 1995). These and other studies (e.g., Chernyshenko & Ones, 1999; Kuncel, Hezlett, & Ones, 2001) indicate that GRE General Test scores are generalizably valid in a modest way for all sorts of measures of graduate performance, especially when selection/admission ratios are taken into account. At the same time, Subject Test scores tend to be better predictors than the General Test scores (Kuncel et al., 2001).

The Educational Testing Service (ETS), located in Princeton, New Jersey, provides a free, online booklet entitled *GRE Information and Registration Bulletin* (www.ets.org/media/tests/gre/pdf/0708_gre_bulletin .pdf; Graduate Record Examinations, 2007), which describes the test and offers examples of the types of questions you can expect to encounter on each section. You can obtain the same information and register for the test by visiting GRE online at www.gre.org. In addition, at this Web site you can order (with a credit card) ETS test preparation books and download preparation software directly onto your home computer.

The test is similar in format to the Scholastic Aptitude Test (SAT) that most of you took prior to college. The three GRE scales are Verbal Reasoning (V), Quantitative Reasoning (Q), and Analytical Writing (AW). The Verbal and Quantitative scales are multiple-choice in format, and scores on the test are based on the number of correct answers selected. Most graduate schools rely on the Verbal and Quantitative scores in evaluating candidates.

The Analytical Writing section, in which you write two essays, is delivered on the computer, and you word-process your responses. For the "Present Your Perspective on an Issue" task, you will choose one of two essay topics selected by the computer from a larger pool of topics. For the "Analyze an Argument" task, you do not have a choice of topics; the computer will present you with a single topic. Your essays are read and scored by two trained raters using a holistic 6-point scale (scoring guidelines can be found at www .gre.org/pracmats.html). Your Analytical Writing (AW) score is reported on the 0–6 scale in half-point increments. Since the AW test is relatively recent, many graduate schools are not yet placing as much emphasis on it as the Verbal and Quantitative scores in admission decisions. But this will surely change in the near future, as graduate admissions committees seek an independent measure of your writing ability.

The GRE General Test is now available only on computer; the traditional paper-and-pencil version was phased out in 1999. This computer-based test always begins with the 75-minute Analytical Writing section: 45 minutes for the Issue essay and 30 minutes for Argument essay. Then follows the 30-minute Verbal section and the 45-minute Quantitative section.

In addition, a pretest section or research section may be included, but answers to these sections do not count toward your score. All told, you will probably spend about 4 hours at the testing center.

When you complete all sections of the GRE at the testing center, you will be asked two questions: Do you want to cancel your scores? To which four graduate schools would you like your test scores sent? If you do *not* cancel your scores, then your Verbal and Quantitative scores are immediately presented on the computer screen. Your Analytical Writing score will arrive by mail in another 4 weeks or so. If you cancel your scores, then you are not provided with those scores.

The testing center consists of multiple cubicles, each containing a computer station. The center may be noisy, so many of our students recommend wearing ear plugs or accepting the offered headphones to minimize the extraneous noise and to enhance your concentration. Some test-takers are unnerved by the presence of cameras in the center (or above the cubicle); these exist only for test security purposes. But knowing in advance will probably decrease your anxiety.

The GRE registration booklet and the free tutorial software (POWER PREP, available at www.ets.org/ powerprep) will familiarize you with the computer-based adaptive format of the Verbal and Quantitative sections. Briefly put, adaptive testing means that your responses to the early items determine the difficulty level of subsequent items and your range of possible scores. As you answer each question, the computer immediately scores that question and your preceding answers to determine which question is presented next. Correct answers lead to increasingly difficult items (and eventually higher test scores); incorrect answers lead to less difficult items (and lower test scores). As a consequence, you may not skip any questions and you may not go back and change a previous answer. An equally important consequence is that you should be very familiar with the test format and computer functions before test day!

TABLE 2-4. Minimum GRE Scores Preferred by APA-Accredited Clinical Psychology Programs

Preferred minimum score	Psy.D. programs		Practice-oriented Ph.D.		Equal-emphasis Ph.D.		Research-oriented Ph.D.		All programs	
	M	SD	M	SD	M	SD	M	SD	M	SD
Quantitative scale	544	40	500	58	580	44	598	36	581	46
Verbal scale	533	50	566	58	583	46	598	36	580	48
Psychology subject test	542	49	601	17	581	48	605	43	587	47

Note. Adapted from Mayne, Norcross, & Sayette (1994) and Turkson & Norcross (1996).

In deciding how much and what type of preparation you will need for this test, ask yourself several questions:

1. What were my SAT scores? These two tests are highly correlated in a positive direction, so this may be your first clue as to how much preparation is ahead of you.
2. How well have I done on multiple-choice tests in college? There is a certain savvy to taking standardized tests, and this is one way to assess yours.
3. How anxious do I become in a testing situation? A moderate amount of test anxiety is optimal: too little anxiety can breed indifference, but too much begets interference. If you tend to approach tests with more than moderate discomfort, you might benefit from additional preparation aimed at relaxing yourself and building your confidence.
4. Can I discipline myself to do the necessary studying? If you are in need of additional preparation, this question is important in deciding what the most appropriate form of preparation will be for you. Be honest with yourself. If you cannot imagine sitting down regularly and studying independently for the GREs, you might be better off taking a preparatory course offered privately in most cities.

Students typically spend an inordinate amount of time worrying about the GREs. The myth exists that clinical applicants need a score of 650 on each of their subscales to be considered seriously. This is simply not the case. Some Psy.D. programs do not even require the GREs. On the other hand, many APA-approved Ph.D. programs prefer GREs of 600 or above. The average GRE score (combined Verbal and Quantitative) of first-year graduate students in psychology master's programs is 1053; in doctoral psychology programs, 1183 (Norcross et al., 2005).

However, even these averages mask considerable variation in preferred minimum GRE scores. In our study of the admission statistics of APA-accredited clinical doctoral programs (Mayne et al., 1994), we found that the preferred minimum scores differed consistently according to the type of program. As shown in Table 2-4, research-oriented clinical Ph.D. programs preferred the highest GRE minimum scores—about 600 each for the Quantitative and Verbal scales. Psy.D. programs were willing to accept lower (but still not low) minimum GRE scores—about 520 to 540 each on the two scales. In between these two poles is the remainder of clinical and counseling psychology doctoral programs, which expect a minimum score of 550 to 560 on each of the scales, on average (Turkson & Norcross, 1996).

Even if your scores are lower than 550, you can bolster other areas of your application to overcome low scores. But if your GRE scores are below 500, then most Ph.D. programs in clinical and counseling psychology will not seriously consider your application. In this case, it will probably be necessary to take them again after completing a preparatory course or after spending time with a study guide. Or you may decide to apply to Psy.D. and master's programs as well.

Overconfidence can be disastrous here. Even if you obtained 700 SATs, aced every multiple-choice exam in college, and are cool-headed in testing situations, you should still familiarize yourself with the test format and complete the practice test offered in the application booklet. It certainly would not hurt to prepare more, but this should be considered the bare minimum.

Many self-study manuals and software packages are sufficient for a disciplined applicant to ready him or herself for the GRE. The books provide helpful test-taking hints, vocabulary and math reviews, and sample tests that the student can self-administer. Many include actual questions given on past GREs that can provide a real flavor for the material likely to be seen on testing day. The software packages administer sample tests and give helpful hints. Sample questions, practice manuals, and downloadable practice software packages can also be found and ordered on the official GRE Web site at www.gre.org. In addition to the official ETS site, several comprehensive and commercial Internet sites provide valuable tips and full-length practice tests. Some of the material is offered for free; some offered for a price. Visit:

- www.princetonreview.com/gre
- www.kaptest.com/Kaplan/3/Psychology/GRE
- www.mygretutor.com/
- 800score.com/gre-index.html
- www.greguide.com/

We heartily recommend taking an online GRE practice test. A practice GRE test serves as a diagnostic tool to assess your abilities, gauges your competitiveness for admission to graduate programs, and identifies areas that need further improvement (Walfish, 2004). Our favorites are the practice GRE tests at www.kaplan.com and www.princetonreview.com. These are free and confidential; use the practice test as a starting point.

Lastly, give yourself *at least* 6 weeks of study time if you decide to use a manual or 8 weeks if you do not have a lot of time to devote solely to studying.

Students feeling less confident, more anxious, or "out of the exam business" should contemplate private courses designed to help you prepare for the GRE. They offer a number of benefits beyond those of study guides:

- A structured time one or more times a week when the material is taught by an impartial instructor who can assess your strengths and weaknesses
- An abundance of study materials and the possibility of individual tutoring
- The chance to take tests under actual test-taking conditions (especially helpful for those with test anxiety)
- Specific work on test-taking skills and the shortcuts that can make problems easier
- Brief introduction to relaxation exercises that can counter test anxiety

The imposed structure on studying and the conscious use of test-taking skills can be very useful. Although these classes cannot guarantee that they will improve your scores, they are undoubtedly the best course of action for some students. Having worked for one of these organizations, we have seen the benefits of this system for many students.

Many students attempt to strengthen their vocabulary for the GRE Verbal section by preparing flashcards or memorizing a vocabulary word each day. The early research on the word-a-day method suggests it can slightly enrich your vocabulary (Prevoznak & Bubka, 1999), but more importantly, it gets you into the swing of GRE preparation and the admissions process. If you are inclined to try this method, consider receiving a word a day from the Web site, www.wordsmith.org, which presents a word with its pronunciation and examples. Or try the vocabulary builders at www.supervoca.com/gre.htm and www.number2.com. They require only a couple of minutes per day.

Scheduling *when* to take your general GRE should be carefully considered. If you do poorly on the test, you can retake it. Consequently, it is prudent to take it at least 6 months before the application deadline, which gives you time to study and prepare for a second administration. For undergraduates planning to apply to graduate school during their senior year, this means taking it during the summer following your junior year or early fall of the senior year. For graduates, this means taking it the spring before you plan to apply. Even if you improve your scores, the current ETS policy is to send to each institution scores from *all* your tests taken during the last 5 years.

We are frequently asked by students in our graduate school workshops if they should retake the GRE General Test if they are dissatisfied with their original scores. Our immediate answer is: it depends. If you studied diligently for the test and if you performed similar to the practice tests, then no—do not retake the test. But if any of the following five factors apply to you, then retaking the test once seems like a good idea (Keith-Spiegel & Wiederman, 2000): (1) You were ill the day you took the GRE; (2) you were immobilized by test anxiety; (3) you did not prepare for the test content; (4) you were unfamiliar with the computer-based format and the adaptive design; (5) your SAT scores were much higher than your GRE scores.

Should you decide to retake the GRE General Test, please be aware of the probable effects of repeating it. The average score gain for repeaters is about 27 points on the Verbal scale and 30 points on the Quantitative scale. Increases of more than 100 points rarely occur, in only 1 or 2% of repeaters (ETS, 1984).

Your GRE score can partially determine where to apply. Low scores suggest applying only to institutions whose minimum scores you surpass. In this way, your GREs can help you make realistic decisions as to your

PREPARING FOR GRADUATE SCHOOL

chances of being accepted at a given school and ultimately whether to apply there.

GRE Psychology Subject Test

The General Test measures knowledge acquired over a long period of time and not indigenous to any specific field of study. By contrast, the Subject Tests—such as the Psychology Subject Test—assume an undergraduate major or extensive background in the specific subject. Consequently, the test may be relatively difficult if you were not an undergraduate psychology major.

Another difference between the General Test and the Subject Test lies in the mode of administration. The General Test is a computer-based test available year-round at over 600 test centers. The Subject Test, by contrast, continues to be a paper-based test offered three times during the academic year.

Table 2-5 summarizes the differences between the GRE General Test and the GRE Subject Test. These profound test differences will lead to different preparation and test-taking strategies on your part.

The GRE Psychology Test consists of about 215 multiple-choice questions. Each item has five options, from which you select the correct or best response.

The total time allotted for the test is 2 hours and 50 minutes.

The GRE Psychology Test yields a total score and two subscores. Virtually all graduate programs, however, concentrate on the total score, not on the subscores. The preferred minimum score is 587 for clinical psychology doctoral programs and 541 for counseling psychology doctoral programs (Mayne et al., 1994; Turkson & Norcross, 1996). That is, most programs will be expecting you to secure a score at or above this number. But here again, as shown in Table 2-4, the preferred minimum ranges from a low of 542 in Psy.D. programs to a high of 605 in research-oriented Ph.D. programs.

The two subscales are an Experimental or natural science orientation and a Social or social science orientation. The Experimental subscore covers questions in learning, cognition, perception, comparative psychology, sensation, and physiological psychology. The Social subscore includes an equal number of questions in personality, clinical, abnormal, developmental, and social psychology.

Percentages of questions devoted to a subject area will vary somewhat from one test administration to

TABLE 2-5. Comparison of the GRE General Test and the GRE Psychology Subject Test

	General Test	Psychology Subject Test
Content assessed	Broad knowledge	Specific knowledge in psychology
Test format	Computer	Paper-and-pencil
Administration schedule	Throughout the year	Three times per year (Oct., Nov., & Apr.)
Recommended test date	Summer of junior year Early Fall of senior year	October for Ph.D./Psy.D. applicants November for master's applicants
Administration format	Individual	Group
Test cost (2007–2008)	$140	$130
Repeat policy	May repeat test once per calendar month up to 5 times per year	May repeat test as often as it is offered
Testing time	2 hours, 45 minutes	2 hours, 50 minutes
Scoring procedure	Adaptive: your early responses determine difficulty level of subsequent questions	Total items answered correctly minus one-fourth the number answered incorrectly
Skipping questions	Not permitted; computer administers one question at a time	Permitted
Scores provided	3 scores (Verbal Reasoning, Quantitative Reasoning, & Analytical Writing)	1 total score, 2 subscores
Scores range	200–800 for Verbal and Quantitative; 0–6 for Analytical Writing	200–990
Scores mean (SD)	500 (100)	540 (100)
Recommended preparation	Intense	Moderate

37

another. Nonetheless, one set of investigators (Waters, Drew, & Ayers, 1988) found these approximate percentages on past tests:

Physiological/comparative psychology	14%
Developmental psychology	12%
Learning and motivation	12%
Sensation and perception	12%
Clinical/abnormal psychology	11%
Personality and social psychology	11%
Cognition and complex human learning	10%
Applied psychology	9%
Research methodology	9%

Scores on the GRE Psychology Test are best predicted by your GRE General Test scores and the number of basic psychology courses completed. The irony is that students can obtain excellent grades in all their psychology courses but still not perform adequately on the Psychology Test if they have not taken the critical courses. A narrow focus on—and many courses in—clinical psychology will probably detract from your score since this one area only accounts for 10 to 12% of the test items. The questions are drawn from courses most commonly offered at the undergraduate level within psychology (ETS, 1995).

A maximum number of "traditional" courses in psychology, as represented in the foregoing list, and a minimum of special topics and "pop" psychology will prepare you best for the GRE Psychology Subject Test. Choose your elective courses for breadth and rigor, not merely your specialized interest.

The GRE Psychology Subject Test is designed to be challenging. Students accustomed to getting 90% correct on in-class exams often worry about the large number of items they miss. The average student answers about half the items correctly, misses about 30%, and omits 20% (Kalat & Matlin, 2000). Because your score is based on the number of questions answered correctly minus one-fourth of the questions answered incorrectly, guessing does *not* lower your score. You are not penalized for guessing; but you are rewarded for eliminating one or two possible answers.

Adequate preparation is essential for this test. We —and others—suggest four steps: (1) obtain the free ETS booklet *A Description of the Advanced Psychology Test;* (2) review a good introductory psychology textbook; (3) volunteer to be a TA (teaching assistant) for the Introduction to Psychology course; and (4) purchase one of the study guides with practice tests. Our favorite study guides are *Practicing to Take the GRE Psychology Test* (2004, published by the GRE board and which can be ordered at the ETS Web site), *Graduate*

Record Examination—Psychology (Raphael & Halpert, 1999; published by Prentice Hall), *GRE Psychology with CD-ROM*—The Best Test Prep for the GRE (Kellogg, 2003; published by Research & Education Association), and *Cracking the GRE Psychology* (2005 by Princeton Review). If these four steps do not suffice, then private courses in preparing for the psychology test are available.

The standard error of measurement for the GRE is quite small, and retaking the General Test in the absence of any *intense* remediation is unlikely to result in a significant change in your score. Your Psychology subject Test scores, however, may be significantly different if intervening study or additional courses occur between the test sessions.

A graduate school may adopt one or more policies in handling cases in which a candidate reports two sets of GRE scores: consider only the most recent one; consider the higher of the two scores; or average the scores. The latter is probably the best alternative, since it creates the least bias and is the most reliable.

Miller Analogies Test

A few clinical and counseling psychology doctoral programs request the MAT, a 50-minute test consisting of 100 word analogies. Your score is the total number correct; the mean for students intending to study psychology in graduate school is 50 to 51 (The Psychological Corporation, 1994). As with the GREs, booklets are available to help improve your scores on the test, and it is useful to take practice tests to familiarize and prepare yourself for the actual event. There are states in which the MAT cannot be administered (e.g., New York) because of test disclosure laws enacted in those states, so be sure to locate the testing center nearest you.

The MATs are rarely required by graduate schools. Because the test can be scheduled at any time, through a network of over 600 testing centers nationwide, consider taking this test after you have received your GRE scores and after you have selected the schools you would like to apply to. You will save time and money if none of the schools that interest you require the test.

Part of the expense of applying to graduate school is the cost of sending test scores. One possible way to reduce costs is to make copies of the test results sent to you and mail them with your application. Any school that is interested in you will request that you have the scores "officially" sent to them. Any school not interested will not need your official scores, and you will have saved the expense of having them forwarded.

Two words of caution must accompany this possibility. First, only do this if you send in your application early. Unless you check with a graduate program before the application deadline to make sure that this procedure will not exclude you as an applicant, you should not send copies. Second, some students send copies of test scores after altering the original document, for example, whiting out poor scores or past scores, putting scores in different columns, and even falsifying scores. *You must never resort to these practices!* These should immediately invalidate your application, and any school that accepts you will need official copies sent anyway.

Finally, low scores on entrance exams do not automatically preclude you from applying to clinical or counseling psychology graduate programs. Rather, low scores mean you will apply to programs that do not emphasize test scores or that accept scores in your range. You can partially compensate in other areas to help offset weak GRE scores. As with each admission criterion, entrance examinations are only one part of the overall picture of a candidate. The best anyone can do is to make his or her application as attractive as possible.

Extracurricular Activities

An applicant's extracurricular pursuits are accorded less weight than GPAs, GRE scores, research competency, and clinical experience. The research reviewed earlier in this chapter clearly bears this point out. However, extracurricular activities, such as Psi Chi membership and campus involvement, are still considered in evaluating the "total person" of the applicant.

The admission implications are thus proscriptive and prescriptive. Strictly in terms of enhancing your candidacy (not in terms of other goals, such as life satisfaction), you should favor good grades and research experience over extracurricular activities. Involvement in a dozen student organizations will not compensate for meager grades and research; doctoral programs will not accept you because you coached youth soccer. When confronted with time conflicts, recall that admissions committees place a premium on variables other than intense campus commitments.

Having stated the obvious but unpleasant facts, we would also urge you to routinely engage in *some* campus and community pursuits. The reasoning here is that clinical and counseling psychology programs seek well-rounded individuals with diverse interests. The "egghead" or "Mr. Peabody" image is to be avoided in the practice of psychology, where your interpersonal skills are as critical as your scientific preparation. Moderate involvement can also better acquaint you with faculty members, who may serve as sources of recom-

mendations, and with the discipline of psychology itself. You can create professional opportunities by simply being involved in departmental activities. "Familiar faces" are frequently given first shots at clinical or research opportunities.

Applicants frequently learn too late that active involvement outside of the classroom is an indispensable education in and of itself. Consider the following student qualities contained in many letter of recommendation forms:

- Academic performance
- Organizational skills
- Interest/enthusiasm
- Interpersonal skills
- Emotional stability
- Communication skills
- Originality/resourcefulness
- Social judgment
- Responsibility/dependability
- Stress tolerance

Most of these dimensions refer to faculty–student interactions *outside* of the classroom, not to your course grades. Many a bright student has sabotaged his or her educational experience, recommendation letters, and career goal by not becoming involved outside of the classroom.

In your extracurricular activities, try to exhibit the chief personality trait which, interacting with intelligence, relates most to vocational success—namely, conscientiousness (Jensen, 1998). Be responsible, dependable, organized, and persistent. This trait applies to every kind of educational and job success. What's more, you want colleagues and friends to document in their letters of recommendation that you are extraordinarily conscientious.

Four specific suggestions come to mind regarding the type of extracurricular activities to pursue. First, join departmental student organizations, such as the Psychology Club, Psi Chi, and the American Psychological Society's Student Caucus. Second, we heartily recommend that you join the American Psychological Association (APA) and/or the American Psychological Society (APS) as a student affiliate. Your APA affiliation brings with it monthly issues of the *American Psychologist,* the flagship journal, and the *APA Monitor,* the association's newspaper. Similarly, APS membership includes subscriptions to the monthly journal *Psychological Science* and the *APS Observer.* Student membership in professional associations reflects favorably on your commitment to the discipline, and this affiliation should be recorded on your curriculum vitae. Your psychology advisor might have applications for student affiliation in his or her office; if not, go online to www.apa.org/membership/forstudents.html and www.psychological science.org/join/.

Third, additional campus and community commitments should be guided by your interests. But those associated with human services, social causes, and artistic endeavors seem to be differentially rewarded. These will obviously vary with the locale; examples include Hand-in-Hand, campus ministries, course tutoring, peer advising, homeless shelters, women's centers, BACHUSS, SADD, theater productions, creative writing, Amnesty International, and the like.

A fourth and invaluable extracurricular experience is to attend a regional or national psychology convention. The benefits are many: socializing you into the profession; learning about current research; discovering how students and professors present research; meeting and hearing nationally known psychologists; adding to your growing professional network; attending and perhaps participating in sessions designed for prospective graduate students (e.g., the Psi Chi sessions and workshops); experiencing the intellectual stimulation; and enjoying the interpersonal camaraderie of fellow students and psychologists (Lubin, 1993; Tryon, 1985). For all these reasons, we have never—and we mean *never*—heard a single graduate school applicant express disappointment about attending his or her first psychology convention.

The challenge for most prospective psychologists is to locate and afford travel to one of the regional or national psychology conferences. To locate upcoming conferences in your area, ask your psychology professors, consult the lists regularly published in *Eye on Psi Chi* and *American Psychologist,* and keep an eye open for announcements and posters on departmental bulletin boards. "Convention season" in psychology is from March to May, when the regional psychological associations hold their annual conventions. These include the Eastern Psychological Association, Midwestern Psychological Association, Rocky Mountain Psychological Association, Western Psychological Association, and Southeastern Psychological Association. The national conventions of APA and APS are annually held in the late spring and summer months. To afford the travel and lodging, consider organizing a convention trip with your fellow students, requesting information on special hotel and registration rates for students, volunteering as a convention assistant, and holding fund-raisers with psychology student organizations to offset your expenses. By hook or crook, definitely plan on expanding your extracurricular horizons by attending a psychology convention.

Extracurricular activities should reflect your active and passionate pursuit of excellence. This is, after all, your chosen profession, your career, your future. Join honor societies, compete for awards, pursue honors, and consider applications for Truman, Rhodes, and Fulbright scholarships. You should be actively investigating undergraduate grants for your research, such as those administered nationally by Psi Chi or those awarded locally in your university. Passivity doesn't cut it in graduate school (or life).

Finally, as part of your preparation, discuss your graduate plans with those people who will be affected by those plans, such as partner, spouse, parents, children, and close friends. The sooner you start discussing your plans, the better. You may move hundreds of miles away and will probably be working 60 hours a week as a graduate student. Your absence—psychological and physical—will likely impact other people close to you. Begin the discussions now, not after you apply (Megargee, 2001).

In this chapter, we reviewed six admission criteria —course work, faculty mentoring, clinical experience, research skills, entrance examinations, and extracurricular activities—and suggested ways to improve in these areas. The material covered in this chapter is concerned with how you as the applicant can improve your credentials or marketability. But the application process goes both ways. In addition to selling yourself, you are also a consumer, evaluating the programs and deciding which ones are for you. The next two chapters help you evaluate characteristics of graduate programs.

CHAPTER 3

GETTING STARTED

Up to this point, we have focused on what you can do to enhance your credentials before beginning the application process. At some point, you must take realistic stock and evaluate where you stand as an applicant. Maybe you have taken your GREs. Perhaps you have signed up for some advanced psychology courses and have a satisfactory GPA. You have been supervised in a clinical setting and have begun research. You have reviewed your credentials and found that you have many strengths but also some weaknesses. You either shore up the deficient areas or make a decision to go ahead with what you have and hope to sell it well. In other words, you are ready to get started with the application process.

Process is an appropriate word to describe the endeavor that you are about to begin. The way you approach this task will greatly influence your chances of gaining admission. Sure, you can simply complete an application and passively wait for an interview. And this may work if your credentials are extremely strong. But for most individuals, an informed approach to the process can make all the difference!

Prospective graduate students frequently become nervous about the application process for several reasons. Perhaps the following remarks sound familiar: "Well, I have good recommendations and a 3.3 GPA, but my GREs are low"; "I have good GREs and spent a year working on a suicide hot line, but I don't have a lot of research experience"; "Although my credentials are excellent, all the schools that I applied to only accept 10 out of 300 applicants." Whichever of these situations applies, simply submitting an application minimizes your chances of acceptance. You can do a great deal to increase your admission probabilities and to decrease your anxiety as you compare yourself to exaggerated standards.

Common Misconceptions

We would like to begin by dispelling three common misconceptions about clinical and counseling psychology programs. The first misconception: there is a direct correlation between a university's undergraduate reputation and the status of its psychology graduate programs. In fact, there is no such correlation. Many of the best undergraduate institutions—Brown, Princeton, and the elite liberal arts colleges, for example—do not even offer graduate studies in clinical or counseling psychology.

A second misconception is that you should apply to a graduate psychology program on the basis of that institution's sports performance. We have met a number of students who have used this selection criterion with unfortunate consequences. Please do not allow your application decisions to rest on whether a university has an excellent football team or whether their basketball team made it to the Final Four of the NCAA tournament! Do not scoff at the reality of this practice; careful research has demonstrated that winning a national championship in a visible college sport consistently translates into increased applications to the winning institution (Toma & Cross, 1998).

A third common misconception is that there is an authoritative list of the finest graduate programs in clinical psychology. In reality, unlike business or law schools, there is no definitive ranking of the "best" psychology graduate programs. The quality of a program depends on what *you* are looking to get out of it.

The best school for someone seeking to become a psychologist conducting psychoanalytic psychotherapy in private practice is probably not going to be the program of choice for someone who has set his or her heart on becoming a psychophysiological researcher at a medical school. Each person could attend the "best" school for psychology in his or her area.

What we want to do is to shift the burden from you trying to meet a school's admissions demands to you finding a school that meets *your* needs. Graduate schools are looking for students with direction and passion. This does not mean you have made an irrevocable commitment to an area of research or type of clinical work. It means that you have an idea of the professional work you would like to do and toward which theoretical orientation(s) you lean.

You are selecting an institution based on your belief that it will mold you in the direction *you* have chosen. Graduate programs will look for this attitude in your statement of purpose. During your interviews, you will be asked about which professors you want to work with and what thoughts you have about their research projects. Even more likely, you will be directly asked, "Why are you applying here instead of someplace else?" By identifying your graduate training goals, you will impress interviewers at your selected programs with your direction and passion.

Acceptance Rates

The most pervasive myth about doctoral psychology programs is that "hardly anyone gets in—only 10%." Like most myths, this one does have a grain of truth. The average acceptance rate for *all* APA-accredited doctoral programs in clinical and counseling psychology is, in fact, 10% (Norcross et al., 2004; Turkson & Norcross, 1996). But in a very real way, the 10% figure is misleading and inaccurate on many counts.

Let's begin our foray into acceptance rates by defining the term. "Acceptance rate" refers to the percentage of applicants accepted for admission into a single graduate program, *not* the percentage of the entire applicant pool to all programs accepted for admission in a given year. The clinical doctoral program at University X may accept only 15 of 150 applicants (10%), but many of the applicants to University X not accepted there will be admitted elsewhere. Although only 10% of the applicants to a single doctoral program might be accepted into that *particular* program, about half of the entire applicant pool will be accepted into *some* clinical or counseling doctoral program. And half a chance isn't that bad.

Note, too, that the 10% figure refers only to acceptance rates of APA-accredited doctoral programs in clinical or counseling psychology. The acceptance rates at *non*-APA-accredited doctoral programs are double that for APA-accredited programs: 20% for nonaccredited Ph.D. programs and 60% for nonaccredited Psy.D. programs (Norcross et al., 2005). The acceptance rates for master's programs are also much higher than those for doctoral programs. The median acceptance rates for master's programs are 49% in clinical psychology and 67% in counseling psychology (Norcross et al., 2005).

Most importantly, the acceptance rates vary tremendously from doctoral program to doctoral program as a function of the research–practice continuum. As shown in the Reports on Individual programs following Chapter 7, acceptance rates at research-oriented clinical Ph.D. programs, such as Yale and Duke, are as low as 3%. The acceptance rates at freestanding Psy.D. programs are often over 50%.

Table 3-1 summarizes the findings of several of our studies on acceptance rates to APA-accredited clinical psychology programs as a function of the type of program. All types of program average between 150 and 200 applications per year. Research-oriented Ph.D. programs accept only 6% of their applicants, on average, whereas the corresponding figures are 10% for equal-emphasis Ph.D. and 12% for practice-oriented Ph.D. programs. University-based Psy.D. programs accept 41% of their applicants on average, and freestanding Psy.D. programs accept 50%. That's quite a

TABLE 3-1. Average Acceptance Rates for APA-Accredited Clinical Psychology Programs

	Freestanding Psy.D.	University-based Psy.D.	Practice-oriented Ph.D.	Equal-emphasis Ph.D.	Research-oriented Ph.D.
Number of applications	186	164	154	170	189
Number of acceptances	93	53	18	21	13
Acceptance rate	50%	41%	10%	10%	6%

Note. Data from Norcross, Castle, Sayette, & Mayne (2004); Norcross & Oliver (2005); and Norcross, Sayette, Mayne, Karg, & Turkson (1998).

range of acceptance rates—6% to 50%—all in APA-accredited doctoral programs in clinical psychology. And that's why we urge caution in tossing around the 10% acceptance rate.

Costs of Applying

Applying to graduate school is an expensive proposition —not only in terms of your valuable time but also in terms of hard money. Application fees average $50 per doctoral program and $35 per master's program (Norcross et al., 2004). Only 7% of graduate schools let you apply for free (Norcross et al., 1996). The fee (in 2008) for the GRE General Test is $140, with a $50 rescheduling fee, and the Psychology Subject Test costs another $130. ETS will electronically transmit your GRE scores free of charge to four graduate schools that you designate in advance; however, each additional score report costs $15 per recipient. Throw in the costs of transcripts, photocopying, postage, and the innumerable telephone calls, and the investment can become quite costly. All told, we estimate that applying to 10–12 schools will run about $1,000 (and that number can increase depending on the cost of traveling to multiple interviews).

Several students challenged our estimate that the graduate application process would cost them $1,000. They protested that our figure was way too high. So, we encouraged them, like good psychologists, to collect data as they proceeded through the process. Here is the breakdown of costs from one typical applicant (Krystle Evans) who applied to 10 doctoral programs in 2004:

Taking the GRE tests	$270
Sending GRE scores	$156
Requesting transcripts	$130
Application fees	$475
Mailing applications	$30

That's a total of $1,061, before traveling to doctoral programs for personal interviews. She now believes the $1,000 estimate is on target.

The good news is that graduate schools are sensitive to financial hardship and that, for many students, the burdensome short-term cost is an excellent long-term investment. Schools build into the application process allowances for students who cannot afford the expense. Even the GRE has a fee waiver for students in dire financial circumstances. One of us was supporting himself on a meager social service salary and was able to keep the cost down to a few hundred dollars.

Moreover, think of the application cost as an investment in yourself and in your career. If you gain acceptance into a doctoral program with tuition remission and a stipend for 4 years, your $1,000 can be converted into a $60,000 to $100,000 payback over the course of your graduate school career.

The bottom line in getting started is this: anticipate the costs of applying to graduate school and plan to have the funds (or waivers) available before you begin completing applications.

Starting Early

Let's discuss timing up front. Applications are typically due from the middle week of December to the second week in February. The sooner you begin preparing, the more advantage you can take of an aggressive, early start to the admission process. As mentioned in earlier chapters and in the Time Line (Appendix A), for undergraduates, ideally this would take place the summer of your junior year. For others, this would best occur the summer of the year before you actually plan to attend graduate school. If it is past that point, you are not too late. You can follow the steps we will describe as late as October of your application year.

Applying to graduate school is like planning a political campaign or a military operation. It is impossible to begin too soon or to be too thorough (Megargee, 1990). Recognize this about the application process and *start almost a year before you expect to begin graduate school.* Completing the application materials in the fall semester alone will consume as much time as a 3-credit course!

Virtually all APA-accredited clinical and counseling psychology programs only accept matriculating students for their fall semesters. As mentioned earlier, in order to be accepted for the fall of 2008, most doctoral programs have application deadlines anywhere from mid-December 2007 to February 2008. The typical deadline for doctoral programs in clinical and counseling psychology is January 15 (Norcross et al., 1996). Accordingly, you will need college transcripts, test scores, and letters of recommendation, not to mention time to prepare yourself before the application deadline. You should expect to begin no later than the fall of the year before you intend to attend graduate school. If you are willing to put in the maximum effort to get into a program, expect to begin the spring before that.

The APA has accredited 232 active doctoral programs in clinical psychology, 67 active doctoral programs in counseling psychology, and 10 active doctoral programs in combined psychology throughout the United States and Canada. Toss in nonaccredited doctoral programs and the mass of master's programs in clinical and counseling psychology and you wind up with roughly 600 graduate programs. How does one proceed in whittling this list to a manageable number?

To begin the selection process, ask yourself, "What kind of research or clinical work do I like? Is there some article I've read or presentation I've heard that really interests me?" There is a certain advantage if you have already conducted research or completed clinical experience as an undergraduate and know something about the field. And if you have completed an honors project or thesis, you may even have a certain amount of expertise. Or you may decide you would like to try something different now.

For example, suppose you have an interest in suicidology, but you are not sure that you want to do research in that area or exactly what that research would entail. Or you think you'd like to specialize in suicide prevention, but you're not sure how psychologists deal with the issue clinically. There are several approaches you can take to familiarize yourself with this area. Ask one of your professors for some readings. Check out a current textbook in the area. Go to a suicide prevention or crisis center and read through their literature. Surf the web. Then decide whether you like the questions being asked and the methods used to answer them.

In summary, have an idea of the field(s) in which you would like to work, either the ones with which you are already familiar or those you are willing to research. Familiarize yourself with the questions being asked and the techniques being used to answer them. Use as many sources as possible to gain information to help you narrow down your interests and educate yourself about them.

In addition to the resources in this book, a number of Internet sites will help you at this stage of the process. You can familiarize yourself with psychology graduate programs in the United States and Canada by accessing a large number of Web sites. Our favorites are:

- www.apa.org/students/
  (APA's site for students includes a list of accredited programs, relevant articles, and other useful materials)
- www.socialpsychology.org/clinical.htm
  (useful page features hyperlinks to 185 departments in the United States offering a Ph.D. in psychology)
- www.clas.ufl.edu/CLAS/american-universities .html#A
  (links for a plethora of American universities)
- www.psychwww.com/resource/deptlist.htm
  (an impressive listing of over 1,000 psychology department Web sites)

- www.petersons.com/gradchannel/
  (brief descriptions of programs offering graduate training in clinical and counseling psychology)
- www.gradschools.com/listings/menus/psych_ clinic_menu.html and
- www.gradschools.com/listings/menus/psych_ cmt_menu.html
  (for searching clinical and counseling psychology programs, respectively, with the added ability to search by geographic region)
- www.jobweb.org/catapult/gguides.htm
  (links to sites about applying to and financing graduate school, and about making the transition to graduate school)

All these—and other—sites enable you to take a virtual tour of graduate programs in professional psychology. Develop an early feel for various departments and begin to sharpen your interests.

Next is the task of putting this knowledge to use. You have interests, and you now need to learn which graduate programs can provide these research or clinical opportunities. Though knowing how much you enjoy research or clinical work may not take a lot of reflection, deciding whether to select a research-oriented, a practice-oriented, or an equal-emphasis program is a question with far-reaching ramifications. This question tends to divide people into three groups: the research oriented (scientists); the practice oriented (practitioners); and the dually committed (scientist–practitioners). The following sections are designed to lead each group in its appropriate direction. These groups tend to follow three rather distinctive career paths in the profession of clinical and counseling psychology (Bernstein & Kerr, 1993; Conway, 1988).

We have repeatedly surveyed the APA-accredited clinical and counseling psychology programs over the past 20 years. Their responses to our questionnaires (e.g., Farry et al., 1995; Mayne et al., 1994; Norcross et al., 1998; Norcross et al., 2004; Norcross, 2005; Oliver et al., 2005; Sayette & Mayne, 1990; Sayette et al., 1999; Turkson & Norcross, 1996) can serve as the basis for your initial selection of graduate programs. By using their responses, we will lead you through an exercise that will provide you with a list that ranks schools by how closely they meet your expectations and interests.

As you review the Reports on Individual Programs, bear in mind that the listings are alphabetical, not geographical. We list the programs alphabetically as they are on the APA (2007; www.apa.org/ed/accreditation/ doctoral.html) materials, but sometimes the order is counterintuitive. For example, the University of Arkansas is not listed under "U," but between Arizona State

University and Auburn University. Thus, you might need to look under two letters to identify specific programs of interest.

For the Research Oriented and Dually Committed

This section gives guidance to those applicants who are centrally focused on research and those with equal practice and research interest. We group these two sorts of applicants together because their initial selection of schools will place more emphasis on the research available at each program and secondarily on the clinical work available. This will allow people with an equal emphasis to cast their nets as widely and as efficiently as possible.

One question we asked of each program in our studies was "In which areas of research are your faculty presently working? Do they presently have a grant in that area?" Appendix E lists all the research areas provided by the graduate programs along with the number of faculty interested in these areas and an indication of whether they have a grant. This information provides you with an index of how intensively each program is pursuing this area of research. Thus, a program with three faculty members researching autism that has a grant supporting their work indicates serious involvement on the part of that faculty.

Find your areas of interest in the appendix; underneath them you will see a list of programs doing that type of research. In addition, you will know the number of professors with whom you could potentially work and whether there is grant money supporting this research.

A few words of caution in interpreting this appendix: not all programs were equally comprehensive in completing the survey. Some schools only included core faculty, whereas others included adjunct faculty. This accounts for what seems to be an overrepresentation of some institutions on the list. Also, some schools had research interests combining two different areas and listed a single grant under both.

Appendix B, entitled "Worksheet for Choosing Programs," is used to select programs to which you will eventually apply. Begin by writing your research interest in the far left-hand column. In the next column, marked "Schools," write the list of schools under that heading in Appendix B. In columns 3 and 4, write down the number of faculty in that area at each school and whether they are grant funded. In addition, some schools merely indicated the presence of grant funding and not the total number of grants. Thus, a "1" in the "Grants" column indicated *at least* one grant. A "0"

indicates no grants, and numbers greater than 1 indicate multiple grants.

There are two worksheets provided in Appendix B, allowing you to explore different areas of interest. If you have more than two main areas of interest, unless they are closely related, you may find the list becoming exceptionally long. In that case, you may wish either to narrow your areas of interest or to complete this worksheet with the aid of a trusted professor who can help you pare down the list of schools to a manageable number. If you have more than one area of interest, put stars next to the programs that have faculty doing research in both of them.

If your interests lean toward research, then you want to pick a programs highly regarded in the area of research you would like to pursue. How do you evaluate the clinical and counseling psychology programs on your list in terms of research? Refer to Table 3-2, which is adapted from the results of the *Social Sciences Citation Index* (SSCI) and *Science Citation Index* (SCI) databases. More than 225 psychology journals from 1998 to 2002 were analyzed to determine the institutions with the most citations. The goal was to identify the institutions employing faculty members who authored the most frequently referenced articles in psychology journals. The table lists, in rank order, the frequency with which articles written by members of a particular institution are cited. Only those institutions with an APA-accredited clinical or counseling program are included on this list. It should also be noted that the list only includes those institutions that produced at least 100 papers over the 5-year span; as a result, several smaller institutions with clinical or counseling psychology programs did not make the list.

Using Table 3-2, write the citation ranking for each school in column 5, labeled "Citation Rank." Be advised that this ranking reflects the psychology department in general, not just the clinical or counseling program. In fact, about 20% of the institutions on the original list of 75 were deleted because they do not have clinical or counseling psychology programs. Inclusion of these nonclinical influences will affect the ranking of the schools you have selected. Still, this will provide you with a rough idea of where each school stands in terms of its research. Our position is that a school that makes it onto this list is probably a strong research-oriented institution. If the school fails to appear on the table, then it may or may not emphasize psychological research. Recognize that only about 20% of APA-accredited programs appear on this list.

Table 3-2 also contains a column headed "Faculty Production Rank." This number represents the rank ordering of APA-accredited clinical psychology programs

TABLE 3-2. Institutions with Most Citations, Most Papers, and Strongest Clinical Faculty Production in Psychology

Citation rank	Institution[a]	Citations	Papers	Faculty production rank
2	University of Michigan	3,999	816	3
4	University of Minnesota	3,231	741	4
5	University of California–Los Angeles	3,211	867	9
6	University of Wisconsin–Madison	2,901	652	5.5
7	University of Illinois at Urbana–Champaign	2,856	690	1
8	Yale University	2,816	585	18.5
9	University of Pittsburgh	2,555	542	10
10	University of Pennsylvania	2,514	582	29
11	Indiana University	2,387	667	7.5
12	University of Washington	2,362	619	13.5
13	Duke University	2,344	453	18.5
14	Pennsylvania State University	2,302	766	11.5
15	University of California–San Diego	2,220	504	—
16	Ohio State University	2,177	617	22
17	Columbia University	2,170	652	29
18	University of Texas at Austin	2,085	551	7.5
19	University of Missouri	2,019	625	26
20	University of Iowa	1,968	495	34.5
21	University of Arizona	1,950	412	—
22	Northwestern University	1,935	449	48.5
23	University of North Carolina at Chapel Hill	1,933	468	31.5
24	University of Maryland College Park	1,921	546	48.5
26	Rutgers State University	1,872	473	18.5
27	University of California–Berkeley	1,862	436	34.5
29	University of Colorado	1,846	476	53.5
30	University of Rochester	1,817	292	15.5
31	New York University	1,775	503	34.5
32	Arizona State University	1,701	526	53.5
33	Vanderbilt University	1,658	340	13.5
34	University of Virginia	1,612	332	—
35	Boston University	1,573	369	—
36	University of Florida	1,498	537	18.5

continued

on the basis of the total number of clinical faculty members trained by that program (Ilardi, Rodriguez-Hanley, Roberts, & Seigel, 2000). Any program that received a ranking in the top 60 has an established track record of producing clinical psychologists who, themselves, later assumed clinical psychology faculty positions. Remember that these lists heavily favor older programs and that no single measure can ever capture the excellence of graduate education. And, again, only about 20% of APA-accredited clinical programs appear on the list. Still, the list does direct students interested in academic careers to programs that have historically excelled in this domain.

As mentioned, any APA-accredited program must provide both clinical and research training. Thus, it is important also to evaluate the clinical opportunities available. As already mentioned, Psy.D. programs by definition emphasize practice and train students to be

TABLE 3-2. Continued

Citation rank	Institution[a]	Citations	Papers	Faculty production rank
38	Emory University	1,470	325	—
39	University of Southern California	1,446	447	34.5
40	Purdue University	1,436	521	22
42	University of Oregon	1,401	241	26
43	University of Georgia	1,362	462	5.5
44	Michigan State University	1,355	411	31.5
45	University of Connecticut	1,308	407	29
48	State University of New York at Buffalo	1,252	322	38
49	Texas A&M University	1,244	399	—
50	Florida State University	1,237	353	22
51	University of Illinois at Chicago	1,231	350	58
52	Washington University	1,224	279	42.5
53	University of Massachusetts at Amherst	1,146	314	42.5
54	City University of New York	1,131	434	48.5
55	University of Miami	1,122	317	58
56	State University of New York at Stony Brook	1,056	285	2
57	University of California–Santa Barbara	1,041	275	—
58	Iowa State University	970	238	—
59	University of Kentucky	970	261	—
60	University of Kansas	944	384	15.5
61	Case Western Reserve University	928	222	—
62	University of Utah	916	256	38
63	University of Alabama	912	381	48.5
67	University of Nebraska	822	354	58
68	Louisiana State University	814	287	42.5
69	Wayne State University	775	281	53.5
71	University of Delaware	669	189	—
72	University of New Mexico	635	173	—
74	Washington State University	626	211	—
75	Yeshiva University	619	158	—

Note. Adapted from 1998–2002 *Social Sciences Citation Index* (SSCI) and *Science Citation Index* (SCI) databases. Also adapted from Ilardi, Rodriguez-Hanley, Roberts, & Seigel (2000).

[a]Institutions without APA-accredited programs in clinical or counseling psychology have been omitted from this table.

practitioners. Although it is possible to obtain research training at a Psy.D. program, this is not the primary emphasis of such programs. Consequently, a student with a clear research orientation should probably choose a Ph.D. program. For the research oriented, this column will be used to cross schools off their application list. Look up each school on your list in the reports on individual programs. If any of these schools offer only Psy.D. programs (see Table 1-4), you can delete that program.

The first column under the "Clinical" section of Appendix B is marked "Orientation." Under each program listed in our reports on individual programs, you will see a list of five theoretical orientations:

- Psychodynamic/psychoanalytic
- Radical behavioral/applied behavioral analysis
- Systems/family systems
- Humanistic/existential
- Cognitive/cognitive-behavioral

If you are clearly committed to (or strongly leaning toward) one of these orientations, then it is important that some faculty share that orientation with you. Check each program on your list and see if a suitable percentage of the faculty shares your orientation. If so, mark the "Orientation" column with a "+" sign. If not, mark it with a "−" sign.

If you are unsure of an orientation, or see yourself as integrative or eclectic, then be sure there is a wide variety of faculty orientations. If there is representation among the faculty in four or more of these orientations, that's a good sign. If the total you get when adding up all the percentages in the different orientations is greater than 100%, this is also a plus. It means some (or most) of the faculty bridge orientations and are integrative themselves. In other words, professors are listed under more than one category. In either case, mark the "Orientation" column with a "+" sign. If the faculty are of one or two orientations and without overlap, then mark this column with a "−" sign.

The second column under "Clinical" is "Res/Clin." Turn to Appendix F, "Specialty Clinics and Practica Sites." This is a list of specialty clinics and practica available at different programs. Specialty clinics focus on a specific clientele, such as depressed or eating-disordered clients. Practica are placements where students will conduct clinical work in their second, third, and/or fourth years of study. Some practica also specialize in a certain clientele. If you have a research interest in a particular population, it is important that the population be available for you to study and that you have the chance to work with that population clinically. For this reason, it is a great help for a researcher to have a specialty clinic or practicum in his or her area.

Look up your research area in Appendix F. If any of the programs on your list in Appendix B has a clinic or practicum in that area, mark the "Res/Clin" column with a plus. You can do likewise using Appendix G Concentrations and Specialty Tracks. Programs offering a formal track or concentration in your area of interest deserve a plus as well.

Again, this is just one indicator and must be kept in perspective. Most programs will have their own psychological training clinic, where a wide range of clinical populations may be seen or made available for research. Additionally, a faculty member may have a research population readily available in the community. And last, a few programs did not include practica placements off campus in the community, thus underrepresenting their practica opportunities. Still, being informed about a clinic or practicum specializing in your population of interest is certainly an advantage in selecting potential graduate programs.

The third column under the "Clinical" section is marked "Rank." Here, we refer to a program's production of students who go on to distinguished careers as clinicians, as measured by becoming ABPP Diplomates and by election as Fellows in APA's Division of Clinical Psychology or Division of Counseling Psychology. The "ABPP" refers to diplomate status awarded by the American Board of Professional Psychology (www.abpp.org), which certifies excellence in 13 fields of psychology, including clinical psychology and counseling psychology. Applicants for ABPP must have at least 5 years of postdoctoral experience, submit examples of their clinical work, and pass an oral examination. The entrance requirements and performance standards are more rigorous than those involved in licensure and represent excellence in applied psychology. Fellowship in APA is based on evidence of unusual and outstanding performance in psychology.

One study (Robyak & Goodyear, 1984) investigated the graduate school origins of ABPP Diplomates and APA Fellows in clinical and counseling psychology. Although older and larger doctoral programs are obviously favored in such a historical study, the results nonetheless give some indication of institutional reputation and their graduates' accomplishments. Table 3-3 presents the top 25 institutional origins of clinical psychology diplomates and fellows as well as the top 12 institutional origins of counseling psychology diplomates and fellows. Clinical psychology diplomates graduated from 153 different universities; fellows from 92. Counseling psychology diplomates graduated from 55 universities; fellows from 46.

If a school is listed in Table 3-3, place a "+" in the "Rank" column in the "Clinical" section. Though many schools not listed on this table provide fine clinical training, this listing indicates that the program is outstanding in terms of its track record for producing excellent professional psychologists.

Finally, there is a column in Appendix B marked "Self-Rating." The first question we asked each program to answer was, "On a 7-point scale, how research or practice oriented would you rate your program?" (1 = practice emphasis; 4 = equal emphasis; and 7 = research emphasis). You will find the school's rating of itself under each individual listing in the reports on individual programs sections. Mark this number under the "Self-Rating" column.

What you now have before you is a list of programs that offer research in your area of interest. You also have the number of faculty in the area that you might work with and whether they presently have grant funding. Finally, you have an approximate rank of that school's research standing.

TABLE 3-3. Institutional Origins of Clinical and Counseling Psychology Diplomates and Fellows

University	Rank order	
	Diplomates	Fellows
Clinical psychology		
New York University	1.5	2.5
Columbia University	2.5	1.5
University of Chicago	3.5	3.5
University of California–Los Angeles	4.5	14.5
University of Michigan	5.5	9.5
University of Iowa	5.5	5.5
University of Minnesota	7.5	6.5
Northwestern University	8.5	7.5
University of California–Berkeley	9.5	15.5
Harvard University	10.5	7.5
Pennsylvania State University	11.5	17.5
Purdue University	12.5	—
Boston University	12.5	17.5
Ohio State University	14.5	4.5
University of Washington	15.5	5.5
University of Southern California	16.5	11.5
Duke University	18.5	—
Stanford University	18.5	10.5
University of Texas	18.5	—
University of Pittsburgh	20.5	11.5
University of Kansas	21.5	—
Case Western Reserve University	23.5	—
University of Illinois at Urbana–Champaign	23.5	—
Yale University	23.5	13.5
University of Pennsylvania	23.5	—
Counseling psychology		
Columbia University	1.5	2.5
Ohio State University	2.5	3.5
University of Minnesota	3.5	1.5
New York University	4.5	4.5
University of Michigan	5.5	—
University of Chicago	6.5	8.5
Stanford University	7.5	7.5
University of Iowa	8.5	7.5
University of Texas	9.5	—
University of Wisconsin	9.5	—
Catholic University	11.5	—
Harvard University	11.5	4.5

Note. From Robyak & Goodyear (1984). © 1984 American Psychological Association. Reprinted by permission.

In clinical terms, you have some sense of whether that school will conform to your theoretical orientation, whether it has clinical training or a formal track in your area of interest, how it ranks in terms of producing outstanding clinicians, and whether it rates itself as emphasizing practice or research.

Given the information before you, you may already want to begin crossing programs off your list. If you're research oriented, and the program is a Psy.D. program or rates itself a 1, 2, or 3 (meaning it is practice oriented), you may choose to delete that school. Alternatively, if your interests reflect equal research and clinical emphasis and you lean toward a psychodynamic orientation, you may want to cross off a school that rates itself as a 7 (very research oriented) or whose faculty is 100% behavioral.

Your revised list of schools can probably satisfy your research and clinical interests. In addition, you have the start of a ranking system, which at this point gives you a rough idea of how well each school conforms to your interests and needs. Unfortunately, this provides you with only half of the information you need to begin writing to schools. The second part of this process asks, "How close do you come to the standards they specify?" This is covered in a later section entitled "Assessing Program Criteria."

For the Practice Oriented

This section gives guidance to those applicants who are centrally focused on psychological practice. These applicants will want to begin to choose their programs based on their theoretical orientation and the availability of clinical opportunities.

Begin by turning to Table 1-4, which lists all the APA-accredited Psy.D. programs. With this list, turn to Appendix B, "Worksheet for Choosing Programs." Under the column marked "School," write the names of the programs found in Table 1-4.

In addition to these programs, you may have a specific population in mind that you are especially eager to work with. Perhaps you already have a sense that you want to work specifically with patients suffering from, say, anxiety disorders. In this case, turn to Appendix F. This appendix, "Specialty Clinics and Practica Sites," lists specialty clinics or practica areas available at different programs. Specialty clinics focus on specific clientele, such as depressed or eating-disordered clients. As mentioned in the previous section, practica are placements where a student will conduct clinical work in his or her second, third, and/or fourth year of study, and some practica also specialize in treating a certain clientele. For a practice-oriented student, it would be especially desirable to be in a program with a specialty clinic in his or her particular area of treatment interest. Therefore, write down the names of programs with specialty clinics or practica in your area of interest on your list in Appendix B.

Do likewise for programs that offer a formal track or concentration in your area of interest. This information can be found in Appendix G, Concentrations and Specialty Tracks.

A word of caution is in order. Most programs will have their own psychology training clinic where a wide range of clinical populations may be seen or made available for research. Practica may also be available in a wide range of settings in the community, providing fertile ground for a rich clinical experience. Still, a clinic or practicum specializing in a population that is of special interest to you is a definite plus and an additional piece of information on which to base your decision. If a program both offers a Psy.D. and has a specialty clinic in your area, put a star next to it.

The next important column for the practice oriented applicant is marked "Orientation." In the Reports on Individual Programs, you will find each school listed, along with information pertaining to its program. Among that information, you will see a list of five theoretical orientations, followed by the percentage of the faculty that subscribes to that orientation:

- Psychodynamic/psychoanalytic
- Radical behavioral/applied behavioral analysis
- Systems/family systems
- Humanistic/existential
- Cognitive/cognitive-behavioral

If you are clearly committed to (or strongly leaning toward) one of these orientations, then it is important that some portion of the faculty share that orientation with you. Check each program on your list and determine if a suitable percentage of the faculty shares your orientation. If so, mark the "Orientation" column with a "+" sign; if not, mark it with a "−" sign.

If you are unsure of your orientation or see yourself as integrative or eclectic, then be sure there is a wide variety of faculty orientations. If there is representation among the faculty in four of these orientations, that's a good sign. If the total you obtain after adding up all the percentages in the different areas is greater than 100%, this is also advantageous. It means some (or most) of the faculty bridge orientations and are integrative themselves. In either case, mark the "Orientation" column with a "+" sign. If you're integrative and the faculty are of one or two orientations and do not overlap, then mark this column with a "−" sign.

The next column is marked "Res/Clin." As we mentioned previously, even if you are looking for a practice oriented program, you still will have to do research: a lengthy professional paper or a clinical dissertation at the very least! Consequently, it is important that someone in your program is conducting research in an area that interests you. With this in mind, look through Appendix E and locate area(s) of research that you find interesting. Under each area, you will find a list of schools that have researchers in that field. If any of the schools on your list in Appendix B is listed here, place a "+" in the column marked "Res/Clin."

The third column under "Clinical" is marked "Rank." Here, we refer to a program's production of students who go on to distinguished careers as clinicians, as imperfectly measured by their becoming ABPP Diplomates and by their election as Fellows in APA's Division of Clinical Psychology and Division of Counseling Psychology. The "ABPP" refers to diplomate status awarded by the American Board of Professional Psychology (www.abpp.org), which certifies excellence in 13 fields of psychology, including clinical psychology and counseling psychology. Applicants for ABPP must have at least 5 years of postdoctoral experience, submit examples of their clinical work, and pass an oral examination. The entrance requirements and performance standards are more rigorous than those involved in licensing and represent excellence in applied psychology. The APA Fellowship is based on evidence of unusual and outstanding performance.

One study (Robyak & Goodyear, 1984) investigated the graduate school origins of ABPP Diplomates and APA Fellows in clinical and counseling psychology. Although older and larger doctoral programs are obviously favored in such a historical study, the results nonetheless give some indication of institutional reputation and their graduates' accomplishments. Table 3-3 presents the top 25 institutional origins of these diplomates and fellows as well as the top 12 institutional origins of counseling psychology diplomates and fellows. Because this list indicates programs that have historically produced outstanding clinicians, place a "+" in this column for any program included in Table 3-3. Though many schools not listed in this table offer fine clinical training, the list provides an indication of the Ph.D. programs (Psy.D. programs are too new to be listed) that are likely to offer the sort of clinical training you seek.

Finally, there is a column in Appendix B marked "Self-Rating." In the reports on individual programs you will find each school's rating of itself (1 = practice emphasis; 4 = equal emphasis; and 7 = research emphasis). Mark this number under the "Self-Rating" column. Though Psy.D. programs are practice oriented by definition, they vary on how much research they expect their students to conduct. Thus, their ratings will allow you to guide your expectations of what each program will expect of you. This self-rating will also help you avoid a Ph.D. program with a specialty clinic in your area that is clearly research oriented.

What you now have before you is a list of programs that are practice oriented and/or that offer a specialty clinic or formal track in your area of interest. You have some sense of whether these schools will conform to your theoretical orientation and whether they have ongoing research in your area of clinical interest. You also have their self-rating of the program's emphasis on practice or research.

Given the information on your worksheet, you may already want to begin crossing programs off your list. If you're practice oriented and a Ph.D. program offers a specialty clinic in your area but rates itself with a 6 or 7 (very research oriented), you may choose to delete that school. Alternatively, if you're very behaviorally oriented, you may want to cross off a school where 100% of the faculty is psychodynamic/psychoanalytic.

Your revised list of schools can provide you with practice oriented training and possibly special clinical training in your population of choice. In addition, you have the start of a ranking system that at this point gives you a rough idea of how well each school conforms to your interests and needs. Unfortunately, this only provides you with half the information you need to begin writing to schools. The second half of this process is related to how closely you come to the specified standards of these programs. This is covered in the "Assessing Program Criteria" section.

For the Racial/Ethnic Minority Applicant

Before continuing to the assessment of program criteria, it is important to discuss the special case of minority applications. "Minority" in this context refers to racial or ethnic background, although with women comprising 70% of all doctoral students in psychology (Pate, 2001), a few graduate student programs are starting to treat men as minority applicants. Ethnic minority students now account for 21% of master's students in psychology and 27% of doctoral students in psychology (Norcross, Kohout, & Wicherski, 2005).

Nearly every APA-accredited program makes special efforts to recruit minority applicants (Munoz-Dunbar & Stanton, 1999; Rogers & Molina, 2006), recognizing the need in our society for well-trained minority professionals. Typical methods for recruiting underrepresented groups to clinical and counseling psychology programs are offers of financial aid, the use of personal contacts, visits to other schools, use of APA's Minority Undergraduate Students of Excellence (MUSE) program, diversity courses, special events, reimbursements of application fees, and preferential screening (Rogers & Molina, 2006; Steinpreis et al., 1992). Programs often make an extra effort to review minority applications to ensure that qualified candidates are given appropriate consideration.

In fact, a study of Psy.D. programs revealed that 82% of them implemented formal minority admissions policies designed to improve racial representation (Young & VandeCreek, 1996). The study found that:

- 94% of the programs gave extra points on ratings of application materials to minority applicants;
- 69% of the programs waived or lowered GRE scores for minority applicants;
- 41% of the programs waived or lowered GPA cut-offs for minority applicants; and
- 21% of the programs interviewed all minority applicants, regardless of the quality of their application materials.

As a consequence, ethnic minorities in the applicant pool are significantly more likely than whites to receive offers of admission (Munoz-Dunbar & Stanton, 1999). Our guidance and the following worksheets in this *Insider's Guide* may thus not accurately reflect a minority applicant's enhanced chances of acceptance. We recommend that you carefully read program descriptions regarding their minority selection procedures and encourage you to apply to programs that are within reach of your credentials.

Several ethnic/racial minority students have written to us over the years and complained that they were neither actively recruited nor accepted for admission into the doctoral psychology programs to which they had applied. So let us be perfectly clear and honest: Most, but not all, doctoral programs have implemented policies (as reviewed above) to recruit and admit underrepresented racial/ethnic minority students. However, that does not mean that all programs will be knocking down your door to interview you. Nor does that mean that most programs will finance your interview. Nor does that mean acceptance is a certainty. Doctoral programs will evaluate all candidates on their GPAs, GREs, letters of recommendation, research experiences, and so on. A modest advantage is just that—an advantage, never a guarantee.

The APA is committed to ensuring that the practice of psychology—and the production of psychologists—is in the vanguard of addressing the needs of culturally diverse populations. The APA's Commission on Ethnic Minority Recruitment, Retention, and Training in Psychology produces several valuable publications in this regard. Go to www.apa.org/pi/oema/careers/book3/page1.html to read APA's guidebook, *For College Students of Color Applying to Graduate & Professional Programs.* Also consult the Web site of *Project 1000,* a national program created to assist students of color applying to graduate school (mati.eas.asu.edu:8421/p1000).

Although the special consideration given minority applicants is advantageous, it also represents a special challenge. One well-qualified minority student we knew was advised by a university career counselor that he would have no problem getting into the school of his choice. He applied to several very competitive programs, and received acceptances and offers of financial aid across the board. Unfortunately, he skipped the process of matching his interests with the strengths of the program. After 1 year, he was looking to transfer to another program that had more faculty conducting research and psychotherapy in his areas of interest.

The moral of the story is: Don't let the potential advantage of being a minority candidate become a disadvantage. Just because you can get into a program doesn't mean that it is the best program for you. A rigorous approach to the application process is the best approach for everyone.

For the LGBT Applicant

Lesbian, gay, bisexual, and transgendered (LGBT) applicants to doctoral programs can face the same social and interpersonal hurdles as ethnic/racial minority applicants. There is, however, a key difference: There are limited federal protections for members of the LGBT community. This fact may lead lesbian, gay, bisexual, and transgendered students to question whether to disclose their sexual orientation ("come out") in the application process, or even to inquire about the atmosphere of inclusivity toward sexual minorities within a particular program. In this section, we review some research and advice on LGBT applicants' selection of graduate programs and present potential strategies for those who elect to come out during the application process.

Before turning to the specifics, let us emphasize this general point: The burden should not be placed on the potentially stigmatized applicant to disclose sexual orientation. Such a burden promotes silence and fear. Rather, each applicant should choose his/her own path, and program faculty should create an inclusive, welcoming atmosphere for all students. The APA accreditation guidelines require doctoral programs to embrace diversity in their students.

Qualitative research (e.g., APA, 2006; Lark & Croteau, 1998; Rader, 2000) indicates that LGBT psychology students screen prospective graduate schools for their gay affirming (or at least, nonhomophobic) position. The typical criteria used for screening prospective programs are (Biaggio et al., 2003):

- Reports of other LGBT students
- Presence of faculty who are openly lesbian/gay or heterosexual allies
- Availability of specific training on LGBT issues and opportunity to work with LGBT clients
- Sensitivity to diversity issues on campus (including the presence of LGBT support and advocacy groups)
- Geographic location of the program (frequently avoiding programs in conservative rural areas)
- Size of the educational institution (larger public institutions being relatively more liberal)

In addition, we recommend that LGBT students look for climate indicators favorable to sexual diversity. Screen prospective programs by

- searching departmental and university homepages for the presence of an LGBT student union and faculty teaching and researching on sexuality
- looking for specific housing policies for LGBT couples (remember, though legally married in one state, another state may not recognize your gay marriage or civil union, and the university may not be legally bound to provide equal access to "married" housing).
- avoiding institutions that require a religious or doctrinal oath and that prohibit LGBT organizations on campus.
- seeking programs with curricula that explicitly integrate LGBT and other diversity issues.
- reviewing APA's list of graduate faculty in psychology interested in lesbian and gay issues (available at www.apa.org/pi/lgbc/publications/lgbsurvey/grad_home.html).
- evaluating the university's mission statement for a formal commitment to diversity of sexual orientation.
- determining if the institution has a coordinator (or office) for lesbian, gay, and bisexual concerns
- considering the state laws concerning equitable treatment of LGBT, such as civil unions, domestic partnership, adoption, health insurance for partners, and the like.

Homophobia and heterosexism persist in the United States and, unfortunately, also in institutions of higher education. Although the situation has improved considerably in recent decades, some institutions remain "tolerant" as opposed to "affirming" of sexual diversity, whereas other institutions may favor an LGBT student to maintain or expand program diversity.

The question, then, is whether to come out during the application process. On one side, there is the risk of being rejected from a program where some discrimination persists. On the other side, there is the potential advantage of being a member of a minority group in a program that actively pursues diversity. In either case, the alternative to not coming out during the application process is to come out later, or to try to hide your sexual orientation for 4 to 6 years.

If and when to disclose sexual orientation in the admissions process is ultimately a personal decision, and it can occur at different stages in the process: in the application itself, during the interview, upon acceptance to the program, or upon the decision to attend the program. As part of your application, you can indicate your sexual orientation in your research interests (e.g., lesbian health), clinical experiences (e.g., working with gay youth), and/or extracurricular activities (e.g., member of the LGBT alliance on campus). More directly, you can incorporate your sexual identity into your personal statement, especially if it has bearing on your choice of clinical or research work, or your decision to pursue psychology as a career. If you do come out in your personal statement, be sure that this fact is integrated into the overall statement and not simply a dangling fact unconnected to the rest of what you've written.

Some applicants choose to come out during the interview process with a simple but straightforward statement: "As a gay man (or lesbian), it's important to me to be in a gay-friendly environment. Would being gay be a concern in this program?" Though it would be a mistake to over-generalize, such questions are typically met with positive responses about program diversity and discussions of resources for LGBT students. If such questions are met otherwise, it serves as a key piece of information in your decision process.

Another strategy is to raise sexual orientation at the point at which an offer of admission is tendered. As discussed in subsequent chapters, once an offer is made, an applicant has some latitude in negotiating issues around admission, tuition remission, funding, and so on. This can be the time to indicate that having a gay-affirmative environment is one of the factors in your decision of which program to accept and to inquire about the atmosphere in that program. Still other

LGBT students elect not to disclose until they are actually matriculated in the program and have begun coursework.

Whatever path you decide to take, your sexual orientation should not be the defining issue of your application; your composite strengths as a potential doctoral student remain the center of your application. [For additional information, consult the *APAGS Resource Guide for LGBT Students in Psychology* (APA, 2006) and *Graduate Faculty in Psychology Interested in Lesbian, Gay, and Bisexual Issues* (at www.apa.org/pi/lgbc/publications/lgbsurvey/grad_home.html)].

For the Disabled Applicant

Organized psychology is increasingly aware that diversity extends beyond gender, ethnicity, and sexual orientation to all individual differences, including disability status. Applicants with disabilities confront many of the same prejudices as other minority populations, including obstacles to graduate applications and interviews. APA's *Resource Guide for Psychology Graduate Students with Disabilities* (www.apa.org/pi/cdip/resources/home.html) presents tips on applying to graduate school, requesting fair accommodations, and preparing for a successful experience. The guide also lists national resources on disability issues; our favorite is Ken Pope's website on accessibility in psychology graduate education and practice (at kpope.com).

When and how to disclose a disability is a complex and personal decision, a decision that you must make after sorting through the choices and perhaps discussing them with a knowledgeable mentor. There are eight different occasions during the admissions process when you might choose to disclose (Khubchandani, 2002):

- In your CV or application form
- When a prospective graduate school contacts you for an interview
- During the interview
- After the interview but before an offer
- After the offer but before an acceptance
- After you start the graduate program
- After a problem on the job
- Never (disclose)

There are pros and cons for each timing of disclosure, but ultimately your decision will be based on what you know about your own needs and what you have learned about the specific graduate program (Khubchandani, 2002). If and when you do disclose a disability, be straightforward and factual about it only

as it affects your specific job functions, as defined by the Americans with Disabilities Act. Specify the type of accommodation that you will require or the work restrictions that are involved. Don't dwell on your disability; rather, be enthusiastic about your skills and resources. Stress that your disability did not interfere with previous performance or attendance.

Your multiple abilities, not select dis-abilities, are what count in graduate school. As with ethnicity and sexual orientation, your disability status should not occupy center stage in your application. Assertively request fair accommodation and accessibility as provided by law, to be sure. But help the admissions committee avoid the stereotype of equating you with your disability. Your application should focus squarely on your credentials and accomplishments.

Assessing Program Criteria

Assessing the criteria clinical and counseling psychology programs use to evaluate applicants is an important step in the process of applying to graduate school. To illuminate this point, we will relate the story of one applicant we knew several years ago. She was an Ivy League graduate, a 3.8 psychology major, who had conducted research with a prominent psychologist. She had fine letters of recommendation and clinical experience with developmentally disabled children, but her GREs were in the low 500s. Thinking that her credentials were excellent, she applied to the most competitive research programs and one practice-oriented program. She was rejected across the board at these top research schools and just barely made it into what she had mistakenly considered her practice-oriented "safety school." Her mistake was to ignore the fact that all the research-oriented schools to which she applied specified minimum GRE scores of 600 or more. Her application was unsuccessful because she ignored one piece of information each school had indicated to be essential. She was nearly rejected in the more practice-oriented program she had felt was a "sure thing" because she did not possess the clinical experience they were looking for. And she was lucky that that particular doctoral program did not have GRE requirements beyond her range!

The moral of the story is twofold: (1) Attend closely to the admission standards of each program. If a school sets standards you cannot realistically meet, you need to work very, very hard to get them to make an exception. In other words, think twice about applying there. (2) Apply to programs with a range of admission criteria, and consider a safety school as one that announces admission requirements that you exceed by a wide margin. This does not guarantee acceptance, but does dramatically increase the probability of making it into their finalist pool.

Now, turn your attention to Appendix C, "Worksheet for Assessing Program Criteria." In Appendix C, you will rate yourself on how well you conform to each school's admission requirements. The aim is that you not waste time and money applying to programs that indicate in no uncertain terms that you do not meet their criteria. There is no reason to feel inadequate because you fall short of these specifications. There may be programs on your list with requirements you do meet or exceed. If you are unable to meet the minimum requirements of any programs on your list, you should seriously consider taking time off to better prepare yourself or applying to less competitive master's programs.

Begin by transferring the name of each school from Appendix B to the "School" column of Appendix C. Simply copy the list from one table to the other. Also copy the number in the "Self-Rating" column from one worksheet to the other. Next, look up the first program on your list in the Reports on Individual Programs. Read through all the information provided just to start familiarizing yourself with that program.

As you begin filling out Appendix C and listing each school's admission criteria, remember that these are simply indications of your strength as an applicant to each school. These scales are not set in stone and do not guarantee that you will be accepted. You may not readily fall into any of the categories listed and will have to make some rough approximations for yourself. Or you may find that you fall between categories and have to add 0.5 point here or subtract 0.5 point there. If you think it is appropriate to modify the categories or scoring systems, by all means do so. *The most important result is not an absolute number but a relative sense of how well you meet each program's admission criteria.*

You may also find that a graduate program does not require certain test scores, or gives no mean GRE scores, or doesn't list preferred or mandatory courses. In this case, simply score a "0" in the appropriate column. When it comes time to total each school's score, this will neither detract from nor add to your ability to meet their requirements.

Now, go to the respective Reports on Individual Programs and look at the prerequisite courses. You will see two questions pertaining to course preparation prior to applying: "What courses are required for incoming students to have completed prior to enrolling?" and "Are there courses you recommend that are not mandatory?" Underneath each question you will find a

list of courses that the particular school assigned to each category. On your list in Appendix C, under the column marked "Courses," score yourself as follows (in this table, "M" indicates "mandatory" and "R" indicates "recommended"):

+2   You have taken all the M and R courses and earned B+ or better in them all.

+1   You have taken all the M courses and/or several of the R courses and earned B+ or better.

0   You have taken all the M courses, but none of the Rs, or earned B– or lower in some M courses.

1   You have not taken one or two of the M courses, or have earned B– or lower in several of them.

–2   You have not taken several or any of the M courses or have received C or lower in some of the M or R courses.

The next section on each "Program" page is marked GREs and GPA. This section gives mean scores for the GREs and GPAs for each program listed.

On your list, under the columns marked "GRE-V" (verbal), "GRE-Q" (quantitative), and "GRE-S" (psychology subject test), score yourself as follows:

+2   You exceed the school's M score by at least 100 points.

+1   You exceed the school's M score by more than 50 but less than 100 points.

0   You meet the school's M minimum or exceed it by less than 50 points.

1   You do not meet the school's M score, but are less than 100 points below it.

–2   You are below the M score by 100 points or more.

For GPA, we asked programs for the mean score of their incoming class and asked if that applied to more than one type of GPA. It is not uncommon for programs to look at cumulative or overall GPA (all undergraduate courses taken), psychology GPA (only psychology courses), and junior/senior GPA (all courses taken in the last 2 years of college). Again, it is wise to review the average GPA of incoming students. Under the column marked "GPA," score yourself as follows:

+2   You exceed the school's M GPA by 0.5 points or more.

+1   You exceed the school's M GPA by less than 0.5 points.

0 You meet the school's M GPA.

1 You do not meet the school's M GPA, but are less than 0.2 below it.

−2 You are below the school's M by more than 0.5 points.

Next, look back to the second column of Appendix C, "Self-Rating." This is how the program rates itself on the practice–research continuum. If a program emphasizes one more than the other, this gives some indication of what it would consider important in an applicant. A school that stresses research will probably desire an applicant to have some amount of research experience. Under the "Research" column in Appendix C, rate yourself as follows:

+2 The school rates itself as a 6 or a 7 and you will have completed an honors thesis or will have at least 2 years of experience in psychology research.

+1 The school rates itself as a 4, 5, 6, or 7 and you will have at least 1 year of experience in psychology research.

0 The school rates itself as a 1, 2, or 3.

1 The school rates itself as a 4 or 5, and you have no research experience.

−2 The school rates itself as a 6 or 7, and you have no research experience.

Similarly, a program emphasizing clinical work will prefer that an applicant enter with some practical experience in human services or health care. Under the "Clinical" column, rate yourself as follows:

+2 The school rates itself as a 1 or a 2, and you will have worked in a full-time (35+ hr./week) clinical position for at least 1 year.

+1 The school rates itself as a 1, 2, 3, or 4 and you will have volunteered part-time (8+ hr./week) at a clinical facility for at least 1 year.

0 The school rates itself as a 5, 6, or 7.

1 The school rates itself as a 3 or 4, and you have no clinical experience.

−2 The school rates itself as a 1 or 2, and you have no clinical experience.

At this point, you should have completed the first nine columns of Appendix C from "School" to "Clinical."

Additional information provided for each program in the Reports on Individual Programs are "How many applications were received in 2007?," "How many applicants were given an admission offer in 2007?,"

and "How many admitted students are incoming?" These give a rough estimate of the competitiveness of a program.

You may be amazed at how high this ratio can become. The average acceptance rates at freestanding Psy.D. programs is now 50% (Norcross et al., 2005). In applying to programs, be realistic and reasonable. You may have a sterling application, but when Yale accepts roughly 1 in 50 applicants, you had best be applying to other places as well.

Bear in mind: Programs accept more applicants than actually end up attending. This makes programs appear more restrictive than they actually are. This is why we added the third item regarding the number of students who will enter the program—a number invariably smaller than the number of accepted students. For example, an applicant gaining acceptance to five programs will ultimately reject four of them. A program planning on an incoming class of six students will accept more than six before gaining their new class. Nonetheless, apply to several schools with a range of competitiveness as a precautionary measure.

In the column marked "Compete" in Appendix C, record the ratio of applications to acceptances. It should be noted that competitiveness is difficult to quantify. Although we have selected the ratio of applicants to acceptances as our measure, other relevant criteria include GRE scores and GPA. Since we have already discussed these criteria, we are using this opportunity to highlight yet another area related to competitiveness.

The last column is marked "Total." Add the numbers under the "Courses," "GRE-V," "GRE-Q," "GRE-S," "GPA," "Research," and "Clinical" columns. This will provide you with a total somewhere between −14 and +14, which is a rough indication of how well you meet each school's admission requirements and expectations.

Now you have a grand list of programs that are performing research or clinical work in the areas you have specified. In addition, you have several indications of how well each school will address your needs and expectations as a graduate student. Finally, you have a rating of yourself as an applicant to each program.

The best way to begin your decision-making process is to select the programs that have admission requirements within your reach. As you look through the "school requirements" part of your list, note any −2s. Unless you can reasonably expect to change these to zeros or better before you complete your applications, you are better off dropping these programs from your list. After that, you will then have to decide for yourself what are reasonable places to apply.

Below is a rating system based on your "Total" column for each school. Although this system may help you decide where to apply, it is by no means definitive. *These are rough approximations,* and ultimately you will have to decide where to apply based on this and any other information to which you are privy. From the "Total" column of Appendix C, evaluate each program as follows:

10 to 14   Your chances are very good. Apply to many of these schools, since your application may be especially strong here.

6 to 9   Your chances are good. These schools are within your reach, as you exceed several of the credentials they value.

4 to 5   Your chances are moderately good here, but be sure to apply to some schools where you rank more highly.

0 to 3   These schools are within your range of abilities. Your application may not be outstanding, but it is somewhere between "adequate" and "more than adequate." Be sure also to apply to several schools in a higher range.

1 to –4   These schools are a stretch for you. Go ahead and apply to a few, but the bulk of your applications should go to schools on which you achieved a higher score.

<–4   These schools are looking for something different from your experience or performance at this time. If you wish to attend a program in this range, take time off or attend a master's program to bolster your research, clinical, and academic performance.

Although this worksheet embodies many of the relevant criteria used by admissions committees, it of course cannot integrate all possible criteria. If a professor has expressed interest in working with you, for example, the worksheet total may underestimate your chances for acceptance. Other useful resources when selecting your list of schools include specific professors, undergraduate psychology advisors, and bulletin boards in the psychology building that display postgraduate brochures. Graduate students at your local university can also be helpful, and a few large universities have even created notebooks on clinical and counseling psychology graduate programs (Todd & Farinato, 1992). Take advantage of all the available information to augment the data provided in the Reports on Individual Programs.

Using the system in Appendix C, delete some of the schools that have admission criteria outside of your present range. This will enable you to begin the next phase: selecting programs that match your expectations in terms of the training you desire.

For the research-oriented applicant, these decisions may be easiest. Look at the schools remaining on your worksheet. Note the number of faculty interested in your research area(s) and whether any of them are funded. Grant funding is a rough indicator of the intensity of the program's commitment to a particular research area. The premise is that a grant-funded area may offer more opportunities to study the issue and may be more likely to generate research. In addition, grant funding has the potential of making assistantship money available. This by no means suggests that a program that does not have a grant in your area is not conducting current research or will not have money available to you. Additionally, a program with several faculty in an area may simply be "between" grants. Thus, the number of faculty alone also can indicate a school's commitment to this area of research.

Next, check the program's productivity ranking and their self-rating as being more practice or research oriented. Again, if you are more research oriented, you may well find yourself crossing those schools off your list that are low on productivity and that are clearly practice oriented. You are going to find that this shortens your list but that you still have a number of schools that cover a wide range of desirability. This is exactly where you want to be at this point! What you desire is a list of 15 to 30 programs for which you will secure additional information. Then, you can begin fine-tuning and selecting the 10 to 20 programs to which you will actually apply.

If you are more strongly inclined toward practice, you will find yourself crossing schools off your list that are research oriented, favor theoretical orientations different from your own, or are too restricted for your needs. The programs highlighting clinical work, and especially those sharing your orientation or providing a specialty clinic in your area, will be the most desirable.

The applicant who equally emphasizes practice and research training is the most challenged. You want a program that is research oriented, but not at the cost of clinical work. But you also want a program that will offer high-quality clinical training without sacrificing high standards in research. Using your list, find the programs that are moderate or high in productivity and that have a number of people interested in your area. Check to see that they rate themselves as a 4 or 5, indicating that they emphasize practice and research nearly equally. Then, check to see if their theoretical orientation conforms to your own and whether they

678 Wilmington Drive
Derby, NY 14047

September 3, 2008

Director of Admissions
Department of Psychology
Bogus University
1234 Monument Square
Upstate, NY 14000

Dear Sir or Madam:

I am interested in applying to your Ph.D. (Psy.D.) program in clinical (counseling) psychology for the fall of 2009. Please send me an application and any information you have available concerning your program. Kindly include financial aid information as well.

Thank you for your time and consideration.

Sincerely yours,

Chris Smith

FIGURE 3-1. Sample E-mail requesting application and information.

have a specialty clinic or formal tracks in your area. Again, you are going to find a range of programs, some conforming to your needs better than others. This is exactly what you want at this point in the process.

You are now ready to gather the detailed information necessary to choose among the 15 to 30 programs you will use for your selection pool. If your number of schools does not fall within these parameters, you should consider modifying your list. The Web site, mailing address, and e-mail address of each program are listed with each entry in the Reports on Individual Programs. At this point, all you need is to spend a few

hours on the Web. Research demonstrates that Web sites provide more information about graduate programs than direct mailings, especially in areas not directly related to graduate applications (Bartsch, Warren, Sharp, & Green, 2003), so feel comfortable in securing the requisite information online.

Instead, you could send a brief letter requesting information and an application. When requesting information, your e-mail or letter should be neat, typed, and focused. Figure 3-1 shows a sample letter or e-mail.

Congratulations! You have taken the first steps in your application process.

CHAPTER 4
SELECTING SCHOOLS

Between late summer and late fall you will spend time on the World Wide Web, or e-mail or "snail mail" a letter similar to the one displayed in Figure 3-1 to a number of graduate programs for information. You will scan Web sites and download files describing each program. You are ahead of the game if you begin during late summer, because most applicants will not be starting this process for another 2 to 3 months. This is an opportunity for you to take advantage of an early start to set yourself apart as an organized and optimal candidate.

When applying for undergraduate study, you probably visited a few colleges to help you decide where to apply. When applying for graduate study, by contrast, visits are rare—at least until you are invited. The exception may be when you live close to a graduate school of special interest. But otherwise, you will only visit doctoral programs "virtually" through online descriptions until invited for a pre-admission interview.

In order to select programs that best suit your needs and interests, we again return to the questions: What is it I want for myself? What is it I'm interested in doing? And where do I want to do it? A firm commitment to a single clinical interest, research area, geographic location, or theoretical orientation is not required at this time; however, the more specific your interests, the more intelligent a choice you are going to make.

In the previous chapter we helped you to get started in narrowing your choices of potential graduate programs. We did so by identifying your interests, comparing your credentials to those required by graduate programs of interest, and by searching for potential matches with the offerings of graduate programs.

In this chapter we will help you by reviewing five critical variables to take into account in narrowing your choices: research interests, clinical opportunities, theoretical orientations, financial aid, and quality of life.

A Multitude of Considerations

Each graduate school applicant is undeniably unique in his or her reasons for applying to particular programs in clinical or counseling psychology. As we advise students and conduct workshops on graduate school admission, we hear a litany of specific restrictions: "I have to stay close to my spouse in Los Angeles," "It must be a Catholic school," "I can only attend if I receive full financial aid," "The program needs to be gay friendly, or have gay faculty mentors," "I am interested solely in cognitive-behavioral programs," "I would really like to be near the mountains," "The program must have lots of women faculty," and so on. There is obviously no single, definitive list of factors to consider in selecting potential schools. Although we will examine in some detail the five most common considerations, we will be unable to canvass the almost infinite range of reasons for selecting programs to which to apply.

In an ideal world, graduate student aspirants would have sufficient funds and freedom to consider any clinical or counseling psychology program in the country. In the real world, however, you may be limited in your choice by financial, family, and geographic considerations. Although we appreciate these very real constraints, we encourage you not to be prematurely limited by your own vision. Try to think broadly and boldly. It is, quite simply, your career at stake.

Geographic location will be a determining factor for some applicants. By this we mean both the area of the country and proximity to significant others in your life, such as parents, spouses/partners, siblings, or lovers. If you do not possess the mobility to relocate to another area of the country, then you might delay applying until your situation changes or apply only to regional schools, even if they are less desirable. Don't spend time, money, and energy on futile missions, in this case applying to programs you will be unable to attend.

At the same time, we heartily encourage you to "get out of town." Far too often students restrict themselves unnecessarily to schools close to their homes or to their undergraduate institution. Yet, graduate programs that better match their needs may be located across the country or four states south. Your future demands that you "look around" the entire country and Canada.

The gender, ethnicity, or sexual orientation composition of programs may be an influential factor for other applicants. If this is the case for you, obtain updated resource directories from the American Psychological Association and apply accordingly. Three examples are APA's *Graduate Faculty Interested in the Psychology of Women* (www.apa.org/pi/wpo/gradfaculty2005.html), *The Directory of Ethnic Minority Professionals in Psychology,* and *Graduate Faculty Interested in Gay and Lesbian Issues in Psychology* (www.apa.org/pi/lgbc/publications/lgbsurvey/grad_home.html). The Reports on Individual Programs also present the percentage of ethnic minority, international, and women students in each clinical, counseling, and combined psychology program. These can be a useful source of direction in your choice.

Our general point is this: think through your personal criteria for applying to certain programs and then be proactive in securing information about those criteria. Even if your choice of programs is limited, make it an informed choice. Accept as you must the restrictions in the range of potential graduate schools, but do not leave your future to chance!

Research Interests

The Web site for most programs will include a list of psychology faculty members in that department and their current research. You are looking to learn something from the faculty, so our advice is to find the professors who are experts in your areas of interest. If you are interested in family therapy, locate those psychologists active in training and research in that field. If you are interested in alcohol studies, find the alcohol

researchers or clinicians. Download the faculty member's Web page, or the description provided by the department. Read their descriptions carefully with a highlighter. What kind of questions are they asking? Have you asked yourself those same questions? Is this the sort of thing you can envision yourself exploring? Have you read a sample of what they have written?

In selecting professors whose interests parallel your own, you are searching for a good *match.* You are looking for mentors—psychologists who will take you on as an apprentice and teach you about your chosen profession. The more similar your views are, the better the match. For example, if you are practice oriented, psychodynamically disposed, and interested in private practice, you might choose to cross off your list a program with professors who operate exclusively from behavioral orientations and research perspectives. This does not mean your interest has to be pinpoint focused. Knowing you would rather investigate or treat psychodynamically may be enough to narrow your list of schools down to a sufficient range. But it is our experience that the more focused you are, the better fit you can find.

As you review the faculty list and other materials, you should begin to get a sense of whom you would like to work with, who is going to have the facilities to allow you to research or treat the population in which you are interested. You should eventually have a list of 10 to 20 programs that have faculty with whom you would like to work and a general idea of what each of them does.

Having created such a list of programs, we suggest that you review some of the articles or books that these professors have written. Most Web sites include a list of each faculty member's recent publications. So examine their bibliographies on the Web, inspect the program brochure, or search the *Psychological Abstracts* on *PsycLIT* for the last 5 to 7 years to locate some recent publications. Then go online and look them up. What methods do they use? What are the specifics of their psychotherapy or research that really hold your attention? If you find yourself quickly getting bored or saying, "So what? OK, so alcoholics tend to smoke more? Who cares?", then you have a valuable piece of information. If you are finding these articles interesting, you are on the right track. This is a time to get excited about your field and where you want to attend graduate school!

Here are some additional bits of information you can gather to whittle down your number of applications in terms of research interests. Consult (1) the data in the Reports on Individual Programs in this book, (2) the program's Web page, (3) correspondence with faculty,

(4) interviews with professors and/or graduate students at your own school about the programs in question, and (5) the CUR Registry of Undergraduate Researchers and Graduate Schools (at www.cur.org/UGRegistry select.html). The latter links undergraduate students who have research experience with graduate programs interested in recruiting such students. Get the necessary information and corroborate it, if possible.

When it comes to your research interests, discover if there is a medical school library or science facilities at your disposal. Library facilities should be a prime consideration, but we have found that medical libraries in particular contain journals and books not usually available elsewhere. Access to journals online through university computer facilities is also essential. An associated medical school or hospital may also offer facilities and populations available for your research. Determine if they are present, and then investigate their relationship to the Psychology Department. In addition, learn more about the research space specific to your area. For example, does someone have the equipment you need, lab or research space, funding? If you desire to conduct research in cardiovascular psychophysiology and you have found a professor who has published several articles, determine if he or she has equipment to monitor cardiac responses. If not, there should be equipment available somewhere in the department.

We realize that this process requires a great deal of time and energy. It may also provoke anxiety in an already nerve-wracking application process. This is one reason why we advocate an early start. Again, we would emphasize that you can get into a program without doing this extra work. This preparation, however, will give you the edge to get into the program of your choice or to overcome any weaknesses in your application.

Clinical Opportunities

Having read articles by the professors with whom you would like to work, you know better which ones you find interesting. However, if your career interest is primarily practice, it is possible you might find that the person you're most interested in working with does not have recent publications in your area(s) of interest. Or you know a program has an alcohol abuse clinic, but you can't figure out which professors treat clients there. Your first recourse should be to search the university's Web site to try to locate this information. If it is not on the psychology program's Web page, it may exist somewhere else within the university's Web site. If all else fails, call the department and ask to speak

with the director of training. Simply ask this person for materials specific to the clinic you would like to work in, or ask to speak with the director of that clinic to determine which faculty are practicing there.

Now, we are going to suggest something that we have found to be a powerful way of making final decisions about where to apply and of increasing your chances of being accepted there. During early fall of the year you apply, contact a *few* of the professors you have been investigating. E-mail the ones whose interests seem most closely aligned to your own. Most program Web sites include faculty e-mail addresses.

There are many reasons to directly contact a faculty member. First, it gives you an opportunity to gain information you probably could not gather in any other way—information about the program, its facilities, and its faculty. Second, these e-mails give you a chance to get to know someone you are genuinely interested in working with. It gives you an opportunity to evaluate how happy you would be in a mentorship with this faculty member. Of course, there must be aspects of this person's research or clinical work that attract you. If you do not know his or her interests or the literature well enough to demonstrate a working knowledge of the individual's contributions, do *not* write to him or her. Professors routinely receive letters from people looking to make contact, and unless you can pique their interest and demonstrate familiarity with their work, you are unlikely to receive a response.

Whether your interests are oriented toward research, practice, or both, you are not looking to take this person or his or her field by storm. You seek to make a contribution in this particular area, a contribution made *after* you have taken the time to learn and gain experience in the field under their mentorship. Or, you are looking to gain experience and clinical training with an experienced practitioner.

Take a moment to look at this relationship from the professor's perspective. If she is a researcher, then she is looking for students to help with that research, for students with the knowledge and drive to run studies. If she is a clinician, then she is looking for individuals eager for supervision who will be able to carry a client load. And that is what you have to offer. You are looking for the best fit of a program and faculty to your interests.

Contacting a professor is not a necessity. Many students are admitted to excellent programs and then take 1 or 2 years to explore, to figure out what they want and where they fit in. In fact, some programs require students to work with several professors during their initial year before selecting an adviser. Nonetheless, it is to your advantage to spend sufficient time deciding

246 Wood Street
Babylon, NY 14000

September 3, 2008

Pat Morris, Ph.D.
Department of Psychology
University of Southern States
13 Peachtree Drive
Wilkesville, VA 15000

Dear Dr. Morris:

I am a psychology senior at Babylon University, where I have been working with Dr. Frances Murrow, studying the effects of self-esteem on math performance anxiety. As I was searching the literature, I read several of your articles concerning the use of relaxation techniques to improve self-esteem and test anxiety.

After reading your paper "The Uses of Relaxation in Schools" (December issue of *School Psychology*), I had some questions I hoped you could answer. We used several of the questionnaires that you used in that study. In looking at our data, we have found that participants responded quite differently to the Test Anxiety Questionnaire at various times in the semester. We found that the further into the semester students progressed, the more their anxiety affected their scores. Have you also found this to be true in your research? Secondly, I have begun to wonder if self-efficacy might not be a factor affecting both test anxiety and self-esteem. I noticed that you had done some early work involving self-efficacy and was wondering what ideas you might have on this subject.

On a related matter, I will soon be applying to clinical psychology doctoral programs that offer research training in performance anxiety. I would be very interested in learning whether you routinely supervise the research of doctoral students at the University of Southern States on this topic and, if so, whether you will be taking any new students in the next academic year.

Thank you for your time and consideration. I look forward to hearing from you.

Sincerely yours,

Chris Smith

FIGURE 4-1. Sample e-mail of introduction—research oriented.

which professors would be best suited for you. Locate programs and professors who seem appropriate; then go ahead and contact a few of them to test the waters.

Figures 4-1 and 4-2 show sample e-mails of introduction, the former for research-oriented applicants and the latter for practice oriented. *These are not forms to copy in which you simply insert your own words!* You may want to show a draft of your letter to a professor to preview how well it is likely to be received.

Some students have asked whether it is acceptable to send letters to more than one faculty member at the same program. Despite the fact that applicants may have multiple research and clinical interests, most faculty (ourselves included) have a negative reaction to learning that the same person has written to more than one faculty member. Remember, there is a certain amount of self-interest involved: We're looking for bright, motivated students to collaborate on research and clinical work. It can be awkward when an admissions committee is discussing an applicant, and two faculty express a desire to work with him/her, only to find that the applicant has been actively expressing in-

246 Wood Street
Babylon, NY 14000

September 3, 2008

Pat Morris, Ph.D.
Department of Psychology
University of Southern States
13 Peachtree Drive
Wilkesville, VA 15000

Dear Dr. Morris:

I am a psychology senior at Babylon University, where I recently completed an upper-level course in clinical/counseling psychology. My professor, Dr. Frances Ellis, discussed your social problem-solving program targeted to elementary school children. Dr. Ellis spoke highly about the manner in which you use your clinical findings to derive theoretical models of problem solving and use these models to guide your interventions.

I am interested in learning more about school-based social problem-solving programs. I have been involved in such a project with Dr. Ellis and wish to continue my education in this area. I am preparing applications for Psy.D. programs and would like to learn more about your particular program. Specifically, what opportunities exist for clinical Psy.D. students to work on your social problem-solving program? My interests lie primarily in the clinical aspects of your school-based program. I would like to help train teachers in imparting social problem-solving skills to students.

I would appreciate any materials that you could send me describing your problem-solving program in greater detail. I am especially interested in the role for Psy.D. students. Thank you for your time and consideration.

Sincerely yours,

Chris Smith

FIGURE 4-2. Sample e-mail of introduction—practice oriented.

terest in *both* of them. Our advice: Don't write to more than one faculty member in any one graduate program.

What if the professor does not respond within a month? Absence of a response does not mean that you will not be able to work with that individual if you are accepted. Most likely the professor received too many queries to respond. Indeed, at some schools, professors are receiving dozens of e-mails during the months leading up to the application deadline. Later, when your application is reviewed, your e-mail may be read.

If the selected professor does write back, then it may be the beginning of a working relationship. Even if you are not accepted to his or her program or ultimately decide not to attend, you are making professional contacts in your field. There is no guideline as

to exactly how to behave from here, since each professor is different. But you should begin getting a sense of whether this is the right person (and program) for you.

If the task of introducing yourself to a professor "cold" seems overly daunting, consider alternatives. Local and regional conferences present prime opportunities for meeting potential mentors and gathering information about graduate programs. Numerous societies hold yearly conferences in which research is presented in specialty areas of psychology. For example, if one of your interests lies in health psychology or behavioral medicine, there is the Society for Behavioral Medicine, the American Psychosomatic Society, and the Society for Psychophysiological Research. If, for another example, your interests lie in psychotherapy, there are the annual conferences of the Society for Psychotherapy Research, the APA Division of Psychotherapy, and the Society for the Exploration of Psychotherapy Integration. Your psychology advisor can probably suggest several societies in each area of psychology.

Student membership in a scientific society brings a number of benefits. For beginners, it will probably provide you with a directory of members (including contact information), which is an easy way of quickly ascertaining who is doing research in your area. Most scientific organizations will invite you to join their electronic listserve. With membership also typically comes a newsletter or a journal, which can give you a sense of the leaders in the field.

Attending a conference can provide a great deal more information, as we have already emphasized in Chapter 2. If you are interested in particular professors, you may have a chance to see them "in action" if they are presenting a poster or a paper. In this way, you can get acquainted with the person and the research without taking the risk of formally introducing yourself. Alternatively, you may approach the professor directly and express your interest in the research or ask your psychology advisor to make the introduction. Many graduate students first met their mentors in these ways.

After you have communicated with a professor, it may be appropriate to ask to tour this person's research lab or clinical facilities. This is a wonderful opportunity, in that you will get a chance to gather all sorts of information if you visit a school ahead of time. Meeting this professor face to face, getting a sense of his or her personal, clinical, and research style, and seeing how you might fit into an ongoing team can be indispensable information. If you do find yourself in the position of visiting a professor before interviews, use the advice in Chapter 6 to help guide you in gathering information during this phase.

Try to determine if this department's psychological clinic serves the surrounding community or only the college community. College students are fine clients with whom to begin, but you will probably desire a greater diversity of populations and disorders. Learn more about the school's affiliated or specialized departmental clinics. Who can work there and when? Who does the supervision? Do you have to be affiliated with a specific professor, or is there a competitive process toward earning that placement? If you're choosing a school in part based on the availability of this clinic, how available will this clinic really be to you?

Table 4-1, "Questions to Ask about Psy.D. Programs," contains questions more specific to Psy.D. and practice oriented Ph.D. applicants. This list was compiled, in part, by surveying the clinical Psy.D. students at the Graduate School of Applied and Professional Psychology at Rutgers University and asking them what questions they had (or wish they had) asked when applying to Psy.D. programs.

Theoretical Orientations

A question related to clinical and research opportunities is whether the graduate program will provide you with training in the desired theoretical orientations. We are *not* recommending that you prematurely affiliate with any theoretical camp; rather, we suggest that you identify those orientations you are interested in learning more about and those you are not. Several programs in the Northeast are strongly committed to a psychoanalytic approach and offer few, if any, training opportunities beyond that. The obvious implication is to avoid applying to programs that will not offer supervised experience in your theoretical approach(es). By the same token, you may scratch programs from your preliminary list that rigidly adhere to, say, a behavioral persuasion if you are disinclined toward behaviorism.

The Reports on Individual Programs provide the approximate percentage of faculty in each program who subscribe to the five most popular theoretical orientations—psychodynamic/psychoanalytic, behavioral analysis/radical behavioral, family systems/systems, existential/phenomenological/humanistic, and cognitive/cognitive-behavioral. Let these figures guide you in ruling out a few programs that fail to address your theoretical predilections or, if you are uncommitted, that neglect exposure to multiple or integrative approaches.

Table 4-2 presents the average percentage of faculty endorsing these five theoretical orientations in APA-accredited clinical and counseling programs. In general, the cognitive/cognitive-behavioral tradition predominates, accounting for half of the faculty members. Radical behaviorism is relatively infrequent, with psychodynamic, systems, and humanistic theories falling in between these two extremes. These global figures do not specifically include the integrative/eclectic orientation, which is the most popular approach of mental health professionals (Norcross & Goldfried, 2005). The fact that the percentages add up to more than 100% indicates that faculty practice across orientations. Note too that the counseling psychology faculty endorse the humanistic/existential orientations much more frequently than do the clinical psychology faculty (28% versus 10%).

These average percentages mask significant differences among programs as a function of their placement along the practice–research continuum. Research-

TABLE 4-1. Questions to Ask about Psy.D. Programs

Is the Psy.D. program freestanding or part of a university?

Is the program owned or operated by a for-profit company?

If the program also has a clinical Ph.D. program, are the "best" practicum opportunities available to Psy.D. students or Ph.D. students? Is it possible to take the Ph.D. courses as well? What is the relationship between the Psy.D. and Ph.D. students?

Will the internship occur in the third or fourth year? Do you complete an internship before or after your clinical dissertation?

What percentage of Psy.D. students receive full financial support? What is the annual tuition?

What is the typical debt level of graduating students?

Does the university offer housing for Psy.D. students? If not, how much are the monthly rents locally?

Are there opportunities for live supervision? Do the full-time faculty perform the clinical supervision?

Does the school offer exposure to a variety of theoretical orientations, or is it dominated by one orientation?

Is it possible to gain experience working with . . . ? With families? With groups?

What types of clinical populations are available?

What percentage of the faculty are full-time? What percent are tenured?

Do the faculty have independent practices?

What percentage of first-year students complete the program? How many years does it typically require to complete the program?

What is the size of the incoming class? How many students are in a typical graduate course?

What percentage of students obtain an APA or APPIC-accredited internship?

---

oriented programs, as a rule, have a higher percentage of cognitive-behavioral faculty, while practice-oriented programs have a higher percentage of psychodynamic faculty (Mayne et al., 1994). These differences are quite large: Fully 64% of faculty members in research-oriented Ph.D. programs are cognitive-behavioral versus 33% in practice-oriented Psy.D. programs. Only 12% of faculty in research-oriented Ph.D. programs are psychodynamic versus 29% in practice-oriented Psy.D. programs (Norcross et al., 2005).

The upshot is to investigate thoroughly the area of psychology (clinical, counseling) and the type of program (practice-oriented to research-oriented) that

regularly provide training in your preferred theoretical orientation(s).

In addition to reviewing the percentages of faculty theoretical orientations in the Reports on Individual Programs, those of you with an intense hankering for training in a particular theoretical orientation may want to peruse specialty directories. A number of professional societies maintain or publish lists of graduate programs that offer training in their theory of choice. The Association for Behavioral and Cognitive Therapies (ABCT), for example, publishes a directory of graduate programs in behavior therapy and experimental clinical psychology (www.aabt.org). The Society for the

---

TABLE 4-2. Theoretical Orientations of Faculty in APA-Accredited Clinical and Counseling Psychology Programs

Orientations	% of clinical faculty	% of counseling faculty
Psychodynamic/Psychoanalytic	24	18
Applied behavioral analysis/Radical behavioral	7	4
Family systems/Systems	19	24
Existential/Phenomenological/Humanistic	10	28
Cognitive/Cognitive-behavioral	51	43

Note. Data from Oliver, Norcross, Sayette, Griffin, & Mayne (2005).

Exploration of Psychotherapy Integration (SEPI), for another example, has pulled together a list of integrative and eclectic training programs throughout North America (visit www.cyberpsych.org/sepi/, Norcross & Kaplan, 1995). The APA Division of Humanistic Psychology, for a final example, cosponsors a directory of graduate programs in humanistic and transpersonal psychology (visit www.westga.edu/~psydept/humanistic directory). Consult your advisors regarding the existence of specialty directories in your field of interest.

The popularity of theories, as with other professional fads, undergoes transformation over time. Extrapolating from historical trends and expert predictions (Norcross, Hedges, & Prochaska, 2002), cognitive-behavioral, eclectic/integrative, family systems, and multicultural theories will be in the ascendancy in the future. By contrast, classical psychoanalysis, humanistic theories, and existentialism are expected to decline. In an era of managed care, theoretical orientations that emphasize brief problem-focused treatments and document their effectiveness will probably thrive.

Financial Aid

The next question, and it is by no means premature, is the availability of financial aid. Unless you can afford to pay for graduate school on your own or you are prepared to take out substantial loans, you require some idea of the probability of support from the graduate program. This is not a suggestion to avoid schools with scarce financial aid. It is a suggestion not to apply only to schools with scarce financial aid.

APA's (2002) *Ethical Principles of Psychologists and Code of Conduct* requires truth in advertising about graduate programs. Standard 7.02 (Description of Programs) stipulates that "Psychologists responsible for education and training programs take reasonable steps to ensure that there is a current and accurate description of program content . . . stipends and benefits, and requirements that must be met for satisfactory completion of the program. This information must be made readily available to all interested parties." Not only is it your perfect right to request such information, but it is also the ethical obligation of the graduate psychology program to provide it.

Yet, research indicates that only a minority of psychology doctoral programs are fully disclosing all of the information required by the APA Commission on Accreditation (Burgess, Keeley, & Blashfield, 2006). Graduate programs need to be more disclosing of these crucial data. A prime objective of this *Insider's Guide* is to present financial aid information in our Reports on Individual Programs.

Figuring the total cost of full-time graduate study must include both academic expenses and living expenses. The academic side includes tuition, fees, supplies, books, and journals. Full-time tuition ranges from a low of $3,000 a year for some in-state Ph.D. students to $25,000 for some private, Psy.D. programs (Pate, 2001). Multiplying the tuition by 4 years gives you some idea of the probable tuition burden. The living side includes rent, transportation, food, clothing, insurance, and entertainment. Health insurance has emerged as a large part of the cost of graduate studies. Some assistantships include health insurance, but others do not. Not surprisingly, most graduate students are relatively poor; at least you will have company in your financial misery (Fretz & Stang, 1980).

Determine the availability of teaching assistantships and research assistantships from the program's home page and the Reports on Individual Programs. In particular, find out the percentage of first-year students who receive assistantships. Is it 100%, 50%, or 0%? Do the assistantships include health insurance? If not, you will either go without insurance or purchase it on your own.

On average, 57% of full-time doctoral students in psychology receive some financial support from the program; the remaining 43% do not. The picture is less encouraging for full-time master's students in psychology: only 23% receive any support (Gehlman, Wicherski, & Kohout, 1995). As you can see, the probability of financial support from the program itself is a very salient consideration in narrowing your choices.

Be wary of online descriptions of doctoral programs that simply declare "all incoming students receive financial aid" unless that same description provides the sources of the aid and the typical monetary stipend. We are aware of several psychology programs that automatically award "fellowships" to every student in the amount of $2,000 but then immediately charge over $20,000 annual tuition! Hence, we have begun to use the phrase *full assistantship* in our Reports on Individual Programs.

These reports provide the percentages of incoming doctoral students who receive full tuition waiver only, full assistantship/fellowship only, and both tuition waiver *and* assistantship for each doctoral program. Table 4-3 summarizes these data across the practice–research continuum for APA-accredited clinical psychology programs. The continuum moves from the freestanding Psy.D. programs on one end, through the equal-emphasis Ph.D. programs in the middle, to the research-oriented Ph.D. programs on the other end. As seen there, the probability of receiving financial assistance in graduate school is a direct function of

TABLE 4-3. Percentage of Students Receiving Financial Aid in APA-Accredited Clinical Psychology Programs

	Free-standing Psy.D.	University-based Psy.D.	Equal-emphasis Ph.D.	Research-oriented Ph.D.
Tuition waiver only	10%	13%	10%	1%
Assistantship only	13%	25%	10%	13%
Waiver and assistantship	3%	10%	63%	81%

Note. Data from Norcross, Castle, Sayette, & Mayne (2004) and Norcross & Oliver (2005).

the type of program (Norcross et al., 2004). Only 3 to 10% of Psy.D. students, on average, will receive both a tuition waiver and a full assistantship, compared to 81% of students in research-oriented Ph.D. programs in clinical psychology. You don't need to perform a *t* test; that is a large, significant difference. The equal-emphasis programs tend to fall in between; about 63% of their students receive both a tuition waiver and a full assistantship.

In other words, higher acceptance rates come at a (tuition and living) cost to the incoming student. More rigorous admission standards and acceptance odds translate into increased probability of substantial financial aid (Kohout, Wicherski, & Pion, 1991; Mayne et al., 1994). In the most extreme comparison (Psy.D. vs. research-oriented Ph.D. programs), students are 5 times more likely to gain acceptance but 10 times less likely to receive full funding (stipend plus tuition waiver). An awareness of these trade-offs among the different types of programs will enable you to make informed choices regarding your graduate applications and career trajectories.

There *is* financial aid available from graduate schools to students possessing sterling credentials, and we wish to reaffirm its existence. Nevertheless, the increasing number of acceptances into clinical and counseling psychology doctoral programs during a period of economic "downsizing" raises difficult questions about internal funding opportunities and federal financial assistance. Our findings (Norcross et al., 2004) on financial aid portend a "pay as you go" expectation for half of all doctoral candidates in clinical and counseling psychology. This is particularly true, as we have seen, in Psy.D. programs. The explicit expectation, as is true in such other practice disciplines as medicine and law, is that graduates will be able to repay their debt after they are engaged in full-time practice. We should note, however, that uncertainties regarding health care—specifically changes in insurance coverage for mental health—in the United States make this expectation difficult to evaluate at the present time.

The debt may be substantial. Research demonstrates that 77% of recent graduates in clinical and counseling psychology have debt related to graduate studies (over and above any debt associated with their undergraduate education; APA, 2003). Graduates of Psy.D. programs report a median debt of $90,000 (Wicherski & Kohout, 2005). The median debt for clinical Ph.D. graduates is $50,000, lower but still substantial. As noted earlier, there is considerable variation here, as some clinical Ph.D. programs—such as those in the APCS—offer full tuition and stipend to nearly all their students, while clinical Ph.D. programs housed in professional schools rarely offer this degree of assistance.

With a median starting salary of approximately $50,000 for new psychology doctorates (Wicherski & Kohout, 2005), graduate school debt represents a heavy financial burden for many years. (Go to the Loan Repayment Calculator at www.finaid.org/calculators/ for a sobering look at repayment schedules.)

In large part, the difference in debt between Psy.D.s and Ph.D.s is attributable to the huge differences in financial aid between Vail-model and Boulder-model programs as pictured in Table 4-3. The APA researchers who compiled the debt figures conclude, "It is important to disseminate this information to students who may be considering a career in psychology—so that their decisions can be fully informed" (Kohout & Wicherski, 1999, p. 10). We wholeheartedly agree.

In fact, we recently completed a study that looked specifically at the financial assistance offered by various types of Psy.D. programs (Norcross et al., 2004). You may recall from Chapter 1 that Psy.D. programs can be housed in three different settings: (1) in a university's Psychology Department; (2) as a separate school or institute in a university; (3) as a private, free-standing institution without affiliation to a comprehensive university. As you have already learned, Psy.D. programs give proportionally less financial assistance to students than Ph.D. programs.

But it gets a bit more complicated because not all Psy.D. programs are created equally with regard to financial assistance. An average of 26% of incoming Psy.D. students to a freestanding program will receive *any* financial support from the program and only 3% of incoming students will receive a full boat (tuition remission plus assistantship). By contrast, an average of 48% of incoming Psy.D. students to a Psychology Department program will receive some financial support and 10% of incoming students a full boat (see Table 4-3). That's a whopping difference. If you desire considerable financial assistance directly from the graduate program, then do not apply to freestanding Psy.D. programs. Your best bet, financially speaking, will be the university-affiliated Psy.D. programs and, of course, the research-oriented Ph.D. programs.

How do students cobble together the necessary funds to pay for doctoral study in psychology? By a mixture of means:

- university-provided financial assistance
- personal savings
- family support
- graduate school loans
- earnings during graduate school
- federal fellowships or traineeships

Many universities provide specific Web pages on these sources of funding graduate school. In addition to general information, they often list school- or program-specific scholarships and fellowships available to incoming students. It is worth the added effort to examine the financial aid pages at each school to search for scholarship programs for which you may be eligible.

In addition to aid provided by the school itself, financial assistance is available from external private and public organizations. This funding comes under various names—self-sought, external, independent—to distinguish it from financial aid provided internally by the university. A variety of scholarships and fellowships is offered annually, but you will need to research those that pertain to your circumstances.

Your local Office of Career Services and Office of Financial Assistance should be able to direct you to potential sources of external support for graduate studies.

We recommend Princeton Review's (2005) *Paying for Graduate School Without going Broke.* Another very useful resource is *Financing Graduate School,* a compact paperback authored by Patricia McWade (1996). The subtitle captures the centrality of the topic—*How to Get the Money for Your Master's or Ph.D.* These two books transverse the entire geography of financial aid—grant applications, loan possibilities, federal and state support, and other sources of money for graduate study.

Peterson also offers a free online cram course in financial aid at www.petersons.com/gradchannel/file.asp?id=1080&path=gr.pfs.overview. Be sure to check out the loads of advice and searchable databases on line at www.finaid.com and at www.studentaid.ed.gov/PORTALSWebApp/students/english/gradstudent.jsp.

Federal funding is also available for psychology graduate students, either in the form of training and research grants to institutions, which then fund graduate assistantships, or in the form of fellowships and dissertation grants awarded directly to students (Bullock, 1997). The National Science Foundation (NSF) funds separate competitions for Graduate Fellowships and for Minority Graduate Fellowships. NSF does not support clinical or counseling research per se, only research directed at elucidating basic functioning, not focused on disease-related processes. The National Institutes of Health (NIH) also fund psychology student awards through the National Institute of Mental Health, the National Institute on Drug Abuse, the National Institute on Alcohol Abuse and Alcoholism, and the Office of AIDS Research. Check out these programs through their Web pages: www.nsf.gov and www.nih.gov.

Several funding directories are also available free of charge from philanthropic and professional organizations. Among the more prestigious (and therefore, more competitive) are the predoctoral fellowships sponsored by the Danforth Foundation, Ford Foundation, and Armed Forces Health Professions Scholarship. The American Psychological Association publishes an online *Directory of Selected Scholarship, Fellowship, and Other Financial Aid Opportunities for Women and Ethnic Minorities in Psychology,* which we highly recommend (forms.apa.org/pi/financialaid/). The APA Minority Fellowship Program is now online at www.apa.org/mfp. APA also offers an online list of resources for financial assistance at www.apa.org/ppo/funding/.

As you can anticipate, the Web has literally exploded with interactive sites devoted to securing financial assistance for graduate school. Many of these are useful and recommended, but be wary of and avoid those that charge you for their services. In addition to the APA sites listed above, we would suggest you visit:

- www.gradview.com/financialaid/
- www.scholarships.com
- www.petersons.com/finaid/
- www.finaid.org/otheraid
- collegeapps.about.com/

Explore all these possibilities early and actively.

Student loans are also available for graduate students, but these are monies that must be repaid. The Federal Family Education Loan (FFEL) Program and the William D. Ford Federal Direct Loan (Direct Loan) Program, generally known as Stafford Loans, are available to assist graduate and professional students. Students may borrow up to $8,500 per academic year through the subsidized Stafford Loan. The interest on these loans is subsidized by the federal government and repayment at reasonable interest rates does not begin until 6 months after graduation, or following withdrawal from the program. In addition to this $8,500, up to an additional $12,500 per academic year can be borrowed through the unsubsidized Stafford Loans. The total amount that can be borrowed, including both subsidized and unsubsidized portions, is currently $138,500. The in-school interest on the unsubsidized Stafford Loans may be paid quarterly or deferred and repaid when principal repayments begin.

Starting in 2006, the government began offering Graduate PLUS Loans, federally sponsored loans for students attending graduate school at least half time. With a Grad PLUS loan, you may borrow up to the full cost of your education, less other financial aid received including Federal Stafford loans. Graduate students should exhaust their federal Stafford loan eligibility before applying for a Graduate PLUS loan because the Staffords charge lower interest.

Some institutions also award Federal Perkins Loans, a long-term loan program with a 5% interest rate available to graduate students demonstrating financial need. Other state loan programs exist; check these out as well. The bottom line is that every full-time graduate student is eligible for loans to finance his or her education, if necessary.

Speaking of loans reminds us to mention loan repayment options and loan forgiveness programs. We recommend that you visit the U.S. Department of Education Web site, www.ed.gov, which describes student loan types and loan repayment options. Three options that can trim loan payments for graduate students are the graduated repayment plans, income-sensitive repayment plans, and the loan consolidation plans. See the Web site for details, but remember that most student loans only permit a single refinancing or consolidation. Clinical and counseling psychologists working in designated underserved areas as part of the National Health Services Corps (NHSC) are also eligible for loan forgiveness (up to $25,000 or $35,000 per year) while receiving a competitive salary. Go to nhsc.bhpr.hrsa .gov for details of the program.

Quality of Life

A fifth and final consideration in selecting graduate schools is the quality of student life. It may be difficult to imagine, but occasionally you will want a break from graduate studies, to relax or engage in some non-psychological pursuit!

You should have a handle on the specifics of your own needs. Can they be met by the university and surrounding community? Do you want museums, fine dining, and professional theater? Then you probably want to live in or near a large city. If not, do you have a car capable of regularly getting you to one? Or do you get away to the mountains, enjoy rock climbing and camping, or find the city distracting? Or do you prefer to work late at night and need a campus that's safe after dark? Then be sure to apply to some rural campuses. Also, consider whether you have friends or family nearby. Having a place to escape to can be important, especially if you do not have the funds to *really* escape. You are not going to base your decisions exclusively on any of these factors. But you can increase the probability of having everything you want by applying to schools you know can provide it all.

The Web is an excellent resource for investigating locations, towns, and cities that are far away and that you may not have the time or finances to visit. Most cities have their own Web pages, which include pictures, maps, lists of attractions, and so on, for potential visitors and residents. Take the time to "virtually" explore the towns and cities of programs on your list. You may find that it is far more (or less) desirable than you had imagined.

The weight accorded to the quality of life in application decisions varies considerably among people. At one extreme are those applicants who give little thought to program location and heavily value the research and clinical opportunities. In the words of one colleague, "I'd live in hell for 4 or 5 years [the time it ordinarily takes to complete a doctorate] to be trained by the best people in my field." At the other extreme are those who will only apply to programs situated near family, friends, or an attractive community. "Five years," they say, "is too long to be away from what I need as a person." We will not be so presumptuous as to advise which position you should adopt for yourself, except to remark that you should carefully weigh personal (location, fit) and professional (reputation, opportunities) considerations.

Putting It All Together

Having seriously reflected on your own interests and having carefully examined the clinical opportunities, research training, theoretical orientations, financial aid, and quality of life of various programs, you are very close to completing applications.

Now is the time to put together all the information you have obtained about yourself and graduate programs in the form of a final list of schools—anywhere from 10 to 20, depending on the specificity of your interests and the strength of your credentials. As you make a final list of the applications you are about to complete, make one last check to insure that you are applying to the programs that best fit your needs. You may do this informally by mentally reviewing the program information you have obtained or you may do this systematically by completing Appendix D.

To complete Appendix D, write the name of each graduate program in the first column. In column 2, "School Criteria," write the total you computed for each school in Appendix C. This is an index of your strength as an applicant and should range from about 5 to 15. For each of the next five columns, you can rate your impressions about each program on a 5-point scale. Create these scales yourself in ways that are personally relevant to you. The important thing is to know where each school rates in these areas in terms of your needs and desires. Below are some examples of rating systems you might model your own after.

In the column marked "Research," rate how strongly you feel toward the professors you have singled out as wanting to work with:

1   I do not know enough about them, but their research is in my area.

3   I like the specifics of their research but do not know enough about their lab or their personalities.

5   I have been in contact with these professors and am impressed by their facilities and by them personally. I would like to work with them.

In the column marked "Clinical," rate each school according to how its opportunities suit your needs.

1   The school has only a psychological training clinic that treats students, and I want more experience.

3   The school has a good psychological training clinic, but it has no practica in the community, and getting various populations may be difficult.

5   The school has many excellent clinical opportunities, including a specialty (e.g., eating disorders) clinic or track in my area of interest.

Or, possibly:

1   The school requires students to find their own clinical placements in the community, and I don't like that system.

3   The school has a college counseling center, but I'm not interested in working only with college students.

5   The school has a good psychological services clinic, and that's all I need.

"Theoretical Orientation" is the following column:

1   The program avers strict adherence to, and training in, a theoretical orientation that is in contrast to mine.

3   The program offers some courses and supervision in my preferred theoretical orientation.

5   The program provides considerable training in my preferred theoretical orientation plus other opportunities.

Next, consider "Financial Aid":

1   There is no funding for first-year students and no mention of outside means of support, and I need it.

3   I am likely to get at least tuition remission and have the possibility of working part-time for the university. It is likely that I could be a resident advisor and get free housing.

5   For the last 5 years, all first-year students have gotten full stipends and full tuition remission.

Or, possibly:

1   There is no funding for first-year students and no mention of outside means of support.

3   I am likely to get at least tuition remission, though only for the first 2 years.

5   The school guarantees tuition remission for 4 years, and that's all I need.

And last, rate the "Quality of Life":

1   This program is located in an unattractive area and seems bereft of culture.

3   I am indifferent to the location, and there is culture within the college community.

5   The area is ideal for me, and there are museums, concert halls, and theaters nearby.

Or, possibly:

1   This university is located in an unsafe section of a large city where I don't know anyone.
3   This university is located in a small city, and a friend of mine also attends.
5   This university is located in a small college town, and I have several close relatives and friends there.

Look at your list. Are you applying to programs within a realistic range of admission criteria? Are you applying to at least some programs where you like the faculty, where the clinical facilities are suitable, where the theoretical orientation is compatible, where financial aid is available, and where you will feel comfortable living? If the answer to all of these is "No," then go back a step. Find at least a few graduate programs where these qualities are present, possibly in abundance, and add them to your list of applications.

Before moving on to the next chapter of this *Insider's Guide* and the next step in the application process, take one final moment to celebrate. You deserve it! You have learned much about graduate training in clinical and counseling psychology, investigated potential graduate programs, assessed your match with those programs, and whittled down your final list. You have already mastered challenges more intense than those associated with many college courses. So, after weeks of arduous and sometimes anxious work, you deserve affirmation and reward. Give them to yourself or, at least, allow us to affirm and reward you from afar.

CHAPTER 5

APPLYING TO PROGRAMS

You are ready to start completing the applications. You have assessed your interests and have located programs that provide the training and mentorship you desire. You have evaluated your own credentials and have chosen programs that will consider you seriously. You have received applications from these programs either by mail or by downloading materials from the 90% of clinical programs with Web pages (Corcoran, Michels, & Ahina, 1999). You have carefully looked at their research offerings, clinical opportunities, theoretical orientations, financial aid, quality of life, and other variables of importance to you. Your task now is to actually apply to these graduate programs.

You should attack this application process with all the drive and commitment you can muster. The rewards of applying are typically in direct proportion to your exertion. Try to emulate the manic zeal of successful medical school applicants. As they will readily inform you, the application itself reflects directly on your potential as a graduate student. In a real sense, your professional future is at stake.

The "application year," as it is known, will probably be intense. We suggest that you take a lighter course load or work schedule during the fall of your application year. Completing applications, securing letters of recommendation, and writing personal statements constitute more work than a typical college course. We also suggest that you inform friends and family members that you will be more preoccupied and distracted than usual. Position yourself for a busy fall.

A completed application will typically consist of the following elements: application form, curriculum vitae, personal statement, letters of recommendation, tran-

scripts, entrance examination scores, and an application fee. This chapter traces the requisite steps of compiling, completing, and transmitting these materials in a coordinated fashion. But before we address the nuts and bolts of doing so, let us touch upon the crucial question of how many programs to apply to.

How Many?

The average number of applications made by students to clinical and counseling psychology programs is about 13. The precise number to which you should apply depends on the strength of your credentials and the competitiveness of the prospective programs; more applications are indicated for weaker credentials and more competitive programs.

Our rule of thumb is to apply to *at least* 10 to 12 programs: five "safe" (you clearly meet or exceed their standards); five "target" or "ambitious" programs (your credentials just make or miss their requirements); and perhaps one or two "reach" or "stretch" programs (where you do not approximate their standards but you have a particular hunch, research compatibility, or personal relationship that has a chance of sweeping you into the finalist pool). We have met industrious students who have applied to over 40 programs and confident students who have applied to just four or five.

But "don't pull a Missar," as we say at the University of Scranton. David Missar was an exceptional undergraduate and good-humored fellow (who gave us permission to use his story as a lesson for others to learn). He had a sky-high GPA, impressive GREs, a practicum to his credit, and even a coauthored publication. He was feeling a bit too confident in applying to only four doctoral programs, all located around his home town of Washington, D.C., which happens to have some of the most competitive programs in the country. Despite his stellar academic credentials, Dave did not receive any acceptances his first year simply because his research interests and strengths did not "match" those of the clinical faculty and institutions to which he applied. Had he applied to a greater number or larger variety of programs, he surely would have been accepted somewhere, as he was easily the next year when he corrected his miscalculations.

Application Form

You have a list of 10 to 20 programs in front of you. The deadlines range from mid-December to mid-February. You have used the late summer and fall months to investigate potential programs—the professors, the orientations, the locations, and the costs. It is now time to start writing.

One of the easiest parts is filling out the application itself. When you download an application from the Web, be sure it is on clean, white, high-quality paper. Some students have found it useful to make a copy of the application and complete a first draft on the photocopy. The completed application reflects on you; keep it as professional and neat as possible.

Slightly more than half of all graduate programs allow you to submit an application through e-mail or the World Wide Web (Norcross et al., 2005). If you have the choice, we advise against doing this. Taking the time to carefully consider (and often change) portions of your application is an important part of the process. Your personal statement requires a great deal of thought and will go through many revisions. By completing the application and reading it over several times before mailing it, you are likely to catch and correct errors or poor choices. This is one of the places where we recommend against taking full advantage of technological advances.

Online applications can be an Internet nightmare. You don't know what your completed application will look like. You don't know where it goes—or where it does not go. You can easily fail to indicate essential information, such as faculty members with whom you desire to work. On the other hand, online applications are quick, potentially less expensive, and the software improving rapidly. So, if you elect to submit an application online, please be careful. Proofread the document several times and try to cut and paste a fully formed personal statement from a word processing file.

Begin the applications at least 1 month before the earliest deadline. Some applicants, particularly under-

graduates in their senior year, wait until the end of the fall semester on the holiday break. *This is too late*—do not wait, lest you be rushed, unprepared, and working on a tight deadline.

Unlike the medical school process, which uses an identical application form for every school, each graduate program in psychology has its own, unique application. Providing the same information over and over again in slightly different formats can become frustrating and time consuming. Several years ago a committee recommended a standardized graduate application form to reduce the paperwork, but comparatively few programs have instituted it. Nonetheless, it provides a good idea of the information that will be requested of you:

- Full name
- Previous and maiden names
- Citizenship status
- Semester of entrance
- Current mailing address
- Permanent home address
- Educational history
- Degree sought
- Field of study
- Relevant courses taken
- Grade point averages
- Academic honors
- Clinical experience
- Special qualifications
- Employment history
- Teaching/research experience
- Career objectives
- References

Submitting applications is worse than filling out income tax returns (Fretz & Stang, 1980). Allow yourself enough uninterrupted time to do it carefully and completely. Illegible handwriting, incorrect spelling, and poor grammar will hurt your chances.

Some additional tips:

- Keep the application forms for each school separated. Individual file folders might help. Since the forms are often poorly marked, you may not otherwise know which forms belong to what school.
- Create a spreadsheet to keep track of your multiple applications—the application deadlines, number of recommendations required, what was sent, what was received, and so on. This method helps to organize the blizzard of paperwork, especially if you are applying to more than a few graduate programs.
- Enclose with each application a self-addressed, stamped postcard that the school can return to

verify receipt of your application. On the back of the card simply type: "Please send to verify receipt of application to _____ University."

- Print a copy or photocopy each application before mailing it. Graduate schools and the postal service have been known to lose—or misplace—entire forms. A hard copy will enable you to quickly re-submit if necessary.

On a side note, completing application forms for graduate school marks a good time to critically examine the impression that your voice- and e-mail are communicating to others. A Dave Matthews tune on your voice mail may entertain fellow students, but probably not the director of clinical training. Cute e-mail addresses, such as bongmeister@gmail.com or hotchick @aol.com, may delight romantic partners, but certainly not the dean of the graduate school. So now may be the time to alter those messages and convey a more professional demeanor.

By the same token, take a few moments to clean up your homepage, blog, and MySpace account. You may believe that your biographical entries and provocative photos are entertaining, but academics may question your judgment. More than one-quarter of employers state that they have researched potential job candidates on the Web (National Association of Colleges and Employers, 2007). We have every reason to believe that members of graduate admission committees do likewise.

Curriculum Vitae

Curriculum vitae means, literally, "the course of your life." The vitae or CV summarizes your academic and employment history in a structured form.

Both resumes and CVs summarize your credentials, but they differ in several ways. A resume is typically for employment, whereas a CV is for graduate school and academic positions. Resumes are brief, typically on a single page, whereas CVs go on for several pages. Resumes always list objectives, such as "To obtain an entry-level position in . . .", but CVs do not. Resumes frequently present personal interests and hobbies; CVs rarely do.

Figures 5-1 and 5-2 present two possible formats for a CV; you will need to adapt these samples to your individual needs. Although the samples are single-spaced and occupy only one page, CVs are *double-spaced* between entries and occupy several pages.

As a general comment, keep the CV honest and positive. Never fabricate, but perhaps "embellish" ap-

propriately. The line to be drawn here is demarcated by whether you can look an interviewer directly in the eye and factually defend an entry that could subsequently be corroborated by a supervisor, professor, or another person. Structured brevity is the key; lengthy expositions of experiences are best left to personal statements or job descriptions.

And this "academic resume" should be positive, upbeat in tone. Avoid any negative features that might red-flag your application. Save confessions and excruciating honesty for the clergy and psychotherapist. Omit sections that do not apply to you, such as "Presentations" or "Publications" if you have had none at this point in your career.

Let's proceed through the different sections of a CV and offer some additional hints. List your legal name, including any suffixes such as "Jr." Distinguish between a current address and a permanent home address, if this applies to your living circumstances. Note any anticipated changes in your address. Include telephone numbers and e-mail addresses at which program directors or professors can easily reach you. If you share voice mail or an answering machine with other people, insure that they will graciously take a message for you and reliably transmit that message to you.

Information on your marital status and dependents is definitely optional. Opinions differ widely on whether you should include this material on your CV: the probable positives are that you are being honest and sharing information about yourself; the likely downsides are that the information may be used against you or lead to illegal considerations in admission decisions. The marital status question is now almost moot since approximately half of all graduate students in psychology are married (Pate, 2001).

Regarding education, list degrees as "anticipated" if they have not yet been awarded. Impressive grade point averages may also be listed here. Honors are listed in chronological order, usually excluding those obtained in high school. If you received an honor specific to a university (e.g., the Lawrence Lennon Memorial Award), then record what it is for. Similarly, specify the disciplines of honor societies. Clinical experiences and research experiences can be listed together or separately, depending on what will strengthen your CV, but in either case indicate position title, relevant dates, number of hours, duties performed, and the supervisor. Include any presentations or publications in APA style, thereby demonstrating your familiarity with the psychologist's publication manual. The names of references should be listed only after you have obtained their permission to do so. *Never list a reference*

November 2008

CURRICULUM VITAE

Name:	Chris Smith
Address:	15 Easy Street
	Babylon, NY 12345
Telephone:	(516) 555-1212
E-mail:	bear@babu.edu
Place of Birth:	Scranton, Pennsylvania
Citizenship:	United States of America

Education:

H.S. Diploma	Cherry Hill High School, City, State, June 2005
B.S. (anticipated)	Psychology, Babylon University, May 2009

Honors and Awards:

New York State Regents Scholarship, 2005–2009
Dean's List, Babylon University, 2008–2009
Psi Chi, 2008
Babylon University Honors Program, 2007–2008
Who's Who Among Students in American Colleges & Universities, 2008

Clinical Experience:

Mental Health Technician, Friendship House, Jackson, Wyoming, June 2007–August 2008. Duties: recreational counseling and supervision of 20 behaviorally and emotionally disturbed children. Supervisor: Doris Day, M.S. 40 hours weekly.

Telephone Counselor, Mesopotamia County Community Crisis Center, Babylon, New York, 2006–2007. Duties: used a crisis intervention model to counsel a wide range of callers. Supervisor: Randal Kaplan, M.A. 4 hours weekly.

Research Experience:

Research Assistant, Babylon University, Department of Psychology, September 2007–June 2008. Duties: word processing, manuscript preparation, and data analyses for Chris Demanding, Ph.D. 15 hours weekly.

Honors Research, Babylon University with Rita Murrow, Ph.D., 2006–2008. Duties: proposed and conducted an original project; data input and analysis using SPSSx; write-up and oral defense.

Professional and Honor Societies:

Psi Chi, National Honor Society in Psychology
American Psychological Association (student affiliate)
Alpha Gamma Epsilon Omega (National Honor Society in Ergonomics)

Presentations and Publications:

Smith, C., & Murrow, F. A. (2007, April). *Self-esteem and math performance: Another look.* Paper presented at the meeting of the Babylon Psychological Association, New York.

Murrow, F. A., & Smith, C. (2008). The effects of self-esteem on math test performance. *Journal of Psychology, 46,* 113–117.

Campus Activities and Leadership:

Psychology Club, member (2007–2008) and president (2007–2008)
University Singers, Babylon University, 2005–2007
Hand-in-Hand, participant (2005–2008) and campus coordinator (2008)

References:

Frances Murrow, Ph.D., Associate Professor, Department of Psychology, Babylon University, Babylon, NY 12345. Voice: 516-555-1212; e-mail: murrow@babu.edu

Theodore Demanding, Ph.D., Professor and Chair, Department of Psychology, Babylon University, Babylon, NY 12345. Voice: 516-555-1212; e-mail: les@babu.edu

Doris Day, M.S., Senior Therapist, Children's House, 78 Oak Street, Jackson, WY 12345. Voice: 307-555-1212

FIGURE 5-1. One format for curriculum vitae.

Chris Smith   November 2008

Personal History:

Business Address:	Department of Psychology
	Babylon University
	Babylon, New York 12345
Phone:	(516) 555-1212
Home Address:	1017 Jefferson Avenue
	Cherry Hill, NJ 08002
Phone:	(609) 555-1212
E-mail:	bear@babu.edu
Birthdate:	March 15, 1987
Citizenship:	United States of America

Educational History:

Babylon University, Babylon, New York
Major: Psychology
Degree: B.S. (anticipated), May 2009
Dean's List, 2006–2008
Who's Who Among Students in American Colleges & Universities, 2008
Honors Thesis: Investigation of the relationship between self-esteem and math performance (Chairperson: Rita Murrow, Ph.D.)

Professional Positions:

1. Telephone Counselor, Mesopotamia County Community Crisis Center, Babylon, New York. Part-time position, 2006–2008. Duties: used a crisis intervention model to counsel a wide range of callers. Supervisor: Randal Kaplan, M.A.
2. Mental Health Technician, Friendship House, Jackson, Wyoming. Full-time summer, 2007. Duties: recreational counseling and supervision of 20 behaviorally and emotionally disturbed children. Supervisor: Doris Day, M.S.
3. Research Assistant, Babylon University. Half-time position, 2007–2008. Duties: word processing, manuscript preparation, and data analysis. Supervisor: Chris Demanding, Ph.D.

Membership in Professional Associations:

Psi Chi (National Honor Society in Psychology)
American Psychological Association (student affiliate)
Alpha Gamma Epsilon Omega (National Honor Society in Ergonomics)

Professional Activities:

President, Babylon University Chapter of Psi Chi, 2007–2008
Member of Program Committee, Babylon University Psychology Conference, 2007

Papers Presented:

Smith, C. E., & Murrow, F. A. (2007, April). *Self-esteem and math performance: Another look.* Paper presented at the meeting of the Babylon Psychological Association, New York.

Publication:

Murrow, F. A., & Smith, C. (2007). The effects of self-esteem on math test performance. *Journal of Psychology, 46,* 113–117.

Campus Activities:

Psychology Club, member (2006-2008) and president (2007–2008)
University Singers, Babylon University, 2006–2008
Hand-in-Hand, participant (2005–2008) and campus coordinator (2008)

References:

Frances Murrow, Ph.D., Associate Professor, Department of Psychology, Babylon University, Babylon, NY 12345. Voice: 516-555-1212; e-mail: murrow@babu.edu

Theodore Demanding, Ph.D., Professor and Chair, Department of Psychology, Babylon University, Babylon, NY 12345. Voice: 516-555-1212; e-mail: les@babu.edu

Doris Day, M.S., Senior Therapist, Children's Hospital, 78 Oak Street, Jackson, WY 12345. Voice: 307-555-1212

Note. Adapted from Hayes & Hayes (1989) with the permission of the authors.

FIGURE 5-2. Another format for curriculum vitae.

on a CV or application form unless you have secured that person's agreement to write a letter in support of your application.

Place the date (month and year) on the upper right-hand corner of the CV. In this way, you can submit an addendum if your credentials significantly improve by, say, having a paper accepted for publication or receiving your department's "student of the year" award. Lay out the information in an attractive and organized manner. Use a consistent format both within each section and between sections. For example, if you opt to list your clinical experiences from the most recent to the past, then maintain this format in all the other sections.

Here is an idea to enhance the CV for students who have developed specific research or computer competencies. List them on your vitae as a separate section. Computer skills might include proficiency with SPSS, SAS, Pascal, Harvard Graphics, Chartmaster, SigmaScan, SigmaPlot, CricketGraph, and Aldus Pagemaker. Research skills might include performing computerized library searching on *PsycLIT* or *Medline,* administering the Wisconsin Card Sorting Test (or another psychological test), or operating an electroencephalograph (EEG). Also include here any special skills, such as fluency in foreign languages or proficiency in American Sign Language. A faculty member screening applications may realize that these competencies are exactly what he or she is looking for in a new graduate assistant or research assistant. So use your CV to highlight your abilities! Omit this optional section if you have none or only one specific competency; in the latter case, describe the special qualification in your personal statement.

What should *not* be put on the CV? Eliminate listings of religion, hobbies, pets, favorite books, and items of that kind (Hayes & Hayes, 1989). They are unnecessary; save them for a resume. Nor is a photograph customary.

Padding of all varieties must be avoided. Padding occurs when a reader reacts to the CV as more form than substance ("Who are they trying to fool?!"). Potentially risky is listing professional projects under way—one or two legitimate research projects may pass but any more will probably be considered suspect. Other signs of padding, and therefore sections to exclude, are conventions attended, journals read, and projects you worked on in a nonprofessional capacity.

Pumping up your past on CVs and application forms is common but inadvisable. A recent survey of 2.6 million job applications discovered that 44% of them contained lies (Kluger, 2002); do not be among the 44%. Once you are caught fibbing on a graduate school application, it is practically impossible to restore your integrity and character at that program. While some of your friends may exhort you to exaggerate your previous positions and to inflate your GPA, we strongly advise honesty.

Proofread the document carefully; review it with an advisor before you print it. It ideally would be produced on a laser printer with a few fonts, but any letter-quality printer will suffice. Staple the pages together when finished (Hayes & Hayes, 1989).

The CV, like personal statements (below), should be printed on standard-sized white or cream stock. Purchase good quality bond paper for these documents. Avoid onionskin paper, goldenrod color, odd-sized papers, memo pads, green or red ink, and other unconventional or "cheap" materials.

Although much of the information contained in the CV is requested on the application form itself, we believe the inclusion of a CV enhances your application—providing it is properly prepared. A CV denotes a scholarly demeanor, highlights your accomplishments, and communicates familiarity with the workings of academia.

Personal Statements

Another bridge you must cross is writing the statement of purpose. Every program will want to know why you chose clinical or counseling psychology and the area within it that you plan to study. Admissions committees will also want to know how you came to this decision and what sorts of goals you have in mind. Each application will ask this question in a slightly different way because each program has different expectations and approaches to training. *Read the instructions carefully.* Do not just word process one statement and submit it to everyone.

Do not misinterpret the meaning of personal in *personal statement.* This essay is not the place to espouse your philosophy of life, to describe your first romance, or to tell the story about your being bitten by the neighbor's dog and subsequently developing an anxiety disorder. Instead, think of the essay as a *professional statement.* Write about your activities and experiences as an aspiring psychologist (Bottoms & Nysse, 1999).

An analysis of 360 essays required as part of the graduate application process demonstrated wide variability in the content requested (Keith-Spiegel, 1991). The most frequent requests were to articulate:

- Career plans
- Clinical experiences

- Interest areas
- Specific faculty of interest
- Research experiences
- Autobiographical statement
- Academic objectives
- Reasons for applying to that particular program
- Educational background

To reiterate: carefully read the question, individualize your response to each program, and respond to all parts of the question posed to you.

Be attentive to what the program requests. If they stress research, highlight your research interests and experience. If they stress clinical work, highlight the development of these interests and your training experiences to date. Show how you started with a question or a clinical observation, how you pursued that question, and how it developed into a greater understanding of the issues at hand and a need to know more. Demonstrate how this program meets your needs and is the ideal place to continue to pursue knowledge. State the goals you wish to attain with this knowledge, the career path you hope to work toward. If you are committed to the Boulder model, indicate how research is useful and how it is clinically applicable.

If you can make this connection in your personal statement, you will impress on the admission committee the integration APA sets forth as its ideal for Boulder-model, Ph.D. programs.

Graduate selection committees value clarity, focus, and "passion" in personal statements (Keith-Spiegel, 1991). Clarity and focus are typically construed as indicators of lucid thought, realistic planning, and self-direction, all valuable assets in a graduate student. At the same time, try to communicate a heartfelt commitment to your chosen career. "Passion" is not too strong a term—even relentless, obsessed, committed, fascinated; in short, what we call "catching the fever!" Your statement might well include such assertions as "I love college and the academic environment," "I am fascinated by counseling psychology and its potential to empower people and change communities," or "Research is a passion, not only a course requirement." Graduate faculty seek students who find it difficult to distinguish between work and pleasure when it comes to academic tasks (Kieth-Spiegel & Wiederman, 2000).

The personal statement is a prime opportunity to induce a match with the research and clinical interests of a faculty member. Many programs, as we have said, attempt to match faculty with incoming graduate students on the basis of mutual interest, for example, family therapy, women's issues, or neuropsychological assessment. This matching strategy is more often employed by research-oriented than practice-oriented programs, but attempt it in all of your personal statements.

To illustrate, consider the clinical admissions process of the University of Ottawa, a program with an equal emphasis on research and practice. Like many programs, they create a finalist pool by eliminating applications with lower GPAs and GRE scores. Then each of the clinical faculty members reviews all the finalist applications in order to locate several possible matches. These applicants then receive interviews. As you can see, and as we have repeated throughout this book, gaining admission into competitive doctoral programs is not limited simply to one's credentials but also includes a match in research and clinical interests.

Here, then, are a few general guidelines for writing personal statements that increase the probability of a match:

- Mention at least two and perhaps up to four of your interests. This obviously covers a wider range than a single interest.
- Cast your interests in fairly broad terms—not administering the Wisconsin Card Sorting Test, but neuropsychological assessment; not a mail survey of counseling psychologists, but the characteristics and practices of psychotherapists.
- Nominate at least two professors with whom you would like to work at that particular graduate program. This, too, enhances the chance of a successful match.
- Integrate the program's training philosophy into you personal statement. For example, "I resonate with Babylon University's goal of producing multiculturally competent psychologists to work directly in the community."

A commonly asked question is, "How personal should I get in my personal statement?" Although there is no universally correct answer, some suggestions can be offered. A personal detail, such as describing how growing up with a handicapped or disturbed sibling has affected your life and decision to enter psychology, is appropriate. However, depicting the situation in intimate detail without relating it to its contribution to your own growth may lead an admissions committee to question your judgment. A rule of thumb is to be introspective and self-revealing without sounding exhibitionistic. For example, it is appropriate for an applicant to state how personal life experiences have contributed to better self-understanding, but it sounds peculiar when the applicant goes into great detail about particular relationships or early life events (Halgin, 1986). Although allusions to your personal psychotherapy in personal statements does not appear to overly stigmatize candidates or lead disproportionately to their rejections (Schaefer, 1995), we recommend against including your personal therapy in written materials. Better to save such intimate disclosures for the personal interview, if appropriate.

Many personal statements are ineffective because, first, the student fails to spend time preparing them and, second, the student fails to be "personal" (Osborne, 1996). Therefore, as an applicant you should devote a substantial amount of time thinking, writing, rethinking, and rewriting the personal statement. Your statement should include personal details that relate to your ability to be a successful graduate student and that demonstrate maturity, adaptation, and motivation—the very characteristics sought by admissions committees.

Another question we are frequently asked is, "How distinctive or unique should my personal statement be?" Our answer is "as distinctive or unique as you are." Some applicants labor under the delusion that personal statements should resemble creative writing samples that magnify their singular accomplishments or that set the world on fire. Set the bar more realistically and aim for a personal statement that tells your own story clearly and convincingly.

A good idea is to show humility. Even if you have golden research and clinical experiences and 1400 GRE scores, you are still entering as a student. You are coming to learn. Mention the areas you hope to develop during your graduate school experience.

Be prepared to back up the claims you make in your personal statements. If you profess a working knowledge of, say, experiential psychotherapy, then be prepared for questions on the work of Carl Whitaker, Leslie Greenberg, and Alvin Mahrer. Similarly, if you claim fluency in Spanish, then expect one of the interviews to be conducted entirely in Spanish (Megargee, 1990).

The "to do's" of personal statements are process suggestions and thus difficult to pinpoint, but the "not to do's" are content oriented and easier to delineate (Whitbourne, 1999). We characterize three such "nots" as the three H's: Humor, Hyperbole, and Hard luck stories. Humor rarely works in a formal written statement; so unless you are an unusually gifted satirist, we recommend you avoid jokes and funny stories about your life. Similarly, hyperbole rarely impresses the admissions committee. References to your "overwhelming childhood trauma" and "triumph over undiagnosed learning disabilities" in personal statements cast doubt on the veracity and accuracy of your judgment. And hard luck stories typically come off feebly. Many stu-

dents financed their undergraduate educations, many survived disastrous relationship choices, and many muddled through two academic majors before finding their niche in psychology. Avoid making adversity the theme of your statement.

Our advice is supported by a recent study on the "kisses of death" in the graduate school application process (Appleby & Appleby, 2004). Eighty-eight chairs of graduate admissions committees provided examples of application materials that caused the admissions committee to draw negative conclusions about the applicant. A prevalent theme among these kisses of death was damaging personal statements that were (a) overly altruistic, (b) excessively disclosing, or (c) professionally inappropriate. Examples of the overly altruistic statements were "I want to help all people live happy lives" and "I want to help people because of how very much I have been helped." Examples of excessive self-disclosure were "being a recovering drug addict daughter of a sexually deviant and alcoholic mother" and excruciating details of an applicant's year-long struggle with painful hemorrhoids! Our favorite example of professional inappropriateness was the applicant who submitted a statement of purpose titled "Statement of Porpoise" that contained drawings of the sea mammal and a description of the applicant frolicking in the ocean with a porpoise on a visit to Florida. As we said, avoid humor, hyperbole, and hard luck in your personal statement.

One way to make your personal statement sparkle is to describe any teaching assistantships or experiences. Talk about how you learned leadership skills and teamwork in this role. Specific examples of how you responsibly handled challenging courses or teaching activities will lead the reader to infer you possess the "right stuff."

Your personal statement should tell a compelling, integrative story of a reflective individual who explicates accomplishments without joking or bragging or sobbing. As a colleague (Whitbourne, 1999) puts it: Don't say it softly or loudly, just say it clearly!

You will be asked in practically every personal statement and personal interview why you chose to apply to *this* particular graduate program in clinical or counseling psychology. Figure 5-3 presents a *portion* of a sample statement, addressing this ubiquitous question, written by one of our undergraduate students in his successful bid for entry into a clinical psychology doctoral program committed to the scientist–practitioner model. His reasons for applying to "Bogus University" are presented only as a single example; your statements will need to be tailored to your interests and credentials as well as the application instructions. Remember

It is my strong desire to attend a doctoral program in clinical psychology. I am seeking a program committed to the Boulder model, training scientist–practitioners able to serve society in a variety of capacities. The program I attend should stress the importance of understanding and integrating the broad field of psychology, as well as providing the knowledge and training specific to clinical psychology.

After a thorough review of more than 50 programs in clinical psychology, I have chosen to apply to Bogus University for a number of reasons. First, your program is known for producing stellar graduates, and has been repeatedly recommended to me by several psychology faculty. Second, Bogus University allows students to immerse themselves in research early in their graduate careers. Third, I am drawn toward several of your faculty members, including Dr. Babe Ruth for her work in substance abuse and cognitive therapy, and Dr. Ty Cobb for his work in sexual health, stress, and coping. I would be pleased to have either of these faculty members as my mentor. Fourth, the available clinical experiences would allow me to work with a population I find of particular interest, such as adults and families at the Psychological Services Center. And fifth, I am looking to attend school in a scenic area of the country where both my fiancé and I think we would be happy.

FIGURE 5-3. Portion of a sample autobiographical statement.

that this is just one part of an entire autobiographical statement.

Nonetheless, his why-I-applied-to-your-program statement illustrates several important points. First, he advances multiple reasons for applying to that particular program. Five reasons sound much more convincing than one or two. Second, his reasons for applying to Bogus U. primarily address his professional match with the program (their reputation, faculty members, clinical opportunities) but nicely concludes with a personal touch (geographic location). Third, he mentions two specific faculty and several potential research interests in an attempt to maximize the chances of a match. Fourth, the statement reflects his careful reading and incorporation of the program's self-description; for example, he cites the opportunity to immerse himself early into research and names the Psychological Services Center. Fifth, the statement is systematically organized and clearly written—indicators of an organized and clear-thinking graduate student!

Compose your personal statement as carefully as you would an important term paper. Write several rough drafts and then set it aside for a few days. Avoid slang words on the one hand, and overly technical or elaborate words on the other. Stick to the information requested; avoid too many "ruffles" and lengthy expositions of your own philosophy (Fretz & Stang, 1980). Write as many drafts as necessary until the statement sounds right to you.

Before you finish your personal statement, have friends read it for grammar, spelling, and typos. Regardless of the content, technical accuracy really makes a difference. Once it is error free, have one or more faculty members read it and make suggestions. Let them know where the statement is going, and they should be able to guide you on form and appropriateness.

For further tips on writing your personal statement, skim Donald Asher's (2000) *Graduate Admissions Essays: How to Write Your Way into the Graduate Program of Your Choice* and visit the following Web sites:

- www.essayedge.com
- www.psywww.com/careers/perstmt.htm
- www.accepted.com/grad/personalstatement.aspx
- www.english.uiuc.edu/cws/wworkshop/writer_resources/writing_tips/personal_statements.htm
- www.indiana.edu/~wts/pamphlets/personal_statement.shtml

We hope that our suggestions in this section guide you in writing your personal statement. It is also our hope that they are not too constraining. This is the part of the application where an admissions committee gets to see you in a more personal, three-dimensional light, an area where "you can be you."

Letters of Recommendation

What do admission committees gain from letters of recommendation? The answer is a personal but objective evaluation of your work from a professional experienced in the field. Admission committees desire a more objective sense of your abilities and experience than what you provide about yourself. Consequently, it is best to have at least two of the people writing your letters be at the doctoral level in psychology or psychology-related disciplines. One fine letter from a master's-level clinician is usually acceptable, but he or she will not be in a position to attest to your ability to complete doctoral studies. By the same token, bachelor's degree recipients, friends, and relatives should never write letters of recommendation to doctoral programs —they simply do not have the experience or knowledge of what it takes to earn a doctorate. Letters from politicians and your psychotherapists typically are inappropriate as well; they tend to write personal and psychological testimonies instead of academic letters of reference.

Choose people with whom you have worked for a long enough period, preferably for a year or more. That typically excludes professor you have taken a single class with, even if you did get an A. If you wrote a particularly strong paper in the class and the professor knows you a bit better, then he or she could serve as a reference, but this reference is still not the most desirable. At best this person can say, "This student was always on time, participated in discussions, attended office hours, and tested very well. On this basis I consider him/her an intelligent student and a good candidate for graduate school."

By contrast, admissions committees want to hear something more detailed, like: "This student has worked with me for 1 year. During that time she scored MMPIs, tested participants using a Grass Model 7 polygraph, analyzed data, and conducted her own honors thesis. She was dependable and worked beyond what was required by the department. Given this student's intelligence, motivation, and responsibility, I think she would make an outstanding doctoral student." Though the above is a strong example, the point is that you want someone to attest to your ability and responsibility.

Table 5-1 lists some of the self-sabotaging things students do to receive neutral letters of recommendation. Although presented for its humor, it also provides sage warnings about interpersonal behaviors that annoy professors.

TABLE 5-1. Professors' Pet Peeves: Avoiding Neutral Letters of Recommendation

Students sometimes are unaware of how the seemingly innocuous things they do and say can annoy their professors. In turn, the professors provide students with less than enthusiastic letters of recommendation. Here are some examples suggested by William W. Nish of Georgia College, reprinted with his kind permission.

Be quick to apply such concise labels as "busy work," "irrelevant," and "boring" to anything you do not like or understand. Not only is this a convenient way of putting the professor down, but also you will not be bothered with the inconvenience of understanding something before you judge it.

Always be ready with reasons why you are an exception to the rules established for the class, such as the dates for submitting written assignments.

Avoid taking examinations at the same time as the rest of the class. Be certain to take it for granted that the professor will give you a make-up exam at your convenience, regardless of your reason for missing the exam.

Be very casual about class attendance. When you see your professor be sure to ask, "Did I miss anything important in class today?" This will do wonders for his or her ego. By all means expect the professor to give a recital of all of the things you missed instead of taking the responsibility for getting the information from another member of the class.

Be consistently late to class and other appointments. This shows other people how much busier you are than they are.

Do not read your assignments in advance of class lecture and discussion. This actually allows you to study more efficiently, for you can take up class time asking about things that are explained in the reading.

Avoid using the professor's office hours or making an appointment. Instead, show up when he or she is frantically trying to finish a lecture before the next class hour and explain that you must see him or her right that minute.

Do not participate in such mundane activities as departmental advising appointments. Instead, wait until the last minute for approval of your schedule, and then expect the professor to be available at your convenience.

Other students receive neutral letters of recommendation through no fault of their own. They experience difficulty in securing detailed letters of recommendation because they:

- Transferred from one college to another college before graduating (which occurs, according to the U.S. Department of Education, to almost one-third of all students);
- Attended a mammoth state university where they only took huge lecture classes and never had the same psychology professor twice; or
- Switched majors relatively late in their college career and did not get to know their psychology professors well.

We are sympathetic to these plights. If you fall into one of these categories, then you need to double your efforts to get involved in clinical experiences, research activities, and departmental matters—and do so quickly.

Graduate programs request three or four letters of recommendation. Try to secure letters that will give the admissions committee the information it desires. At a practice-oriented program, two letters from clinical supervisors and one from a research advisor might be prudent. At a research-oriented school, two letters from research advisors and one from a clinical supervisor would probably be better. All things being equal, it is preferable to have your "research" letters come from faculty. However, if you believe that a letter from an employer would be significantly more helpful than that of a professor with whom you are not well acquainted, then it is probably a good idea to use the employer.

Our general advice was confirmed by an interesting study (Keith-Spiegel & Wiederman, 2000) that asked members of admissions committees to rank sources of recommendation letters. Raters were asked to assume that the letters from these different sources were equally positive so that rating variations were due solely to the referee's characteristics. The most valuable sources of letters of recommendation were (in descending order): (1) A mentor with whom the applicant has done considerable work; (2) the applicant's professor, who is also a well-known and highly respected psychologist; (3) an employer in a job related to the applicant's professional goals; (4) the chair of the academic department in which the applicant is majoring; (5) a professor from another department from whom the applicant has taken a relevant upper-division course. By contrast, a letter from a graduate teaching assistant was rated, essentially, as no help.

And a letter from one's personal therapist was rated negatively!

Very important: First ask the person writing the letters whether he or she can write you a good one. Ask this direct and specific question: "Can you write a good letter of recommendation for me?" If the person is hesitant or gives any indication of having reservations, *ask someone else!* A bad letter of recommendation is deadly. Better to have one brief letter from a professor who gave you an "A" than from someone who might express reservations about your abilities. "I don't know" is better than "I know, but I have reservations."

The way you approach professors for a recommendation is an underappreciated topic. You will ask specifically, "Can you write a good recommendation for me?" If the person responds in the affirmative, we strongly recommend that you provide that person with a letter similar to that shown in Figure 5-4. The person writing a letter of recommendation needs adequate information in order to produce a credible and informative letter. You can be powerful in shaping a professor's letter of recommendation!

This letter—and the attendant course listing and CV—will promote accuracy and detail. These are essential characteristics of strong letters of recommendation in that the admissions committee looks for positive tone *and* detail. A two-paragraph laudatory letter on the order of "Great student, fine person" simply doesn't make the detailed case for your admission into competitive doctoral programs.

What admissions committees also find useless in letters are duplicate and irrelevant information. One set of researchers (Elam et al., 1998) queried members of admissions committees and discovered the five *least* helpful aspects of letters of recommendation:

- Repetition of information from the application (e.g., repeating grades, honors, and scores available elsewhere on the application)
- Unsubstantiated superlatives or vague generalities
- Detailed descriptions of grades in one particular course
- Lack of strong relationship between applicant and letter writer
- Inclusion of irrelevant information, such as religious beliefs or hearsay

Put another way, give your referees sufficient data to render informed and positive letters about your personal characteristics, academic strengths, and interpersonal skills so that they do not resort to filling your recommendations with irrelevant content.

246 Wood Street
Babylon, NY 14000

November 2008

Leslie Jones, Ph.D.
Department of Psychology
East Coast University
1200 Faculty Building
Hausman, MD 43707

Dear Dr. Jones:

Thank you for agreeing to write a letter of recommendation on my behalf. I hereby waive (or do not waive) my right to inspect the letter of recommendation written for me and sent to the designated schools of my choice. I am applying to (master's, doctoral) programs in clinical (counseling) psychology. My earliest deadline is ____ _____.

Here are the courses I have taken from you.

Fall 2006	Abnormal Psychology	A–
Spring 2007	Clinical Psychology	B+
Fall 2008	Undergraduate Research	

Here are other activities in which I have participated.

| 2007–2008 | Research Assistant |
| 2006–2007 | Vice President of Psi Chi |

My latest GRE scores were 580 Verbal, 590 Quantitative, and 5.0 Analytical Writing. My Psychology Subject Test score was 610.

Finally, I attach a copy of my current vitae and a list of psychology courses for any additional information that might prove useful. Please feel free to call me at 555-1212 or to e-mail me at Chris_smith@phonyemail.com. Thanks again.

Sincerely yours,

Chris Smith

Encls.

FIGURE 5-4. Sample letter to request a letter of recommendation.

Here's how one doctoral program (University of Rhode Island) attempts to translate the content of recommendation letters into numerical categories.

1 Summary recommendations in all three letters are neutral or negative. Positive and negative assessments are listed. Overall evaluation in all three is neutral.

2 Letters meet criteria between anchor points 1 and 3.

3 Summary recommendations in all three letters are positive and general. Positive

statements from all three letters. Statements are general in nature.

4 Letters meet criteria between anchor points 3 and 5.

5 Summary recommendations in all three letters are excellent and detailed. Positive statements from all three letters are very favorable and very detailed in their support.

Note, again, that the emphasis is on positive tone *and* supportive detail. This is the desired result of your extra work in providing references with factual information and assertive requests for letters of recommendation. A "liability letter" is one that communicates limited knowledge of the applicant, leading an admissions committee to conclude that the person was only minimally connected to professors in his or her undergraduate or master's department (Halgin, 1986).

Many universities provide their own form for recommendations as part of the application package. Your institution will probably have one of two ways of handling these forms. One way is to provide your professor with these forms and stamped envelopes addressed to the schools to which the forms are to be sent. This is a small but crucial precaution—do not take the chance that postage will delay return of the letter. It is also courteous: Your professor is doing you a favor taking considerable time and contemplation to write a strong letter. Another way is to provide your professor with these forms; he or she will then complete them and return them to the Office of Career Services/Planning for processing and mailing. Ask your reference which method he or she prefers.

A growing proportion of graduate schools are requesting that letters of recommendation be submitted electronically through their homepages or admission portals. In this case, you list the names, positions, and e-mail addresses of people writing you letters of recommendation on your application. The graduate schools then directly contact your referees via e-mail and provide them with the URL and a password to electronically submit their letters of recommendation to your application file. Online submission of recommendations will streamline the entire process and will become the rule in the near future.

The recommendation forms from graduate schools may appear to be quite different at first glance; however, closer inspection will reveal that they request essentially the same information. The forms typically ask the people writing the letters to note the length of time they have known you and in what capacities. Then the referees are asked to rate your research ability, originality, writing skills, organizational ability, maturity,

interpersonal skills, persistence, and similar qualities on a structured grid. Typical forms request an appraisal of the applicant in terms of 10 qualities in comparison with others applying for graduate study whom the referees have known in the applicant's proposed field of study. The rating grid offers responses of top 3%, next 10%, next 20%, middle third, lowest third, and unable to judge. On most forms, an open space is then presented for a narrative description of your strengths and weaknesses. The forms usually conclude with a request for a summary rating: a check mark on a continuum from "not recommended" to "highly recommended" or a numerical value representing an overall ranking of this student to others taught in the past or some similar estimate.

Researchers have identified the most frequent applicant characteristics that recommenders were requested to rate on the forms (Appleby, Keenan, & Mauer, 1999). The resulting list—based on the analysis of 143 recommendation forms—describes the characteristics that psychology graduate programs value in their applicants. In descending order of frequency, the top dozen are as follows:

- Motivated and hardworking
- High intellectual/scholarly ability
- Research skills
- Emotionally stable and mature
- Writing skills
- Speaking skills
- Teaching skills/potential
- Works well with others
- Creative and original
- Strong knowledge of area of study
- Character or integrity
- Special skills, such as computer or lab

One important lesson to be learned is that graduate school aspirants should make a concerted effort to behave in ways that allow them to acquire relevant skills (research, writing, speaking, computer) and to be perceived by at least three of their professors as motivated, bright, emotionally stable, capable of working well with others, and possessing integrity (Appleby et al., 1999).

Recommendation forms, by law, will contain a waiver statement asking whether you do or do not waive your right to inspect the completed letter of reference. The Family Education Rights and Privacy Act of 1974 (the so-called Buckley Amendment) mandated that students over age 18 be given access to school records unless they waive this right. This is a complicated topic, but we advise applicants to waive their right of access *providing,* as previously discussed, the person writing the letter knows the student well and has unhesitantly agreed to serve as a reference. Do not waive access—or better yet, do not request letters—from persons you do not trust or do not know.

A confidential letter carries more weight. By waiving your right to access, you communicate a confidence that the letters will be supportive, and you express trust in your reference. In fact, over 90% of health profession schools prefer letters of recommendation that are waived by the student (Chapman & Lane, 1997). Our experiences and naturalistic studies (e.g., Ceci & Peters, 1984; Shaffer & Tomarelli, 1981) suggest that professors' honest evaluations will be compromised when you have access to what they have written. By waiving the right, you are communicating an intent to have the "truth" told. Otherwise, admissions committees may lump the letter with all the other polite and positive testimonials (Halgin, 1986).

In making your choice of whether to waive or not to waive, be clear about the law. Most students correctly know that if they waive their rights they may never see the letter. However, many students erroneously think that choosing not to waive their rights means that they can see their letter if they do not get accepted or that they have a right to preview the letter before it is sent (Ault, 1993). These are common fallacies, but fallacies nonetheless.

The relevant laws do not dictate that professors must show students the completed letter. One study (Keith-Spiegel, 1991) of college faculty found that 17% never show students their letters of recommendation, 46% usually do not, 8% only to students they know well, 15% only if students ask, and 14% routinely show students their letters. Nor does the law guarantee a student access to letters if the student is rejected from a graduate program; in fact, students may inspect their files at a graduate school only after they have been accepted at and enrolled in that graduate school (Ault, 1993).

Going one step further, contrary to some students' beliefs, faculty do *not* have to write letters of recommendation for students. Letters are a common and voluntary courtesy, not a job requirement.

Why might faculty members decline to write a letter for a student? The single most common reason is that they don't know the student well enough (Keith-Spiegel, 1991). Other frequent reasons given by faculty are that they question the student's motivation level, emotional stability, academic credentials, or professional standards. If faculty defer on your request for a letter, politely inquire about their reasoning and graciously thank them for their candor.

One creative study asked psychologists how they would handle requests for a letter of recommendation from a student exhibiting specific problems (Grote, Robiner, & Haut, 2001). The majority indicated that they would *not* write a letter for a student who was abusing substances or who had shown unethical behavior. For most of the other student problems—interpersonal problems, lack of motivation, paucity of responsibility, marginal clinical skills—psychologists routinely would tell the student about their reservations, then write the letter including the negative information. If faculty members tell you that they have reservations about your behavior, then they will probably include the negative evaluation in their letter of recommendation. Politely inquire if their reservation will in fact appear in the letter. If so, thank them for their candor and withdraw your request for a letter.

Play it safe and provide the reference form at least 6 weeks before the deadline. Completing your recommendation may not be the top priority of the person you have asked to write it, or he or she may be out of town prior to the deadline. Do not take any chances that a letter will be late. Allow 3 weeks and ask if the letter has been sent. Be politic: do not pester, but do follow up.

If you seek additional information on requesting letters of recommendation, then we suggest the pointers offered by the following Web sites:

- gradschool.about.com
  (click on All About Recommendation Letters)
- www.uwm.edu/People/ccp2/work/recletter.html
- www.psychwww.com/careers/lettrec.htm

Transcripts and GRE Scores

An application file will not be complete—and probably not even considered by the admissions committee—unless the required academic transcripts and entrance examination scores have been received. Your task here consists of requesting the appropriate organizations to transmit official copies of these materials to the graduate schools of your choice and then ensuring that the schools have received them.

With respect to transcripts, you must request that the Registrar's Office of all attended colleges and universities mail an *official* copy of your transcript directly to the graduate school. An official copy will contain the seal, stamp, and authorized signature of the institution. The cost of transcripts varies from place to place, but it averages $3 to $10 per copy. Submit transcript requests at least 1 month before the application deadline. Many universities take 2 weeks during the semester to process these requests. The college form requesting a transcript will most likely accompany the transcript itself and thereby enter your graduate application file. Accordingly, this request form or mailing address should be typed or printed neatly.

Virtually all graduate programs continue to require hard copies of transcripts mailed from academic institutions. Online transcript exchange has been difficult to establish and is still uncommon. However, online transcripts will become more common with the advent of companies such as the recently formed National Transcript Center to provide secure electronic transmissions among institutions (Fauber, 2006).

A reminder: request an unofficial copy of your own transcript in September or October prior to applying. Inspect it closely for errors and omissions. Horror stories abound regarding erroneous transcript entries misleading admissions committees—an initial grade of I (incomplete) becoming an F (failure), honors credits not registered, unpaid term bills delaying transcripts, and so on. Don't leave it to chance; check it out yourself.

One creative researcher (Landrum, 2003) surveyed graduate admissions directors about the impact of transcripts and withdrawals in the admissions process. Results show that your transcript will get a careful review in practically all programs and will be reviewed by more than one member of the admissions committee in about 87% of the programs. With respect to the effects of course withdrawals (dropping a course after mid-semester) on transcripts, less than 4% of programs indicated that a withdrawal from a single course would hurt an applicant's chance of admission into the graduate program. But more than 20% of the programs indicated that two or more withdrawals hurt a student's entry into their graduate program. Thus, our advice to students contemplating a course withdrawal is that one is probably not hurtful, but that two or more withdrawals, especially from required courses such as statistics and research methods, may well have a negative impact.

With respect to GREs, score reports will automatically be mailed to you and electronically submitted to the four graduate schools you listed when you completed the GRE testing. The mailing date for the score reports is approximately 6 weeks after the test date for paper-based testing (Psychology Subject Test) and 2 weeks for computer-based testing (General Test). Your copy of the score report is intended only for your information; official reports are sent directly by ETS to the score recipients you designate. This procedure—as with the registrar transmitting an official transcript—"is

intended to ensure that no questions are raised about the authenticity of a score report" (GRE, 2001, p. 16).

You will probably be applying to more than the four schools you designated for score reports. Toward this end, you can use the "Phone Service for Additional Score Reports" by dialing 1-888-GRE-SCORE. The charge is $6.00 per call plus $15.00 for each report requested, charged to your credit card. Your scores will be mailed within 5 working days. Or, you can submit an "Additional Score Report Request Form," published by ETS and obtainable at your Career Services Office, and remit your payment of $15.00 for *each* score recipient listed. ETS pledges in writing to "make every effort to send your score reports within 10 working days after receipt of your request" (GRE, 2001), but you should allow for at least 1 month. You may have your GRE scores transmitted at any time during the 5-year period after they are initially reported.

Remember: only send *un*official copies of your GRE scores if you are applying well before the deadline, and telephone to be sure that this will not impede your application.

Unsolicited Documents

A frequently asked question is, "What if a program doesn't ask for something that I'd like to send?" Some examples are the curriculum vitae, a research paper, and job descriptions. If a program does not want additional documents, it will state so clearly on the application. In that case, do as the program requests. But even then, you may be able to make additional documents a part of your application if you have come to know a professor at the school and have shared any of these documents with him or her. In general, it is a good idea to send a curriculum vitae, research paper, and/or job descriptions if they are applicable.

If you have relevant work and clinical experiences but can only use one for a letter of reference, then include a curriculum vitae or job description. One benefit is that these allow you to spend less time focusing on the details of these work experiences in your personal statement. You can relate how the experiences influenced you without wasting space explaining exactly what you did.

As a professional, you will need a CV eventually, and we recommend you begin one even if you do not use it in every application. Start a vitae file and toss notes and memos into it regarding assistantship duties, noteworthy activities, committee assignments, professional associations—in short, everything you need to update your vitae (Hayes & Hayes, 1989).

A job description details your duties and responsibilities. When asking a supervisor to write a job description, ask him or her to focus on your specific tasks and how well you performed them rather than asserting how well suited you are to graduate school. This allows you to spend less time describing what you did and how well you did it when writing your personal statement. For example, prior to graduate school, one of us worked with a psychotherapist conducting a social skills group for preadolescents. In his personal statement he was simply able to speak about how that experience had affected him. By referring to the "enclosed job description," the personal statement did not get bogged down in the details of this experience. Further, if you performed well at this job, having a supervisor's positive assessment allows you to be more modest in your personal statement.

If you have a large number of work experiences, be careful not to overwhelm admissions committees with paperwork. Choose two experiences that showcase your diversity and that highlight characteristics not likely tapped by those writing your letters of recommendation. If you send more job descriptions than this, you may weaken their impact and increase the chances that the most laudatory ones will not be read (or at least not carefully).

If you have written a thesis or a research paper and have received feedback that it is well written, then include it. If there is someone whose research corresponds with your own, this may open a door for you. However, if there is a question as to your paper's quality, then do not to send it. A questionable paper may do more harm than good.

Application Fees

Last but unfortunately not least, most schools require application fees. These fees range from $0 to $100 per school, and average $50 for doctoral programs and $35 for master's programs (Norcross et al., 2005). For paper applications, send a personal check or a cashier's check (never cash). Online applications will require a credit card, typically Visa, Master Card, or Discover.

If you are in financial need or are experiencing trouble meeting application expenses, read the application instructions carefully. There is usually a statement allowing fees to be waived because of financial hardship. Go to the school's application Web site, or call and ask how to have the application fee waived. That some students cannot afford the fees is the reason schools make the allowance in the first place. Graduate schools are sensitive to the impoverished status of many applicants, so please feel no compunction about requesting a fee waiver if it applies to you.

Check and Recheck

At this point, you have completed the application forms, requested letters of recommendation (and seen to it they were sent), written your personal statement, asked to have transcripts and GREs transmitted, and copied the unsolicited documents you plan to include in your applications. Once again, before you actually submit the material, have one of your professors check that it is accurate and well written. Have friends review it for typos and spelling. All material should be typed or word processed: it should look neat, error-free, and professional. It represents you in a very real way. Anything handwritten or tattered can convey the message that you are careless and unprofessional. Submission of materials should reflect a meticulous attention to detail. Finally, make sure your personal statement is not among those we see each year that carelessly includes the name of a different university when explaining why it is a perfect match!

After all this effort, make certain your application is submitted on time. We suggest (if you can afford the extra expense) that you send your application via FedEx, UPS, Express, or certified mail. Each of these systems will allow you to track your materials to ensure they have arrived and to have the name of the person to whom they were delivered. However, our suggestion does not imply that you should wait until the last minute to express mail your application, implying procrastination (not a positive quality in a graduate student). Do express mail, but do it well ahead of the deadline.

One of the most frustrating experiences in the graduate application process is ascertaining that the respective programs have in fact, received all of your materials. Your application, transcripts, GREs, letters of recommendation—all need to be received, processed, and filed correctly by the graduate admissions office. Horror stories abound about application materials being lost or misfiled or sent to the wrong department. It happened to one of us!

Recently, one of our students shared a similar story. The ETS claimed that her GRE scores were electronically transmitted to and downloaded at a major Midwest university. The university, which required two official sets of GRE scores, claimed that they never received either set. The student was caught in the middle between two opposing claims. She telephoned ETS again and the university's graduate admissions office repeatedly. The GREs had to be resent, at the student's expense.

We estimate that 50% of graduate programs will send a letter or e-mail apprising you of the application materials they have received on your behalf. Another 20% to 25% of graduate programs will post an application status page on their Web site where you can check yourself. That leaves 25% of the graduate programs that you can either blindly trust (which we *do not* recommend) or that you can contact (which we *do* recommend).

Call or e-mail the admissions office and verify that the material has been received. Some students prefer to include a self-addressed postcard to verify receipt, as discussed earlier, whereas others prefer the telephone. In either case, you have invested too much sweat, time, and money to leave the application to chance. Do not rely on graduate schools to keep you apprised; take personal responsibility.

CHAPTER 6
MASTERING THE INTERVIEW

The applications have been electronically submitted or mailed and are now out of your hands. Following the short-lived relief of finishing the applications, this period can be a nerve-wracking time. You have sold yourself on paper, and now it is up to the programs to decide which applicants to contact for further consideration and probable interviews.

The doctoral admissions process has been characterized as "multiple hurdles," with some of the hurdles applied sequentially (King, Beehr, & King, 1986). The initial hurdle in most programs is the GRE and GPA score minimums. The second hurdle is rating of applications on such criteria as clinical experience, research skills, letters of recommendation, and the like. Being invited for an interview means you have successfully leaped these early hurdles, and this is a great compliment in and of itself. The final and determining hurdle for most programs is the personal interview.

Not all programs require personal interviews, and they will most likely state in the application if they do not. Make a note of this so that you do not become distressed when you are not invited. We wonder which is worse: the disappointment of not being asked to interview or the stress of being asked!

Our research on APA-accredited clinical, counseling, and combined psychology programs found that 93% of them required some type of preadmission interview (Oliver et al., 2005). As shown in Figure 6-1, 62% of APA-accredited programs strongly preferred an interview in person but were willing to accept a telephone interview. Another 27% of the programs absolutely required a face-to-face interview. Four percent required only a telephone interview. All told, only 7%

of programs did not require an interview before admission into the program.

Nearly all clinical and counseling psychology programs, then, require some type of personal interview, be it by phone or in person, prior to acceptance. Since some programs absolutely insist on interviews in person, do *not* apply to distant programs requiring an in-person interview unless you can afford it. Only in very rare instances will programs reimburse the applicant for all interview costs, and only 10% of the programs reimburse for some of the costs (Kohout et al., 1991). In other words, 90% of the programs expect you to absorb all the interview expenses personally.

Expect to hear from interested doctoral programs that require interviews from mid-January through early

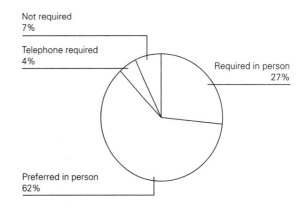

FIGURE 6-1. Preadmission interview policies of APA-accredited programs. Data from Oliver, Norcross, Sayette, Griffin, & Mayne (2005).

March. Programs rarely contact students in the finalist pool after March 30 because the first round of offers usually goes out on April 1. It is still possible to be contacted, however, if you are on the alternate or wait list.

Interview Strategically

The simple situation occurs when you are invited on a couple of interviews, the dates of the interviews do not conflict, and you have set aside enough money to travel to all the interviews. If only life were so simple! Instead, some applicants will not receive any interview offers, some will be invited to interview on a day they are already scheduled elsewhere for an interview, and still others will have depleted their funds and cannot afford interview travel.

How to handle these complex situations? In a word, strategically. Think through your options, discuss them with your mentor, and consider the following strategies.

If you have not received an interview request or a rejection letter by the middle of March, then calmly e-mail or telephone the doctoral program and inquire about the status of your application. If you have been rejected, politely thank the person. You never know, you may apply there again or have professional contact with the people in that program in the future. If your application is still being considered, it is permissible to ask when you might expect a decision. Just be careful not to be rigid or demanding.

If you are offered a personal interview at two doctoral programs on the very same day, not to worry. Should you be so blessed, we recommend that you (1) inquire if the programs have alternative interview days (and schedule one program on the alternative day). If not, then (2) ask if you can complete a video-conference interview or telephone interview at the less-preferred program. Remember that approximately two-thirds of programs will accept a telephone interview. If you value both programs equally, then (3) accept the interview at the least expensive program or the program with the highest likelihood of acceptance.

If you have depleted your funds for interview travel, then honestly inform the program and respectfully request a phone interview. Your email might read: "I am very interested in your program and initially planned to attend your interview day on February 15th. Unfortunately, my personal finances do not allow me to travel to Bogus University on that day. I am hopeful that you will permit me to conduct a phone interview on a day that is convenient for you. Thanks very much for understanding; I do wish that I could visit in person."

Many applicants obtain strategic information on interview invitations and admission offers from online message boards. The last few years have witnessed an increase in the number and popularity of these message boards devoted to doctoral programs in psychology (Fauber, 2006). Three examples spring to mind: Psych Grad.org, the Student Doctor Network (psychology), and Yahoo Message Board. These and other online boards are particularly valuable for notifying everyone the moment interview invitations are extended and admission offers are delivered. They also provide peer support through the taxing application process. However, we have read much online advice that is questionable, even downright wrong. Thus, use the free online boards to secure strategic information and timely support from peers but be wary of the proffered advice.

The Dual Purpose

The interview provides a critical opportunity for information gathering, not only for the program but also for you. That is, the dual purpose of an interview is for the program to check you out and for you to check the program out. Perhaps right now it seems outrageous to contemplate evaluating a doctoral program—you're probably delighted just to be asked! But a few interviews and an acceptance or two will reorient your perspective.

If you go on more than one interview, these interactions will give you the decisive information in choosing which program to attend. You will find out about clinical training, faculty members, student life, program fit, research facilities, and the like. Interviewers will be looking at your social skills, your emotional stability, your professional maturity, your focus, and your goals. The interviewers may want to see the development of your pursuits, the connection between your research and clinical work, or perhaps your adherence to the Boulder or Vail model. You may be asked pointed questions and will be expected to ask probing questions about the program.

Although the interview often generates anxiety for an applicant, it need not. As with anything else in the application process, the more you prepare, the more confident and less nervous you will feel.

A few basic observations about the interview process will contribute to your preparation. The interview is highly charged for the applicants and programs alike. *Both* wish to be evaluated positively and to achieve the best match. You are not alone in trying to put your best foot forward! Interview styles, moreover, vary tremendously—from a conversational tone to grueling questions, from casual to formal, from mundane content to intrusively personal content. Be prepared for all styles, and remember that all count equally in the final analysis.

That final analysis is the program's unenviable task of deciding which of the interviewees they will eventually select for admission. Programs ordinarily interview two to three times as many students as they can admit. The pool must be whittled down from, say, 200 applicants, from which 25 are selected for interviews, and from which 10 to 15 will be tendered an offer to obtain 7 confirmed acceptances.

Rehearsal and Mock Interviews

Rehearse the interview beforehand with a professor, a career counselor, or a knowledgeable friend. Although the research-oriented schools are usually less personal and invasive in their interviews, it may behoove you to get accustomed to being asked personal questions without being thrown. Such practice is invaluable, especially for preparing you to think on your feet. Rehearsing also will desensitize you to some degree, take the edge off of your anxiety, and add to your comfort with the process. During the interview, you are on stage, selling yourself, and knowing what the interview is all about can only help you.

In keeping with the dual purpose of the interview, rehearsing will also afford you practice in the interview style you seek to convey. A respectful and curious tone—"I am wondering about the chances of receiving an assistantship if I am fortunate enough to be accepted?"—is preferable to a blunt and forceful disposition—"How much will you pay me if I come?" How you phrase a question is important. The interviewer will be more impressed with your eagerness to learn if you ask how many courses in an area are *offered* as opposed to how many are *required* (Megargee, 1990).

Rehearsing should also entail preparation for frequently asked questions of applicants. Table 6-1 presents common interview questions to anticipate and prepare for. *We strongly recommend that you have a concise and thoughtful response ready for each of these.* An "I haven't really given that question much thought" answer hurts. Role-play these questions with a professor or, better yet, undergo a "mock interview" at your career services center. During this pretend experience, request that the interviewer ask several of the questions in Table 6-1 and videotape the encounter.

Beneath the dozens and dozens of possible questions that an interviewer could ask you, career experts say they all boil down to only a few basic questions. The people making the final decisions really want to know (Bolles, 2006):

- Why are you *here?* (As opposed to another graduate program; in other words, how well do you fit with us?)

TABLE 6-1. Common Interview Questions to Anticipate

1. Why do you want to be a psychologist?
2. What qualifications do you have that will make you a successful psychologist?
3. What attracts you to *our* program?
4. Will you tell me a little about yourself as a person?
5. Do you think your undergraduate grades (or GRE scores) are valid indicators of your academic abilities?
6. What do you see as your strengths and weaknesses?
7. What do you bring into the program? What are your special attributes?
8. Have you ever had personal therapy? If yes, what sort of issues did you work on? If no, why not?
9. What are your research interests? Tell me about your research project/honors thesis.
10. What is your theoretical orientation?
11. Which of our faculty members do you think you would work with?
12. Where else have you applied or interviewed?
13. Can you tell me about a recent clinical encounter? How did you conceptualize or treat your last client?
14. What are your hobbies, avocations, favorite books, and interests outside of psychology?
15. What are your future plans and goals as a psychologist?
16. What questions do you have for me?

- What can you do for us? (How can your skills, knowledge, and experience enhance our program?)
- What kind of person are you? (Are you reliable and personable? Can we trust you with our research projects and/or our clinic patients?)
- What distinguishes you from 20 other people who can do the same tasks? (What makes you different from the other qualified applicants we are interviewing? Do you work better, harder, longer, more thoroughly?)
- Can we get you here? (If we accept you into our program, what is the probability that you will attend? How much will it cost us—in tuition remission or an assistantship, for example?)

Of course, you cannot anticipate all possible questions. Some interviewers pride themselves on avoiding stock questions and instead asking novel questions, thus precluding rehearsed and polished replies. The rationale behind these queries, such as "Who are your heroes?" and "What was the best day in your life?" is that they give a glimpse into your natural response style and tap into spontaneous information processing. One method to handle novel queries is to delay thoughtfully, remark that it is one you have not been asked before, request a moment of contemplation, and then respond forthrightly.

Similar to novel questions are behavior-based interview questions. These are increasingly being asked to assess an applicant's behavioral repertoire and actual experiences. The behavioral questions rely on the familiar psychological dictum, "Past behavior is the best predictor of future behavior," to glean something about your future behavior in their doctoral program. Four examples are:

- Tell me about an instance when someone asked you to do something that you considered ethically or morally wrong. How did you respond?
- Describe the biggest challenges you faced in the past year and how you handled it.
- Tell me about a work or school situation where you had to do creative problem solving.
- Relate a recent situation in which you had to persuade someone to accept your idea or proposal.

Your answers will enable you to concretely demonstrate integrity, resilience, creativity, and persuasion as opposed to simply saying you possess the traits. Insure that your responses communicate a successful ending, both for you and the other party involved in the situation.

Interview Attire

Your interview rehearsal should direct attention to your physical attire, which will be an influential factor in attributions made about you. For men, we recommend a conservative two-piece suit or a jacket and slacks, white or light shirt, and contrasting tie. Three-piece suits and "funeral outfits" are out. Wear shined brown or black shoes that are well maintained; as your parents have probably told you, the way you take care of your shoes communicates a lot about you. Dark socks only; save your white socks for work-outs. Hair should be trimmed and neatly groomed.

For women, we recommend a pant suit or a suit with a skirt, dark in color or muted plaid, with medium heels in matching color. Wear a simple style blouse, white or soft color. Interview professionals suggest a "no distraction" hairstyle, tasteful makeup, and clear or light nail polish. One pair of small earrings should suffice. For both men and women, plan your interview clothes, try them on, and lay them out well before the interview to assure that they fit, are clean, and are in good repair.

Attire should err on the side of conservative and formal; better to be overdressed and loosen a tie or remove a scarf than to be underdressed for the occasion. Avoid flashy colors and loud fashions. Jewelry should be conservative and understated; go light on the perfume and cologne. Leave the piercings at home.

Some applicants complain to us that many faculty interviewers are wearing business casual, and thus ask why they (the applicants) can't wear business casual as well. Our answer is clear: You are an applicant trying to make a stellar impression as a serious, motivated candidate for a competitive graduate program. You are trying to distinguish yourself as one of the premier students, not one of the underdressed herd. We urge you to "dress for success" in interviews, not in business casual. You can wear casual clothes after you are admitted to the program for most of your graduate life. But during the interview, you never have a second chance to make a first impression.

Questions about the program and other written material should be held in a professional attaché or briefcase. The location and weather will influence your choice of clothing. Reliable answers about expected attire can be provided by graduate students with whom you may stay prior to the interview itself.

Travel Arrangements

While preparing and rehearsing for the interviews, you will simultaneously be making arrangements to travel to the interviews. The costs of travel vary wildly—from a few bucks for parking at a local university on interview day to more than $500 for a 3-day jaunt across the nation involving air travel, rental car, and hotel. Our intent in the following paragraphs is to save you hassle and money in getting to the interviews.

As a general rule, you can save a great deal of money by booking early and paying promptly for air travel, but you must pay a stiff penalty if you make any changes in your reservation. So begin early to find those bargains. Start by calling the airlines on their toll-free numbers to ask for their best rates. Then use your computer and go online to seek the best fares through that airline's Web site. Airlines typically post special discounted fares on their Web sites. Before booking, take a quick look at expedia.com, travelocity.com, and other commercial sites that promise the lowest possible fares. Compare the schedules and fares from all three sources—the airline agents, the airlines' Web site, and commercial Web sites—and then make a decision.

Being flexible in your travel schedule will probably save you money. It may save you money to leave from a different city than the one closest to you. We have saved hundreds of dollars on airfare by simply driving an extra hour to another airport. Or it may save you money to fly to a different city and then drive an hour or two to the interview. Try inserting nearby alternative cities in your computer search and see what fare comes up. One applicant flew out of Washington, D.C. instead of his home airport of Norfolk, Virginia, and reduced his ticket price from over $1,000 to $278 (Megargee, 2001).

Another way of being flexible is changing when you fly. As most business travelers return home on the weekend, airlines typically offer deep discounts on trips that extend over a Saturday night. The cost of another night at the hotel might save you hundreds in airfare. And consider flying on the "red eye" or "night owl" flights that criss-cross the country overnight. In order to fill otherwise empty seats, airlines frequently offer reduced fares at unpopular (and ungodly) hours (Megargee, 2001).

Booking an airline ticket with multiple destinations (circle trips) can also ease the toll on your credit card. You can fly from Chicago to an interview in Denver and then onto an interview in Dallas before returning to Chicago. This circle ticket often costs less than a separate round trip to each destination.

Some doctoral programs coordinate rides from the airport to the university for applicants, but most do not. You are on your own. In advance of your arrival, check out bus and train routes. The university's home-page will typically have public transportation routes and driving directions from the local airport to the campus. If public transportation is unavailable, you will need to rent a car at the airport. You will find, again, that the rental costs vary widely. And you will, again, investigate the costs early and aggressively to locate the best fare. Rely on the three traditional sources—the rental company's toll free number, its Web site, and the commercial travel Web sites—for two or three rental companies.

Renting a car on your own will require at least three things: a valid driver's license; a major credit card in your name; and a chronological age over the minimum, typically 25 years of age. The latter can be a huge hassle if you are still an undergraduate; be aware of the company's age policy in advance. Most companies will charge an extra daily fee for renters age 21 to 24—typically about $25 per day.

Most doctoral programs will extend you an invitation to room with a graduate student in the program the night before the interview. If possible, take advantage of this opportunity. It will allow you to save money, acquire masses of information, and gain a sense of student life and the campus community from people in a position to know. If you reside with a graduate student, ask for a tour the day or night before the interview. Ask to see the psychology building, the training clinic, the library, and some of the labs. If possible, get comfortable with the rooms where the interviews will be held.

Unfortunately, not all programs offer or provide a free place to sleep. In these cases, unless you have a large extended family, you will spend an evening or two in a hotel. Your task here is to secure a safe, convenient location at a reasonable rate. Use the AAA tour book and the Web for preliminary reconnaissance. If you have wheels, you can often save money by staying at one of the less expensive places on the edge of town or near an Interstate exit. In particular, if you are on a tight budget, be sure to check out places with the code word "Inn" in their names, as in Comfort Inn, Days Inn, Fairfield Inn, Hampton Inn, Hobo Inn, and Red Roof Inn (Megargee, 2001).

Even these inns may have negotiated rates. Ask the person scheduling your interview if the university has negotiated special rates with any local hotels. When booking your room, ask what discounts are available—for students, AAA members, government employees, and so on.

Whether you spend the night in a hotel or with a graduate student, you may well be invited to dinner. Be sociable and friendly, but do not drink heavily or party hearty the night before (even though you may be invited!). Get a solid night's sleep, arise on time, and eat a sensible breakfast.

Although we discussed attire and appearance in the previous section, it is worth a few more sentences as applied to travel. You may well experience some delays in your flight itinerary or in your driving time to the interview. As a consequence, you may not have that expected hour or two to clean up and change clothes before the interview. Or you may well meet other applicants en route and faculty members at the airport. The moral: do not travel in cutoffs, warm-up suits, or t-shirts unless you are prepared to interview in that outfit. Dress and travel like a professional.

Interview Style

The objective of your interview style is to present yourself as a confident, knowledgeable, and genuine person—an imperfect human, to be sure, but one without major interpersonal deficits or gross psychopathology. Even if you are anxious, try to appear relaxed, calm, confident. Any anxiety you may be experiencing is understandable and should be dealt with maturely. Strive to be as mature and natural as possible.

The interview is designed for the interviewer to get to know you as a person—your interpersonal skills, career goals, and clinical acumen. One of the few empirical studies on the role of the personal interview in the psychology admission process found that the rating of an applicant's clinical potential was the most highly weighted measure among all the interview data. Ratings of verbal skills and research skills also contributed to the prediction equation, but ratings of clinical potential contributed most to discriminating among groups of accepted applicants, alternates, and rejected applicants (Nevid & Gildea, 1984). In one way or another, you must impress the interviewers as someone they would be comfortable sending a member of their own family to for professional services.

The following factors have been found to lead to rejection of an applicant during interviews (Fretz, 1976):

- Poor personal appearance
- Overbearing, overaggressive, know-it-all style
- Inability to express yourself clearly—poor voice, diction, grammar
- Inadequate interest and enthusiasm—passive, indifferent
- Lack of confidence and poise—nervousness, appearing ill at ease

- Making excuses, evasiveness, hedging on unfavorable factors in record
- Lack of tact and maturity
- Condemnation of past professors
- Little sense of humor
- Emphasis on whom you know
- Inability to take criticism
- Failure to ask questions about the program

The last point is worth emphasizing. Each interviewer will want to get to know you as a person and will expect you to ask questions. Nothing is tougher on an interviewer than the person who does not ask questions or simply responds "Yes" or "No."

So even if it has been a long day, when the fifth interviewer asks you if you have any questions, don't reply, "No, all my questions have already been answered." And respond to the questions of the fifth interviewer with the same enthusiasm as you showed to the first interviewer (Megargee, 1990).

At the same time that you are conveying clinical potential and a mature interpersonal presence, you want to acquire the factual program information necessary to make informed decisions. Table 6-2 presents questions you can ask when you interview. You should ask some of these questions during the interview, others before, and others after. Some should be asked of professors, because they are best suited to answer them and asking can make you look prepared and informed. Some questions should be asked of first-year students because they have recently been through the process and are closest to your situation. Some questions are better asked of fourth-year students because they are about to leave and may have less investment in hiding the program's shortcomings.

The best questions to ask are those that indicate initiative, curiosity, and responsibility (Hersh & Poey, 1984). Try to communicate motivation to learn and eagerness to participate in many activities; avoid questions that promote a speculation that you are demanding, complaining, or single-minded.

A caveat: never ask for information that is available in the program description or the graduate catalog. These questions make you appear unprepared for the interview and uninterested in the program.

Alternatively, link your specific question to general information sent to you. Examples might include: "I read that all of your first-year students receive an assistantship and tuition remission. Is this also true of second-year students?" "Your graduate catalogue lists a Couples Therapy course, a special interest of mine, but it does not indicate if clinical supervision in that area is

TABLE 6-2. Interview Questions an Applicant Might Ask

Clinical

Is training available in different theoretical orientations?

Is the supervision individual or group? Is it live supervision?

Do the full-time faculty conduct the clinical supervision?

What type of supervision will I receive?

When do I actually begin clinical work?

How many practica are offered?

What are your off-campus clinical practica like? Where are they located?

What types of patient populations are available?

Are specialty clinics available?

Do the faculty have active private practices?

Do faculty serve as clinicians or consultants at local mental health facilities?

Research

What is the student–faculty ratio?

About how many dissertations and master's theses are chaired by each faculty member?

When and how am I assigned an advisor?

Does this person have weekly research meetings?

Could I sit in on a lab meeting?

How many of the core faculty are actively involved in research projects (e.g., regularly publishing)?

How many research grants finance graduate students?

If I wanted to change my mentor or advisor, is that allowed?

How many lab computers are available to graduate students?

Are computers readily available? Is photocopying free?

Is SAS or SPSS available?

What is the relationship with the medical or law school?

Finances

What percentage of students receive full financial support (assistantship plus tuition waiver)?

What types of fellowships are available?

What types of research and teaching assistantships are available?

What is the average amount of a 9-month assistantship?

Who gets tuition remission? What are my chances?

Do the stipends cover the costs of living in this area? How are the rents?

What percentage of students receive funding during the summer?

Do any of the assistantships include health insurance?

What percentage of students have taken out student loans?

Quality of Life

What is it like to live around campus? Is it safe? Expensive?

What is the surrounding city/town like?

Is graduate housing available? Do most students live on campus?

What is the off-campus housing situation like? The neighborhoods?

Where can I go to get a housing application today?

Are there theaters, movies, decent restaurants nearby?

Is there public transportation, or do I need a car?

What are some of the campus events and clubs?

Is the Graduate Student Association active?

Do the students socialize frequently?

How is the student cohesion?

Do students and faculty attend the colloquia?

Department and Politics

Do students and faculty have good relationships with each other?

Do graduate students have a role in departmental policy and admission decisions?

In your experience, what are the best and worst features of this program? (ask of graduate students)

What are one or two things you wished you knew before attending this program? (ask of graduate students)

What is the standing of the psychology department within the university?

How do the different branches of psychology interact?

What are the professional goals of the current students?

How many fifth-, sixth-, seventh- . . . year students are there?

Is there a sense of competition or cooperation among the students?

How much emphasis is put on course work and grades?

How common are grades of C?

Do professors tend to collaborate on projects?

Do I get a master's degree along the way? When is this usually done?

Can the program be undertaken on a part-time basis? What percentage of the student body is part-time?

When do I take the qualifying exams? What are they like? How many people fail? Can they be retaken?

Could I see a course schedule for next (or last) year?

Are teaching opportunities available for graduate students?

For applicants who already have a master's: Once accepted, how are transcripts evaluated regarding credits?

Outcomes

Where do your students complete their internships?

What percentage of your students obtains an APPIC or APA-accredited internship?

What is the average length of the program (including internship)?

What percentage of your incoming students eventually earn their doctorates here?

Do dissertations usually get published?

In what type of settings do most of your graduates eventually find employment—academic, private practice, clinics?

available." "While reading about your impressive Psychological Services Clinic, I wondered how many of the full-time clinical faculty provide supervision there." And so on.

The intent is to get beyond the gloss and formality of the published program descriptions to the lived and personal experiences of the program participants. Virtually all descriptions of clinical and counseling psychology programs, for example, will allude to ample opportunities for practical experience in off-campus placements. But when you directly ask students, "What is your clinical placement like?" their answers may diverge substantially from the published information. Their responses may indeed be positive, but it is not uncommon to learn that some of the placements are 50 miles away, do not offer any stipend, and are very competitive. To be sure, be tactful in your questioning, but also be assertive in securing crucial data.

Program directors (e.g., Hersh & Poey, 1984) have nominated certain questions to *avoid* asking. These unwittingly annoy interviewers or communicate an undesirable impression: questions regarding the typical length of a graduate-student week, which may indicate fear of hard work or a long week; persistent inquiries regarding an area of interest that the graduate program only minimally provides; questions reflecting resistance to learning the major theoretical orientation offered by that program; and antagonistic questions concentrating on the perceived limitations of the program, be they financial, faculty, or geographical.

Bring your list of questions with you to the interview, but do not constantly have it in plain sight to check off. Your task is to ask the questions of the most appropriate individuals in a respectful manner. On a similar note, many people have "palm pilots" to help organize personal information. Though you might use one to make an important note at the *end* of an interview, keep them away during the interview itself. And on that note, cell phones and beepers should be turned off during the interview. Having one beep or buzz will be disruptive, and checking a pager or taking a call would be seen as *extremely* unprofessional and rude.

Extreme ideologies—religious, sociopolitical, or clinical—do not bode well in interviews. One interesting study (Gartner, 1986) mailed mock graduate school applications to professors of clinical psychology. The results showed that professors were more likely to admit an applicant who made no mention of religion than they were to admit an otherwise identical applicant who was identified as a fundamentalist Christian. Do not deny your beliefs, of course, but try to avoid expressions of rigid extremes. Academics favor informed pluralism and critical open-mindedness.

Bernard Lubin (1993), a former national president of Psi Chi and a veteran of conducting admission interviews, enjoins applicants to present themselves as *knowledgeable* and *collaborative* during the interview. Being familiar with the research interests and productivity of the program faculty can go a long way. Carefully reading the program's guide and identifying faculty publications through *PsycLIT* are direct evidence of a mature and scholarly attitude. This leads to presenting yourself as a potential collaborator: welcoming opportunities to work with faculty members and fellow students, displaying an affirming and positive attitude toward interdependent activities.

A final piece of advice on interview style concerns your nonverbal behavior. Some applicants are so preoccupied with asking questions and trying to impress the interviewer that they neglect the way they present themselves nonverbally. But interviewer impressions of candidate personality depend heavily on nonverbal behaviors (Anderson & Shackleton, 1990). Maintaining eye contact, making changes in posture, and varying facial expressions strongly contribute to an image as a mature and enthusiastic person. The research consistently advises interviewees to keep high levels of eye contact with the interviewer and to display frequent positive facial expressions to maximize their chances of success. Your mock and actual interviews should strive for an interpersonally engaging style that creates personal liking and that cultivates an impression of interpersonal and intellectual skill.

Literally hundreds of Web sites offer advice on interviewing skills. Although they are no substitute for live rehearsals and mock interviews, they are a source of considerable information and examples. Some even offer virtual interviews. Our favorite sites are:

- www.quintcareers.com
- www.quintcareers.com/behavioral_interviewing
  .html
  (specifically on behavioral interviewing)
- www.content.monster.com/interview/home.aspx
- www.glencoe.com/sec/careers/career_city/index
  .html
- www.nextstep.org

Stressful Questions

This brings us to consider a prominent fear, namely, being placed on the spot with intensely personal questions. You may have heard stories about applicants being asked intimate questions about their families of origin, romantic relationships, and personal history they would prefer not to share. You should be prepared to answer personal questions about such relationships and self-perceptions. Answering these questions in a straightforward manner contributes to the interviewer's positive evaluation of an applicant.

The nature of these questions varies with the interviewer's style as well as the program's theoretical orientation. Applying to a research-oriented behavioral program, however, is no guarantee that you will not be interviewed by a psychodynamic member of their faculty. Questions pertaining to family conflict or to your personal therapy could arise. Anticipating such questions can help you to determine how to handle them most comfortably and to decide how much information you are willing to disclose. Knowing where to set your boundaries will lead to a smoother interview.

Speaking of boundaries, the APA Ethics Code (APA, 2002, p. 1068) does not require students to disclose sensitive information regarding their "sexual history, history of abuse and neglect, psychological treatment, and relationships with parents, peers, and spouses or significant others" unless the training program has clearly identified this requirement ahead of time. Thus, unless the program sent you a specific notice of such a requirement for the interview, you are not ethically obliged to reveal such personal information. Our advice is to balance your need for privacy with the program's need for information about your personal history and psychological dynamics.

One stressful but popular question concerns your personal weaknesses. Applicants naturally wonder how honest to be about their deficits and try to balance the need for honesty with the need to leave a favorable impression.

We have found three strategies useful in approaching this question. One is to minimize an existing limitation: showing your awareness of it but not articulating the full severity or manifestation. If being taken advantage of frequently is your perceived weakness, for example, you might reply on the order of "Occasionally I find myself being taken advantage of by others in small but consistent ways." A second strategy is to turn the weakness into a possible strength. Following the same example, you might remark that "I give to a fault on occasion and find some people will take advantage of my tendency to look for the best in people." A third possible strategy is to express your awareness of the weakness and your efforts to remediate it; this reply demonstrates both introspective and corrective attitudes. "I've been working to become more conscious of how people, especially personality-disordered clients, can take advantage of me. My overtrusting nature is slowly giving way as I attend more closely to this relationship pattern." Whatever strategy—or combination

of strategies—you elect, the response must be consistent with who you are. A phony or inauthentic response can immediately strike an applicant from further consideration.

One stressful situation necessitates your careful preparation. A few programs and faculty use what is called a "stress interview." In this interview, the faculty member intentionally acts inappropriately and tries to intimidate applicants, simply to see how they handle the stress of the situation. This can come in many forms: long silences after you answer questions; asking overly intimate questions; disagreeing violently with your position or answer; feigning disinterest in you as an applicant; or even giving you coffee in one hand, a powdered donut without a napkin in the other, and then handing you an article to browse! Knowing ahead of time that this can happen is crucial, because you can remind yourself that it is not personal but simply part of the process. In a few programs, the professors place all the applicants in an empty room and suggest they speak with each other while the professors observe the interpersonal process: no other directions, no other structure. This all serves to compound the students' anxiety.

Stress interviews are designed to assess how comfortably you behave under such interpersonally challenging conditions. The interviewers deliberately arrange situations or ask questions that you cannot predict, for examples, "How would you redesign a giraffe?" or "Where is Oregon?" The particular answer you give is not as important as the manner in which you answer. Here your interpersonal savvy and presence can triumph. The interviewer is testing your reaction to stress: do you react to stress with humor, anxiety, self-denigration, anger? The stress interview is an ambiguous, semi-projective device.

Our advice is to remain calm and polite, yet assertive. Generally, it is not wise to become entangled in a verbal battle or retreat into an apologetic or defensive stance. In the face of an inappropriately personal question, a "I wonder how that question relates to my admission here?" will demonstrate both your personal boundaries and your willingness to broach a difficult topic. In the face of continuing conflict, a polite "we respectfully disagree" can suffice, and leave it at that (Heppner & Downing, 1982).

Practicing stress interviews with professors or peers may sufficiently desensitize you to keep your head and field the situation without too much ego bruising. Another way to prepare yourself is to stay overnight before the interview and take the opportunity to ask graduate students which professors might conduct such an interview, allowing you to know ahead of time that this person is likely to intentionally try to stress you. Foreknowledge and preparation are the best defenses.

Group Interviews

Admission interviews in clinical and counseling psychology differ markedly from one program to another. At one extreme, a few programs invite you for a single, 2-hour interview with a senior faculty member. That's it—no tour, no group interview, no program orientation, and no interaction with current graduate students.

At the other extreme, a number of programs invite selected applicants for an entire admissions weekend. At the University of Pittsburgh, for example, invitees to the clinical program's weekend spend a full day (about 7 hours) interviewing with faculty and graduate students. In addition, there are clinical and research information sessions, laboratory tours, evening parties, and a poster session featuring research projects. Many of the applicants arrive on Friday and leave Sunday morning.

In between these two approaches are intensive 1-day sessions. For instance, at Fordham University's counseling psychology program (Kopala et al., 1995), the interview process entails a brief orientation to the program, individual interviews with a faculty member and a graduate student, a videotaped group experience, a 30-minute writing sample, an open session with graduate students, and then a closing session with the director of training.

Virtually all programs will arrange for at least one individual interview with a faculty member and for some interactions with current doctoral students. A healthy proportion of programs will also include admission interviews featuring multiple candidates in the same room at the same time. This group interview may be conducted in the interest of sheer efficiency, of observing your interpersonal style, or both.

Our advice on your interview style and objectives in these group interviews remains essentially the same as for the individual interviews, but there are a couple of twists. First of all, strive to be pleasant and honest with the other interviewees. Share your experiences, never denigrate their credentials, and treat them like future colleagues (which they may very well be). A negativistic or superior attitude is likely to be held against you in the final deliberations of the admission committee.

Second of all, since it is a group situation, try to present yourself as an admirable facilitator. Don't be a group psychotherapist or a control maniac, but a respectful cofacilitator of the interview process. If you have already asked a few questions about the pro-

gram, for instance, you might say that you have additional questions but would first like other people to have an opportunity to have their questions answered. As they say in the social psychology literature, try to manifest both a high task orientation and a high social orientation.

Additional Tips

Whether it is an individual interview or a group interview, here are additional tips regarding the interview.

- Arrive at least 15 minutes early on interview day. Find the offices, acclimate to the building, and get settled.
- Be compulsive and double-check your interview schedule. Being late or missing an interview (even when it is not your fault) can reflect poorly on you.
- Greet each interviewer in a friendly, open manner. Your handshake should be firm and your eye contact frequent.
- Demonstrate your active listening skills: wait to answer until the interviewer has completed asking the question and give complete answers to the question posed to you.
- Keep your answers to 1.5 to 2 minutes long. Use good grammar and diction. Say "No," not "nah."
- Avoid all irritating hiccups in your answers. On the short list are the irritating "you know," "like," and "okay."
- Always bring extra copies of your CV. Every interviewer may have not received a copy or may have not yet reviewed it, so bring along copies to present and leave with people (Megargee, 1990).
- Take cash along in case you are invited to lunch or dinner with graduate students.
- Conclude each interview by thanking the interviewer for her time and information. Wrap it up with a cordial and pleasant tone.

Our collective experience in conducting interviews also generates a list of *don'ts:*

- Don't call faculty members by their first names until (or if) they offer. The default option is to call them "Dr." or "Professor."
- Don't whine or complain about the interview arrangements. Accept the free housing with gratitude; be agreeable about the food; act flexibly about interview dates. Nobody, including admissions committees, likes a fussbudget.
- Don't accept offers of coffee or other beverages during the interview itself. It tends to be messy,

distracting, and awkward for you as the interviewee. Wait until after the interviews are complete and then graciously accept the offer.

- Don't ask about or negotiate financial assistance before receiving an offer of admission. The nitty-gritty of finances can wait until later.
- And don't ask questions during the interview that are answered in the materials sent to you or posted on the program Web site. We have already made this point earlier in the chapter, but it is important enough to reiterate it here.

If you follow these steps, you will find it easier to relax during the interview. The more prepared you are, the more confident and at ease you will feel.

Telephone Interviews

Two situations may dictate a telephone interview. In the first, you are asked to visit the school for an interview, but you cannot afford to do so. This is no reason to be embarrassed, and the more straightforward you are about it the better. You can request a phone interview if you do not have the resources for an actual visit. In the second situation, you receive the dreaded,

unannounced phone interview. At least one of your prospective programs will probably call without prior notice and ask to speak with you on the spot.

Luckily, if you anticipate telephone interviews, you have nothing to worry about. One strategy is to rarely or never take a phone interview "cold." Consider telling the caller, "I'm sorry, but I was just leaving for an appointment. Could you leave a number and arrange for me to call you back?" This buys you time to review your information on that program and to prepare for the interview. However, you do not want to communicate disinterest in the program.

Another strategy is to prepare phone cards, palm pilot notes, or computer files. You make index cards or short files for each program to which you applied. On it, record a few reasons for your interest in that graduate program and the name(s) of the professor(s) you are interested in working with, a little about their research areas, and questions you may have about clinical training or facilities (many of the questions in Table 6-2). Figure 6-2 is an example of such a card. Keep a stack of these by the phone, or on a computer by the phone and in moments you will find the card for a particular school and not be caught unaware! This little extra effort can prevent a serious detraction

---

University of Alexandria

Reasons for my interest: Great reputation in child psychopathology and psychotherapy; specific professors (Smith, Adams); geographic location; has specialty clinic in behavioral medicine.

Key professors:

Dr. Smith: child psychopathology; substance abuse

I read your May [2007] article in *Journal of Bogus Psychology,* in which you found offspring of alcoholics to be more receptive to the anxiety-reducing effects of alcohol than control subjects. Do you expect to continue this line of research next year? Is an assistantship available?

Dr. Adams: behavioral medicine; psychotherapy

I was impressed that you have a separate clinic in behavioral medicine. What type of clients do you most often treat? What opportunities are there for clinical experience?

Other professors with potential interest:

Dr. Jones: prevention

Dr. Watson: forensic psychology

Program questions: [Refer to Table 6-2 for representative listing]

When do I begin seeing clients in the training clinic?

What percentage of incoming students are financially supported?

What are the research opportunities in child psychopathology?

FIGURE 6-2. Sample telephone card.

246 Wood Street
Babylon, NY 14000

March 16, 2008

Patricia Jones, Ph.D.
Director of Clinical Training
Department of Psychology
University of Western States
13 Orangegrove Drive
Wilksville, CA 98765

Dear Dr. Jones:

I want to thank you for interviewing me for a position in your clinical psychology doctoral program. I enjoyed meeting with your faculty and staff and learning more about the program. My enthusiasm for the program was particularly strengthened as a result of my interactions with Drs. Timothy Hogan, Elizabeth Cannon, and Carole Buchanan.

I want to reiterate my strong interest in attending your program; the University of Western States offers a great deal that appeals to me. Please feel free to call me at (123) 456-7890 or e-mail me at csmith@uofs.edu if I can provide you with any additional information.

Again, thank you for the interview and your consideration.

Sincerely yours,

Chris Smith

FIGURE 6-3. Sample letter of appreciation to an interviewer.

from your application. If you receive one of these telephone calls and cannot remember which professors are at that school, their areas of research, or their facilities, it tells the interviewer that you are not serious about his or her program. This could place you lower than someone who has this information off the top of his or her head.

A Note of Thanks

Once you have completed an interview, whether by telephone or in person, a brief note of thanks to the interviewer is in order. This gesture serves multiple purposes: it demonstrates your social skills, communicates your gratitude to the faculty and students involved, reaffirms your interest in the program, and keeps your name alive in the admission process. Seldom will such a brief note do so much for you.

The "who" and "what" of these thank-you letters are almost entirely dependent on your interview experiences. The "who" should certainly include anyone who has shown you special attention, such as a graduate student you roomed with the night before or after the interview, a professor who personally escorted you around a lab or clinic, or a faculty member who offered an unscheduled interview. Letters to several people are often called for. If the interview was less personal, then at a minimum send the Director of Training a letter of appreciation. A sample letter is displayed in Figure 6-3. An e-mail note of appreciation may suffice, but we definitely prefer an ordinary letter by mail, because it will probably be placed in your application file for all to see and appreciate.

The "what" of the letter must be individualized to your particular experiences, but will probably contain at least three components: an expression of gratitude for the interview, an enumeration of your favorable impressions of the program, and a reiteration of your interest in attending that program. Try to personalize each letter by referring to specific topics or experiences; for instance, recall your discussion of potential research studies or mention the friendliness of the graduate students. There is no definitive list of do's and don't's, but don't send a generic, impersonal letter and don't promote your candidacy. Do sound appreciative and personal. As with all written materials, insure that your letter communicates an image of sincerity and professionalism. Most of the letters should probably be word-processed, but a neat, handwritten note is appropriate if an interview was relatively informal and personal.

The Wait

Once you have finished the interviews and mailed the thank-you letters, it is a waiting game. But not for the programs, which still have a finalist pool of students much larger than they are able to accept! The interview process has probably weeded out a few, but the faculty are left with too many finalists, all of whom have acceptable GPAs, GREs, and letters of recommendation.

What, then, are the *final* selection criteria? This pivotal question was addressed in a study by Keith-Spiegel, Tabachnick, and Spiegel (1994), who had 113 faculty members actively involved in selecting psychology Ph.D. students rate criteria used in making the last cuts in admission decisions. (Results of this study should *not* be generalized to Psy.D. programs.) The faculty members were asked to imagine that they were left with a pool of finalists, three times the size of the number they can accept, all of whom had strong undergraduate GPAs, GRE scores, and letters of recommendation. They then rated 31 final variables in terms of importance.

Congruent with this book's advice and earlier studies, the top-rated criteria in clinical programs pertained to student match with the program and its faculty, research experience resulting in a journal article or a paper presentation, and the clarity and focus of the applicant's statement of purpose. Considered to be somewhat to very important in assisting selection committees with their final admission decisions were research assistant experience; reputation of the student's referees; relevant clinical experience; membership in an underrepresented ethnic minority group; knowledge and interest in the program; number of statistics, methodology, and hard science courses completed; prestige of the psychology faculty in the student's undergraduate department; reputation of the undergraduate institution itself; and honors bestowed on the student by that undergraduate institution. Rated as not important or minimally important were such variables as the student's geographic residence, Psi Chi membership, and a close relationship between the student and former graduates of that program.

Demand always exceeds supply in competitive clinical and counseling psychology programs. The three primary criteria used to evaluate applicants by doctoral selection committees—grade point averages, GREs, and letters of recommendation—typically fail to narrow the applicant pool to the small number of slots available. At that point, research skills, clinical experiences, "good match" factors, and writing skills come to the fore (Keith-Spiegel et al., 1994). Bear these considerations in mind as you approach your interview—just as we have in preparing this book.

And now you wait until contacted with the final decision of the admissions committee. Until the week before April 1, it is probably not a good idea to contact a program and ask where you stand. Applicants who make repeated calls or e-mails may appear overly anxious and irritate the staff (Mitchell, 1996). The one exception is if you have received other offers, and the program you would most like to attend has not contacted you—a situation covered in Chapter 7.

This brings us to the last step in the application process and the final chapter of the *Insider's Guide*.

CHAPTER 7
MAKING FINAL DECISIONS

As with any realm of human affairs, good decisions regarding graduate school require time, preparation, and knowledge (Scott & Silka, 1974).

By April 1, all APA-accredited clinical, counseling, and combined psychology programs will make their first round of acceptance offers. At this point you will have 2 weeks to make your final decision as to where you want to go to school. By APA regulations, you have the right to consider offers until April 15, at which time an offer may be withdrawn. So you must be thoughtful but decisive in these 2 weeks.

To protect applicants from making hasty, premature decisions, all APA-accredited programs and most others have agreed to allow candidates until April 15 for a final decision (or the first Monday after April 15, if April 15 falls on a weekend). This is in accordance with a policy adopted by the Council of Graduate Schools in the United States in 1965 and renewed in 2004. It was endorsed by the Council of Graduate Departments of Psychology in 1981 and again in 2000. The Resolution Regarding Graduate Scholars, Fellows, Trainees and Assistants (www.cgsnet.org/portals/0/pdf/cgsresolutionjune2005.pdf) reads as follows:

> Acceptance of an offer of financial aid (such as graduate scholarship, fellowship, traineeship, or assistantship) for the next academic year by a prospective or enrolled graduate student completes an agreement that both student and graduate school expect to honor. In that context, the conditions affecting such offers and their acceptance must be defined carefully and understood by all parties.
>
> Students are under no obligation to respond to offers of financial support prior to April 15; earlier

deadlines for the acceptance of such offers violate the intent of this Resolution. In those instances in which the student accepts the offer before April 15 and subsequently desires to withdraw that acceptance, the student may submit in writing a resignation of the appointment at any time through April 15. However, an acceptance given or left in force after April 15 commits the student not to accept another offer without first obtaining a written release from the institution to which the commitment has been made. Similarly, an offer by an institution after April 15 is conditional on presentation by the student of the written release from any previously accepted offer. It is further agreed by the institutions and organizations subscribing to the above Resolution that a copy of this Resolution should accompany every scholarship, fellowship, traineeship, and assistantship offer.

Acceptances and Rejections

What do you do when one program makes you an offer and you are still waiting to hear from another program you would prefer to accept? To begin with, *don't say yes to any graduate program until you are certain that this is where you want to go!* Once you say "yes," that is it. You are committed. Saying yes to another program can endanger your acceptance at both places. If you have any reservations, do not feel pressured to say yes. Thank the person and say that you have been made other offers and you need a few days to consider this crucial decision.

If you have received offers but have not heard from the programs that most interest you, telephone or e-mail them. Explain that you are considering offers

TABLE 7-1. Student Reasons for Choosing a Clinical Psychology Doctoral Program

Reason	Mean rating	Rank
Reputation of the program	4.29	1
Amount of clinical supervision	4.27	2
Training facilities available	4.21	3
Appropriate mentors available	4.19	4.5
Emotional atmosphere of the program	4.19	4.5
Tuition waiver available	4.10	6
Amount of stipend offered	4.07	7
Theoretical orientation	4.04	8
Diversity of program	4.00	9
Specific specialty training available	3.89	10
Research experience available	3.85	11
Expected length of program	3.82	12
Amount of research supervision	3.80	13
Success of previous graduates	3.79	14
Specificity of the training program	3.66	15
Geographic location	3.60	16
Specific professor to work with	3.57	17
Family/significant others in area	3.00	18
Recreational activities available	2.69	19
Number of minority members in program	2.48	20
Break required during program	2.30	21

Note. From Walfish, Stenmark, Shealy, & Shealy (1989). © 1989 American Psychological Association. Reprinted by permission.

but that you do not want to act on them until you know what your status is there. It's OK to say, "I've been accepted at University X and Y, but I am most interested in your program. Can you give me an indication where my application stands, or at least whether it is still being considered?"

The "Guidelines for Graduate School Offers and Acceptances," adopted by the Council of University Directors of Clinical Psychology (1993), specifically encourage directors of training (or admissions) to apprise students of their position on the alternate list. Typically this entails a placement of high, middle, or low on the alternate list. If such a designation is used, the operational definition of "high on the alternate list" is that, in a normal year, the student would receive an offer of admission (but not necessarily funding) prior to the April 15 decision date.

Earlier, we emphasized the point that you should not accept an offer until you are certain that is the program you want to attend. On the other hand, if you have been accepted at three programs, and one of them is obviously less suited to your needs, be considerate of other applicants and decline that offer. The program

can then make their offer to someone else who may very much want to attend that school. *Only keep two offers alive at any one time.* Otherwise, a huge "logjam" or "bottleneck effect" will occur across the country, with each program waiting for a few students to decide.

As long as there is a possibility that you may attend a certain program, be careful not to decline prematurely. As other students decline at these schools, you may be offered a better financial package if you have not yet made a formal commitment.

When all is said and done, how will you decide on which offer to accept? This is a difficult question to answer because of the multiple factors involved and because the final determinant will be how you, as an individual, weigh those various factors.

One study (Walfish, Stenmark, Shealy, & Shealy, 1989) had 201 first-year graduate students rate the reasons for their final selection of a doctoral clinical program. Their average ratings are shown in Table 7-1, where a rating of 1 was "very unimportant" and 5 was "very important." As seen there, the most important factors were the reputation of the program, the amount of clinical supervision, the training facilities, availability of mentors, and the emotional atmosphere of the program. We have emphasized throughout the preceding chapters the importance of the first four factors, but not the last.

The emotional and interpersonal ambience of a program should not be underestimated. Seriously consider interactions with faculty and graduate students in your decision. The faculty–student relationship may be the single most important factor in your intellectual and professional development, and this relationship may be formal or informal, distant or close. Concurrently, the vast majority of graduate student time is spent with other students rather than with faculty members. You are likely to retain these personal contacts and professional relationships over the years. Moreover, fellow students are essential sources of encouragement, companionship, and inspiration. You want a good, lasting "fit" with the program (Scott & Silka, 1974).

In choosing a graduate program, all students place a premium on general factors such as program quality, training opportunities, emotional atmosphere, and financial aid. At the same time, ethnic minority applicants rate the relevance of multicultural factors higher than do white students (Bernal et al., 1999; Toia, Herron, Primavera, & Javier, 1997). These considerations include minority students in the program, presence of minority faculty, research on minority topics, and opportunity to work with multicultural clients. Be particularly attentive to the program's diversity as it relates to your interests and goals.

The expected length of the doctoral program is a fairly important reason for choosing a particular program, as seen in the middle of Table 7-1. You may recall from Chapter 1 that clinical Ph.D. students take an average of 6.2 years to complete their doctorates, including the 1-year internship. Psy.D. students take an average of 5.1 years, a consistent difference of 1 to 1.5 years less. On the one hand, the shorter training period favors the Psy.D. programs. But, on the other hand, the financial aid favors the Ph.D. programs. As you have learned, far more Ph.D. students are receiving tuition waivers and assistantship stipends than Psy.D. students, most of whom are footing the entire bill for their doctoral education. Use the Reports on Individual Programs to consider the expected length of the program in the context of probable financial aid from the program.

The reasons for choosing a clinical psychology program, as shown in Table 7-1, are largely self-evident, but two reasons *not* listed in that table deserve some consideration. *Attrition rates* refer to the percentage of students not completing the program. Attrition has

been characterized as a "hidden crisis in graduate education" (Lovitts & Nelson, 2000). About 20% of full-time psychology students, on average, formally leave programs without completing their doctorates (Fennell & Kohout, 2002). Attrition in graduate programs is not solely related to academic ability; life problems, financial difficulties, interpersonal conflicts, and program dissatisfaction enter into the equation. Doctoral programs in which more than 25% of the students fail to graduate should be carefully screened when you make your final decision.

Our Reports on Individual Programs provide the attrition rates for each doctoral program, as reported by that program's director of training. The attrition rate is calculated for the past 7 years as the number of matriculated students who have left the program for any reason divided by the total number of students matriculated in the program. Again, pay close attention to any program in which a quarter or more of students have left the program.

Preliminary or qualifying examinations, another consideration in the complexities of your choice, are a series of structured tests that some programs require at the end of their first or second year. These examinations assume many forms, but they all test a candidate's knowledge of a wide range of areas in psychology—research methodology, learning, development, motivation, history, social, and personality. In some programs, only one attempt may be permitted to pass this examination (Scott & Silka, 1974). You should learn if the program requires "prelims" or "quals," whether multiple attempts are provided, and what percentage of students pass, before you make your final decision.

You should now be well acquainted with the importance of the decision criteria presented in Table 7-1 in your own life and well informed about the program's attractiveness on these criteria. If not, immediately request additional information on any of these for which you lack knowledge prior to making an informed choice of the program to attend.

The Financial Package

Note in Table 7-1 that the sixth and seventh most important selection factors are financial (tuition waiver and stipend amount). For many applicants, the financial aid offered by the school will probably assume an even higher priority in making final decisions. When an offer is made, establish if the program is offering financial assistance. If so, does it cover tuition remission? Is it guaranteed for 4 years? Is it considered taxable at that institution? Does it provide health insurance? If you have a teaching or research assistantship, how

TABLE 7-2. Median Tuition Costs in Psychology by Institution Type and Degree Level

	Institution type		Degree level	
	Public	Private	Doctoral	Master's
State residents	$3,178	$16,596	$5,362	$2,776
Nonstate residents	$8,416	$16,596	$11,824	$7,217

Note. Adapted from Pate (2001).

many hours per week will it entail? Are you allowed to earn additional outside income?

On average, private universities are more expensive than public or state universities. Typically, the "in-state" versus "out-of-state" cost difference that operates in undergraduate education is not as salient in graduate education. That is because (1) once you begin study, you can establish residency there and pay in-state tuition after the first year, and (2) many financial aid packages include a tuition remission.

But graduate training is expensive, and external sources of financial support are slowly drying up. Consider, for instance, the average stipends and accumulated loans for Ph.D. psychology students over the years (Golding, Lang, Eymard, & Shadish, 1988). Back in the 1960s and 1970s the average graduate stipend was higher, and the typical student's accumulated loan lower, than in the 2000s, adjusted for inflation. In fact, the average stipend amount decreased 36% (controlled for inflation) over the past 30 years. About three-quarters of psychology doctoral candidates carry loans. Support is still available but not to the degree it once was—which accounts, in part, for your professors' fond memories of their "good ol' graduate days."

Federal support for graduate training has been eroding in all fields, including psychology. In the 1970s, for instance, almost 30% of Ph.D. recipients in clinical psychology reported that federal grants and traineeships provided the major support for their graduate training (Coyle & Bae, 1987). Thirty years later, federal sources supported less than 4% of full-time graduate students in psychology (Wicherski & Kohout, 2005). Federal sources have slipped as a primary source of support for psychology graduate students and, to compensate for these shrinking resources, students have had to look elsewhere, to personal resources, student loans, and university financial assistance.

Research supports the conclusion that today's graduate students are being asked to shoulder a larger share of their education costs. This is particularly true in Psy.D. programs, which fund proportionally fewer graduate students than Boulder-model Ph.D. programs.

Refer to the Reports on Individual Programs for the percentage of a program's students who receive partial or full funding.

Table 7-2 shows the median tuition costs for psychology graduate students. The numbers demonstrate that tuition is largely a function of three variables: institution type, state residence, and degree level. Private universities uniformly charge higher graduate tuition than public institutions, just as is the case on the undergraduate level. Tuition at private institutions per academic year is four times higher than state tuition at public institutions. Psy.D. programs, routinely charge between $15,000 and $25,000 per year for tuition. Although your state residence does not influence tuition at private universities, it definitely reduces your tuition at public universities—from a median of $8,416 for non-state residents to $3,178 for state residents per year. Predictably, too, tuition is higher for doctoral programs than for master's programs. So, your annual tuition can range from $0 if you secure tuition remission, to $3,000 if you are a resident attending your state university, to $16,000 if you attend a Ph.D. program at a private university with no financial assistance, all the way up to $25,000 if you attend a freestanding Psy.D. program.

Table 7-3 presents the assistantship stipends for psychology graduate students in 2004. As seen there, the median 9-month stipends for teaching and research assistantships averaged $5,000 for master's students and $10,000 for doctoral students (Norcross et al., 2005). The typical hours worked per week for an assistantship are 15 to 16. Stipends for doctoral students are consistently higher than those for master's students (Fennell & Kohout, 2002).

Financial considerations include the tuition cost, available stipend, and living costs. The latter cannot be ignored: although tuition costs may be equivalent in New York City and Kansas, the living costs are certainly not.

Once accepted into a doctoral program, you will naturally be eager to learn about the status of your financial assistance, but you will hear from institutions

TABLE 7-3. Median Assistantship Stipends in Psychology

	Doctoral students	Master's students
Teaching assistantship	$10,617	$5,000
Research assistantship	$10,065	$5,000
Fellowship/scholarship	$11,500	$2,000
Traineeship	$13,658	$6,000

Note. Data from Norcross, Kohout, & Wicherski (2005).

at different times depending on the form of the financial assistance. If it is department-controlled financial assistance, then you will ordinarily hear when you are accepted or shortly thereafter. If it is university financial assistance, not directly controlled by the psychology department or school, then it may well be weeks after you are accepted. Examples in this category are fellowships from the Graduate School, resident assistantships from Student Affairs, or a Graduate Assistantship in the Admission Office. If it is financial assistance from a government agency, such as the National Science Foundation (NSF) or National Institutes of Health (NIH), then you will hear on or before their published notification dates. Finally, if it is financial assistance in the form of loans, then you will hear from the bank, Sally Mae, or the lending institution on their (painfully slow) schedule.

The Alternate List

Your fervent hope is to receive an e-mail or telephone call in March from the director of admissions offering you acceptance into your top-rated program with generous financial aid. But this glorious dream may not happen; instead, the sobering reality is that many applicants will be rejected from several programs, will secure offers from programs lower on their list, or will receive offers without financial assistance. Many will also receive calls informing them that they have been "wait listed"—that is, placed on the alternate list.

As mentioned previously, ask the director of admissions where you stand on the alternate list—high, middle, or low. For your planning purposes, be politely assertive in probing further: "In typical years, what percentage of students with this position on the alternate list receive an admission offer? What percentage of the students admitted from the alternate list receive funding?" Without answers to these questions, you cannot render an informed decision on your other offers.

The admissions directors will, in all likelihood, arrange for you to be kept abreast of your admissions status until April 15th. They may email you or you may email them on occasion to determine the probability of admission.

When speaking with the program representative try to impress upon him or her three key ideas. First, you are keenly interested in attending that program. Second, express your availability by stating you have not accepted another offer of admission. And third, if you have received another offer, inform the program accordingly; most schools desire people who are attractive to others. Enthusiasm, availability, and attractiveness frequently move students up the alternate list.

The tricky part of this process is how frequently an alternate should contact (by telephone or e-mail) the program representative. Too much contact will appear aggressive or desperate; too little, passive or complacent. Strike a balance by asking the program representative how often you may contact him or her without being irritating.

Decision Making

The choice of which offer to accept and which program to attend is a momentous one indeed. You, like 86% of students enrolling in graduate programs, will quickly discover that the decision-making process boils down to your sense of fit with a program (Kyle, 2000). A few fortunate souls may receive an early offer with excellent financial aid from their number one program. But most graduate school applicants will ultimately select the program that makes the "best" offer—an offer that needs to be seriously weighed on a host of the aforementioned and often conflicting considerations.

The "April madness" abounds with such quandaries as: "Should I take Program X with the best training but with no financial aid or Program Y with solid training and half tuition remission for 4 years?"; "Two programs have offered the same money, but the one that I prefer is 600 miles from my partner. What should I do?"; "My top program guaranteed me a teaching assistantship that requires 15 hours a week. My fourth choice is offering tuition remission and a fellowship. Any advice?"

Our advice centers on using systematic decision making. Begin by gathering all the salient data by interviewing program faculty and students, consulting published materials, and speaking with your mentors. Prioritize your primary reasons for selecting one program over another. Then develop a decision-making grid that will assist you in ranking your choices.

Two practical articles describe in detail how to apply decision-making techniques to choosing psychology programs and internships. Jacob's (1987) decision grid asks candidates to evaluate training programs along criteria that are important to them. You weigh those criteria that are more important to you correspondingly higher. You then tally the ratings for each training program to make the final decision. While it may sound a bit over-intellectual, in practice we have found that the decision grid forces students to identify the criteria that they value most highly.

Stewart and Stewart (1996) describe a paired-comparison ranking technique, a method originally traced back to psychophysiological methods developed by Gustav Fechner. The first step of this technique is to select the relevant personal, professional, and practical criteria that you will use in comparing programs to one another. Consult the preceding pages to identify these criteria; more importantly, conduct an honest self-evaluation to determine which of these lie in your heart. The second step involves prioritizing these selection criteria. Do this by writing the name of each criterion on a single index card or piece of paper, and then forcing yourself to rank them in order. The third step entails generating a list of programs that will be compared to one another. We suggest that you use those programs that have accepted you or which have placed you on their waiting list.

The fourth step of the technique involves the actual pairwise comparison of the programs. Write the names of the graduate programs along one side of a large piece of paper and the selection criteria on the other side. Which of the training programs most clearly satisfies your criteria? Make a choice and allow no ties. For each criterion, put a hash mark across from the program that wins. The hash marks will be counted to determine your choice.

Although the final result will generally agree with what you expected, the more productive outcome of these two decision-making techniques may be that they force you to view your selection decision from multiple perspectives and to prioritize numerous criteria. To be sure, this is a complex method for a complex decision, but one that we and our students have repeatedly found surprisingly effective for making "impossible" choices more thoughtfully and systematically.

Finalizing Arrangements

An offer must eventually be formalized and specified in writing. Verbal offers and verbal acceptances are binding, but your acceptance of the offer should be in writing at the end of the process. Likewise, assistantships, tuition waivers, and stipends should be guaranteed in the written offer; respectfully insist that the financial arrangements be specified so that misunderstandings do not ensue. Should the offer be "contingent on expected funding," determine the odds of the funding coming through. No position is absolutely certain in life, but some are more certain than others.

Weighing offers, negotiating financial aid, and dealing with rejections make this a heady period. Be careful not to get caught up in the experience and forget the most important point: accept one offer and confirm it in writing!

One of our students (the affable Jean Willi) was offered admission to a prestigious doctoral program, with financial assistance. He carefully considered alternative offers, negotiated with other programs, leading to predictable delays. He awoke one morning in a cold sweat, realizing that he had turned down all other offers but had not formally accepted the offer of admission and financial package from his school of choice. He was in graduate school purgatory! Although the school was understanding and everything eventually worked out for Jean, because he missed the deadline, the school had the option of changing the financial aid package, or even revoking the offer of admission. The moral of the story: don't pull a Willi! Be clear and decisive and put it in writing.

Figure 7-1 presents a representative letter of acceptance. Note that the letter should explicitly mention any conditions of your acceptance, including financial assistance.

Once you have formally accepted an offer of admission in writing, two small matters of etiquette remain: (1) informing other programs who have accepted you, and (2) expressing your appreciation to those mentors who wrote letters of recommendation on your behalf and on their own time. Figure 7-2 offers a sample letter declining an offer of admission. It should be succinct yet polite. Thereafter, send a brief e-mail or thank-you note to those who have assisted you through your graduate application journey. They will

246 Wood Street
Babylon, NY 14000

March 25, 2008

Annika Jones, Ph.D.
Director, Admissions Committee
Department of Psychology
University of Western States
13 Orangegrove Drive
Wilksville, CA 98765

Dear Dr. Jones:

I am pleased to accept your offer of admission to the University of Western State's Ph.D. program in counseling psychology as a full-time matriculated student beginning in the Fall 2009 term. My acceptance is predicated on the conditions outlined in your letter of March 20th (attached), including full tuition remission for three years. I appreciate your confidence in me and very much look forward to joining the counseling psychology program.

Sincerely yours,

Chris Smith

FIGURE 7-1. Sample letter of acceptance.

be interested in the outcome of your application process and may well join the ensuing celebration!

If Not Accepted

What happens if you are not accepted anywhere? The grim truth is that about one-third of the entire applicant pool to APA-accredited clinical and counseling psychology programs will *not* make it in a given year. There are at least five alternatives:

1. *Contact the APA Education Directorate in early May to view the "Graduate School Openings List."* This document contains a list of graduate programs in psychology that still have openings for students in the fall. Although there are no APA-accredited clinical or counseling doctoral programs and only a few nonclinical doctoral programs on the list, you may find other programs of interest to you. To review the listings, go to the APA Web site in May at www.apa.org/ed/graduate/homepage.html.

2. *Apply to master's programs in clinical or counseling psychology.* Master's degrees are frequent stepping stones to the doctorate in psychology. Although taking your master's at one institution and transferring to another for the doctorate is not as efficient as being admitted directly into a doctoral program, there are advantages nonetheless. One is that the acceptance odds are more favorable—49% for master's programs in clinical psychology and 67% for master's in counseling psychology on average (Norcross, Kohout, & Wicherski, 2005). A second advantage is that a few years of graduate training in psychology can improve your grade point average, GRE Psychology Test score, clinical acumen, and research skills. A third plus is an opportunity to confirm that psychology is the career for you. A cruel irony of baccalaureate recipients admitted directly into doctoral programs is that they have little direct contact with the field they claim as their lifelong career! A fourth advantage is exposure to twice the number of faculty supervisors and theoretical orientations. A fifth and final advantage is the flexible

246 Wood Street
Babylon, NY 14000

March 25, 2008

Annika Jones, Ph.D.
Director, Admissions Committee
Department of Psychology
University of Western States
13 Orangegrove Drive
Wilksville, CA 98765

Dear Dr. Jones:

I was pleased to receive your March 19th letter offering me admission to the Psy.D. program in clinical psychology at the University of Western States. I thoroughly enjoyed speaking with you and your colleagues and appreciated your generous offer of financial assistance. Unfortunately, I can only accept one admission offer, and I must regrettably decline your attractive offer. Please extend my genuine thanks and best wishes to the entire admissions committee.

Sincerely yours,

Chris Smith

FIGURE 7-2. Sample letter declining an admission offer.

course offerings—part-time study and, frequently, night courses are available in master's programs (Actkinson, 2000).

Selecting a *quality* master's program in psychology may be a key to eventual admission into a doctoral clinical program. By all means try to avoid master's programs that have come to be pejoratively called "money mills." These programs exhibit most or all of the following features: accepting a very high percentage (80% plus) of applicants; offering courses only in the evening or largely by part-time faculty; providing no funded graduate assistantships; being reluctant or unwilling to state what percentage of their graduates go on to doctoral programs; declaring openly their disinterest in research; requiring little undergraduate preparation in psychology; and communicating greater interest in filling classroom seats than in attracting qualified students.

By contrast, quality terminal master's programs in psychology can be roughly assessed by three criteria: exhibiting few of the aforementioned characteristics of "money mills"; holding a favorable reputation among the psychological community; and faculty producing

published research. Gordon (1990) lists 20 American master's programs ranked highest in productivity in 15 APA journals; interested students are directed to that article.

In addition to the foregoing research-based article, we heartily recommend that you consult an extensive compilation of master's programs in psychology. The classic is APA's (2007) *Graduate Study in Psychology*, which lists hundreds of master's (and doctoral) programs in psychology throughout the United States and Canada. To order, go to APA's Web site where you can purchase a hard copy or purchase a three-month electronic access. Another source, consisting of over 260 master's programs, is *Master's Programs in Psychology and Counseling Psychology* (Buskist & Mixon, 1998). To order, call 1-800-278-3525 or e-mail ablongwood @aol.com.

3. *Apply to doctoral programs that are not accredited by APA.* In general these programs fit into one of two categories. They may be credible institutions that simply have not been around long enough to gain APA approval. Programs cannot apply for accreditation

until they have graduated students, which takes several years. Usually these programs are planning on applying for accreditation as soon as they are eligible.

However, there is a second category of institution not accredited by APA. These programs usually do not conform to APA standards and often do not even attempt to gain accreditation. The quality of these programs is often considerably lower than those of the APA-accredited programs. Because of their status, non-APA-accredited programs typically provide greater probabilities for acceptance. If you do apply to such programs, by all means determine why they are not accredited, and whether their students are able to gain admission into credible internships and, later, to become licensed psychologists. You should refer to the most recent edition of APA's *Graduate Study in Psychology* to explore these and other programs.

4. *Decide against a doctorate in clinical or counseling psychology.* If your goal is to become a researcher or a practitioner, psychology is not your only option. Reexamine the other choices listed in Chapter 1 and consult your advisors to see if one of these options is suited to your needs.

5. *Apply again in a year or two to APA-accredited programs.* Knowing the criteria used by graduate schools, take a realistic look at what seem to be the limitations in your application. Many students continue to resubmit the same rejected application year after year to no avail; "doing more of the same" typically results in more of the same misery.

Another year can be an opportunity to remediate your weaknesses. Were your GREs low? Take a professional preparation course and retake the test. Was your GPA a bit low? Then take some additional courses or retake some old courses in which you did not perform your best to improve it. Take some graduate courses in psychology on a nonmatriculating basis to demonstrate your ability. Were you short on research skills? Then take 1 or 2 years and acquire a research position, paid or volunteer, in a psychology or psychiatry department. Did you lack significant clinical experience? Then spend a night or two a week working for a suicide hot line or find a job at a women's shelter. Were your letters of recommendation tepid or brief? Then acquaint yourself better with potential referees so they can write a positive and detailed letter.

Another year can also provide an opportunity to enhance your interview style or to acquire better matches with graduate faculty members. Some applicants find themselves in the position of perennial "bridesmaids" or "best men," not because their credentials were inadequate, but because their interview style or matching potential was a tad weak. Spend the extra months improving your interpersonal presentation and investigating programs that promise to be better fits with your interests.

The so-called gap year is not intended as a vacation or a "year off." Instead, it is a year dedicated to improving your credentials and working hard at what interests you. When friends or parents ask what you are doing on your purported "year off," we believe the appropriate response is to proudly reply, "Preparing for my career in clinical/counseling psychology!"

In summary, reread this text and conduct a rigorous self-assessment of where you are and where you want to be. If you're still set on a career in clinical or counseling psychology, be prepared to take the time and energy to make yourself a better applicant. Especially if you are still in college and had planned to go straight on to graduate school, take time to gain some life experiences. Age and experience can work in your favor, and they will certainly help you better define your goals next time through the application process.

Two Final Words

Realism and persistence. Be realistic about your credentials, capacities, and acceptance odds. Some applicants refuse to accept the hard facts of the admission process and tragically resubmit the identically flawed application year after year to no avail. An honest evaluation of your credentials, perhaps with the assistance of an experienced professor, will enable you to strengthen your application, select more appropriate programs, or reevaluate your career decisions. This is not to dissuade or discourage you; it is realistic encouragement.

And be persistent! Many successful psychologists have required two or three tries to get into a doctoral program. Thousands of clinical and counseling psychologists have earned a master's degree at one institution before moving on to receive a doctorate at a different university. There is no shame in reaching for the stars; the real loss is not to reach at all.

We hope the information and suggestions contained in this *Insider's Guide* have been helpful to you. We wish you the best success in the application process and in graduate school.

REPORTS ON COMBINED
PSYCHOLOGY PROGRAMS

University at Buffalo/State University of New York (Ph.D.)

(counseling/school)
Department of Counseling, School, & Educational Psychology
Buffalo, NY 14260
phone#: (716) 645-2484
e-mail: r@acsu.buffalo.edu
Web address: www.gse.buffalo.edu/DC/CEP/CP.html

1	2	**3**	4	5	6	7
Practice oriented		Equal emphasis			Research oriented	

Percentage of faculty subscribing to each of the following orientations:

Psychodynamic/Psychoanalytic	0%
Applied behavioral analysis/Radical behavioral	50%
Family systems/Systems	25%
Existential/Phenomenological/Humanistic	5%
Cognitive/Cognitive-behavioral	25%

Courses required for incoming students to have completed prior to enrolling:
Most students have a B.S. in psychology.

Recommended but not mandatory courses:
None

GRE mean
Verbal 602   Quantitative 618   Analytical Writing 5.0

GPA mean
Overall GPA 3.7

Number of applications/admission offers/incoming students in 2007
Not reported

% of students receiving:
Full tuition waiver only: 0%
Assistantship/fellowship only: 0%
Both full tuition waiver & assistantship/fellowship: 100%

Approximate percentage of students who are
Women: 85% **Ethnic Minority:** 20% **International:** 0%

Average years to complete the doctoral program (including internship): 5 years

Personal interview
Required in person

Attrition rate in past 7 years: 0%

Percentage of students applying for internship last year accepted into APPIC or APA internships: 82%

Formal tracks/concentrations: none

Research areas	# Faculty	# Grants
assessment	4	0
family therapy	1	0
health psychology	4	3
multicultural psychology	1	0
rehabilitation psychology	2	0
vocational psychology	2	0

Clinical opportunities
Very diverse, including schools, community agencies, and hospitals in urban, suburban, and rural areas.

University of California–Santa Barbara (Ph.D.)

(clinical/counseling/school)
Department of Counseling, Clinical and School Psychology
Santa Barbara, CA 93106
phone#: (805) 893-3375
e-mail: mfurlong@education.ucsb.edu, cosden@education.ucsb.edu
Web address: education.ucsb.edu/ccsp/

1	2	3	4	5	**6**	7
Practice oriented		Equal emphasis			Research oriented	

Percentage of faculty subscribing to each of the following orientations:

Psychodynamic/Psychoanalytic	30%
Applied behavioral analysis/Radical behavioral	20%
Family systems/Systems	30%
Existential/Phenomenological/Humanistic	20%
Cognitive/Cognitive-behavioral	60%
Developmental	30%
Feminist	20%

Courses required for incoming students to have completed prior to enrolling:
None

Recommended but not mandatory courses:
Human development, personality or abnormal psychology, research design or statistics, biopsychology

GRE mean
Verbal 600   Quantitative 650

GPA mean
Junior/Senior GPA 3.71

Number of applications/admission offers/incoming students in 2007
331 applied/28 admission offers/19 incoming

% of students receiving:
Full tuition waiver only: 5%
Assistantship/fellowship only: 35%
Both full tuition waiver & assistantship/fellowship: 60%

Approximate percentage of incoming students with a B.A./B.S. only: 50% Master's: 50%

Approximate percentage of students who are
Women: 89% **Ethnic Minority:** 50% **International:** 1%

Average years to complete the doctoral program (including internship): 6 years

Personal interview
Preferred in person but telephone acceptable

Attrition rate in past 7 years: 5%

Percentage of students applying for internship last year accepted into APPIC or APA internships: 100%

Formal tracks/concentrations: counseling, clinical, school

Research areas

autism	neuropsychological
career counseling	assessment
counseling LGBT clients	psychological assessment
cross-cultural counseling	psychotherapy
family violence	school (violence/safety/
learning disabilities	bullying)
mental health services for	substance abuse
high-risk families,	
children	

Clinical opportunities

autism	inpatient psychiatric
career counseling	hospital
child abuse	neuropsychological
community LGBT agency	personality assessment
community mental health	school interventions
eating disorders	university counseling
family therapy	

Florida State University (Ph.D.)

(counseling/school)
Psychological Services in Education Program
Department of Educational Psychology and Learning Systems
307 Stone Building
Tallahassee, FL 32306-4453
phone#: (904) 644-8796
e-mail: pfeiffer@coe.fsu.edu
Web address: www.epls.fsu.edu/general/programs.htm

1	2	3	4	**5**	6	7
Practice oriented		Equal emphasis			Research oriented	

Percentage of faculty subscribing to each of the following orientations:

Psychodynamic/Psychoanalytic	10%
Applied behavioral analysis/Radical behavioral	15%
Family systems/Systems	50%
Existential/Phenomenological/Humanistic	10%
Cognitive/Cognitive-behavioral	100%

Courses required for incoming students to have completed prior to enrolling:

None required; core psychology (e.g., statistics, research) highly recommended

Recommended but not mandatory courses:

Core psychology recommended

GRE mean

Verbal 570   Quantitative 610
Analytical Writing 4.5–5.0

GPA mean

Junior/Senior GPA 3.65

Number of applications/admission offers/incoming students in 2007
65 applied/8 admission offers/8 incoming

% of students receiving:
Full tuition waiver only: 0%
Assistantship/fellowship only: 0%
Both full tuition waiver & assistantship/fellowship: 100%

Approximate percentage of incoming students with a B.A./B.S. only: 33%   **Master's:** 67%

Approximate percentage of students who are Women: 60%   **Ethnic Minority:** 20%
International: not reported

Average years to complete the doctoral program (including internship): 6.5 years

Personal interview
Very strongly encouraged; telephone acceptable under unique circumstances

Attrition rate in past 7 years: 10–15%

Percentage of students applying for internship last year accepted into APPIC or APA internships: 100%

Formal tracks/concentrations: counseling and school psychology

Research areas	# Faculty	# Grants
career development	2	2
counseling/psychotherapy	4	1
school/community interventions	3	1
gifted/talent development	2	2

Clinical opportunities

adult learning and evaluation center (diagnose learning disabilities and prescribe treatments to young adults)
full-service career center
human services center (general psychological services to 5-county area)
community placements in variety of mental health, medical and behavioral health care agencies
university counseling center

Hofstra University (Ph.D.)

(clinical)
Department of Psychology
Hempstead, NY 11549
phone#: (516) 463-5662
e-mail: Psyjtc@hofstra.edu
Web address: www.hofstra.edu/clinicalpsy

1	2	3	**4**	5	6	7
Practice oriented		Equal emphasis			Research oriented	

Percentage of faculty subscribing to each of the following orientations:

Psychodynamic/Psychoanalytic	2%
Applied behavioral analysis/Radical behavioral	45%
Family systems/Systems	3%
Existential/Phenomenological/Humanistic	0%
Cognitive/Cognitive-behavioral	50%

Courses required for incoming students to have completed prior to enrolling:
Statistics, research design

Recommended but not mandatory courses:
Yes

GRE mean
Verbal 603   Quantitative 683
Advanced Psychology 654
Analytical Writing 5.0

GPA mean
Overall GPA 3.76

Number of applications/admission offers/incoming students in 2007
203 applied/24 admission offers/14 incoming

% of students receiving:
Full tuition waiver only: 19%
Assistantship/fellowship only: 81%
Both full tuition waiver & assistantship/fellowship: 0%

Approximate percentage of incoming students with a B.A./B.S.only: 75%   **Master's:** 25%

Approximate percentage of students who are Women: 70%   **Ethnic Minority:** 20%   **International:** 10%

Average years to complete the doctoral program (including internship): 5.5 years

Personal interview
Required in person

Attrition rate in past 7 years: 10.9%

Percentage of students applying for internship last year accepted into APPIC or APA internships: 0%
Not used by program until 2009–10 when it is required for all students

Formal tracks/concentrations: none

Research areas	# Faculty	# Grants
addictive behaviors (smoking, obesity, etc.)	3	1
anger disorders	2	0
attitudes and attitude change	1	0
behavior analysis	3	0
behavior modification (in industry, professional sports, depression, anxiety, social skills)	2	0
biofeedback	1	0
body image	2	0
communication of emotions	1	0
cross-cultural psychology	2	0
depression	1	0
family process/therapy	1	0
human error	1	0
infant/toddler development	1	0
normal and abnormal personalities	2	0
prevention of childhood disorders	2	0
psychotherapy for anger, guilt, fear, and anxiety	1	2
quantitative research methods	2	0
rational-emotive/behavior therapy for marital therapy	1	0
schizophrenia	2	1
self-report validity	1	0
sexual dysfunctions	1	0
verbal behavior	1	0
work attitudes and scholarly activities	1	0

Clinical opportunities
Professional services are offered to the community and to Hofstra University students. Placement throughout the New York City metro area.

James Madison University (Psy.D.)
(clinical/school)
Department of Graduate Psychology
Harrisonburg, VA 22807-7401
phone#: (540) 568-7857
e-mail: henriqgx@jmu.edu
Web address: www.psyc.jmu.edu/cipsyd/

1	2	3	4	5	6	7
Practice oriented		Equal emphasis			Research oriented	

Percentage of faculty subscribing to each of the following orientations:

Psychodynamic/Psychoanalytic	20%
Applied behavioral analysis/Radical behavioral	0%
Family systems/Systems	40%
Existential/Phenomenological/Humanistic	20%
Cognitive/Cognitive-behavioral	20%

Courses required for incoming students to have completed prior to enrolling:
Students are required to have a master's degree in a psychology-related field.

Recommended but not mandatory courses:
Master's degree and professional experience

GRE mean
Verbal 530   Quantitative 620
Advanced Psychology 600
Analytical Writing 4.5

GPA mean
Master's GPA 3.8

Number of applications/admission offers/incoming students in 2007
55 applied/6 admission offers/6 incoming

% of students receiving:
Full tuition waiver only: 0%
Assistantship/fellowship only: 0%
Both full tuition waiver & assistantship/fellowship: 100%

Approximate percentage of incoming students with a B.A./B.S. only: 0%   **Master's:** 100%

Approximate percentage of students who are Women: 86%   **Ethnic Minority:** 33%   **International:** 15%

Average years to complete the doctoral program (including internship): 3.8 years

Personal interview
Required

Attrition rate in past 7 years: 10%

Percentage of students applying for internship last year accepted into APPIC or APA internships: 100%

Formal tracks/concentrations: none

Research areas	# Faculty	# Grants
attachment theory	1	0
integrative theory	4	0
beliefs and values	3	2
clinical training processes	3	0
depression and suicide	1	0
biofeedback	1	1
family processes	2	0
international/cultural issues	4	1
parent–child interaction	2	0
social motivation and affect	1	0
social/skill development	4	0
supervision and leadership	1	0
theoretical unification	1	0
traumatic brain injury	1	0
treatment outcomes	1	0

Clinical opportunities

child/family therapy
counseling and
   psychological clinic
forensic assessment
inpatient/hospital practice
learning disabilities
multidisciplinary assessment
neuropsychology
outpatient private practice
school assessment
supervision/leadership

Northeastern University (Ph.D.)

(counseling/school)
Department of Counseling and Applied Educational Psychology
Bouve College of Health Sciences
203 Lake Hall
Boston, MA 02115
phone#: (617) 373-2708
e-mail: w.purnell@neu.edu
Web address:
www.bouve.neu.edu/programs/combined/index.php

1	2	3	4	5	6	7

Practice oriented   Equal emphasis   Research oriented

Percentage of faculty subscribing to each of the following orientations:

Psychodynamic/Psychoanalytic	10%
Applied behavioral analysis/Radical behavioral	10%
Family systems/Systems	30%
Existential/Phenomenological/Humanistic	20%
Cognitive/Cognitive-behavioral	30%

Courses required for incoming students to have completed prior to enrolling:
We require a master's degree in a field (applied preferred) of psychology

Recommended but not mandatory courses:
None

GRE mean
Verbal 500   Quantitative 500
Analytic Writing not reported

GPA mean
Overall GPA 3.0   Psychology GPA 3.0

Number of applications/admission offers/incoming students in 2007
70 applied/10 admission offers/7 incoming

% of students receiving:
Full tuition waiver only: 25%
Assistantship/fellowship only: 25%
Both full tuition waiver & assistantship/fellowship: 25%

Approximate percentage of incoming students with a B.A./B.S. only: 10%   **Master's:** 90%

Approximate percentage of students who are Women: 70%   **Ethnic Minority:** 20%
International: not reported

Average years to complete the doctoral program (including internship): 5.5 years

Personal interview
Required

Attrition rate in past 7 years: 10%

Percentage of students applying for internship last year accepted into APPIC or APA internships: 100%

Formal tracks/concentrations: school psychology, counseling psychology

Research areas	# Faculty	# Grants
consultation with telecommunication	1	1
counseling needs of minorities	1	1
early intervention	1	1
eating disorders	1	1
forensics in juvenile crime	1	1
impact of managed care on clinical training	1	0
leadership development	3	1
neuropsychological function	1	0
spatial ability and cognitive transfer	2	0

Clinical opportunities
Students have the opportunity to work with families, women, men, psychotics, chronically ill, autistic, etc. Training settings in the Boston area include all manners of ethnic and cultural diversity, medical, mental health, and private care facilities.

Ontario Institute for Studies in Education (Ph.D.)

(clinical/school)
Department of Human Development and Applied Psychology
OISE/University of Toronto
252 Bloor Street West
Toronto, Ontario M5S 1V6 Canada
phone#: (416) 923-6641, ext. 2492
e-mail: kscott@oise.utoronto.ca
Web address:
hdap.oise.utoronto.ca/pages/schoolClnChldPsych.html

1	2	3	4	5	**6**	7
Practice oriented		Equal emphasis			Research oriented	

Percentage of faculty subscribing to each of the following orientations:

Psychodynamic/Psychoanalytic	11%
Applied behavioral analysis/Radical behavioral	11%
Family systems/Systems	11%
Existential/Phenomenological/Humanistic	0%
Cognitive/Cognitive-behavioral	22%
Other-Psychoeducational	45%

Courses required for incoming students to have completed prior to enrolling:
6 six credit courses (or its equivalent) in psychology, 3 of which must be at a senior level; at least 3 credit courses in research methods

Recommended but not mandatory courses:
History and systems in psychology, developmental psychology, biological, social, and cognitive/affective bases of behavior.

GRE mean
We do not require GRE scores.

GPA mean
Students must have the equivalent of at least an A– (3.7) at the University of Toronto to be considered for the program, but most have an A average.

Number of applications/admission offers/incoming students in 2007
450 applied/27 admission offers/24 incoming
Admission numbers include the 6 students who are proceeding from the M.A. to the Ph.D.

% of students receiving:
Full tuition waiver only: 0%
Assistantship/fellowship only: 0%
Both full tuition waiver & assistantship/fellowship: 100%

Approximate percentage of incoming students with a B.A./B.S. only: 62% **Master's:** 38%

Approximate percentage of students who are Women: 91% **Ethnic Minority:** 33% **International:** 10%

Average years to complete the doctoral program (including internship): 5 years

Personal interview
Not required as part of admission process

Attrition rate in past 7 years: 4%

Percentage of students applying for internship last year accepted into APPIC or APA internships: 50%

Formal tracks/concentrations: none

Research areas	# Faculty	# Grants
ADHD	4	9
anxiety disorders	2	2
behavioral/cognitive behavioral intervention	2	2
child epilepsy	1	1
child maltreatment	2	1
cognition (critical thinking, intentional learning)	2	2
cross-cultural psychology	3	3
developmental psychopathology	4	5
emotions	3	3
fetal alcohol disorder	1	1
gender identity disorder	1	1
hypothyroidism	1	1
learning disabilities	4	4
math and technology	2	1
parenting	3	3
peer relations	2	2
reading/literacy	5	7
social cognition (theory of mind, moral development)	3	2
young offenders/children's rights	2	1

Clinical opportunities

ADHD	Hospital for Sick Children
anxiety/mood	learning disabilities
autism	mental retardation
Centre for Addiction and Mental Health	OISE/University of Toronto, Integra
developmental	physical disabilities
family	psychoeducational
family life center	Surrey Place
fire setting	traumatic brain injury
gender identity	TREADD

Pace University (Psy.D.)

(school/clinical)
Department of Psychology
New York, NY 10038
phone#: (212) 346-1506
e-mail: bmowder@pace.edu
Web address:
www.pace.edu/dyson/psychology/psydgi.html

1	**2**	3	4	5	6	7
Practice oriented		Equal emphasis			Research oriented	

Percentage of faculty subscribing to each of the following orientations:

Psychodynamic/Psychoanalytic	33%
Applied behavioral analysis/Radical behavioral	0%
Family systems/Systems	22%
Existential/Phenomenological/Humanistic	11%
Cognitive/Cognitive-behavioral	33%

Courses required for incoming students to have completed prior to enrolling:
General psychology, experimental psychology, statistics, developmental psychology, learning, personality, psychopathology

Recommended but not mandatory courses:
None

GRE mean
Verbal + Quantitative 1300
Analytical Writing not reported

GPA mean
Overall GPA 3.6

Number of applications/admission offers/incoming students in 2007
273 applied/66 admission offers/24 incoming

% of students receiving:
Full tuition waiver only: 25% partial tuition waiver
Assistantship/fellowship only: 25%
Both full tuition waiver & assistantship/fellowship: 0%

Approximate percentage of incoming students with a B.A./B.S. only: 88% **Master's:** 12%

Approximate percentage of students who are Women: 85% **Ethnic Minority:** 38% **International:** 5%

Average years to complete the doctoral program (including internship): 5.7 years (varies from year to year)

Personal interview
Required in person (on occasion grant telephone interviews)

Attrition rate in past 7 years: 5–10%

Percentage of students applying for internship last year accepted into APPIC or APA internships: 75%

Formal tracks/concentrations: none

Research areas	# Faculty	# Grants
community psychology	1	0
gender	2	0
infant and early childhood	3	0
learning disabilities	1	0
learning	1	0
multicultural	2	0
posttraumatic stress disorder	1	0
psychometric	3	0

Clinical opportunities
early childhood   neuropsychological assessment
psychotherapy   many, varied opportunities available

Utah State University (Ph.D.)

(clinical/counseling/school)
Department of Psychology
Logan, UT 84322-2810
phone#: (435) 797-1460
e-mail:PsyDept@cc.usu.edu
Web address:
www.coe.usu.edu/psyc/programs/phd_combined/index.html

1	2	3	4	5	6	7
Practice oriented			Equal emphasis			Research oriented

Percentage of faculty subscribing to each of the following orientations:
Psychodynamic/Psychoanalytic	10%
Applied behavioral analysis/Radical behavioral	10%
Family systems/Systems	10%
Existential/Phenomenological/Humanistic	20%
Cognitive/Cognitive-behavioral	50%

Courses required for incoming students to have completed prior to enrolling:
General psychology, developmental psychology, learning, elementary statistics, personality, physiological, abnormal

Recommended but not mandatory courses:
Introduction to counseling, cognitive psychology, social psychology

GRE mean
Verbal 540   Quantitative 680
Verbal + Quantitative 1220
Analytical Writing not reported

GPA mean
Junior/Senior GPA 3.83

Number of applications/admission offers/incoming students in 2007
68 applied/12 admission offers/6 incoming

% of students receiving:
Full tuition waiver only: 0%
Assistantship/fellowship only: 85%
Both full tuition waiver & assistantship/fellowship: 15%

Approximate percentage of incoming students with a B.A./B.S. only: 80% **Master's:** 20%

Approximate percentage of students who are Women: 80% **Ethnic Minority:** 15% **International:** 5%

Average years to complete the doctoral program (including internship): 6 years

Personal interview
Preferred in person but telephone acceptable

Attrition rate in past 7 years: 5%

Percentage of students applying for internship last year accepted into APPIC or APA internships: 86%

Formal tracks/concentrations: child clinical/school, health/neuropsychology

Research areas	# Faculty	# Grants
addiction/substance abuse	1	0
ADHD	1	0
behavioral medicine/health psychology	3	2
child behavior problems	4	2
childhood/adolescent depression	2	0
Native American mental health	1	0
rural mental health	2	1
school behavioral assessment	1	0

Clinical opportunities

behavioral medicine
cardiac rehabilitation
chronic mental health
community mental health
disabilities
early intervention
eating disorders

Head Start
minority mental health
neuropsychology
pediatric psychology
student counseling center
student wellness center

Yeshiva University (Psy.D.)

(clinical/school)
Ferkauf Graduate School of Psychology
Bronx, NY 10461
phone#: (718) 430-3945
e-mail: givner@aecom.yu.edu
Web address:
www.yu.edu/ferkauf/page.aspx?id=733&ekmensel=
242_submenu_290_btnlink

1	2	3	4	5	6	7

Practice oriented   Equal emphasis   Research oriented

Percentage of faculty subscribing to each of the following orientations:

Psychodynamic/Psychoanalytic	50%
Applied behavioral analysis/Radical behavioral	10%
Family systems/Systems	20%
Existential/Phenomenological/Humanistic	0%
Cognitive/Cognitive-behavioral	40%

Courses required for incoming students to have completed prior to enrolling:

Statistics, abnormal psychology, child development

Recommended but not mandatory courses:

None

GRE mean

Verbal 593   Quantitative 680
Analytical Writing 5.0

GPA mean

Overall GPA 3.51

Number of applications/admission offers/incoming students in 2007

185 applied/45 admission offers/23 incoming

% of students receiving:

Full tuition waiver only: 5%
Assistantship/fellowship only: 50%
Both full tuition waiver & assistantship/fellowship: 5%

Approximate percentage of incoming students with a B.A./B.S. only: 75%   Master's: 25%

Approximate percentage of students who are

Women: 70%   Ethnic Minority: 18%   International:

Average years to complete the doctoral program (including internship): 5.0 years

Personal interview

Required in person

Attrition rate in past 7 years: not reported

Percentage of students applying for internship last year accepted into APPIC or APA internships: 85%

Formal tracks/concentrations: child psychotherapy

Research areas	# Faculty	# Grants
ADHD	2	0
adolescence	2	0
assessment	3	0
attachment	3	0
behavioral interventions	3	0
early childhood	2	0
fathering	2	0
learning disabilities	3	0
multicultural issues	3	1
nontraditional families	2	0
professional issues	3	0
social-emotional correlates	2	1
symbolic play	1	0

Clinical opportunities

bilingual/multicultural
child/adolescence
early childhood

family–school collaboration
parent training
school age

REPORTS ON INDIVIDUAL CLINICAL PSYCHOLOGY PROGRAMS

Adelphi University (Ph.D.)

Derner Institute of Advanced Psychological Studies
Garden City, NY 11530
phone#: (516) 877-4800
fax#: (516) 877-4805
email: Ross@adelphi.edu
Web address: derner.adelphi.edu/doctoral

1	2	3	4	5	6	7
Practice oriented		Equal emphasis			Research oriented	

Percentage of faculty subscribing to each of the following orientations:

Psychodynamic/Psychoanalytic	90%
Applied behavioral analysis/Radical behavioral	15%
Family systems/Systems	10%
Existential/Phenomenological/Humanistic	10%
Cognitive/Cognitive-behavioral	20%

Courses required for incoming students to have completed prior to enrolling:
Statistics, experimental methods, developmental psychology, abnormal psychology

Recommended but not mandatory courses:
none

GRE mean
Verbal 620   Quantitative 660
Analytical Writing not reported
Advanced Psychology 660

GPA mean
Overall GPA 3.50   Psychology GPA 3.6

Number of applications/admission offers/incoming students in 2007
235 applied/45 admission offers/23 incoming

% of students receiving:
Full tuition waiver only: 0%
Assistantship/fellowship only: 100%
Both full tuition waiver & assistantship/fellowship: 0%

Approximate percentage of incoming students with a B.A./B.S. only: 67%   **Master's:** 33%

Approximate percentage of students who are Women: 80%   **Ethnic Minority:** 15%   **International:** 10%

Average years to complete the doctoral program (including internship): not reported

Personal interview
Required in person

Attrition rate in past 7 years: 7.5%

Percentage of students applying for internship last year accepted into APPIC or APA internships: 90%

Formal tracks/concentrations: child psychotherapy

Research areas	# Faculty	# Grants
change processes	2	0
creativity	1	1
developmental	1	1
developmental (lifespan)	1	1
equity in personal relationships	1	1
group process	2	0
health psychology	1	1
marriage	1	1
psychoanalysis	8	3
psychotherapy process	3	2
unconscious processes and motivation	1	0

Clinical opportunities

psychoanalytic psychotherapy
addiction
child, adolescent, and family
group therapy
psychotherapy integration
short-term psychotherapy
neuropsychological assessment

Adler School of Professional Psychology (Psy.D.)

65 East Wacker Place, #2100
Chicago, IL 60601-7203
phone#: (312) 201-5900
admissions: (312) 201-5900 ext 222
e-mail: admissions@adler.edu
Web address:
www.adler.edu/academics/4211DoctorofPsychologyin ClinicalPsychologyPsyD.asp

1	2	3	4	5	6	7
Practice oriented		Equal emphasis			Research oriented	

Percentage of faculty subscribing to each of the following orientations:

Psychodynamic/Psychoanalytic	10%
Applied behavioral analysis/Radical behavioral	0%
Family systems/Systems	10%
Existential/Phenomenological/Humanistic	40%
Cognitive/Cognitive-behavioral	40%

Courses required for incoming students to have completed prior to enrolling:
Advanced abnormal psychology, general psychology, psychometrics, theories of personality, and others to total 18 credits

Recommended but not mandatory courses:
none

GRE mean
not reported

GPA mean
not reported

Number of applications/admission offers/incoming students in 2007
262 applied/131 admission offers/59 incoming

% of students receiving:
Full tuition waiver only: 0%
Assistantship/fellowship only: 10%
Both full tuition waiver & assistantship/fellowship: 0%

Approximate percentage of incoming students with a B.A./B.S. only: 75%   **Master's:** 25%

**Approximate percentage of students who are
Women:** 79.6%   **Ethnic Minority:** 28.8%
International: 2%

**Average years to complete the doctoral program
(including internship):** 5.1 years

Attrition rate in past 7 years: 15.5%

**Percentage of students applying for internship last
year accepted into APPIC or APA internships:**
67% APPIC
26% APA/CPA

Formal tracks/concentrations: Adlerian psychotherapy,
clinical neuropsychology, child & adolescence, group
psychotherapy, primary care psychology, substance abuse
treatment, marriage & family

Personal interview
Required in person

Research areas	# Faculty	# Grants
adult human development	1	0
disabled children and coping	2	0
neuropsychology of offenders	4	1
community clinical	1	1

Clinical opportunities

Department of Corrections	schools
developmental disabilities	hospitals
halfway release programs for sex offenders	community mental health centers

University of Alabama at Birmingham (Ph.D.)

Department of Psychology
CH 415
1530 3rd Avenue South
Birmingham, AL 35294-1170
phone#: (205) 934-8723
e-mail: medpsych@uab.edu
Web address: www.psy.uab.edu/medpsych.htm

1	2	3	**4**	5	6	7

Practice oriented   Equal emphasis   Research oriented

**Percentage of faculty subscribing to each of the
following orientations:**

Psychodynamic/Psychoanalytic	30%
Applied behavioral analysis/Radical behavioral	0%
Family systems/Systems	0%
Existential/Phenomenological/Humanistic	0%
Cognitive/Cognitive-behavioral	70%
Health psychology	100%

**Courses required for incoming students to have
completed prior to enrolling:**
At least 18 credit hours of psychology, including statistics;
at least 18 credit hours of life sciences (the number of
hours are recommended, not required)

Recommended but not mandatory courses:
Psychopathology, learning, cognitive psychology, social
psychology

GRE mean
Verbal 560   Quantitative 700
Analytical Writing & Subject Test not required for admission

GPA mean
Overall GPA 3.75

**Number of applications/admission offers/incoming
students in 2007**
56 applied/10 admission offers/7 incoming

% of students receiving:
Full tuition waiver only: 0%
Assistantship/fellowship only: 100%
Both full tuition waiver & assistantship/fellowship: 100%

**Approximate percentage of incoming students with a
B.A./B.S. only:** 100%   **Master's:** 0%

**Approximate percentage of students who are
Women:** 86%   **Ethnic Minority:** 14%   **International:** 0%

**Average years to complete the doctoral program
(including internship):** 6 years

Personal interview
Preferred in person but telephone acceptable

Attrition rate in past 7 years: 9%

**Percentage of students applying for internship last
year accepted into APPIC or APA internships:** 100%

Formal tracks/concentrations: medical/clinical
psychology, neuropsychology, pediatric psychology,
geropsychology

Research areas	# Faculty	# Grants
aging	3	6
behavioral medicine	2	2
developmental disabilities	6	16
eating disorders	1	1
neuropsychology	3	2
psychophysiology	1	1
substance abuse	3	5

Clinical opportunities
behavioral medicine
neuropsychology

University of Alabama at Tuscaloosa (Ph.D.)

Department of Psychology
P. O. Box 870348
Tuscaloosa, AL 35487-5083
phone#: (205) 348-1919
e-mail: mbhubbard@as.ua.edu
Web address:
psychology.ua.edu/academics/graduate/clinical/clinical
.html

1	2	3	4	**5**	6	7

Practice oriented   Equal emphasis   Research oriented

Percentage of faculty subscribing to each of the following orientations:

Psychodynamic/Psychoanalytic	0%
Applied behavioral analysis/Radical behavioral	10%
Family systems/Systems	10%
Existential/Phenomenological/Humanistic	10%
Cognitive/Cognitive-behavioral	80%

Courses required for incoming students to have completed prior to enrolling:
Undergrad statistics, research methods, abnormal psychology

Recommended but not mandatory courses:
None

GRE mean
Verbal 675   Quantitative 660
Advanced Psychology 675
Analytical Writing 4.6

GPA mean
Overall GPA 3.6 Psychology GPA 3.7
Junior/Senior GPA 3.7

Number of applications/admission offers/incoming students in 2007
189 applied/17 admission offers/10 incoming

% of students receiving:
Full tuition waiver only: 0%
Assistantship/fellowship only: 90%
Both full tuition waiver & assistantship/fellowship: 80%

Approximate percentage of incoming students with a B.A./B.S. only: 90%   Master's: 10%

Approximate percentage of students who are Women: 80%   Ethnic Minority: 16%   International: 0%

Average years to complete the doctoral program (including internship): 6 years

Personal interview
Preferred in person but telephone acceptable

Attrition rate in past 7 years: 10%

Percentage of students applying for internship last year accepted into APPIC or APA internships: 100%

Formal tracks/concentrations: health, child, geropsychology, psychology & law

Research areas	# Faculty	# Grants
adult psychopathology	3	2
affective disorders/depression	1	0
aging	5	3
assessment	1	0
behavioral medicine	3	2
biofeedback	0	0
child clinical	4	3
clinical judgment	0	0
cross-cultural psychology	2	2
forensic	4	0
pain management	1	1
professional issues	2	0
psychotherapy process and outcome	2	0
social skills	2	1
violence/abuse	2	2

Clinical opportunities
autism
conduct disorder
factitious disorder
forensic psychology
gerontology
health promotion behavior
pain management
parent–child interaction
anxiety
chronic mental illness
neuropsychological assessment
sleep disorders

University at Albany/State University of New York (Ph.D.)
Department of Psychology
1400 Washington Avenue
Albany, NY 12222
phone#: (518) 442-4820
e-mail: forsyth@albany.edu
Web address: www.albany.edu/psy/gradclinical.html

1	2	3	4	5	6	7
Practice oriented		Equal emphasis			Research oriented	

Percentage of faculty subscribing to each of the following orientations:

Psychodynamic/Psychoanalytic	0%
Applied behavioral analysis/Radical behavioral	30%
Family systems/Systems	0%
Existential/Phenomenological/Humanistic	0%
Cognitive/Cognitive-behavioral	70%

Courses required for incoming students to have completed prior to enrolling:
18 semester hours in psychology, including classes in statistics and experimental design

Recommended but not mandatory courses:
None

GRE mean
Verbal 643   Quantitative 669
Advanced Psychology 669   Analytical Writing 5.1

GPA mean
Overall GPA 3.5   Psychology GPA 3.7

Number of applications/admission offers/incoming students in 2007
182 applied/10 admission offers/8 incoming

% of students receiving:
Full tuition waiver only: 0%
Assistantship/fellowship only: 0%
Both full tuition waiver & assistantship/fellowship: 100%

Approximate percentage of incoming students with a B.A./B.S. only: 90%   Master's: 10%

Approximate percentage of students who are Women: 82%   Ethnic Minority: 26%   International: 2%

Average years to complete the doctoral program (including internship): 6.1 years

Personal interview
Preferred in person but telephone acceptable

Attrition rate in past 7 years: 11%

Percentage of students applying for internship last year accepted into APPIC or APA internships:

Formal tracks/concentrations: none

Research areas	# Faculty	# Grants
anxiety disorders	1	0
autism/developmental disabilities	1	3
behavioral medicine	2	0
children	4	1
eating disorders	1	1
neuropsychology	1	0
psychopathology	1	0
substance abuse/addiction	2	2

Clinical opportunities

addictive disorders
adolescents
anxiety disorders
autism/developmental
   disabilities
health psychology
children
cross-cultural issues
eating disorders
neuropsychology

Alliant International University–Fresno (Ph.D.)

5130 East Clinton Way
Fresno, CA 93727
phone#: (866) 825-5426
e-mail: admissions@alliant.edu
Web address: www.alliant.edu/cspp

1	2	3	4	**5**	6	7
Practice oriented			Equal emphasis			Research oriented

Percentage of faculty subscribing to each of the following orientations:

Psychodynamic/Psychoanalytic	10%
Applied behavioral analysis/Radical behavioral	10%
Family systems/Systems	40%
Existential/Phenomenological/Humanistic	10%
Cognitive/Cognitive-behavioral	30%

Courses required for incoming students to have completed prior to enrolling:
If no BA in psychology or score is below the 80th percentile on the Advanced Psychology GRE, then the following are required: statistics, tests & measurements, abnormal psychology and one of the following: experimental psychology or physiological psychology or learning theory.

Recommended but not mandatory courses:
Refer to above.

GRE mean
GRE scores are not used as part of the standard admissions process.

GPA mean
Overall 3.5

Number of applications/admission offers/incoming students in 2007
25 applied/9 admission offers/7 incoming

% of students receiving:
Full tuition waiver only: 0%
Assistantship/fellowship only: 5%
Both full tuition waiver & assistantship/fellowship: 0%

Approximate percentage of incoming students with a B.A./B.S. only: 79%   **Master's:** 21%

Approximate percentage of students who are Women: 75%   **Ethnic Minority:** 18%   **International:** 7%

Average years to complete the doctoral program (including internship): 6 years

Personal interview
Preferred in person but telephone available

Attrition rate in past 7 years: 6%

Percentage of students applying for internship last year accepted into APPIC or APA internships: 100%

Formal tracks/concentrations: clinical forensic, child, health psychology

Research areas	# Faculty	# Grants
child/family	2	not reported
clinical forensics	1	
health psychology	4	
multicultural psychology	4	
play therapy	1	

Clinical opportunities
Over 125 field placements in almost all areas of psychology, including inpatient, outpatient, and residential treatment programs for children, adolescents, and adults.

Alliant International University–Fresno (Psy.D.)

5130 East Clinton Way
Fresno, CA 93727
phone#: (866) 825-5426
e-mail: admissions@alliant.edu
Web address: www.alliant.edu/cspp

1	**2**	3	4	5	6	7
Practice oriented			Equal emphasis			Research oriented

Percentage of faculty subscribing to each of the following orientations:

Psychodynamic/Psychoanalytic	10%
Applied behavioral analysis/Radical behavioral	10%
Family systems/Systems	20%
Existential/Phenomenological/Humanistic	10%
Cognitive/Cognitive-behavioral	50%

Courses required for incoming students to have completed prior to enrolling:

If no BA in psychology or score is below the 80th percentile on the Advanced Psychology GRE then the following are required: statistics, tests & measurements, abnormal psychology and one of the following: experimental psychology or physiological psychology or learning theory.

Recommended but not mandatory courses:
Please refer to above.

GRE mean
GRE scores are not used as part of the standard admissions process

GPA mean
3.42

Number of applications/admission offers/incoming students in 2007
131 applied/53 admission offers/43 incoming

% of students receiving:
Full tuition waiver only: 0%
Assistantship/fellowship only: 5%

Approximate percentage of incoming students with a B.A./B.S. only: 85%   Master's: 15%

Approximate percentage of students who are
Women: 75%   Ethnic Minority: 21%   International: 5%

Average years to complete the doctoral program (including internship): 4.6 years

Personal interview
Preferred in person but telephone available

Attrition rate in past 7 years: 8%

Percentage of students applying for internship last year accepted into APPIC or APA internships: 90%
10% accepted into CAPIC-member internships.

Formal tracks/concentrations: clinical forensic emphasis, ecosystemic child emphasis, health psychology emphasis

Research areas	# Faculty	# Grants
child and family	3	not reported
clinical forensics	1	
health psychology	6	
integrative psychology	1	
multicultural psychology	3	
play therapy	2	
psychology of women	3	

Clinical opportunities
inpatient
outpatient
residential treatment
  programs for children/
  adolescents/adults
behavioral health/
  neuropsychological
  populations

college counseling centers
mental health centers
forensic
ethnic minority populations
women
gay/lesbians
disabled

Alliant International University–Los Angeles (Ph.D.)

1000 South Fremont Avenue, Unit 5
Alhambra, CA 91803-1360
Phone: (866) 825-5426
e-mail: admissions@alliant.edu
Web address: www.alliant.edu/cspp

1	2	3	4	5	6	7
Practice oriented		Equal emphasis			Research oriented	

Percentage of faculty subscribing to each of the following orientations:
Psychodynamic/Psychoanalytic	15%
Applied behavioral analysis/Radical behavioral	0%
Family systems/Systems	15%
Existential/Phenomenological/Humanistic	0%
Cognitive/Cognitive-behavioral	15%
Research	50%

Courses required for incoming students to have completed prior to enrolling:

If no BA in psychology or score is below the 80th percentile on the Advanced Psychology GRE, then the following are required: statistics, tests & measurements, abnormal psychology and one of the following: experimental psychology or physiological psychology or learning theory.

Recommended but not mandatory courses:
Refer to above.

GRE mean
GRE scores are not used as part of the standard admissions process.

GPA mean
Overall 3.53

Number of applications/admission offers/incoming students in 2007
75 applied/36 admission offers/23 incoming

% of students receiving:
Full tuition waiver only: 0%
Assistantship/fellowship only: 5%
Both full tuition waiver & assistantship/fellowship: 0%

Approximate percentage of incoming students with a B.A./B.S. only: 75%   Master's: 25%

Approximate percentage of students who are
Women: 81%   Ethnic Minority: 34%   International: 2%

Average years to complete the doctoral program (including internship): 6.8 years

Personal interview
Preferred in person but telephone acceptable

Attrition rate in past 7 years: 4%

Percentage of students applying for internship last year accepted into APPIC or APA internships: 15%

Formal tracks/concentrations: family/couple, health psychology, multicultural community

Research areas	# Faculty	# Grants
chemical dependency	1	not reported
family and couple	2	
health psychology	4	
integrative psychology	1	
multicultural/community	3	
psychology of women	3	
trauma and PTSD	1	

Clinical opportunities
We have over 125 field placements in almost all areas of psychology including inpatient, outpatient, and residential treatment programs for children, adolescents, and adults

---

Alliant International University– Los Angeles (Psy.D.)

1000 South Fremont Avenue, Unit 5
Alhambra, CA 91803-1360
Phone: (866) 825-5426
e-mail: admissions@alliant.edu
Web address: www.alliant.edu/cspp

1	**2**	3	4	5	6	7

Practice oriented	Equal emphasis	Research oriented

Percentage of faculty subscribing to each of the following orientations:

Psychodynamic/Psychoanalytic	50%
Applied behavioral analysis/Radical behavioral	0%
Family systems/Systems	30%
Existential/Phenomenological/Humanistic	10%
Cognitive/Cognitive-behavioral	10%

Courses required for incoming students to have completed prior to enrolling:
If no BA in psychology or score is below the 80th percentile on the Advanced Psychology GRE then the following are required: statistics, tests & measurements, abnormal psychology and one of the following: experimental psychology or physiological psychology or learning theory.

Recommended but not mandatory courses:
Please refer to above.

GRE mean
GRE scores are not used as a part of the standard admissions process.

GPA mean
3.22

Number of applications/admission offers/incoming students in 2007
198 applied/86 admission offers/70 incoming

% of students receiving:
Full tuition waiver only: 0%
Assistantship/fellowship only: 5%
Both tuition waiver & assistantship/fellowship: not reported

Approximate percentage of incoming students with a B.A./B.S. only: 82%   **Master's:** 18%

Approximate percentage of students who are Women: 80%   **Ethnic Minority:** 39%   **International:** 3%

Average years to complete the doctoral program (including internship): 4.0 years

Personal interview
Preferred in person but telephone acceptable

Attrition rate in past 7 years: 2%

Percentage of students applying for internship last year accepted into APPIC or APA internships: 8%
92% accepted into CAPIC-member or equivalent internships.

Formal tracks/concentrations: family/couple, health psychology, multicultural community

Research areas	# Faculty	# Grants
depression and anxiety	1	not reported
family and couple	6	
health psychology	4	
interpersonal processes	3	
multicultural and community	6	
pediatric psychology	1	
trauma and PTSD	2	

Clinical opportunities
We have over 125 field placements that specialize in almost all areas of psychology including inpatient, outpatient, and residential treatment programs for children, adolescents, and adults, hospitals specializing in behavioral health and neuropsychological populations, college counseling centers, mental health centers, forensic sites, and placements specializing in the treatment of specific ethnic minority populations, women, gay/lesbians, and the disabled.

Alliant International University– San Diego (Ph.D.)

10455 Pomerado Road
San Diego, CA 92131-1799
phone#: (866) 825-5426
e-mail: admissions@alliant.edu
Web address: www.alliant.edu/cspp

1	2	3	**4**	5	6	7

Practice oriented	Equal emphasis	Research oriented

Percentage of faculty subscribing to each of the following orientations:

Psychodynamic/Psychoanalytic	15%
Applied behavioral analysis/Radical behavioral	31%
Family systems/Systems	38%
Existential/Phenomenological/Humanistic	0%
Cognitive/Cognitive-behavioral	16%

Courses required for incoming students to have completed prior to enrolling:
If no BA in psychology or score is below the 80th percentile on the Advanced Psychology GRE, then the following are required: statistics, tests & measurements,

abnormal psychology and one of the following: experimental psychology or physiological psychology or learning theory.

Recommended but not mandatory courses:
Refer to above.

GRE mean
GRE scores are not used as part of the admissions process.

GPA mean
Overall 3.46

Number of applications/admission offers/incoming students in 2007
117 applied/47 admission offers/31 incoming

% of students receiving:
Full tuition waiver only: 0%
Assistantship/fellowship only: 5%
Both full tuition waiver & assistantship/fellowship: 0%

Approximate percentage of incoming students with a B.A./B.S. only: 73% **Master's:** 27%

Approximate percentage of students who are Women: 84% **Ethnic Minority:** 23% **International:** 2%

Average years to complete the doctoral program (including internship): 5.9 years

Personal interview
Required in person (telephone interviews may be considered).

Attrition rate in past 7 years: 5%

Percentage of students applying for internship last year accepted into APPIC or APA internships: 8%

Formal tracks/concentrations: family/child emphasis, family track, forensic psychology emphasis, health track, multicultural emphasis, psychodynamic emphasis

Research areas	# Faculty	# Grants
behavioral assessment	3	not reported
clinical forensics	1	
family/child	6	
health psychology	5	
multicultural	4	
pediatric and child psychology	4	
trauma and PTSD	4	

Clinical opportunities
We have over 85 field placements in almost all areas of psychology, including inpatient, outpatient, and residential treatment programs for children, adolescents, and adults

Alliant International University–San Diego (Psy.D.)

10455 Pomerado Road
San Diego, CA 92131-1799
phone#: (866) 825-5426
e-mail: admissions@alliant.edu
Web address: www.alliant.edu/cspp

1	2	3	4	5	6	7
Practice oriented		Equal emphasis			Research oriented	

Percentage of faculty subscribing to each of the following orientations:

Psychodynamic/Psychoanalytic	35%
Applied behavioral analysis/Radical behavioral	10%
Family systems/Systems	25%
Existential/Phenomenological/Humanistic	5%
Cognitive/Cognitive-behavioral	25%

Courses required for incoming students to have completed prior to enrolling:
If no BA in psychology or score is below the 80th percentile on the Advanced Psychology GRE, then the following are required: statistics, tests & measurements, abnormal psychology and one of the following: experimental psychology or physiological psychology or learning theory.

Recommended but not mandatory courses:
Refer to above.

GRE mean
GRE scores are not used as part of the admissions process.

GPA mean
Overall 3.38

Number of applications/admission offers/incoming students in 2007
124 applied/54 admission offers/46 incoming

% of students receiving:
Full tuition waiver only: 0%
Assistantship/fellowship only: 5%
Both full tuition waiver & assistantship/fellowship: 0%

Approximate percentage of incoming students with a B.A./B.S. only: 85% **Master's:** 15%

Approximate percentage of students who are Women: 76% **Ethnic Minority:** 15% **International:** 4%

Average years to complete the doctoral program (including internship): 5.5 years

Personal interview
Required in person (telephone interviews may be considered).

Attrition rate in past 7 years: 4%

Percentage of students applying for internship last year accepted into APPIC or APA internships: 4%

Formal tracks/concentrations: family/child emphasis, family track, forensic psychology emphasis, integrative psychology emphasis, multicultural emphasis, psychodynamic emphasis

Research areas	# Faculty	# Grants
behavioral assessment	1	not reported
chemical dependency	3	
child and adolescent	4	
couples and family	4	
forensic psychology	3	

health psychology	3
integrative psychology	1
multicultural and community	5

Clinical opportunities

We have over 85 field placements in almost all areas of psychology, including inpatient, outpatient, and residential treatment programs for children, adolescents, and adults

Alliant International University–San Francisco (Ph.D.)

One Beach Street, Suite 100
San Francisco, CA 94133
phone#: (866) 825-5426
e-mail: admissions@alliant.edu
Web address: www.alliant.edu/cspp

1	2	3	**4**	5	6	7
Practice oriented			Equal emphasis			Research oriented

Percentage of faculty subscribing to each of the following orientations:

Psychodynamic/Psychoanalytic	30%
Applied behavioral analysis/Radical behavioral	0%
Family systems/Systems	60%
Existential/Phenomenological/Humanistic	20%
Cognitive/Cognitive-behavioral	50%

Courses required for incoming students to have completed prior to enrolling:

If no BA in psychology or score is below the 80th percentile on the Advanced Psychology GRE, then the following are required: statistics, tests & measurements, abnormal psychology and one of the following: experimental psychology or physiological psychology or learning theory.

Recommended but not mandatory courses:
Refer to above.

GRE mean
GRE scores are not used as part of the admissions process.

GPA mean
Overall 3.44

Number of applications/admission offers in 2007
83 applied/45 admission offers/28 incoming

% of students receiving:
Full tuition waiver only: 0%
Assistantship/fellowship only: 5%
Both full tuition waiver & assistantship/fellowship: 0%

Approximate percentage of incoming students with a B.A./B.S. only: 90%   Master's: 10%

Approximate percentage of students who are
Women: 75%   Ethnic Minority: 30%   International: 5%

Average years to complete the doctoral program (including pre-doc internship): 6.6 years

Personal interview
Preferred in person but telephone acceptable

Attrition rate in past 7 years: 5%

Percentage of students applying for internship last year accepted into APPIC or APA internships: 25%

Formal tracks/concentrations: family/child/adolescent psychology, gender studies, health psychology, multicultural/community psychology, program evaluation, organizational assessment and consultation

Research areas	# Faculty	# Grants
chemical dependency	2	not reported
family/child/adolescent	3	
gender studies and LGBT	6	
health psychology	3	
multicultural and community	4	
program evaluation	1	
psychology of women	3	

Clinical opportunities

inpatient	mental health centers
outpatient	forensic
residential treatment	ethnic minority populations
behavioral health/	women
neuropsychology	gay/lesbians
college counseling centers	disabled

Alliant International University–San Francisco (Psy.D.)

One Beach Street, Suite 100
San Francisco, CA 94133
phone#: (866) 825-5426
e-mail: admissions@alliant.edu
Web address: www.alliant.edu/cspp

1	**2**	3	4	5	6	7
Practice oriented			Equal emphasis			Research oriented

Percentage of faculty subscribing to each of the following orientations:

Psychodynamic/Psychoanalytic	26%
Applied behavioral analysis/Radical behavioral	0%
Family systems/Systems	21%
Existential/Phenomenological/Humanistic	15%
Cognitive/Cognitive-behavioral	5%

Courses required for incoming students to have completed prior to enrolling:

If no BA in psychology or score is below the 80th percentile on the Advanced Psychology GRE, then the following are required: statistics, tests & measurements, abnormal psychology and one of the following: experimental psychology or physiological psychology or learning theory.

Recommended but not mandatory courses:
Refer to above.

GRE mean
GRE scores are not used as part of the admissions process.

GPA mean
Overall 3.29

Number of applications/admission offers in 2007
218 applied/131 admission offers/63 incoming

% of students receiving:
Full tuition waiver only: 0%
Assistantship/fellowship only: 5%
Both full tuition waiver & assistantship/fellowship: 0%

Approximate percentage of incoming students with a B.A./B.S. only: 76% **Master's:** 24%

Approximate percentage of students who are Women: 83% **Ethnic Minority:** 28% **International:** 4%

Average years to complete the doctoral program (including internship): 5.2 years

Personal interview
Preferred in person but telephone acceptable

Attrition rate in past 7 years: 3%

Percentage of students applying for internship last year accepted into APPIC or APA internships: 24%

Formal tracks/concentrations: child & family track, family/child emphasis, forensic family/child track, gender studies emphasis, health psychology emphasis, multicultural community emphasis, psychodynamic/adult psychotherapy emphasis

Research areas	# Faculty	# Grants
chemical dependency	5	not reported
child and family forensics	2	
family/child	7	
gender studies and LGBT Issues	6	
health psychology	4	
multicultural and community issues	11	
psychodynamics	3	

Clinical opportunities
We have over 225 field placements in almost all areas of psychology, including inpatient, outpatient, and residential treatment programs for children, adolescents, and adults

American University (Ph.D.)

Department of Psychology
Washington, DC 20016
phone#: (202) 885-1726
e-mail: cweissb@american.edu
Web address:
www.american.edu/cas/psych/clinicalprog.html

1	2	3	**4**	5	6	7
Practice oriented		Equal emphasis			Research oriented	

Percentage of faculty subscribing to each of the following orientations:

Psychodynamic/Psychoanalytic	15%
Applied behavioral analysis/Radical behavioral	0%
Family systems/Systems	0%
Existential/Phenomenological/Humanistic	15%
Cognitive/Cognitive-behavioral	70%

Courses required for incoming students to have completed prior to enrolling:
none

Recommended but not mandatory courses:
psychology major, including experimental psychology and statistics

GRE mean
Verbal 668   Quantitative 676   Advanced Psychology 697
Analytical Writing 5.0

GPA mean
Overall GPA 3.6   Psychology GPA 3.5

Number of applications/admission offers/incoming students in 2007
219 applied/12 admission offers/6 incoming

% of students receiving:
Full tuition waiver only: 0%
Assistantship/fellowship only: 0%
Both full tuition waiver & assistantship/fellowship: 83%

Approximate percentage of incoming students with a B.A./B.S. only: 67% **Master's:** 33%

Approximate percentage of students who are Women: 67% **Ethnic Minority:** 16%
International: not reported

Average years to complete the doctoral program (including internship): 6.5 years

Personal interview
Required in person

Attrition rate in past 7 years: 1%

Percentage of students applying for internship last year accepted into APPIC or APA internships: 100%

Formal tracks/concentrations:

Research areas	# Faculty	# Grants
addiction	2	2
anxiety disorders	1	0
child	1	0
coping	1	0
depression	1	0
eating disorders	1	0
treatment cost effectiveness	1	0

Clinical opportunities
cognitive-behavior therapy   psychological testing
person-centered therapy   neuropsychological testing
psychodynamic therapy   externships

Antioch University New England (Psy.D.)

Department of Clinical Psychology
40 Avon Street
Keene, NH 03431
phone#: (603) 357-3122
e-mail: rpeterson@antiochne.edu
Web address: www.antiochne.edu/cp/

1	2	**3**	4	5	6	7
Practice oriented			Equal emphasis			Research oriented

Percentage of faculty subscribing to each of the following orientations:

Psychodynamic/Psychoanalytic	30%
Applied behavioral analysis/Radical behavioral	10%
Family systems/Systems	10%
Existential/Phenomenological/Humanistic	10%
Cognitive/Cognitive-behavioral	20%
Integrative	20%

Courses required for incoming students to have completed prior to enrolling:
Undergraduate or graduate degree in psychology is preferred, at a minimum at least 15 credits of relevant coursework is required.

Recommended but not mandatory courses:
None

GRE mean
Verbal 520   Quantitative 567

GPA mean
Overall GPA 3.25

Number of applications/admission offers/incoming students in 2007
101 applied/64 admission offers/36 incoming

% of students receiving:
Full tuition waiver only: 0%
Assistantship/fellowship only: 18% (small stipends)
Both full tuition waiver & assistantship/fellowship: 0%

Approximate percentage of incoming students with a B.A./B.S. only: 53%   Master's: 47%

Approximate percentage of students who are
Women: 81%   Ethnic Minority: 6%   International: 2%

Average years to complete the doctoral program (including internship): 7 years

Personal interview
Required in person

Attrition rate in past 7 years: 12.8%

Percentage of students applying for internship last year accepted into APPIC or APA internships: 76.9%

Formal tracks/concentrations: child clinical, assessment, adult psychotherapy, and heath psychology

Research areas	# Faculty	# Grants
community services	2	2
children	2	0
health psychology	1	1
graduate training	2	0
group	1	0
multicultural psychology	1	0
outcome evaluation	2	0
women's issues	2	0

Clinical opportunities

assessment	gay and lesbian
battering/abuse	group therapy
behavioral medicine	health psychology
child clinical psychology	neuropsychology/
cognitive/behavioral therapy	rehabilitation
conduct disorders	personality disorders
community services	psychodynamic
counseling center	rural psychology
family therapy	school based: substance
forensic	abuse, supervision

Argosy University–Atlanta Campus (Psy.D.)

Formerly—Georgia School of Professional Psychology
980 Hammond Drive, Suite 100
Atlanta, GA 30328
phone#: (770) 671-1200 or (888) 671-4777
e-mail: tcbrown@argosy.edu
Web address: www.argosy.edu/atlanta

1	**2**	3	4	5	6	7
Practice oriented			Equal emphasis			Research oriented

Percentage of faculty subscribing to each of the following orientations:

Psychodynamic/Psychoanalytic	33%
Applied behavioral analysis/Radical behavioral	0%
Family systems/Systems	25%
Existential/Phenomenological/Humanistic	8%
Cognitive/Cognitive-behavioral	33%

Courses required for incoming students to have completed prior to enrolling:
General psychology, abnormal psychology, and statistics/research methods

Recommended but not mandatory courses:
Tests and measurement, physiological psychology, and personality theory

GRE mean
Verbal 500   Quantitative 500
Advanced Psychology not reported
Analytical Writing not reported

GPA mean
Overall GPA 3.25   Psychology GPA 3.25
Junior/Senior GPA 3.25

Number of applications/admission offers/incoming students in 2007
155 applied/73 admission offers/52 incoming

% of students receiving:
Full tuition waiver only: 0%
Assistantship/fellowship only: 20%
Both full tuition waiver & assistantship/fellowship: 0%

Approximate percentage of incoming students with a B.A./B.S. only: 95%   Master's: 5%

Approximate percentage of students who are
Women: 80%   Ethnic Minority: 20%   International: 2%

Average years to complete the doctoral program (including internship): 6 years

Personal interview
On-campus interview preferred; minimal requirement is telephone interview.

Attrition rate in past 7 years: 12%

Percentage of students applying for internship last year accepted into APPIC or APA internships: 92%

Formal tracks/concentrations: child/family, adult clinical, health psychology, neuropsychology/geropsychology

Research areas	# Faculty	# Grants
geropsychology	0	0
multicultural issues	3	0
neuropsychology	3	0
pediatric psychology	2	0
psychological assessment	4	0
short-term, dynamic therapy	1	0
teenage sexuality	2	0

Clinical opportunities

assessment
adult psychotherapy
child & adolescent
    psychotherapy
crisis intervention
educational assessments
    and consultation
forensic psychology
health psychology
inpatient and outpatient
    clinical services
neuropsychology
rehabilitation medicine
substance abuse
    rehabilitation

Argosy University, Chicago Campus (Psy.D.)
(formerly the Illinois School of Professional Psychology)
350 N. Orleans Street
Chicago, IL 60654
phone#: (312) 777-7600 or (800) 626-4123
e-mail: lhorvath@argosy.edu
Web address: www.argosy.edu/colleges/psychology-behavioral-sciences/Default.aspx

1	2	3	4	5	6	7
Practice oriented		Equal emphasis			Research oriented	

Percentage of faculty subscribing to each of the following orientations:
Psychodynamic/Psychoanalytic 40%
Applied behavioral analysis/Radical behavioral 0%
Family systems/Systems 14%
Existential/Phenomenological/Humanistic 20%
Cognitive/Cognitive-behavioral 26%

Courses required for incoming students to have completed prior to enrolling:
Introductory psychology, abnormal psychology, statistics, tests and measures, personality

Recommended but not mandatory courses:
None

GRE mean
Not reported

GPA mean
Overall GPA 3.3   Psychology GPA 3.3
Junior/Senior GPA 3.3

Number of applications/admission offers/incoming students in 2007
327 applied/163 admission offers/68 incoming

% of students receiving:
Full tuition waiver only: 0%
Assistantship/fellowship only: 14%
Both full tuition waiver & assistantship/fellowship: 0%

Approximate percentage of incoming students with a B.A./B.S. only: 56%   **Master's:** 44%

Approximate percentage of students who are Women: 74%   **Ethnic Minority:** 27%
International: 17%

Average years to complete the doctoral program (including internship): 5.9 years

Personal interview
Preferred in person but telephone acceptable (international students only)

Attrition rate in past 7 years: 11.4%

Percentage of students applying for internship last year accepted into APPIC or APA internships: 70%

Formal tracks/concentrations: child/adolescent psychology, client-centered/experiential psychotherapies, diversity/multicultural psychology, family psychology, forensic psychology, health psychology, organizational consulting, psychoanalytic psychology, psychology & spirituality

Research areas	# Faculty	# Grants
adolescence and delinquency	1	0
behavioral medicine	4	3
diverse students' needs	3	1
eating disorders	1	0
gay men adult development	2	0
international psychology	1	0
parenting	1	0
person-centered interventions	2	0
personality disorders	1	0
play therapy	1	0
romantic relationships	1	0
substance abuse	1	0
therapist development	2	1
therapy of severe mental illness	1	0
trauma recovery	1	0
women's career choices	1	0

Clinical opportunities

behavioral medicine
child and adolescent
    psychology
chronic mental illness
cognitive-behavioral
    psychotherapy
neuropsychology
person-centered and
    experiential psychotherapy
personality disorders
prevention
psychoanalytic psychotherapy

community psychology	refugee populations/trauma
couples	and torture survivors
eating disorders	rehabilitation
emergency crisis	religiously committed clients
ethnic-racial psychology	school-based programs
family psychology	sexual abuse
forensic psychology	short-term psychotherapy
gay/lesbian/bisexual	sports psychology
gerontology	substance abuse
group therapy	victim/abuse/battering

Argosy University, Honolulu Campus (Psy.D.)

400 ASB Tower, 1001 Bishop Street
Honolulu, HI 96813
phone#: (808) 536-5555
e-mail: hawaii@argosy.edu
Web address:
www.argosy.edu/honolulu/programdegrees
.asp?plid=54

1	**2**	3	4	5	6	7
Practice oriented		Equal emphasis			Research oriented	

Percentage of faculty subscribing to each of the following orientations:

Psychodynamic/Psychoanalytic	0%
Applied behavioral analysis/Radical behavioral	0%
Family systems/Systems	28%
Existential/Phenomenological/Humanistic	36%
Cognitive/Cognitive-behavioral	36%

Courses required for incoming students to have completed prior to enrolling:
abnormal psychology, tests and measurements, personality, research methods, statistics

Recommended but not mandatory courses: None

GRE mean
Not reported

GPA mean
Overall 3.7

Number of applications/admission offers/incoming students in 2007
117 applied/86 admission offers/34 incoming

% of students receiving:
Full tuition waiver only: 0%
Assistantship/fellowship only: 5%
Both full tuition waiver & assistantship/fellowship: 0%

Approximate percentage of incoming students with a B.A./B.S. only: 75% **Master's:** 25%

Approximate percentage of students who are Women: 85% **Ethnic Minority:** 50% **International:** 3%

Average years to complete the doctoral program (including internship): 5.72 years (mean)

Personal interview
Preferred in person but telephone acceptable

Attrition rate in past 7 years: 1.8%

Percentage of students applying for internship last year accepted into APPIC or APA internships: 83%

Formal tracks/concentrations: child/family, diversity, health psychology

Research areas	# Faculty	# Grants
diversity education	9	0
gay/lesbian relationships	2	0
health psychology	1	0
neuropsychology	2	0
children	3	0

Clinical opportunities

child and adolescent	outpatient treatment centers
day treatment and hospice programs	psychiatric, medical, and veterans hospitals
community mental health centers	public and private schools
developmental evaluation clinics	state courts, prisons
	substance abuse

Argosy University–Phoenix Campus (Psy.D.)

American School of Professional Psychology
2233 West Dunlap Avenue, Suite 150
Phoenix, AZ 85021
phone#: (602) 216-2600
e-mail: cpinnell@argosy.edu
Web address:
www.argosy.edu/phoenix/programdegrees
.asp?plid=136

1	**2**	3	4	5	6	7
Practice oriented		Equal emphasis			Research oriented	

Percentage of faculty subscribing to each of the following orientations:

Psychodynamic/Psychoanalytic	0%
Applied behavioral analysis/Radical behavioral	9%
Family systems/Systems	9%
Existential/Phenomenological/Humanistic	0%
Cognitive/Cognitive-behavioral	36%

Courses required for incoming students to have completed prior to enrolling:
Personality, abnormal psychology, test and measurement, psychological assessment, statistics or research methods.

Recommended but not mandatory courses:
none

GRE mean
not reported

GPA mean
Overall 3.52

Number of applications/admission offers/incoming students in 2006–2007
137 applied/67 admission offers/48 incoming

% of students receiving:
Full tuition waiver only: 0%
Assistantship/fellowship only: 0%
Both full tuition waiver & assistantship/fellowship: 0%

Approximate percentage of incoming students with a B.A./B.S. only: 75%   **Master's:** 25%

Approximate percentage of students who are Women: 80%   **Ethnic Minority:** 16%
International: not reported

Average years to complete the doctoral program (including internship): 5 years

Personal interview
Preferred in person but telephone acceptable

Attrition rate in past 7 years: not reported

Percentage of students applying for internship last year accepted into APPIC or APA internships: 91%

Formal tracks/concentrations:

Research areas	# Faculty	# Grants
diversity	5	0
learning disability/ADHD	1	0
neuropsychology	1	0
psychopharmacology	1	0
geopsychology	1	0
health	2	0

Clinical opportunities
None as a part of the school, but we do offer a diverse array of practicum placement in specialty clinics, including but not limited to sexual offender treatment, substance abuse, pain management, neuropsychology, surgical centers, schools and specialty schools, inpatient and outpatient psychotherapy, HIV/AIDS, and culturally diverse sites.

Argosy University–San Francisco Bay Area Campus (Psy.D.)

American School of Professional Psychology
1005 Atlantic Avenue
Alameda, CA 94501
Telephone number: 1-866-215-2777
Fax: (510) 217-4800
Email address: jstfan@argosy.edu or
alrappaport@argosy.edu
Website:
www.argosy.edu/colleges/ProgramDetail.aspx?ID=732

1	2	3	4	5	6	7
Practice oriented		Equal emphasis			Research oriented	

Percentage of faculty subscribing to each of the following orientations:
Psychodynamic/Psychoanalytic   50%
Applied behavioral analysis/Radical behavioral   10%
Family systems/Systems   30%
Existential/Phenomenological/Humanistic   5%
Cognitive/Cognitive-behavioral   5%

Courses required for incoming students to have completed prior to enrolling:
abnormal, tests & measures, statistics or research methods, personality

Recommended but not mandatory courses:
psychology major

GRE mean
not reported

GPA mean
not reported

Number of applications/admission offers/incoming students in 2007
196 applied/124 admission offers

% of students receiving:
Full tuition waiver only: not reported
Assistantship/fellowship only: not reported
Both tuition waiver & assistantship/fellowship: not reported

Approximate percentage of incoming students with a B.A./B.S. only: Master's:

Approximate percentage of students who are Women:82%   **Ethnic Minority:** 32%   **International:** 5%

Average years to complete the doctoral program (including internship): 4 years

Personal interview
Preferred in person, but telephone acceptable.

Attrition rate in past 7 years: not reported

Percentage of students applying for internship last year accepted into APPIC or APA internships: 26%

Formal tracks/concentrations: none

Research areas	# Faculty	# Grants
HIV	1	0
substance Abuse	1	0

Clinical opportunities
family therapy
forensic agencies
neuropsychological assessment
severely disordered clients
substance abuse treatment
University counseling departments
cultural diversity (including Spanish and Asian dialects)
disability-focused agencies
school-based agencies

Argosy University–Schaumburg Campus (Psy.D.)

(Illinois School of Professional Psychology)
Rolling Meadows, IL 60008
phone#: (847) 290-7400
e-mail: admissionscnw@argosy.edu
Web address: www.argosy.edu/schaumburg

1	2	3	4	5	6	7
Practice oriented		Equal emphasis			Research oriented	

Percentage of faculty subscribing to each of the following orientations:

Psychodynamic/Psychoanalytic	17%
Applied behavioral analysis/Radical behavioral	0%
Family systems/Systems	17%
Existential/Phenomenological/Humanistic	25%
Cognitive/Cognitive-behavioral	25%

Courses required for incoming students to have completed prior to enrolling:

Abnormal psychology, tests and measurement (or intro to psychological assessment), personality theory, introductory statistics

Recommended but not mandatory courses:
none

GRE mean
not reported

GPA mean
not reported

Number of applications/admission offers/incoming students in 2007
not reported

% of students receiving:
Full tuition waiver only: 0%
Assistantship/fellowship only: 25%
Both full tuition waiver & assistantship/fellowship: 0%

Approximate percentage of incoming students with a B.A./B.S. only: 51%   Master's: 49%

Approximate percentage of students who are Women: 78%   Ethnic Minority: 14%
International: not reported

Average years to complete the doctoral program (including internship): 5.2 years

Personal interview
Required in person

Attrition rate in past 7 years: not reported

Percentage of students applying for internship last year accepted into APPIC or APA internships: not reported

Formal tracks/concentrations: none

Research areas	# Faculty	# Grants
ADHD and child externalizing	1	0
cultural bias in psychological testing	2	0
effectiveness of process	2	1
experiential therapy	3	1
family therapy effectiveness	1	0
men's perception of psychotherapy	1	0
multicultural training	2	1
psychotherapy process and outcome	2	1
stigma in mental illness identity	1	1
substance abuse program evaluation	1	1
treatment of domestic violence	2	0

Clinical opportunities
Numerous sites available; more than 200 practicum sites in greater Chicago area. Specialization sites include:
  child and pediatric psychology
  college counseling center
  community mental health
  correctional psychology
  family and marital counseling
  forensics
  health and medical psychology
  inpatient psychiatric hospital, adult and adolescent
  neuropsychological assessment
  rehabilitation
  severely mentally ill
  substance abuse

Argosy University–Twin Cities Campus (Psy.D.)
Clinical Psychology Program
Graduate Admissions
Argosy University/Twin Cities
1515 Central Parkway
Eagan, MN 55121
phone#: (888) 844-2004
e-mail: tcadmissions@argosy.edu
Web address: www.argosy.edu

1	2	3	4	5	6	7
Practice oriented		Equal emphasis			Research oriented	

Percentage of faculty subscribing to each of the following orientations:

Psychodynamic/Psychoanalytic	35%
Applied behavioral analysis/Radical behavioral	0%
Family systems/Systems	20%
Existential/Phenomenological/Humanistic	20%
Cognitive/Cognitive-behavioral	25%

Courses required for incoming students to have completed prior to enrolling:
4 psychology courses and 1 statistics course

Recommended but not mandatory courses:
none

GRE mean
not reported

GPA mean
3.55 for students applying with a BA; 3.26 for students applying with an MA

Number of applications/admission offers/incoming students in 2007
183 applied/93 admission offers/59 incoming

% of students receiving:
Full tuition waiver only: 0%
Assistantship/fellowship only: 35%
Both full tuition waiver & assistantship/fellowship: 0%

Approximate percentage of incoming students with a B.A./B.S. only: 70%   Master's: 30%

Approximate percentage of students who are
Women: 75%   **Ethnic Minority:** 15%
International: < 5%

Average years to complete the doctoral program (including internship): 5 years

Personal interview
Required in person

Attrition rate in past 7 years: 6.7%

Percentage of students applying for internship last year accepted into APPIC or APA internships: 75%

Formal tracks/concentrations: forensic psychology, health psychology, psychology and trauma, child clinical

Research areas	# Faculty	# Grants
properties of Rorschach	2	0
psychotherapy outcome	2	0
attachment disorders	1	0
multicultural competence	2	0

Clinical opportunities
Over 100 practicum sites in the greater Twin Cities area

Argosy University–Washington, DC Campus (Psy.D.)

1550 Wilson Boulevard, Suite 600
Washington, DC 22209
phone#: 703-526-5800
e-mail: rbarrett@argosy.edu
Web address: www.argosy.edu

1	2	3	4	5	6	7

Practice oriented   Equal emphasis   Research oriented

Percentage of faculty subscribing to each of the following orientations:

Psychodynamic/Psychoanalytic	57%
Applied behavioral analysis/Radical behavioral	0%
Family systems/Systems	21%
Existential/Phenomenological/Humanistic	36%
Cognitive/Cognitive-behavioral	64%

Courses required for incoming students to have completed prior to enrolling:
Statistics or research methods, abnormal psychology, plus two other psychology courses

Recommended but not mandatory courses:
None

GRE mean
not reported

GPA mean
Overall 3.25

Number of applications/admission offers/incoming students in 2007
345 applied/166 admission offers/83 incoming

% of students receiving:
Full tuition waiver only: 0%
Assistantship/fellowship only: 11%
Both full tuition waiver & assistantship/fellowship: 11%

Approximate percentage of incoming students with a B.A./B.S. only: 51%   **Master's:** 45%

Approximate percentage of students who are
Women: 81.5%   **Ethnic Minority:** 31%
International: not reported

Average years to complete the doctoral program (including internship): 5 years

Personal interview
Preferred in person but telephone acceptable

Attrition rate in past 7 years: 4%

Percentage of students applying for internship last year accepted into APPIC or APA internships: 87%

Formal tracks/concentrations: forensic concentration, child and family concentration, health and neuropsychology concentration, diversity concentration

Research areas	# Faculty	# Grants
cognitive attributions	1	0
multicultural competence	1	0

Clinical opportunities

anxiety disorders/OCD	sexual orientation
child abuse	school mental health
children's hospitals	substance abuse
forensic hospitals/prisons	university counseling center
gerontology	community mental health
neuropsychology	centers
posttraumatic stress disorder	

University of Arizona (Ph.D.)

Department of Psychology
Psychology Building
Tucson, AZ 85721
phone#: (520) 621-1867
e-mail: varda@u.arizona.edu
Web address:
psychology.arizona.edu/programs/g_each/clinical.php

1	2	3	4	5	6	7

Practice oriented   Equal emphasis   Research oriented

Percentage of faculty subscribing to each of the following orientations:

Psychodynamic/Psychoanalytic	0%
Applied behavioral analysis/Radical behavioral	5%
Family systems/Systems	30%
Existential/Phenomenological/Humanistic	5%
Cognitive/Cognitive-behavioral	60%

Courses required for incoming students to have completed prior to enrolling:
B.A. or B.S. in psychology; abnormal psychology; statistics and methods.

137

Recommended but not mandatory courses:
Social, biological psychology, cognitive, and developmental

GRE mean
Verbal 626   Quantitative 691
Advanced Psychology 701

GPA mean
Overall GPA 3.6

Number of applications/admission offers/incoming students in 2007
205 applied/8 admission offers/6 incoming

% of students receiving:
Full tuition waiver only: 0%
Assistantship/fellowship only: 0%
Both full tuition waiver & assistantship/fellowship: 100%

Approximate percentage of incoming students with a B.A./B.S. only: 80%   **Master's:** 20%

Approximate percentage of students who are Women: 60%   **Ethnic Minority:** 22%
International: 15%

Average years to complete the doctoral program (including internship): 6 years

Personal interview
Preferred in person but telephone acceptable

Attrition rate in past 7 years: 6%

Percentage of students applying for internship last year accepted into APPIC or APA internships: 80-90%

Formal tracks/concentrations: none

Research areas	# Faculty	# Grants
clinical neuropsychology	2	2
depression	2	2
family systems	2	4
health psychology	6	6
mental health policy	2	1
sleep disorders	1	2
treatment outcome	3	4

Clinical opportunities

individual therapy	depression
empirically supported	gerontology
treatments	neuropsychology/
behavioral medicine	rehabilitation
community psychology	sleep disorders
couple and family therapy	

Arizona State University (Ph.D.)

Department of Psychology
Tempe, AZ 85287-1104
phone#: (480) 965-7606
e-mail: Manuel.Barrera@asu.edu
Web address:
www.asu.edu/clas/psych/gprogram/clinical/

1	2	3	4	5	**6**	7
Practice oriented		Equal emphasis			Research oriented	

Percentage of faculty subscribing to each of the following orientations:

Psychodynamic/Psychoanalytic	0%
Applied behavioral analysis/Radical behavioral	5%
Family systems/Systems	30%
Existential/Phenomenological/Humanistic	0%
Cognitive/Cognitive-behavioral	65%

Courses required for incoming students to have completed prior to enrolling:
B.A. in psychology or equivalent

Recommended but not mandatory courses:
None

GRE mean
Verbal 651   Quantitative 687
Analytical Writing 5.14

GPA mean
Overall GPA 3.83

Number of applications/admission offers/incoming students in 2007
270 applied/16 admission offers/7 incoming

% of students receiving:
Full tuition waiver only: 0%
Full assistantship/fellowship only: 0%
Both full tuition waiver & assistantship/fellowship: 100%

Approximate percentage of incoming students with a B.A./B.S. only: 90%   **Master's:** 10%

Approximate percentage of students who are Women: 75%   **Ethnic Minority:** 27%   **International:** 2%

Average years to complete the doctoral program (including internship): 6.6 years

Personal interview
Preferred in person but telephone acceptable

Attrition rate in past 7 years: 19%

Percentage of students applying for internship last year accepted into APPIC or APA internships: 87.5%

Formal tracks/concentrations: child clinical, community/ prevention, health

Research areas	# Faculty	# Grants
aging/gerontology	2	2
behavioral medicine/health psychology	7	6
child clinical	5	15
community psychology	6	11
family interactions	4	4
gender roles	1	1
hispanic studies	3	6
minority mental health	6	11
personality assessment	1	0
prevention	6	9
psychoneuroimmunology	3	3
substance abuse	2	4

Clinical opportunities

behavioral analysis
behavioral medicine
child clinical psychology
child health psychology
family therapy
geropsychology

individual therapy
intellectual and academic
  assessment
marital/couples therapy
parenting groups
prevention programs

University of Arkansas (Ph.D.)

Department of Psychology
216 Memorial Hall
Fayetteville, AR 72701
phone#: (479) 575-4256
e-mail: tcavell@uark.edu
Web address: www.uark.edu/depts/psyc/clinical.htm

1	2	3	4	**5**	6	7

Practice oriented   Equal emphasis   Research oriented

Percentage of faculty subscribing to each of the following orientations:

Psychodynamic/Psychoanalytic	0%
Applied behavioral analysis/Radical behavioral	30%
Family systems/Systems	50%
Existential/Phenomenological/Humanistic	15%
Cognitive/Cognitive-behavioral	100%

Courses required for incoming students prior to enrolling:
Core courses in the science of psychology.

Courses recommended but not mandatory:
18 semester hours in psychology including statistics, learning, and experimental psychology

GRE mean
Verbal 581   Quantitative 649
Analytical Writing 5.28

GPA mean
Overall GPA 3.77

Number of applications/admission offers/incoming students in 2007
109 applied/9 admission offers/5 incoming

% of students receiving:
Full tuition waiver only: 0%
Assistantship/fellowship only: 0%
Both full tuition waiver & assistantship/fellowship: 100%

Approximate percentage of incoming students with a B.A./B.S. only: 80%   **Master's:** 20%

Approximate percentage of students who are Women: 70%   **Ethnic Minority:** 15%   **International:** 0%

Average years to complete the doctoral program (including internship): 6 years

Personal interview

Attrition rate in past 7 years: 7%

Percentage of students applying for internship last year accepted into APPIC or APA internships: 89%

Formal tracks/concentrations: none

Research areas	# Faculty	# Grants
aggression & victimization	3	1
child and family interventions	2	0
cognitive vulnerability to anxiety and depression	2	0
emotion regulation and psychopathology	3	0
family, parent, couples relationships	3	0
science and psuedoscience in psychological practice	1	0
substance abuse/addictions	2	2

Clinical opportunities

ADHD clinic
community mental health
developmental pediatrics

school-based mental health
substance abuse
neuropsychological assessment

Auburn University (Ph.D.)

Department of Psychology
226 Thach
Auburn, AL 36849
phone#: (334) 844-6471
e-mail: bryangt@mail.auburn.edu
Web address:
www.cla.auburn.edu/psychology/gs/prospective/clinical/index.htm

1	2	3	**4**	5	6	7

Practice oriented   Equal emphasis   Research oriented

Percentage of faculty subscribing to each of the following orientations:

Psychodynamic/Psychoanalytic	10%
Applied behavioral analysis/Radical behavioral	20%
Family systems/Systems	45%
Existential/Phenomenological/Humanistic	10%
Cognitive/Cognitive-behavioral	100%

Courses required for incoming students to have completed prior to enrolling:
Strong foundation in theoretical or experimental psychology and quantitative methods

Recommended but not mandatory courses:
History of Psychology, second course in statistics

GRE mean
Verbal + Quantitative 1200

GPA mean
Overall GPA 3.7

Number of applications/admission offers/incoming students in 2007
165 applied/12 admission offers/9 incoming

% of students receiving:
Full tuition waiver only: 0%
Assistantship/fellowship only: 0%
Both full tuition waiver & assistantship/fellowship: 100%

Approximate percentage of incoming students with a B.A./B.S. only: 75% **Master's:** 25%

Approximate percentage of students who are Women: 70% **Ethnic Minority:** 13% **International:** 4%

Average years to complete the doctoral program (including internship): 6 years

Personal interview
Required in person

Attrition rate in past 7 years: 15%

Percentage of students applying for internship last year accepted into APPIC or APA internships: 100%

Formal tracks/concentrations: clinical child psychology

Research areas	# Faculty	# Grants
anxiety disorders	2	0
child clinical/psychopathology	3	1
developmental disabilities	1	1
personality assessment	1	0
sexuality/deviation/dysfunction	1	1
marital relations	1	0

Clinical opportunities

anxiety disorders	posttraumatic stress disorder
disorders in adolescence	substance abuse
ADHD/LD	Autism spectrum disorder

Azusa Pacific University (Psy.D.)

Department of Psychology
901 East Alosta Avenue
Azusa, CA 91702-7000
phone#: (626) 815-5008
e-mail: rwelsh@apu.edu
Web address:
www.apu.edu/bas/graduatepsychology/psyd

1	2	3	4	5	6	7

Practice oriented	Equal emphasis	Research oriented

Percentage of faculty subscribing to each of the following orientations:

Psychodynamic/Psychoanalytic	42%
Applied behavioral analysis/Radical behavioral	0%
Family systems/Systems	58%
Existential/Phenomenological/Humanistic	25%
Cognitive/Cognitive-behavioral	33%

Courses required for incoming students to have completed prior to enrolling:
Master's-level courses: child abuse (7 hours), family therapy, human sexuality/sex therapy, clinical practice, psychological testing, psychopathology, cultural diversity, theories of personality and psychotherapy.
Bachelor's-level courses: Abnormal psychology, human development, theories of personality, statistics

Recommended but not mandatory courses:
none

GRE mean
Verbal 495   Quantitative 557
Analytical Writing 4.7

GPA mean
Overall GPA Master's 3.7   Bachelor's 3.34

Number of applications/admission offers/incoming students in 2007
106 applied/40 admission offers/26 incoming

% of students receiving:
Full tuition waiver only: 0%
Assistantship/fellowship only: 11%
Both full tuition waiver & assistantship/fellowship: 0%

Approximate percentage of incoming students with a B.A./B.S. only: 76% **Master's:** 24%

Approximate percentage of students who are Women: 68% **Ethnic Minority:** 35% **International:** 3%

Average years to complete the doctoral program (including internship): 5 years

Personal interview
Preferred in person but telephone acceptable

Attrition rate in past 7 years: 14%

Percentage of students applying for internship last year accepted into APPIC or APA internships: 85%

Formal tracks/concentrations: family psychology, forensic psychology

Research areas	# Faculty	# Grants
family psychology	2	0
diversity/multiculturalism	2	0
child and adolescent	2	1
counseling skills	2	1
psychological assessment	2	0
forensics	3	1
homelessness/HIV	1	0
moral development	2	1
religion/spirituality	4	1
school-based interventions	2	1
neuropsychology	1	0

Clinical opportunities

behavior medicine	geriatric
children and family	HIV/AIDS
chronically mentally ill	inpatient: acute and chronic
community clinics	school-based
forensics	substance abuse
general population	university counseling

Baylor University (Psy.D.)

Department of Psychology
P.O. Box 97334
Waco, TX 76798-7334
phone#: (254) 710-2961; 254-757-0535
e-mail: Gary_Elkins@baylor.edu
Web address:
www.baylor.edu/psychologyneuroscience/index.php?id=21323

1	2	3	4	5	6	7
Practice oriented		Equal emphasis			Research oriented	

Percentage of faculty subscribing to each of the following orientations:

Psychodynamic/Psychoanalytic	15%
Applied behavioral analysis/Radical behavioral	0%
Family systems/Systems	15%
Existential/Phenomenological/Humanistic	15%
Cognitive/Cognitive-behavioral	55%

Courses required for incoming students to have completed prior to enrolling:
none

Recommended but not mandatory courses:
developmental psychology, psychopathology, statistics, biopsychology, personality, social

GRE mean
Verbal 663   Quantitative 673
Analytical Writing Data not available

GPA mean
Overall GPA 3.73   Psychology GPA 3.7
Junior/Senior GPA 3.7

Number of applications/admission offers/incoming students in 2007
157 applied/7 admission offers/7 incoming

% of students receiving:
Full tuition waiver only: 0%
Assistantship/fellowship only: 0%
Both full tuition waiver & assistantship/fellowship: 100%

Approximate percentage of incoming students with a B.A./B.S. only: 71%   Master's: 29%

Approximate percentage of students who are
Women: 71%   Ethnic Minority: 14%
International: Data not available

Average years to complete the doctoral program (including internship): 5 years

Personal interview
Required in person

Attrition rate in past 7 years: 8.7%

Percentage of students applying for internship last year accepted into APPIC or APA internships: 100%

Formal tracks/concentrations:

Research areas	# Faculty	# Grants
behavioral medicine	1	0
child psychopathology	2	0
cognitive therapy	3	0
depression	3	0
group therapy	1	0
personality assessment	3	0

Clinical opportunities

alcohol and drug dependence	impulse control mood disorders
anxiety disorders	neuropsychology
behavioral medicine	personality disorder

child psychotherapy	play therapy
community psychology	rural psychology
crisis intervention	schizophrenia/psychoses
eating disorders	school/educational
family therapy	sexual offenders
gerontology	suicide prevention
group dynamics	suicide risk assessment and
group therapy	treatment
health psychology	victim/battering/abuse

Binghamton University/State University of New York (Ph.D.)
Department of Psychology
Vestal Parkway East
Binghamton, NY 13902-6000
phone#: (607) 777-2334
e-mail: clinpsyc@binghamton.edu
Web address:
psychology.binghamton.edu/Clinical/index.html

1	2	3	4	5	6	7
Practice oriented		Equal emphasis			Research oriented	

Percentage of faculty subscribing to each of the following orientations:

Psychodynamic/Psychoanalytic	10%
Applied behavioral analysis/Radical behavioral	10%
Family systems/Systems	0%
Existential/Phenomenological/Humanistic	0%
Cognitive/Cognitive-behavioral	80%

Courses required for incoming students prior to enrolling:
Equivalent of a psychology major, with knowledge of experimental psychology and research methods

Courses recommended but not mandatory:
Physiological psychology

GRE mean
Verbal 580   Quantitative 664
Analytical Writing 5.0   Advanced Psychology 630

GPA mean
Overall GPA 3.8

Number of applications/admission offers/incoming students in 2007
215 applied/15 admission offers/8 incoming

% of students receiving:
Full tuition waiver only: 0%
Assistantship/fellowship only: 0%
Both full tuition waiver & assistantship/fellowship: 100%

Approximate percentage of students who are
Women: 77%   Ethnic Minority: 12%   International: 5%

Average years to complete the doctoral program (including internship): 6.25 years

Personal interview
Strongly preferred in person but telephone possible

Attrition rate in past 7 years: 13%

Percentage of students applying for internship last year accepted into APPIC or APA internships: 100%

Formal tracks/concentrations: none

Research areas	# Faculty	# Grants
adult psychopathology	8	2
anxiety disorders	2	1
assessment	4	0
autism spectrum disorders	1	1
behavioral medicine	1	1
child clinical	2	2
depression	1	1
developmental disabilities	1	2
hypnosis	1	1
learning disabilities	1	1
marital process and therapy	1	1
memory construction	2	0
neuropsychology	1	2
pain management	1	1
pediatric psychology	1	1
personality disorders	1	1
posttraumatic stress disorder/trauma	2	0
prevention	3	1
psychophysiology	2	0
social skills	1	0
substance abuse	1	1

Clinical opportunities

adolescent delinquency	disorders of childhood
adult psychopathology	family therapy
anxiety disorders	learning disabilities
autism spectrum disorders	neuropsychology
behavioral medicine	pain management
conduct disorder	psychotherapy supervision
correctional facility	schizophrenia
couples therapy	school consultation
depression	substance abuse

Biola University (Ph.D.)
Rosemead School of Psychology
13800 Biola Avenue
La Mirada, CA 90639
phone#: (562) 903-4752
e-mail: admissions@biola.edu
Web address: www.rosemead.edu/programs/phd.cfm

1	2	**3**	4	5	6	7
Practice oriented		Equal emphasis			Research oriented	

Percentage of faculty subscribing to each of the following orientations:

Psychodynamic/Psychoanalytic	54%
Applied behavioral analysis/Radical behavioral	0%
Family systems/Systems	15%
Existential/Phenomenological/Humanistic	8%
Cognitive/Cognitive-behavioral	23%

Courses required for incoming students to have completed prior to enrolling:
Statistics, experimental psychology, abnormal psychology, personality, learning

Recommended but not mandatory courses:
Social psychology, history of psychology, physiological psychology, biology/zoology, developmental psychology

GRE mean
Verbal + Quantitative 1275
Analytical Writing not reported

GPA mean
3.6

Number of applications/admission offers/incoming students in 2007
153 applied/15 admission offers/7 incoming

% of students receiving:
Full tuition waiver only: 2%
Assistantship/fellowship only: 60%
Both full tuition waiver & assistantship/fellowship: 0%

Approximate percentage of incoming students with a B.A./B.S. only: 78% **Master's:** 32%

Approximate percentage of students who are Women: 67% **Ethnic Minority:** 35%
International: 25%

Average years to complete the doctoral program (including internship): 6 years

Personal interview
Required in person

Attrition rate in past 7 years: 10%

Percentage of students applying for internship last year accepted into APPIC or APA internships: 100%

Formal tracks/concentrations: none

Research areas	# Faculty	# Grants
cross-cultural adjustment	4	0
grief	1	0
neuropsychology	1	0
object relations	4	0
parenting behaviors	3	0
spirituality	4	2

Clinical opportunities

cultural and individual diversity	individual outpatient/inpatient
family/child	therapy and spirituality

Biola University (Psy.D.)
Rosemead School of Psychology
13800 Biola Avenue
La Mirada, CA 90639
phone#: (562) 903-4752
e-mail: admissions@biola.edu
Web address: www.rosemead.edu/programs/psyd.cfm

1	**2**	3	4	5	6	7
Practice oriented		Equal emphasis			Research oriented	

Percentage of faculty subscribing to each of the following orientations:

Psychodynamic/Psychoanalytic	54%
Applied behavioral analysis/Radical behavioral	0%
Family systems/Systems	15%
Existential/Phenomenological/Humanistic	8%
Cognitive/Cognitive-behavioral	23%

Courses required for incoming students to have completed prior to enrolling:
introductory psychology, statistics, experimental psychology, abnormal psychology, personality, learning

Recommended but not mandatory courses:
social psychology, history of psychology, physiological psychology, biology/zoology, developmental psychology

GRE mean
Verbal + Quantitative 1100
Analytical Writing not reported

GPA mean
3.5

Number of applications/admission offers/incoming students in 2007
153 applied/17 admission offers/11 incoming

% of students receiving:
Full tuition waiver only: 5%
Assistantship/fellowship only: 60%
Both full tuition waiver & assistantship/fellowship: 0%

Approximate percentage of incoming students who entered with a B.A./B.S. only: 60% **Master's:** 40%

Approximate percentage of students who are Women: 65% **Ethnic Minority:** 25% **International:** 12%

Average years to complete the doctoral program (including internship): 6 years

Personal interview
Required in person

Attrition rate in past 7 years: 10%

Percentage of students applying for internship last year accepted into APPIC or APA internships: 75%

Formal tracks/concentrations: none

Research areas	# Faculty	# Grants
cross-cultural adjustment	4	0
gender issues	2	1
grief	1	0
neuropsychology	1	1
object relations	4	0
parenting behaviors	3	0
spirituality	4	2

Clinical opportunities
cultural and individual diversity
family/child
individual
outpatient/inpatient
therapy and spirituality

Boston University (Ph.D.)
Department of Psychology
64 Cummington Street
Boston, MA 02215
phone#: (617) 353-2587
e-mail: nclement@bu.edu
Web address: www.bu.edu/psych/graduate/clinical/

1	2	3	**4**	5	6	7

Practice oriented   Equal emphasis   Research oriented

Percentage of faculty subscribing to each of the following orientations:

Psychodynamic/Psychoanalytic	5%
Applied behavioral analysis/Radical behavioral	0%
Family systems/Systems	17%
Existential/Phenomenological/Humanistic	0%
Cognitive/Cognitive-behavioral	70%
Eclectic	10%

Courses required for incoming students to have completed prior to enrolling:
Statistics, abnormal/clinical psychology, experimental

Recommended but not mandatory courses:
Broad liberal arts and science

GRE mean
Verbal + Quantitative 1300
Analytical Writing 4.5

GPA mean
Overall GPA 3.6

Number of applications/admission offers/incoming students in 2007
577 applied/17 admission offers/13 incoming

% of students receiving:
Full tuition waiver only: 0%
Assistantship/fellowship only: 0%
Both full tuition waiver & assistantship/fellowship: 92%

Approximate percentage of incoming students with a B.A./B.S. only: 80% **Master's:** 20%

Approximate percentage of students who are Women: 85% **Ethnic Minority:** 25% **International:** 10%

Average years to complete the doctoral program (including internship): 6.5 years

Personal interview
Required in person

Attrition rate in past 7 years: 3.8%

Percentage of students applying for internship last year accepted into APPIC or APA internships: 100%

Formal tracks/concentrations: adult clinical, child clinical, neuropsychology

Research areas	# Faculty	# Grants
affective disorders	2	2
anxiety disorders	7	5
behavioral genetics	1	1
community psychology	2	0
emotion	3	1
family	2	1
gender	1	0
gerontology	2	2
minority	2	0
neuropsychology	3	2
personality disorders	1	0
schizophrenia	1	1
substance abuse and addiction	1	1
victim/abuse	1	0
women's emotional health	1	0

Clinical opportunities

abuse/battering
adolescents
affective disorders
behavioral medicine
community psychology
couples therapy
dissociative disorders
eating disorders
family therapy
gerontology
neuropsychology
schizophrenia

Bowling Green State University (Ph.D.)

Department of Psychology
Bowling Green, OH 43403
phone#: (419) 372-2301
e-mail: pwatson@bgsu.edu
Web address:
www.bgsu.edu/departments/psych/page31041.html

1	2	3	**4**	5	6	7

Practice oriented   Equal emphasis   Research oriented

Percentage of faculty subscribing to each of the following orientations:

Psychodynamic/Psychoanalytic	20%
Applied behavioral analysis/Radical behavioral	0%
Family systems/Systems	30%
Existential/Phenomenological/Humanistic	20%
Cognitive/Cognitive-behavioral	65%

Courses required for incoming students to have completed prior to enrolling:
none

Recommended but not mandatory courses:
science, math, statistics, introductory and advanced psychology courses, abnormal, psychology lab courses

GRE mean
Verbal 578   Quantitative 645
Analytical Writing not used for admissions decisions

GPA mean
Overall GPA 3.84   Psychology GPA 3.84

Number of applications/admission offers/incoming students in 2007
119 applied/13 admission offers/6 incoming

% of students receiving:
Full tuition waiver only: 0%
Assistantship/fellowship only: 0%
Both full tuition waiver & assistantship/fellowship: 100%

**Approximate percentage of students who are
Women:** 84%   **Ethnic Minority:** 17%   **International:** 7%

Average years to complete the doctoral program (including internship): 5.5 years

Personal interview
Preferred in person but telephone acceptable

Attrition rate in past 7 years: 2%

Percentage of students applying for internship last year accepted into APPIC or APA internships: 100%

Formal tracks/concentrations: behavioral medicine, child clinical psychology, community psychology

Research areas	# Faculty	# Grants
alcohol and substance abuse	1	0
child clinical psychology	2	1
community psychology	1	1
family	2	0
health psychology	2	1
psychology of religion	2	1

Clinical opportunities

behavioral medicine
child clinical psychology
clinical health psychology
community mental health
community psychology
family
school-based assessment/
  intervention

Brigham Young University (Ph.D.)

Department of Psychology
284 TLRB
Provo, UT 84602
phone#: (801) 422-4050
e-mail: sally_barlow@byu.edu
Web address:
fhss.byu.edu/psych/Graduate/Clinical/CPHD.html

1	2	**3**	4	5	6	7

Practice oriented   Equal emphasis   Research oriented

Percentage of faculty subscribing to each of the following orientations:

Psychodynamic/Psychoanalytic	20%
Applied behavioral analysis/Radical behavioral	20%
Family systems/Systems	10%
Existential/Phenomenological/Humanistic	50%
Cognitive/Cognitive-behavioral	70%

Courses required for incoming students prior to enrolling:
psychological statistics, research design, abnormal psychology, personality, learning or cognition, tests and measurements

Courses recommended but not mandatory:
Additional coursework in areas of interest may be helpful

GRE mean
Verbal 600   Quantitative 670
Analytical Writing Data 5.0

GPA mean
Overall GPA not reported Junior/Senior GPA 3.80

Number of applications/admission offers/incoming students in 2007
60 applied/9 admission offers/9 incoming

% of students receiving tuition waiver & assistantship/fellowship:
All 1st-year students receive assistantships and a waiver for part of their tuition. All 2nd-, 3rd-, and 4th-year students are funded in work settings, which are coordinated by the department, and they also receive a waiver for part of their tuition.

Approximate percentage of incoming students with a B.A./B.S. only: 80%   **Master's:** 20%

Approximate percentage of students who are Women: 42%   **Ethnic Minority:** 23%   **International:** 17%

Average years to complete the doctoral program (including internship): 5.5 years

Personal interview
In-person interview preferred, but telephone possible

Attrition rate in past 7 years: 3%

Percentage of students applying for internship last year accepted into APPIC or APA internships: 92%

Formal tracks/concentrations: neuropsychology, child/adolescent

Research areas	# Faculty	# Grants
autism	1	1
child/adolescent development	3	1
clinical assessment	2	0
cultural diversity/gender issues	2	1
depression and cognitive-behavioral therapy	1	1
eating disorders	1	1
group therapy, process and outcome	3	1
health psychology/behavioral medicine	2	1
individual therapy, process, outcome	4	1
measurement	3	1
neuropsychology	2	4
psychopathology	2	0

Clinical opportunities
adolescent residential treatment facilities
community mental health centers
neuropsychology rehabilitation units
private general hospitals—behavioral medicine, psychiatric units
private practices
residential facilities for eating disorders
school districts
state hospital
state prison
university counseling centers

University of British Columbia (Ph.D.)
Department of Psychology
2316 West Mall
Vancouver, British Columbia V6T 1Z4, Canada
phone#: (604) 822-2755
e-mail: gradsec@psych.ubc.ca
Web address: www.psych.ubc.ca/grad-pgm/
areasspec.psy?contid=101306171911

1	2	3	4	5	6	7
Practice oriented		Equal emphasis			Research oriented	

Percentage of faculty subscribing to each of the following orientations:

Psychodynamic/Psychoanalytic	10%
Applied behavioral analysis/Radical behavioral	0%
Family systems/Systems	0%
Existential/Phenomenological/Humanistic	0%
Cognitive/Cognitive-behavioral	90%

Courses required for incoming students prior to enrolling:
None

Courses recommended but not mandatory:
Statistics, abnormal behavior, and a cross-section of other psychology courses

GRE mean
Verbal 610   Quantitative 704   Analytical 704

GPA mean
Overall GPA M = 86%

Number of applications/admission offers/incoming students in 2007
125 applied/7 admission offers/4 incoming

% of students receiving:
Full tuition waiver only: 0%
Assistantship/fellowship only: 100%
Both full tuition waiver & assistantship/fellowship: 0%

Approximate percentage of incoming students with a B.A./B.S. only: 100%   **Master's:** 0%

Approximate percentage of students who are Women: 90%   **Ethnic Minority:** 12%
International:

Average years to complete the doctoral program (including internship): 7.2 years

Personal interview
Telephone required

Attrition rate in past 7 years: 12%

Percentage of students applying for internship last year accepted into APPIC or APA internships: 100%

Formal tracks/concentrations: none

Research areas	# Faculty	# Grants
anxiety disorders	3	5
attention-deficit disorder	1	3
behavioral medicine	1	3
health psychology	0	0
sexual dysfunction	1	1

Clinical opportunities

assessment
behavioral medicine
child and adult

forensic psychology
hospital settings

University at Buffalo/State University of New York (Ph.D.)

Department of Psychology
Park Hall
Buffalo, NY 14260
phone#: (716) 645-3650, ext. #235
e-mail: ccolder@buffalo.edu
Web address:
www.psychology.buffalo.edu/graduate/phd/clinical

1	2	3	4	5	**6**	7
Practice oriented		Equal emphasis			Research oriented	

Percentage of faculty subscribing to each of the following orientations:

Applied behavioral analysis/Radical behavioral	25%
Family systems/Systems	0%
Existential/Phenomenological/Humanistic	0%
Cognitive/Cognitive-behavioral	75%

Courses required for incoming students prior to enrolling:
Research methods, statistics

Courses recommended but not mandatory:
Good science background, abnormal psychology, cognitive psychology, social psychology, developmental psychology

GRE mean
Verbal 562   Quantitative 650   Analytical Writing 5.0
Advanced Psychology 690

GPA mean

Number of applications/admission offers/incoming students in 2007
181 applied/24 admission offers/14 incoming

% of students receiving:
Full tuition waiver only: 0%
Assistantship/fellowship only: 0%
Both full tuition waiver & assistantship/fellowship: 100%

Approximate percentage of incoming students with a B.A./B.S. only: 93%   **Master's:** 7%

Approximate percentage of students who are Women: 73%   **Ethnic Minority:** 18%   **International:** 6%

Average years to complete the doctoral program (including internship): 6 years

---

Personal interview
Telephone required

Attrition rate in past 7 years: .08%

Percentage of students applying for internship last year accepted into APPIC or APA internships: 80%

Formal tracks/concentrations: none

Research areas	# Faculty	# Grants
addictions	5	8
anxiety disorders	3	1
attention-deficit disorder	2	10
behavioral medicine	2	2
childhood risk of psychopathology	3	1
depression	2	0
assessment/psychometrics	1	0

Clinical opportunities

ADHD
anxiety disorders
child/adolescent
externalizing behavior

depression
parent training
psychological services
center

University of California–Berkeley (Ph.D.)

Department of Psychology
Berkeley, CA 94720-1650
phone#: (510) 643-8114
e-mail: psychapp@berkeley.edu
Web address:
psychology.berkeley.edu/graduate/cl_program.html

1	2	3	4	5	**6**	7
Practice oriented		Equal emphasis			Research oriented	

Percentage of faculty subscribing to each of the following orientations:

Psychodynamic/Psychoanalytic	0%
Applied behavioral analysis/Radical behavioral	0%
Family systems/Systems	30%
Existential/Phenomenological/Humanistic	0%
Cognitive/Cognitive-behavioral	70%

Courses required for incoming students to have completed prior to enrolling:
None

Recommended but not mandatory courses:
Research design and methods, breadth in psychology

GRE mean
Verbal 654   Quantitative 705
Advanced psychology not required
Analytical Writing 5.5

GPA mean
Overall GPA 3.71

Number of applications/admission offers/incoming students in 2007
320 applied/9 admission offers/6 incoming

% of students receiving:
Full tuition waiver only: 0%
Assistantship/fellowship only: 0%
Both full tuition waiver & assistantship/fellowship: 95%

Approximate percentage of incoming students with a B.A./B.S. only: 80%   **Master's:** 20%

Approximate percentage of students who are Women: 72%   **Ethnic Minority:** 28%
International: < 1%

Average years to complete the doctoral program (including internship): 6.75 years

Personal interview
Preferred in person but telephone acceptable

Attrition rate in past 7 years: 0.6%

Percentage of students applying for internship last year accepted into APPIC or APA internships: 100%

Formal tracks/concentrations: none

Research areas	# Faculty	# Grants
ADHD externalizing behavior	1	2
emotion and aging	1	1
emotion and marriage	1	1
emotion and dementia	1	1
emotion, cognition, and schizophrenia	1	2
emotion and depression	1	0
insomnia	1	1
bipolar disorder	1	1
temperament, internalizing, and externalizing behavior	1	1
culture and mental health	1	1
stigma and mental illness	1	1

Clinical opportunities

University of California–Los Angeles (Ph.D.)

Department of Psychology
1285 Franz Hall, Box 951563
Los Angeles, CA 90095-1563
phone#: (310) 825-2617
e-mail: gradadm@psych.ucla.edu
Web address:
www.psych.ucla.edu/Grads/Areas/clinical.php

1	2	3	4	5	6	**7**
Practice oriented		Equal emphasis			Research oriented	

Percentage of faculty subscribing to each of the following orientations:

Psychodynamic/Psychoanalytic	0%
Applied behavioral analysis/Radical behavioral	0%
Family systems/Systems	25%
Existential/Phenomenological/Humanistic	0%
Cognitive/Cognitive-behavioral	75%

Courses required for incoming students prior to enrolling:
Elementary statistics; two of the following: learning, physiological, or perception/information processing; two of the following: developmental, social, or personality/abnormal; one course in biology or zoology; two physical science courses at least one math course; statistics

Courses recommended but not mandatory:
Research design and methods, psychology research labs, independent research courses; a broad background in the mathematical, biological and social sciences

GRE mean
Verbal 662   Quantitative 720
Analytical Writing 5.3   Advanced Psychology 726

GPA mean
Overall GPA 3.75

Number of applications/admission offers/incoming students in 2007
385 applied/19 admission offers/13 incoming

% of students receiving:
Full tuition waiver only: 0%
Assistantship/fellowship only: 0%
Both full tuition waiver & assistantship/fellowship: 80%–90%

Approximate percentage of incoming students with a B.A./B.S. only: 98%   **Master's:** 2%

Approximate percentage of students who are Women: 62%   **Ethnic Minority:** 46%   **International:** 2%

Average years to complete the doctoral program (including internship): 6.2 years

Personal interview
Preferred in person but telephone acceptable

Attrition rate in past 7 years: 6%

Percentage of students applying for internship last year accepted into APPIC or APA internships: 100%

Formal tracks/concentrations: no formal tracks, but there is focused training in severe adult psychopathology, child/adolescent psychopathology, clinical-health psychology, minority mental health, and couples and families

Research areas	# Faculty	# Grants
anxiety disorders and treatment	1	4
family issues	2	2
marital and couple	2	3
medical issues	5	12
minority health issues	4	8
mood disorders	2	3
schizophrenia	3	5
school mental health	1	1

Clinical opportunities
adoptions, families
child and adult affective disorders
child and adult anxiety disorders
community psychology, community mental health
couples/marital
developmental disabilities/autism

family/child
major mental illness
minority populations
psychotherapy supervision
school mental health

California Institute of Integral Studies (Psy.D.)

Psychology Doctoral Program
1453 Mission Street, San Francisco, CA 94103 (Mailing Address)
1390 Market Street, Suite 111, San Francisco, CA 94102 (Physical Address)
phone#: (415)-575-6210
e-mail: dtownes@ciis.edu (Admissions Counselor) or kmcgovern@ciis.edu (Psy.D. Program Director)
Web address: www.ciis.edu/academics/psyd.html

1	2	3	4	5	6	7
Practice oriented		Equal emphasis			Research oriented	

Percentage of faculty subscribing to each of the following orientations:

Psychodynamic/Psychoanalytic 59%
Applied behavioral analysis/Radical behavioral 0%
Family systems/Systems 16%
Existential/Phenomenological/Humanistic 25%
Cognitive/Cognitive-behavioral 0%

Courses required for incoming students to have completed prior to enrolling:

abnormal psychology, lifespan development, and statistics

Recommended but not mandatory courses: none

GRE mean

Verbal 512   Quantitative 551
Advanced Psychology not reported
Analytical Writing 4.4

GPA mean

Overall GPA 3.35

Number of applications/admission offers/incoming students in 2007

139 applied/74 admission offers/30 incoming

% of students receiving:

Full tuition waiver only: 0%
Assistantship/fellowship only: 9%
Both full tuition waiver & assistantship/fellowship: 0%

Approximate percentage of incoming students with a B.A./B.S. only: 66%   Master's: 34%

Approximate percentage of students who are
Women: 75%   Ethnic Minority: 26%   International: 9%

Average years to complete the doctoral program (including internship): 5 years

Personal interview: Preferred in person but telephone acceptable in extenuating circumstances

Attrition rate in past 7 years: 9%

Percentage of students applying for internship last year accepted into APPIC or APA internships: 38%

Formal tracks/concentrations: none

Research areas	# Faculty	# Grants
biofeedback	1	1
spirituality and psychospirituialy	4	1
music apperception test	1	0
test development and validation (MMPI)	1	1
therapists' conceptions of their work	1	0
Jungian and feminist topics	1	0
relational psychoanalysis	2	0
sexuality	1	0

Clinical opportunities

community mental health
children and adolescents
families
crisis screening/evaluation
psychosis, SED, chronic mental illness
addiction and chemical dependency
college counseling
psychotherapy with GLBTQ clients
psychotherapy with people living with AIDS
geropsychology
forensics (violent crime offenders and victims)
neuropsychology
behavioral medicine
Spanish speaking clients
individuals with physical limitations

Carlos Albizu University–Miami Campus (Psy.D.)

2173 NW 99th Avenue
Miami, FL 33172-2209
phone#: (305) 593-1223, ext. 129
e-mail: croca@albizu.edu
Web address:
mia.albizu.edu/web/academic_programs/psychology/doctor_of_psychology_in_clinical_psychology.asp

1	2	3	4	5	6	7
Practice oriented		Equal emphasis			Research oriented	

Percentage of faculty subscribing to each of the following orientations:

Psychodynamic/Psychoanalytic 20%
Applied behavioral analysis/Radical behavioral 0%
Family systems/Systems 10%
Existential/Phenomenological/Humanistic 20%
Cognitive/Cognitive-behavioral 50%

Courses required for incoming students to have completed prior to enrolling:

Research methodology, abnormal psychology, and statistics

Recommended but not mandatory courses: none

GRE mean
not required for admission

GPA mean
3.42

Number of applications/admission offers/incoming students in 2007
247 applied/89 admission offers/60 incoming

% of students receiving:
Full tuition waiver only: 0%
Assistantship/fellowship only: 5%
Both full tuition waiver & assistantship/fellowship: 0%

Approximate percentage of incoming students with a B.A./B.S. only: 60%   **Master's:** 40%

Approximate percentage of students who are Women: 77%   **Ethnic Minority:** 78%
International: 0.5%

Average years to complete the doctoral program (including internship): 4.5 years

Personal interview
Preferred in person but telephone acceptable

Attrition rate in past 7 years: 3.1%

Percentage of students applying for internship last year accepted into APPIC or APA internships: 75%

Formal tracks/concentrations: child psychology, neuropsychology, forensic psychology

Research areas	# Faculty	# Grants
children and adolescents	3	0
depression	3	0
elderly	1	0
forensic psychology	1	0
multicultural	6	0
neuropsychology	2	0
positive psychology	1	0
psychotherapy	6	0

Clinical opportunities
In-house training clinic where students work with multi-ethnic populations of various ages, including children.

Carlos Albizu University–San Juan Campus (Ph.D. Clinical Psychology)

P.O. Box 9023711
San Juan, PR 00902-3711
Phone#: (787) 725-6500, ext. 1129
E-mail: ssayers@albizu.edu
Web address: sju.albizu.edu/code/doctoral_programs/phd_in_clinical_psychology.asp

1	2	3	**4**	5	6	7
Practice oriented		Equal emphasis			Research oriented	

Percentage of faculty subscribing to each of the following orientations:

Psychodynamic/Psychoanalytic	25%
Applied behavioral analysis/Radical behavioral	12%
Family systems/Systems	12%
Existential/Phenomenological/Humanistic	12%
Cognitive/Cognitive-behavioral	37%
Integrative	12%

Courses required for incoming students to have completed prior to enrolling:
Experimental psychology and laboratory, physiological psychology and laboratory, abnormal psychology, introductory statistics, personality theories

Recommended but not mandatory courses:
none

GRE mean:
not reported

GPA mean:
not reported

Number of applications/admission offers/incoming students in 2007:
32 applied/26 admission offers/26 incoming

% of students receiving:
Full tuition waiver only: 0%
Assistantship/fellowship only: 0%
Both full tuition waiver & assistantship/fellowship: 0%

Approximate percentage of incoming students who entered with a B.A./B.S. only: 92%   **Master's:** 8%

Approximate percentage of students who are:
Women: 76%   **Ethnic Minority:** 99%   **International:** 0%

Average years to complete the doctoral program (including internship): 7 years

Personal interview:
Required in person

Attrition rate in past 7 years: 16%

Percentage of students applying for internship last year accepted into APPIC or APA internships: 16%

Formal tracks/concentrations: none

Research areas	# Faculty	# Grants
attention-deficit disorder	2	1
child abuse and neglect	1	0
elderly	2	1
high risk children/adolescents	4	1
HIV/AIDS	1	0
impulsion-aggressive children	3	0
instrument validation	2	0
social skills	2	1
sport psychology	1	0

Clinical opportunities:
domestic violence program

Carlos Albizu University–San Juan Campus (Psy.D.)

San Juan, PR 00902-3711
phone#: (787) 725-6500, ext. 1552
e-mail: galtieri@prip.edu
Web address: sju.albizu.edu/code/doctoral_programs/
psyd_in_clinical_psychology.asp

1	2	**3**	4	5	6	7
Practice oriented		Equal emphasis			Research oriented	

Percentage of faculty subscribing to each of the following orientations:

Psychodynamic/Psychoanalytic	0%
Applied behavioral analysis/Radical behavioral	10%
Family systems/Systems	30%
Existential/Phenomenological/Humanistic	10%
Cognitive/Cognitive-behavioral	50%

Courses required for incoming students to have completed prior to enrolling:

Experimental psychology and laboratory, physiological psychology and laboratory, abnormal psychology, introductory statistics, personality theories

Recommended but not mandatory courses:

GRE mean

not required for admission

GPA mean

3.25

Number of applications/admission offers/incoming students in 2007

60 applied/47 admission offers/44 incoming

% of students receiving:

Full tuition waiver only: 0%
Assistantship/fellowship only: 10%
Both full tuition waiver & assistantship/fellowship: 10%

Approximate percentage of incoming students with a B.A./B.S. only: not reported **Master's:** not reported

Approximate percentage of students who are Women: 70% **Ethnic Minority:** 100% **International:**

Average years to complete the doctoral program (including internship): 6 years

Personal interview

Required in person

Attrition rate in past 7 years: 10%

Percentage of students applying for internship last year accepted into APPIC or APA internships: 18%

Formal tracks/concentrations: none

Research areas	# Faculty	# Grants
health and well-being in elderly	2	0
sexual behavior	2	0
sport anxiety	2	0
forensic	3	0

Clinical opportunities

domestic violence	sexual disorders
forensic psychology	sports psychology
sexual abuse victims	victims of crime
sex abuse therapy	

Case Western Reserve University (Ph.D.)

Department of Psychology
Mather Memorial Building
11220 Bellflower Road
Cleveland, OH 44106
phone#: (216) 368-2686
e-mail: psychdept@case.edu
Web address: www.case.edu/artsci/pscl/clinical.htm

1	2	3	**4**	5	6	7
Practice oriented		Equal emphasis			Research oriented	

Percentage of faculty subscribing to each of the following orientations:

Psychodynamic/Psychoanalytic	50%
Applied behavioral analysis/Radical behavioral	5%
Family systems/Systems	25%
Existential/Phenomenological/Humanistic	5%
Cognitive/Cognitive-behavioral	50%

Courses required for incoming students to have completed prior to enrolling:

General undergraduate psychology courses

Recommended but not mandatory courses:

psychology major

GRE mean

Verbal + Quantitative 1274

GPA mean

Overall GPA 3.7

Number of applications/admission offers/incoming students in 2007

124 applied/7 admission offers/5 incoming

% of students receiving:

Full tuition waiver only: 18%
Assistantship/fellowship only: 0%
Both full tuition waiver & assistantship/fellowship: 57%

Approximate percentage of incoming students with a B.A./B.S. only: 100% **Master's:** 0%

Approximate percentage of students who are Women: 96% **Ethnic Minority:** 25% **International:** 0%

Average years to complete the doctoral program (including internship): 6.8 years

Personal interview

Preferred in person but telephone acceptable

Attrition rate in past 7 years: 19%

What percentage of students applying for internship last year was accepted into APPIC or APA internships?

100%

Formal tracks/concentrations: child/pediatric psychology, adult psychology

Research areas	# Faculty	# Grants
aging	2	1
behavioral medicine/ health psychology	1	1
chronic mental illness	1	0
developmental disabilities	1	1
learning disabilities	1	1
memory	2	0
parent–child interaction	2	0
personality disorders	1	6
self-psychology	1	0
temperament	1	1

Clinical opportunities

ADHD	juvenile bipolar disorder
affective disorders	obsessive–compulsive
aging and dementia	disorders
anxiety disorders	personality disorders
gerontology/Alzheimer's	schizophrenia/psychosis

Catholic University of America (Ph.D.)

Department of Psychology
620 Michigan Avenue, NE
Washington, DC 20064
phone#: (202) 319-5729
e-mail: cua-psychology@cua.edu
Web address:
psychology.cua.edu/graduate/phdclprog.cfm

1	2	3	**4**	5	6	7
Practice oriented		Equal emphasis			Research oriented	

Percentage of faculty subscribing to each of the following orientations:

Psychodynamic/Psychoanalytic	50%
Applied behavioral analysis/Radical behavioral	25%
Family systems/Systems	50%
Existential/Phenomenological/Humanistic	75%
Cognitive/Cognitive-behavioral	85%

Courses required for incoming students to have completed prior to enrolling:
introductory psychology, statistics, research methods

Recommended but not mandatory courses:
research experience in psychology; abnormal psychology; personality; developmental psychology; social psychology

GRE mean
Verbal 690   Quantitative 687
Advanced Psychology 709
Analytical Writing 5.17

GPA mean
Overall GPA 3.50

Number of applications/admission offers/incoming students in 2007
181 applied/13 admission offers/6 incoming

% of students receiving:
Full tuition waiver only: 35%
Assistantship/fellowship only: 9%
Both full tuition waiver & assistantship/fellowship: 56%

Approximate percentage of incoming students with a B.A./B.S. only: 90%   **Master's:** 10%

Approximate percentage of students who are Women: 80%   **Ethnic Minority:** 18%   **International:** 0%

Average years to complete the doctoral program (including internship): 6.9 years

Personal interview
Required in person

Attrition rate in past 7 years: 4.6%

Percentage of students applying for internship last year accepted into APPIC or APA internships: 100%

Formal tracks/concentrations: adult clinical, children, family, and multicultural

Research areas	# Faculty	# Grants
adolescence	3	1
adult psychopathology	3	1
anxiety	1	0
anxiety disorders	2	1
attachment	2	0
child clinical	4	1
clinical training	1	0
cognition	3	0
community context	1	2
couples	1	1
developmental	4	1
developmental psychopathology	4	1
emotions	2	0
emotion regulation	1	0
family	2	1
interpersonal processes	2	0
language development	1	1
mood disorders	2	0
parent–child interactions	2	1
psychotherapy integration	2	0
psychotherapy outcome	3	0
psychotherapy practice	3	0
psychotherapy process	3	0
self-efficacy	1	0
social anxiety	2	0
sport psychology	1	0
stress and coping	3	1
suicide	2	1
violence	1	1

Clinical opportunities

adult psychotherapy	family therapy
assessment batteries	group therapy
child and adult assessment	minority mental health
couples therapy	neuropsychology

University of Central Florida (Ph.D.)

4000 Central Florida Blvd, Psychology Building
Orlando, Florida, 32816-1390

phone#: (407) 823-4344
e-mail: psyinfo@mail.ucf.edu
Web address:
www.cas.ucf.edu/psychology/graduate_degrees
_clinicalphd.php

1	2	3	4	5	6	**7**
Practice oriented		Equal emphasis			Research oriented	

Percentage of faculty subscribing to each of the following orientations:

Courses required for incoming students to have completed prior to enrolling:
a minimum of 18 semester hours of undergraduate psychology courses is required prior to matriculation.

Recommended but not mandatory courses:
Research experience is heavily weighted during admissions

GRE mean
Quantitative 667   Verbal 542
Psychology Advanced Test not reported
Analytical Writing not reported

GPA mean
Overall GPA 3.6

Number of applications/admission offers/incoming students in 2007
128 applied/8 admission offers/7 incoming

% of students receiving:
Full tuition waiver only: 0%
Assistantship/fellowship only: 0%
Both full tuition waiver & assistantship/fellowship: 100%

Approximate percentage of incoming students with a B.A./B.S. only: 100%   **Master's:** 0%

Approximate percentage of students who are Women: 67%   **Ethnic Minority:** 16%   **International:** 0%

Average years to complete the doctoral program (including internship): 6 years

Personal interview
Required in person

Attrition rate in past 7 years: 4%

Percentage of students applying for internship last year accepted into APPIC or APA internships: 100%

Formal tracks/concentrations: clinical child, adult

Research areas	# Faculty	# Grants
alcohol and substance abuse	1	
child/pediatric psychology	1	
developmental psychopathology	1	
ADHD/cognition	1	
eating behavior and body image	2	
multicultural	1	
prevention	1	
schizophrenia	1	

Clinical opportunities

children's learning clinic
clinical neuroscience
eating, appearance, & health
family
substance use

Central Michigan University (Ph.D.)
Department of Psychology
Mt. Pleasant, MI 48859
phone#: (989) 774-6463
e-mail: Reid.Skeel@cmich.edu
Web address:
www.chsbs.cmich.edu/Clinical_psychology/

1	2	3	**4**	5	6	7
Practice oriented		Equal emphasis			Research oriented	

Percentage of faculty subscribing to each of the following orientations:
Psychodynamic/Psychoanalytic — 10%
Applied behavioral analysis/Radical behavioral — 10%
Family systems/Systems — 25%
Existential/Phenomenological/Humanistic — 10%
Cognitive/Cognitive-behavioral — 70%

Courses required for incoming students to have completed prior to enrolling:
none

Recommended but not mandatory courses:
statistics, experimental psychology, developmental psychology, abnormal psychology, personality theory, measurement theory

GRE mean
Verbal 611   Quantitative 741
Analytical Writing 4.7

GPA mean
Overall GPA 3.53   Psychology GPA 3.68

Number of applications/admission offers/incoming students in 2007
125 applied/8 admission offers/4 incoming

% of students receiving:
Full tuition waiver only: 0%
Assistantship/fellowship only: 0%
Both full tuition waiver & assistantship/fellowship: 100%

Approximate percentage of incoming students with a B.A./B.S. only: 100%   **Master's:** 0%

Approximate percentage of students who are Women: 50%   **Ethnic Minority:** 0%   **International:** 0%

Average years to complete the doctoral program (including internship): 6 years

Personal interview
Interview not required

Attrition rate in past 7 years: 3%

Percentage of students applying for internship last year accepted into APPIC or APA internships: 100%

Formal tracks/concentrations: none

Research areas	# Faculty	# Grants
anxiety disorders	1	1
assessment	1	0
children	1	2
diversity and sexual deviance	1	0
health psychology	1	1
neuropsychology	1	1
severe psychopathology	1	1
violence and agression	1	0

Clinical opportunities

adult clinical
behavior therapy
child clinical
cognitive-behavioral therapy
forensic psychology
neuropsychology/
   rehabilitation

parent–child interaction
   therapy
psychodynamic therapy
psychological assessment
school-based interventions

Chestnut Hill College (Psy.D.)

Department of Professional Psychology
9601 Germantown Avenue
Philadelphia, PA 19118-2693
phone#: (215)-248-7020
email: mashettj@chc.edu
Web address:
www.chc.edu/page_template.asp?section=3&file=325
_psyd

1	2	3	4	5	6	7
Practice oriented		Equal emphasis			Research oriented	

Percentage of faculty subscribing to each of the following orientations:

Psychodynamic/Psychoanalytic	40%
Applied behavioral analysis/Radical behavioral	0%
Family systems/Systems	30%
Existential/Phenomenological/Humanistic	10%
Cognitive/Cognitive-behavioral	20%

Courses required for incoming students to have completed prior to enrolling:
Abnormal psychology, statistics

Recommended but not mandatory courses:
Developmental psychology, research design

GRE mean
Verbal 602   Quantitative 520
Analytical Writing 4.6
Advanced Psychology not reported

GPA mean
Overall GPA 3.6

Number of applications/admission offers/incoming students in 2007
135 applied/41 admission offers/25 incoming

% of students receiving:
Full tuition waiver only: 0%
Assistantship/fellowship only: 10%
Both full tuition waiver & assistantship/fellowship: 0%

Approximate percentage of incoming students with a B.A./B.S. only: 52%   **Master's:** 48%

Approximate percentage of students who are Women: 70%   **Ethnic Minority:** 10%   **International:** 2%

Average years to complete the doctoral program (including internship): 6.5 years

Personal interview
Required in person

Attrition rate in past 7 years: 7.1%

Percentage of students applying for internship last year accepted into APPIC or APA internships: 67%

Formal tracks/concentrations: psychological assessment, family therapy

Research areas	# Faculty	# Grants
step-families	1	1

Clinical opportunities
not reported

Chicago School of Professional Psychology (Psy.D.)

325 N Wells
Chicago, IL 60610
phone#: (312) 329-6666
e-mail: admissions@thechicagoschool.edu
Web address:
www.thechicagoschool.edu/content.cfm/clinical
_psychology_doctoral_program_psyd

1	2	3	4	5	6	7
Practice oriented		Equal emphasis			Research oriented	

Percentage of faculty subscribing to each of the following orientations:

Psychodynamic/Psychoanalytic	36%
Family systems/Systems	50%
Existential/Phenomenological/Humanistic	43%
Cognitive/Cognitive-behavioral	46%

Courses required for incoming students to have completed prior to enrolling:
18 hours in psychology, including statistics, lifespan/human development, abnormal psychology

Recommended but not mandatory courses:
none

GRE mean
Verbal + Quantitative 1130
Analytical Writing Data not available

GPA mean
Overall GPA 3.56

Number of applications/admission offers/incoming students in 2007
539 applied/201 admission offers/82 incoming

% of students receiving:
Full tuition waiver only: 0
Assistantship/fellowship only: 2%
Both full tuition waiver & assistantship/fellowship: 0

Approximate percentage of incoming students with a B.A./B.S. only: 61%   **Master's:** 39%

Approximate percentage of students who are Women: 74.5%   **Ethnic Minority:** 22.9%
International: 4.7%

Average years to complete the doctoral program (including internship): 5 years

Personal interview
Required in person

Attrition rate in past 7 years: not reported

Percentage of students applying for internship last year accepted into APPIC or APA internships: 89%

Formal tracks/concentrations: child/adolescent, health, multicultural/community, forensic

Research areas	# Faculty	# Grants
behavioral intervention	1	0
diversity and cultural competence training	9	1
forensic psychology	2	0
latino early education	1	0
multigenerational health	1	0
pediatric obesity	1	0
trauma	1	0

Clinical opportunities

child and adolescent
college counseling center
community mental health
community psychology
correctional/forensic settings
creative and expressive arts
cross-cultural/international
early education/head start
forensic
health
inner city and rural populations
inpatient/outpatient/partial hospitalization
mental health administration
private and group practice
organizational
school based intervention
sexual orientation and gender identity
teaching
veterans

University of Cincinnati (Ph.D.)

Department of Psychology
429 Dyer Hall
Cincinnati, OH 45221-0376
phone#: (513) 556-5580
e-mail: Paula.Shear@uc.edu
Web address:
asweb.artsci.uc.edu/psychology/grad/clinical.cfm

1	2	3	4	5	6	7

Practice oriented   Equal emphasis   Research oriented

Percentage of faculty subscribing to each of the following orientations:

Psychodynamic/Psychoanalytic	20%
Applied behavioral analysis/Radical behavioral	10%
Family systems/Systems	5%
Existential/Phenomenological/Humanistic	10%
Cognitive/Cognitive-behavioral	55%

Courses required for incoming students prior to enrolling:
Preference given to applicants with coursework in psychology

Courses recommended but not mandatory:
Abnormal, statistics, research methods

GRE mean
Verbal 523   Quantitative 619
Analytical Writing 4.5
Advanced Psychology (optional) 670

GPA mean
Overall GPA 3.7

Number of applications/admission offers/incoming students in 2007
194 applied/9 admission offers/8 incoming

% of students receiving:
Full tuition waiver only: 0%
Assistantship/fellowship only: 0%
Both full tuition waiver & assistantship/fellowship: 100%

Approximate percentage of incoming students with a B.A./B.S. only: 86%   **Master's:** 14%

Approximate percentage of students who are Women: 75%   **Ethnic Minority:** 25%
International: not reported

Average years to complete the doctoral program (including internship): 6 years

Personal interview
In person interview strongly preferred

Attrition rate in past 7 years: 10%

Percentage of students applying for internship last year accepted into APPIC or APA internships: 80%

Formal tracks/concentrations: human factors, neuropsychology, heath psychology, general clinical

Research areas	# Faculty	# Grants
addictive behaviors	4	4
adolescence	5	3
adult development	2	0
child clinical	3	2
health psychology	5	3
neuropsychology	6	5
serious mental illness	4	3

Clinical opportunities

addictive behaviors
child clinical psychology
clinical neuropsychology
community mental health
developmental disorders
health psychology
serious mental illness
university counseling center

City University of New York at City College (Ph.D.)

Department of Psychology
138th Street and Covenant Avenue
New York, NY 10031
phone#: (212) 650-5672/5674
e-mail: EJurist@gc.cuny.edu
Web address:
web.gc.cuny.edu/Psychology/clinical/index.html

1	2	**3**	4	5	6	7

Practice oriented   Equal emphasis   Research oriented

Percentage of faculty subscribing to each of the following orientations:

Psychodynamic/Psychoanalytic	60%
Applied behavioral analysis/Radical behavioral	0%
Family systems/Systems	30%
Existential/Phenomenological/Humanistic	10%
Cognitive/Cognitive-behavioral	20%

Courses required for incoming students to have completed prior to enrolling:

15 credits: intro, experimental, statistics, and abnormal

Recommended but not mandatory courses:

None

GRE mean

Verbal 615   Quantitative 640 Analytic 5.0
Advanced Psychology 610
Analytical Writing not reported

GPA mean

Overall GPA 3.7   Psychology GPA 3.8
Junior/Senior GPA 3.8

Number of applications/admission offers/incoming students in 2007

308 applied/14 admission offers/12 incoming

% of students receiving:

Full tuition waiver only: 10%
Assistantship/fellowship only: 20%
Both full tuition waiver & assistantship/fellowship: 35%

Approximate percentage of incoming students with a B.A./B.S. only: 70%   Master's: 30%

Approximate percentage of students who are Women: 65%   Ethnic Minority: 40% International: 20%

Average years to complete the doctoral program (including internship): 6.5 years

Personal interview

Preferred in person but telephone acceptable (if student is out of country)

Attrition rate in past 7 years: 1%

Percentage of students applying for internship last year accepted into APPIC or APA internships: 100%

Formal tracks/concentrations: health psychology, psychology and law, women and gender studies

Research areas	# Faculty	# Grants
African American adolescents	1	0
attachment	3	1
object relations	4	1
social policies in mental health	1	0
racism	1	0
psychotherapy outcome	3	0

Clinical opportunities

adult clinic
child clinic
family clinic

Clark University (Ph.D.) (2006 data)

Frances L. Hiatt School of Psychology
950 Main Street
Worcester, MA 01610
phone#: (508) 793-7269
e-mail: maddis@clarku.edu
Web address: www.clarku.edu/departments/
psychology/grad/gradclinical.cfm

1	2	3	4	**5**	6	7

Practice oriented   Equal emphasis   Research oriented

Percentage of faculty subscribing to each of the following orientations:

Psychodynamic/Psychoanalytic	40%
Applied behavioral analysis/Radical behavioral	40%
Family systems/Systems	40%
Existential/Phenomenological/Humanistic	0%
Cognitive/Cognitive-behavioral	60%

Courses required for incoming students to have completed prior to enrolling:

Statistics, research design, abnormal psychology

Recommended but not mandatory courses:

Psychology major, substantial research experience

GRE mean

Verbal 640   Quantitative 680
Advanced Psychology 680

GPA mean

Overall GPA 3.5

Number of applications/admission offers/incoming students in 2006

135 applied/9 admission offers/4 incoming

% of students receiving:

Tuition waiver only: 0%
Assistantship/fellowship only: 0%
Both tuition waiver & assistantship/fellowship: 100%

Approximate percentage of incoming students with a B.A./B.S. only: 75%   Master's: 25%

Approximate percentage of students who are Women: 75%   Ethnic Minority: 25% International: Data not available

Average years to complete the doctoral program (including internship): 7 years

Personal interview
Required in person

Attrition rate in past 7 years:

Percentage of students applying for internship last year accepted into APPIC or APA internships:

Formal tracks/concentrations: none

Research areas	# Faculty	# Grants
adult psychopathology	2	1
affective disorders	1	1
assessment/diagnosis/classification	1	0
child abuse and children at-risk	1	1
child clinical/child psychopathology	2	1
family research/therapy	3	2
gender roles/sex differences	1	0
motivation	1	1
parent–child interaction	3	1
personality disorders	1	0
prevention	3	0
psychotherapy process and outcome	1	0
social learning	1	0

Clinical opportunities

child therapy/assessment
couples/family therapy
preventive interventions
school-based interventions

University of Colorado at Boulder (Ph.D.)

Department of Psychology
345 UCB
Boulder, CO 80309-0345
phone#: (303) 492-8805
e-mail: whisman@colorado.edu
Web address: psych.colorado.edu/~clinical/

1	2	3	4	5	6	7

Practice oriented   Equal emphasis   Research oriented

Percentage of faculty subscribing to each of the following orientations:
Psychodynamic/Psychoanalytic	10%
Applied behavioral analysis/Radical behavioral	10%
Family systems/Systems	30%
Existential/Phenomenological/Humanistic	0%
Cognitive/Cognitive-behavioral	90%

Courses required for incoming students to have completed prior to enrolling:
Psychology or the equivalent (30 semester hours in psychology)

Recommended but not mandatory courses:
Abnormal, statistics, research methods, psychological assessment, psychotherapy, developmental, social/personality, biological psychology

GRE mean
Verbal 630   Quantitative 680
Psychology Subject 700
Analytical Writing 5.3

GPA mean
Overall GPA 3.6

Number of applications/admission offers/incoming students in 2007
192 applied/6 admission offers/6 incoming

% of students receiving:
Full tuition waiver only: 0%
Assistantship/fellowship only: 0%
Both full tuition waiver & assistantship/fellowship: 100%

Approximate percentage of incoming students with a B.A./B.S. only: 89%   **Master's:** 11%

Approximate percentage of students who are Women: 75%   **Ethnic Minority:** 20%   **International:** 7%

Average years to complete the doctoral program (including internship): 6 years

Personal interview
Required in person

Attrition rate in past 7 years: 6%

Percentage of students applying for internship last year accepted into APPIC or APA internships: 100%

Formal tracks/concentrations: behavioral genetics certification, joint clinical psychology/neuroscience Ph.D.

Research areas	# Faculty	# Grants
adult psychopathology	4	3
affective disorders	3	3
assessment/diagnosis/classification	2	1
child clinical	3	2
developmental	3	1
eating disorders	0	0
family research	2	1
genetics	1	1
personality disorders	0	0
prevention	3	0
psychotherapy outcome/process	4	2
substance abuse	2	2
violence/abuse	2	0

Clinical opportunities

assessment
behavioral activation therapy
behavior therapy
cognitive therapy
family therapy
group therapy
interpersonal psychotherapy
marital/couple therapy
mindfulness
psychodynamic therapy
substance abuse

Concordia University (Ph.D.)

Department of Psychology, PY 119-2
7141 Sherbrooke Street West
Montreal, Quebec H4B 1R6 Canada
phone#: (514) 848-2424 ext. 2205
e-mail: Shirley.Black@concordia.ca
Web address:
psychology.concordia.ca/Grads/admissionsPhD.html

1	2	3	4	**5**	6	7
Practice oriented		Equal emphasis			Research oriented	

Percentage of faculty subscribing to each of the following orientations:
Psychodynamic/Psychoanalytic   15%
Applied behavioral analysis/Radical behavioral   0%
Family systems/Systems   25%
Existential/Phenomenological/Humanistic   0%
Cognitive/Cognitive-behavioral   60%

Courses required for incoming students to have completed prior to enrolling:
honors (B.A./B.S.) in psychology

Recommended but not mandatory courses:
none

GRE mean
Verbal 496   Quantitative 641
Advanced Psychology 697
(Note: GRE's are recommended, but optional.)

GPA mean
Overall GPA 3.81
(Note: Based on Concordia's scale of 4.3)

Number of applications/admission offers/incoming students in 2007
246 applied/28 admission offers/19 incoming

% of students receiving:
Full tuition waiver only: 0%
Assistantship/fellowship only: 78%
Both full tuition waiver & assistantship/fellowship: 22%

Approximate percentage of incoming students with a B.A./B.S. only: 95%   Master's: 5%

Approximate percentage of students who are Women: 89%   Ethnic Minority: 22%
International: Data not available

Personal interview
Preferred in person but telephone acceptable

Attrition rate in past 7 years: 2%

Percentage of students applying for internship last year accepted into APPIC or APA internships: 60%

Formal tracks/concentrations: behavioral neuroscience, clinical health, human development, cognitive science

Research areas	# Faculty	# Grants
anxiety	2	3
behavioral medicine	1	1
developmental/infancy	8	10
developmental psychopathology	3	5
gender roles	2	1
health psychology	1	0
major mental disorder	2	1
neuropsychology	2	5
neuroscience/psychobiology	9	12
perception/cognition	4	5
social competence	1	1

Clinical opportunities
adult
child/adolescent
cognitive/cognitive-behavioral

couples
family
psychodynamic

University of Connecticut (Ph.D.)
Department of Psychology
406 Babbidge Road, Unit 1020
Storrs, CT 06269-1020
phone#: (860) 486 2057 (Admissions information)
e-mail: debra.vardon@uconn.edu
Web address: web.uconn.edu/psychology/

1	2	3	4	**5**	6	7
Practice oriented		Equal emphasis			Research oriented	

Percentage of faculty subscribing to each of the following orientations:
Psychodynamic/Psychoanalytic   8%
Applied behavioral analysis/Radical behavioral   17%
Family systems/Systems   33%
Existential/Phenomenological/Humanistic   0%
Cognitive-behavioral   90%

Courses required for incoming students to have completed prior to enrolling:
None

Recommended but not mandatory courses:
abnormal, research methods

GRE mean
Verbal 614   Quantitative 670
Analytical Writing 5.4 Advanced Psychology 567

GPA mean
Overall GPA 3.70

Number of applications/admission offers/incoming students in 2007
311 applied/11 admission offers/7 incoming

% of students receiving:
Full tuition waiver only: 0%
Assistantship/fellowship only: 0%
Both full tuition waiver & assistantship/fellowship: 100%

Approximate percentage of incoming students with a B.A./B.S. only: 90%   Master's: 10%

Approximate percentage of students who are Women: 83%   Ethnic Minority: 15%   International: 4%

Average years to complete the doctoral program (including internship): 5.6 years

Personal interview
Preferred in person but telephone acceptable

Attrition rate in past 7 years: 6%

Percentage of students applying for internship last year accepted into APPIC or APA internships: APPIC 92%; APA 83%

Formal tracks/concentrations: child clinical, neuropsychology, health psychology

Research areas	# Faculty	# Grants
adult psychopathology	5	2
aging	1	0
anxiety disorders	2	0
autism	3	3
child psychopathology	7	3
developmental psychopathology	7	3
domestic violence	1	0
health psychology	3	2
multicultural psychology	2	1
neuropsychological assessment	4	3
trauma	3	0
depression	3	2

Clinical opportunities

autistic children
childhood psychopathology
chronic mental illness
health psychology
multicultural psychology
neuroimaging
neuropsychological assessment
traumatic brain injury
traumatic stress disorders
anxiety disorders
substance abuse

University of Delaware (Ph.D.)

Department of Psychology
Newark, DE 19716
phone#: (302) 831-2271
e-mail: ahayes@psych.udel.edu
Web address:
psych.udel.edu/graduate/clinical/index.asp

1	2	3	4	5	6	7
Practice oriented		Equal emphasis			Research oriented	

Percentage of faculty subscribing to each of the following orientations:

Psychodynamic/Psychoanalytic	11%
Applied behavioral analysis/Radical behavioral	0%
Family systems/Systems	55%
Existential/Phenomenological/Humanistic	0%
Cognitive/Cognitive-behavioral	89%

Courses required for incoming students to have completed prior to enrolling:
None

Recommended but not mandatory courses:
Statistics, biopsychology, abnormal psychology, history and systems, cognitive, developmental, research design

GRE mean
Verbal 630   Quantitative 685
Analytical Writing 5.0

GPA mean
Overall GPA 3.6

Number of applications/admission offers/incoming students in 2007
168 applied/4 admission offers/3 incoming

% of students receiving:
Full tuition waiver only: 0%
Assistantship/fellowship only: 0%
Both full tuition waiver & assistantship/fellowship: 100%

Approximate percentage of incoming students with a B.A./B.S. only: 90%   **Master's:** 10%

Approximate percentage of students who are Women: 77%   **Ethnic Minority:** 17%   **International:** 9%

Average years to complete the doctoral program (including internship): 6 years

Personal interview
Required in person

Attrition rate in past 7 years: 14%

Percentage of students applying for internship last year accepted into APPIC or APA internships: 100%

Formal tracks/concentrations: clinical-developmental

Research areas	# Faculty	# Grants
anxiety, stress, and coping	3	3
attachment theory	2	2
child clinical	4	3
developmental risk	5	4
emotions	2	1
foster care	1	2
psychophysiology	3	1
psychotherapy research	2	2
couples research	1	1

Clinical opportunities

anxiety disorders
child assessment
conduct disorder
developmental disabilities/ autism
family therapy
child maltreatment
depression
couple therapy
coping with cancer

University of Denver (Ph.D.)

Department of Psychology
University Park
Denver, CO 80210
phone#: (303) 871-3803
e-mail: phoughta@nova.psy.du.edu
Web address:
www.du.edu/psychology/research/child_clinical.htm

1	2	3	4	5	6	7
Practice oriented		Equal emphasis			Research oriented	

Percentage of faculty subscribing to each of the following orientations:

Psychodynamic/Psychoanalytic	12
Applied behavioral analysis/Radical behavioral	25%
Family systems/Systems	25%
Existential/Phenomenological/Humanistic	12%
Cognitive/Cognitive-behavioral	87%

Courses required for incoming students prior to enrolling:
None

Courses recommended but not mandatory:
Statistics

GRE mean
Verbal + Quantitative 1345
Analytical Writing not reported

GPA mean
Overall GPA 3.7

Number of applications/admission offers in 2007
230 applied/10 admission offers/6 incoming

% of students receiving:
Full tuition waiver only: 0%
Assistantship/fellowship only: 0%
Both full tuition waiver & assistantship/fellowship: 100%

Approximate percentage of incoming students with a B.A./B.S. only: 90% **Master's:** 10%

Approximate percentage of students who are Women: 84% **Ethnic Minority:** 27% **International:** 0%

Average years to complete the doctoral program (including internship): 6 years

Personal interview
Preferred in person but telephone acceptable

Attrition rate in past 7 years: 14%

Percentage of students applying for internship last year accepted into APPIC or APA internships: 100%

Formal tracks/concentrations: child clinical

Research areas	# Faculty	# Grants
adolescent psychopathology	5	2
behavioral genetics	1	1
child psychopathology	3	0
close relationships	3	5
community	1	4
developmental disabilities	1	1
family	2	5
marital	2	5
multicultural	2	2
neuropsychology	1	1
poverty	1	1
prevention	2	5
psychotherapy	2	4
sexual abuse	1	1
trauma	3	3

Clinical opportunities

developmental disorders	minority/cross-cultural
family	neuropsychology
inpatient adolescents	pediatrics
marital/couples	

University of Denver (Psy.D.)
Graduate School of Professional Psychology
2460 South Vine Street
Denver, CO 80208-0208
phone#: (303) 871-3873
e-mail: gsppinfo@du.edu
Web address: www.du.edu/gspp

1	2	3	4	5	6	7
Practice oriented		Equal emphasis			Research oriented	

Percentage of faculty subscribing to each of the following orientations:

Psychodynamic/Psychoanalytic	40%
Applied behavioral analysis/Radical behavioral	20%
Family systems/Systems	20%
Existential/Phenomenological/Humanistic	10%
Cognitive/Cognitive-behavioral	10%

Courses required for incoming students prior to enrolling:
Statistics, learning, personality, experimental, child, abnormal, history of psychology

Courses recommended but not mandatory:
Physiological psychology

GRE mean
Verbal 550   Quantitative 550
Advanced Psychology 660
Analytical 4.5

GPA mean
Overall GPA 3.5

Number of applications/admission offers/incoming students in 2007
379 applied/79 admission offers/39 incoming

incoming % of students receiving:
Full tuition waiver only: 2%
Assistantship/fellowship only: 35%
Both full tuition waiver & assistantship/fellowship: 5%

Approximate percentage of incoming students with a B.A./B.S. only: 60% **Master's:** 39%

Approximate percentage of students who are Women: 76% **Ethnic Minority:** 11% **International:** 5%

Average years to complete the doctoral program (including internship): 4 years

Personal interview
Required in person

Attrition rate in past 7 years: 6%

Percentage of students applying for internship last year accepted into APPIC or APA internships: 90%

Formal tracks/concentrations: child clinical, forensic, international disaster psychology, sport and performance

Research areas	# Faculty	# Grants
behavioral medicine	1	0
cognitive issues	1	0
couples and family therapy	2	0
forensic	2	0
multicultural	1	0

Clinical opportunities

assessment	hypnosis
behavioral medicine	international disasters
cognitive therapy	psychodynamic therapy
group therapy	psychotherapy supervision

159

DePaul University (Ph.D.)

Department of Psychology
2219 North Kenmore
Chicago, IL 60614
phone#: (773) 325-7787
e-mail: gradpsych@depaul.edu
Web address: condor.depaul.edu/~psych/clwebsite/

1	2	3	**4**	5	6	7
Practice oriented		Equal emphasis			Research oriented	

Percentage of faculty subscribing to each of the following orientations:

Psychodynamic/Psychoanalytic	0%
Applied behavioral analysis/Radical behavioral	22%
Family systems/Systems	55%
Existential/Phenomenological/Humanistic	0%
Cognitive/Cognitive-behavioral	33%

Courses required for incoming students prior to enrolling:

24 semester hours in psychology, 3 semester hours of statistics, and 3 semester hours in experimental psychology

Courses recommended but not mandatory:

science, computer, and math courses

GRE mean

Verbal 613   Quantitative 690
Analytical Writing not reported
Psychology Subject 682

GPA mean

Overall GPA 3.66

Number of applications/admission offers/incoming students in 2007

288 applied/9 admission offers/6 incoming

% of students receiving:

Full tuition waiver only: 0%
Assistantship/fellowship only: 0%
Both full tuition waiver & assistantship/fellowship: 100%

Approximate percentage of incoming students with a B.A./B.S. only: 66%   Master's: 33%

Approximate percentage of students who are Women: 57%   Ethnic Minority: 43%   International: 7%

Average years to complete the doctoral program (including internship): 8 years

Personal interview

Preferred in person but telephone acceptable

Attrition rate in past 7 years: not reported

Percentage of students applying for internship last year accepted into APPIC or APA internships: 100%

Formal tracks/concentrations: child clinical, community

Research areas	# Faculty	# Grants
adolescent depression	2	2
child abuse and neglect	1	1
chronic fatigue syndrome	1	3
disability	2	2
HIV/AIDS prevention	1	3
minority mental health	3	1
parent–child interaction	1	1
program evaluation	3	1
smoking cessation	1	1
social support	1	1
teenage pregnancy	2	1
violence prevention		

Clinical opportunities

assessment	family therapy
child and adolescent	group therapy
community psychology	minority/diversity

University of Detroit–Mercy (Ph.D.)

Department of Psychology
4001 W. McNichols Road
Detroit, MI 48221-3038
phone#: (313) 578-0570
e-mail: mccownja@udmercy.edu
Web address:
liberalarts.udmercy.edu/psychology/pycphd.html

1	2	**3**	4	5	6	7
Practice oriented		Equal emphasis			Research oriented	

Percentage of faculty subscribing to each of the following orientations:

Psychodynamic/Psychoanalytic	75%
Applied behavioral analysis/Radical behavioral	10%
Family systems/Systems	10%
Existential/Phenomenological/Humanistic	10%
Cognitive/Cognitive-behavioral	25%

Courses required for incoming students prior to enrolling:

Statistics, research methods, personality, abnormal, research course

Courses recommended but not mandatory:

Physiological psychology

GRE mean

Verbal 492   Quantitative 640
Analytical Writing 4.85

GPA mean

Overall GPA 3.6

Number of applications/admission offers/incoming students in 2007

67 applied/14 admission offers/10 incoming

% of students receiving:

Full tuition waiver only: 0%
Assistantship/fellowship only: 100%
Both full tuition waiver & assistantship/fellowship: 100%
(all students in first 2 years of program)

Approximate percentage of incoming students with a B.A./B.S. only: 90%   **Master's:** 10%

Approximate percentage of students who are Women: 80%   **Ethnic Minority:** 10% **International:** 30%

Average years to complete the doctoral program (including internship): 6 years

Personal interview
Required in person

Attrition rate in past 7 years: 1%

Percentage of students applying for internship last year accepted into APPIC or APA internships: 100%

Formal tracks/concentrations: none

Research areas	# Faculty	# Grants
alcohol abuse	1	1
critical incident response	2	0
helping behavior	1	0
identity development	2	0
intellectual assessment using human figure drawings	1	0
marital and family relationships	2	0
perception and eye movement	1	1
posttraumatic stress disorder	2	0
psychiatric diagnosis, ethnicity, and clinical judgment	1	0
psychotherapy process and outcome	4	0
self-esteem/body image	2	0
spirituality	3	0

Clinical opportunities
Practica and internships are completed at one of over 30 agencies in the metropolitan area

Drexel University (Ph.D.)

Department of Psychology
Main Campus Office
3141 Chestnut Street
Philadelphia, PA 19104
phone: (215) 895-1895
e-mail: lamia.p.barakat@drexel.edu
Web address: www.psychology.drexel.edu

1	2	3	**4**	5	6	7
Practice oriented		Equal emphasis			Research oriented	

Percentage of faculty subscribing to each of the following orientations:

Psychodynamic/Psychoanalytic	0%
Applied behavioral analysis/Radical behavioral	0%
Family systems/Systems	5%
Existential/Phenomenological/Humanistic	0%
Cognitive/Cognitive-behavioral	95%

Courses required for incoming students to have completed prior to enrolling:
none

Recommended but not mandatory courses:
foundational courses in psychology

GRE mean
Verbal 618   Quantitative 678   Analytical 616
Advanced Psychology 703
Analytical Writing not reported

GPA mean
Overall GPA 3.72

Number of applications/admission offers/incoming students in 2007
525 applied/15 admission offers/13 incoming

% of students receiving:
Full tuition waiver only: 0%
Assistantship/fellowship only: 0%
Both full tuition waiver & assistantship/fellowship: 100% for 1st-year class; students in subsequent years receive at least a tuition waiver and additional support.

Approximate percentage of incoming students with a BA/BS only: 85%   **Master's:** 15%

Approximate percentage of students who are: Women: 80%   **Ethnic Minority:** 17%   **International:** 8%

Average years to complete the doctoral program (including internship): 5.8 years

Personal interview
Preferred in person but telephone acceptable

Attrition rate in past 7 years: 2.4%

Percentage of students applying for internship last year accepted into APPIC or APA internships: 88%

Formal tracks/concentrations: health, forensic, neuropsychology

Research areas	# Faculty	# Grants
child abuse/neglect	1	0
childhood illness/family coping	1	2
childhood loss	2	2
chronic illness and coping	1	0
conscious/unconscious processes	1	0
divorce	1	0
family systems	2	1
family violence	2	2
health psychology	2	2
homeless families	1	0
inner-city children	4	2
low birthweight children	1	0
neuropsychology	6	4
peer relations/social skills	2	2
personality disorders	2	0
psychotherapy research	5	1
schizophrenia	0	0
social competence in children	2	0
substance abuse	2	2
television violence	0	0

Clinical Opportunities

forensic	cognitive-behavioral
health	adult
neuropsychology	child and family

161

Duke University (Ph.D.)

Department of Psychology
Durham, NC 27708
phone#: (919) 660-5716
e-mail: lkc@duke.edu
Web address: pn.aas.duke.edu/graduate/clin/index.htm

1	2	3	4	5	**6**	7

Practice oriented	Equal emphasis	Research oriented

Percentage of faculty subscribing to each of the following orientations:

Psychodynamic/Psychoanalytic	15%
Applied behavioral analysis/Radical behavioral	0%
Family systems/Systems	15%
Existential/Phenomenological/Humanistic	0%
Cognitive/Cognitive-behavioral	70%

Courses required for incoming students to have completed prior to enrolling:
statistics

Recommended but not mandatory courses:
broad background, personality, and research design

GRE mean
Verbal 665   Quantitative 711
Analytical Writing 5.3

GPA mean
Overall GPA 3.73

Number of applications/admission offers/incoming students in 2007
283 applied/10 admission offers/7 incoming

% of students receiving:
Full tuition waiver only: 0%
Assistantship/fellowship only: 0%
Both full tuition waiver & assistantship/fellowship: 100%

Approximate percentage of incoming students with a B.A./B.S. only: 94%   **Master's:** 6%

Approximate percentage of students who are Women: 81.9%   **Ethnic Minority:** 33%
International: not reported

Average years to complete the doctoral program (including internship): 5.5 years

Personal interview
Required in person

Attrition rate in past 7 years: 5%

Percentage of students applying for internship last year accepted into APPIC or APA internships: 100%

Formal tracks/concentrations: child clinical, adult clinical, health psychology

Research areas	# Faculty	# Grants
affective disorders	4	4
behavioral medicine	4	6
conduct disorders	2	3
eating disorders	1	1
developmental psychopathology	5	5
neuropsychology	1	1
posttraumatic stress disorder	0	0
school/educational	2	2
sexual abuse	0	0
social cognition	3	2
social skills	0	0
stress and coping	4	4

Clinical opportunities

adolescents	eating disorders
affective disorders	neuropsychology
behavioral cardiology	pediatric psychology
behavioral medicine	public sector treatment
behavior disorders of	school/educational
children	substance abuse
child abuse	
cognitive/dialectical	
behavior therapy	

Duquesne University (Ph.D.)

Department of Psychology
Pittsburgh, PA 15282-1753
phone#: (412)-396-6000
email: burston@duq.edu
Web address: www.gradpsych.duq.edu/index.html

1	2	3	**4**	5	6	7

Practice oriented	Equal emphasis	Research oriented

Percentage of faculty subscribing to each of the following orientations:

Psychodynamic/Psychoanalytic	65%
Applied behavioral analysis/Radical behavioral	0%
Family systems/Systems	18%
Existential/Phenomenological/Humanistic	91%
Cognitive/Cognitive-behavioral	18%

Courses required for incoming students to have completed prior to enrolling:
none

Recommended but not mandatory courses:
general breadth, development, social, abnormal, personality, research methods

GRE mean
Verbal 590   Quantitative 630
Analytical Writing not reported
Advanced Psychology not reported

GPA mean
Overall GPA 3.75

Number of applications/admission offers/incoming students in 2007
82 applied/7 admission offers/7 incoming

% of students receiving:
Full tuition waiver only: 0%
Assistantship/fellowship only: 0%
Both full tuition waiver & assistantship/fellowship: 100%

Approximate percentage of incoming students with a B.A./B.S. only: not reported **Master's:** not reported

Approximate percentage of students who are Women: 50% **Ethnic Minority:** 18% **International:** 18%

Average years to complete the doctoral program (including internship): 8.6 years

Personal interview
Required in person

Attrition rate in past 7 years: not reported

Percentage of students applying for internship last year accepted into APPIC or APA internships: 100%

Formal tracks/concentrations: none

Research areas	# Faculty	# Grants

Clinical opportunities
Psychology Clinic (offers psychotherapy to Duquesne's students, faculty, and staff as well as the public)

Eastern Michigan University (Ph.D.)

Department of Psychology
Ypsilanti, MI 48197
phone#: (734)-487-1155
email: ksaules@emich.edu
Web address: www.emich.edu/psychology/programs-grad.html

1	2	3	**4**	5	6	7
Practice oriented		Equal emphasis			Research oriented	

Percentage of faculty subscribing to each of the following orientations:
Psychodynamic/Psychoanalytic — 10%
Applied behavioral analysis/Radical behavioral — 20%
Family systems/Systems — 20%
Existential/Phenomenological/Humanistic — 10%
Cognitive/Cognitive-behavioral — 40%

Courses required for incoming students to have completed prior to enrolling:
Statistics, experimental abnormal, 20 undergraduate credits in psychology

Recommended but not mandatory courses:
Personality, learning, history and systems

GRE mean
Verbal 551   Quantitative 628
Analytical Writing 4.69
Advanced Psychology not reported

GPA mean
Overall GPA 3.71

Number of applications/admission offers/incoming students in 2007
126 applied/12 admission offers/8 incoming

% of students receiving:
Full tuition waiver only: 0%
Assistantship/fellowship only: 0%
Both full tuition waiver & assistantship/fellowship: 100%

Approximate percentage of incoming students with a B.A./B.S. only: 75% **Master's:** 25%

Approximate percentage of students who are Women: 70% **Ethnic Minority:** 4% **International:** 6%

Average years to complete the doctoral program (including internship): 6 years

Personal interview
Preferred in person but telephone acceptable

Attrition rate in past 7 years: 15%

Percentage of students applying for internship last year accepted into APPIC or APA internships: 100%

Formal tracks/concentrations: applied behavioral analysis

Research areas	# Faculty	# Grants
anxiety disorders (PTSD)	2	1
child and family	3	0
neuropsychology	2	1
personality disorders	1	0
substance abuse	1	0
applied behavioral analysis	2	0
behavioral medicine	1	0
sexual deviance	1	0
multicultural issues	2	0

Clinical opportunities
anxiety disorders and PTSD
depression
neuropsychology evaluations
traumatic brain injury
behavioral medicine clinic—chronic pain and migraine
inpatient hospital for children and adolescents

Emory University (Ph.D.)

Department of Psychology
Kilgo Circle
Atlanta, GA 30322
phone#: (404) 727-7456
e-mail: paula.mitchell@emory.edu
Web address:
psychology.emory.edu/clinical/index.html

1	2	3	4	5	**6**	7
Practice oriented		Equal emphasis			Research oriented	

Percentage of faculty subscribing to each of the following orientations:
Psychodynamic/Psychoanalytic — 10%
Applied behavioral analysis/Radical behavioral — 10%
Family systems/Systems — 30%
Existential/Phenomenological/Humanistic — 0%
Cognitive/Cognitive-behavioral — 40%

Courses required for incoming students to have completed prior to enrolling:
None

Recommended but not mandatory courses:
Statistics, methodology, psychopathology, personality

GRE mean
Verbal 570   Quantitative 650   Analytical 680
Analytical Writing 5.5

GPA mean
Overall GPA 3.5

Number of applications/admission offers/incoming students in 2007
238 applied/20 admission offers/12 incoming

% of students receiving:
Full tuition waiver only: 0%
Assistantship/fellowship only: 0%
Both full tuition waiver & assistantship/fellowship: 100%

Approximate percentage of incoming students with a B.A./B.S. only: 97%   **Master's:** 3%

Approximate percentage of students who are Women: 97%   **Ethnic Minority:** 1%   **International:** 2%

Average years to complete the doctoral program (including internship): 5 years

Personal interview
Required in person upon invitation from faculty

Attrition rate in past 7 years: 0.2%

Percentage of students applying for internship last year accepted into APPIC or APA internships: 100%

Formal tracks/concentrations: none

Research areas	# Faculty	# Grants
adolescent psychopathology	2	1
attention-deficit disorder	1	1
behavior control	1	0
behavioral genetics	2	1
eating disorders	1	0
infant development	1	2
neuropsychology	1	0
personality and personality disorders	3	2
schizophrenia	2	1

Clinical opportunities

assessment	interpersonal therapy
behavioral medicine	neuropsychology
behavior therapy	psychodynamic therapy
cognitive therapy	

Fairleigh Dickinson University (Ph.D.)
School of Psychology T-WH1-01
Teaneck–Hackensack Campus
1000 River Road
Teaneck, NJ 07666
phone#: (201) 692-2315
e-mail: mcgrath@fdu.edu
Web address: ucoll.fdu.edu/psychology/psyphd.html

1	2	3	**4**	5	6	7
Practice oriented		Equal emphasis			Research oriented	

Percentage of faculty subscribing to each of the following orientations:

Psychodynamic/Psychoanalytic	50%
Applied behavioral analysis/Radical behavioral	10%
Family systems/Systems	40%
Existential/Phenomenological/Humanistic	20%
Cognitive/Cognitive-behavioral	60%

Courses required for incoming students to have completed prior to enrolling:
18 credits in psychology including statistics, developmental, experimental, social

Recommended but not mandatory courses:
Psychopathology, physiological, assessment

GRE mean
Verbal 585   Quantitative 677   Analytical 680
Advanced Psychology 686
Analytical Writing 5.0

GPA mean

Number of applications/admission offers/incoming students in 2007
191 applied/26 admission offers/11 incoming

% of students receiving:
Full tuition waiver only: 0%
Assistantship/fellowship only: 100%
Both full tuition waiver & assistantship/fellowship: 0%

Approximate percentage of incoming students with a B.A./B.S. only: 73%   **Master's:** 27%

Approximate percentage of students who are Women: 81%   **Ethnic Minority:** 18%   **International:** 2%

Average years to complete the doctoral program (including internship): 5.5 years

Personal interview
Required in person

Attrition rate in past 7 years: 3%

Percentage of students applying for internship last year accepted into APPIC or APA internships: 91%

Formal tracks/concentrations: none

Research areas	# Faculty	# Grants
assessment	6	2
behavioral medicine	3	0
child clinical	2	0
community psychology	3	0
depression	0	0
eating disorders	0	0
ethical issues	2	0
forensic	2	1
minority issues	2	0
relationship	4	0
sexual abuse	3	0
statistics	2	0
stress—disasters	2	0
women's studies	3	0

Clinical opportunities

anxiety disorders	gerontology
assessment	minority populations
behavioral medicine	neuropsychology
community psychology	substance abuse
family therapy	

Fielding Graduate University (Ph.D.)

School of Psychology
2112 Santa Barbara Street
Santa Barbara, CA 93105
phone#: (800) 340-1099
e-mail: admission@fielding.edu
Web address: www.fielding.edu/psy/index.htm

1	2	3	**4**	5	6	7
Practice oriented		Equal emphasis			Research oriented	

Percentage of faculty subscribing to each of the following orientations:

Psychodynamic/Psychoanalytic	32%
Applied behavioral analysis/Radical behavioral	0%
Family systems/Systems	0%
Existential/Phenomenological/Humanistic	12%
Cognitive/Cognitive-behavioral	56%

Courses required for incoming students to have completed prior to enrolling:
A bachelor's degree is the minimum. Strong psychological background recommended.

Recommended but not mandatory courses:
Only appropriate for adult students with professional experience.

GRE mean
Not used

GPA mean
Data not available

Number of applications/admission offers/incoming students in 2007
378 applied/108 admission offers/86 incoming

% of students receiving:
Full tuition waiver only: 0%
Assistantship/fellowship only: 7%
Both full tuition waiver & assistantship/fellowship: 0%

Approximate percentage of incoming students with a B.A./B.S. only: 20% **Master's:** 80%

Approximate percentage of students who are Women: 72% **Ethnic Minority:** 25% **International:** 4%

Average years to complete the doctoral program (including internship): 8.4 years

Personal interview
Required in person

Attrition rate in past 7 years: 8.6%

Percentage of students applying for internship last year accepted into APPIC or APA internships: 46%

Formal tracks/concentrations: health psychology, neuropsychology, forensic psychology

Research areas
health psychology
neuropsychology
prevention and control of violence
parent-infant mental health

Clinical opportunities
Cognitive-behavioral, psychoanalytic/psychodynamic, and TA-Gestalt training tracks

University of Florida (Ph.D.)

Department of Clinical and Health Psychology
Box 100165 University of Florida Health Science Center
Gainesville, FL 32610
phone#: (352) 273-6455
e-mail: jhj@phhp.ufl.edu
Web address:
chp.phhp.ufl.edu/programs/doctoral/index.html

1	2	3	**4**	5	6	7
Practice oriented		Equal emphasis			Research oriented	

Percentage of faculty subscribing to each of the following orientations:

Psychodynamic/Psychoanalytic	10%
Applied behavioral analysis/Radical behavioral	10%
Family systems/Systems	60%
Existential/Phenomenological/Humanistic	20%
Cognitive/Cognitive-behavioral	80%

Courses required for incoming students to have completed prior to enrolling:
Statistics, abnormal

Recommended but not mandatory courses:
Experimental, developmental, social, personality, physiological, perception, statistics

GRE mean
Verbal 611   Quantitative 675
Analytical Writing not reported
Advanced Psychology not reported

GPA mean
3.78

Number of applications/admission offers/incoming students in 2007
378 applied/19 admission offers/15 incoming

% of students receiving:
Full tuition waiver only: 0%
Assistantship/fellowship only: 0%
Both full tuition waiver & assistantship/fellowship: 95%

Approximate percentage of incoming students with a B.A./B.S. only: 80% **Master's:** 20%

Approximate percentage of students who are Women: 78% **Ethnic Minority:** 20% **International:** 6%

Average years to complete the doctoral program (including internship): 6 years

Personal interview
Preferred in person but telephone acceptable

Attrition rate in past 7 years: 3.6%

Percentage of students applying for internship last year accepted into APPIC or APA internships: 100%

Formal tracks/concentrations: clinical health psychology, clinical child/pediatric psychology, neuropsychology, neurorehabilitation, and clinical neuroscience

Research areas	# Faculty	# Grants
anxiety disorders and emotions	2	3
child clinical psychology	3	3
clinical/medical psychology	3	3
functional neuroimaging	2	3
neuropsychology	6	4
obesity treatment	1	1
pain	2	3
pediatric psychology	2	4
rural health	1	2

Clinical opportunities

anxiety
child clinical psychology fear
forensic psychology
inpatient consultation/liaison
medical psychology
neuropsychology

pain and stress
parent training
pediatric consultation
rural behavioral health
weight loss

Florida Institute of Technology (Psy.D.)

School of Psychology
150 West University Boulevard
Melbourne, FL 32901
phone#: (407) 674-8104
e-mail: relmore@fit.edu
Web address: cpla.fit.edu//clinical/index.htm

1	2	**3**	4	5	6	7
Practice oriented		Equal emphasis			Research oriented	

Percentage of faculty subscribing to each of the following orientations:

Psychodynamic/Psychoanalytic	10%
Applied behavioral analysis/Radical behavioral	10%
Family systems/Systems	20%
Existential/Phenomenological/Humanistic	20%
Cognitive/Cognitive-behavioral	40%

Courses required for incoming students to have completed prior to enrolling:
Statistics, learning, personality, physiological, abnormal, social

Recommended but not mandatory courses:
Data not available

GRE mean
Verbal + Quantitative 1054
Analytical Writing 4.5

GPA mean
Overall GPA 3.63

Number of applications/admission offers/incoming students in 2007
101 applied/59 admission offers/29 incoming

% of students receiving:
Full tuition waiver only: 0%
Assistantship/fellowship only: 58%
Both full tuition waiver & assistantship/fellowship: 0%

Approximate percentage of incoming students with a B.A./B.S. only: 60% **Master's:** 40%

Approximate percentage of students who are Women: 78% **Ethnic Minority:** 16% **International:** 1%

Average years to complete the doctoral program (including internship): 5 years

Personal interview
Preferred in person but telephone acceptable

Attrition rate in past 7 years: 10%

Percentage of students applying for internship last year accepted into APPIC or APA internships: 94%

Formal tracks/concentrations: family/child psychology, neuropsychology, clinical health, forensic

Research areas	# Faculty	# Grants
aging	1	2
eating disorders	1	0
family psychology	2	0
health psychology	3	0
neuropsychology	2	1
personality assessment	3	0
sexual abuse	1	1
supervision	1	0
PTSD (Vietnam veterans)	1	0

Clinical opportunities

behavioral medicine/health psychology
eating disorders
family and marital therapy

forensic settings
neuropsychology
sexual abuse
Vietnam veterans

Florida State University (Ph.D.)

Department of Psychology
Tallahassee, FL 32306-1051
phone#: (850) 644-2499
e-mail: dilworth@psy.fsu.edu
Web address: www.psy.fsu.edu

1	2	3	4	5	6	**7**
Practice oriented		Equal emphasis			Research oriented	

Percentage of faculty subscribing to each of the following orientations:

Psychodynamic/Psychoanalytic	0%
Applied behavioral analysis/Radical behavioral	0%
Family systems/Systems	0%
Existential/Phenomenological/Humanistic	15%
Cognitive/Cognitive-behavioral	100%

Courses required for incoming students to have completed prior to enrolling:
Undergraduate degree

Recommended but not mandatory courses:
None

GRE mean
Verbal 653   Quantitative 723
Analytical Writing 4.9

GPA mean
Junior/Senior GPA 3.9

Number of applications/admission offers/incoming students in 2007
Not reported

% of students receiving:
Full tuition waiver only: 0%
Assistantship/fellowship only: 0%
Both full tuition waiver & assistantship/fellowship: 100%

Approximate percentage of incoming students with a B.A./B.S. only: 80%   **Master's:** 20%

Approximate percentage of students who are Women: 81%   **Ethnic Minority:** 23%   **International:** 2%

Average years to complete the doctoral program (including internship): 7 years

Personal interview
Preferred in person but telephone acceptable

Attrition rate in past 7 years: 5%

Percentage of students applying for internship last year accepted into APPIC or APA internships: 100%

Formal tracks/concentrations: none

Research areas	# Faculty	# Grants
addictive behavior	2	1
anxiety	1	4
conduct disorder and antisocial	1	1
bulimia nervosa	3	3
developmental psychopathology	3	3
early intervention	2	1
epidemiological psychology	1	1
prediction of criminal behavior	1	0
problematic social interactions	1	1
suicide	1	0

Clinical opportunities

adolescent delinquency	juvenile felony offenders
anxiety disorders	migrant workers
behavioral health	state psychiatric hospital
child problems	

Fordham University (Ph.D.)

Department of Psychology
Fordham Road and Southern Boulevard
Bronx, NY 10458
phone#: (718) 817-3782
fax#: (718) 817-3785
e-mail: cboyle@fordham.edu

Web address:
www.fordham.edu/academics/colleges__graduate_s/
graduate__profession/arts__sciences/gsas_academics/
psychology/clinical_psychology/

1	2	3	4	**5**	6	7
Practice oriented			Equal emphasis			Research oriented

Percentage of faculty subscribing to each of the following orientations:

Psychodynamic/Psychoanalytic	15%
Applied behavioral analysis/Radical behavioral	10%
Family systems/Systems	15%
Existential/Phenomenological/Humanistic	10%
Cognitive/Cognitive-behavioral	50%

Courses required for incoming students to have completed prior to enrolling:
Statistics, experimental

Recommended but not mandatory courses:
An undergraduate background in psychology is expected, but not required.

GRE mean
1385

GPA mean
3.58

Number of applications/admission offers/incoming students in 2007
375 applied/19 admission offers/11 incoming

% of students receiving:
Full tuition waiver only: 20%
Assistantship/fellowship only: 0%
Both full tuition waiver & assistantship/fellowship: 75%

Approximate percentage of incoming students with a B.A./B.S. only: 80%   **Master's:** 20%

Approximate percentage of students who are Women: 66%   **Ethnic Minority:** 30%   **International:** 10%

Average years to complete the doctoral program (including internship): 7.1 years

Personal interview
No preference given

Attrition rate in past 7 years: 6%

Percentage of students applying for internship last year accepted into APPIC or APA internships: 89%

Formal tracks/concentrations: child/family, health/neuropsychology, forensic

Research areas	# Faculty	# Grants
adolescent development	1	0
assessment	3	0
attachment in couples	1	0
clinical child psychology	2	0
family systems	1	0
health psychology/behavioral medicine	2	2
MMPI	3	0

neuropsychology	2	1
parent–child relationships	2	0
personality disorders	2	1
prevention	1	0
social support	2	0
stress and coping	2	1
substance abuse	2	1

Clinical opportunities

Clinical externships available at numerous inpatient and outpatient specialty clinics in the New York metropolitan area. Appropriate training sites can be found in any area, including highly specialized.

Forest Institute of Professional Psychology (Psy.D.)

2885 West Battlefield Road
Springfield, MO 65807
phone#: (417) 823-3477 or (800) 424-7793
e-mail: admissions@forest.edu
Web address: www.forest.edu

1	2	3	4	5	6	7
Practice oriented		Equal emphasis			Research oriented	

Percentage of faculty subscribing to each of the following orientations:

Psychodynamic/Psychoanalytic	40%
Applied behavioral analysis/Radical behavioral	10%
Family systems/Systems	20%
Existential/Phenomenological/Humanistic	10%
Cognitive/Cognitive-behavioral	20%

Courses required for incoming students to have completed prior to enrolling:

Psy.D.: 18 hours of psychology, abnormal, statistics, development, biological sciences
M.A.: 12 hours of psychology

Recommended but not mandatory courses:

History and systems, personality

GRE mean

Verbal 550   Quantitative 490
Analytical Writing Data not available

GPA mean

Not reported

Number of applications/admission offers/incoming students in 2007

Not reported

% of students receiving:

Full tuition waiver only: 0%
Assistantship/fellowship only: 6%
Both full tuition waiver & assistantship/fellowship: 0%

Approximate percentage of incoming students with a B.A./B.S. only: 54%   **Master's:** 46%

Approximate percentage of students who are Women: 60%   **Ethnic Minority:** 15%
International: not reported

Average years to complete the doctoral program (including internship): 4–5 years

Personal interview

Required in person

Attrition rate in past 7 years: 4%

Percentage of students applying for internship last year accepted into APPIC or APA internships: 90%

Formal tracks/concentrations: marriage & family therapy, child & adolescent, forensic, neuropsychology

Research areas	# Faculty	# Grants
autoimmune disorders and psychological indices	2	1
depression	2	1
electro-stimulation and stress	2	1
pain management	2	1

Clinical opportunities

biofeedback	multicultural center
child therapy	neuropsychology
corrections/forensics	pain management
integrated healthcare	psychopharmacology
marriage and family therapy	underserved populations

Fuller Theological Seminary (Ph.D. & Psy.D.)

(Part of Fuller Theological Seminary)
180 North Oakland Avenue
Pasadena, CA 91101
phone#: (626) 584-5500
e-mail: lwagener@fuller.edu
Web address:
www.fuller.edu/admiss/degrees/phdpsy.asp and
http://www.fuller.edu/admiss/degrees/psyd.asp

1	2	3	**4**	5	6	7
Practice oriented		Equal emphasis			Research oriented	

Percentage of faculty subscribing to each of the following orientations:

Psychodynamic/Psychoanalytic	20%
Applied behavioral analysis/Radical behavioral	10%
Family systems/Systems	30%
Existential/Phenomenological/Humanistic	10%
Cognitive/Cognitive-behavioral	30%

Courses required for incoming students to have completed prior to enrolling:

6 courses in psychology and a B.A. from an accredited school

Recommended but not mandatory courses:

Abnormal, developmental, experimental, physiological, social, statistics, testing, learning, motivation, personality

GRE mean

Verbal + Quantitative 1180

GPA mean

Psychology GPA 3.6

Number of applications/admission offers/incoming students in 2007
111 applied/70 admission offers/40 incoming

% of students receiving:
Full tuition waiver only: 0%
Assistantship/fellowship only: 10%
Both full tuition waiver & assistantship/fellowship: 0%

Approximate percentage of incoming students with a B.A./B.S. only: 76% **Master's:** 24%

Approximate percentage of students who are Women: 70% **Ethnic Minority:** 35% **International:** 6%

Average years to complete the doctoral program (including internship): 6 years

Personal interview
Preferred in person but telephone acceptable

Attrition rate in past 7 years: not reported

Percentage of students applying for internship last year accepted into APPIC or APA internships: 77% in APA internships, 92% in APPIC

Formal tracks/concentrations: Family (Ph.D. & Psy.D.), Leadership (Psy.D. only)

Research areas	# Faculty	# Grants
biopsychosocial	3	2
child clinical	3	1
cognition	1	0
cross-cultural psychology	2	0
depression	1	0
developmental	3	1
family	2	1
group processes	1	0
health psychology/behavioral medicine	3	0
marriages	4	0
neuropsychology	2	0
posttraumatic stress disorders	2	0
relaxation/biofeedback	1	0
religion	7	0
stress and coping	1	0
substance abuse	1	0

Clinical opportunities

assessment	inpatient adult population
child/adolescent therapy	interpersonal psychotherapy
chronic mental illness	marital/couples therapy
family therapy	neuropsychology/
forensic population	rehabilitation
gerontology	supervision
group therapy	victim/battering

Gallaudet University (Ph.D.)

Department of Psychology
8th and Florida Avenue, NE
Washington, DC 20002-3695
phone#: (202) 651-5540
e-mail: Patrick.Brice@Gallaudet.edu
Web address: www.gallaudet.edu/x718.xml

1	2	**3**	4	5	6	7
Practice oriented		Equal emphasis			Research oriented	

Percentage of faculty subscribing to each of the following orientations:

Psychodynamic/Psychoanalytic	60%
Applied behavioral analysis/Radical behavioral	20%
Family systems/Systems	0%
Existential/Phenomenological/Humanistic	20%
Cognitive/Cognitive-behavioral	40%

Courses required for incoming students to have completed prior to enrolling:
Major or minor in undergraduate psychology including statistics, experimental, abnormal, and child development

Recommended but not mandatory courses:
Social psychology, personality, learning, cognition, perception

GRE mean
Verbal 485   Quantitative 512
Advanced Psychology not required
Analytical Writing 4.0

GPA mean
Overall GPA 3.3   Psychology GPA 3.5

Number of applications/admission offers/incoming students in 2005
20 applied/7 admission offers/7 incoming

% of students receiving:
Full tuition waiver only: 20%
Assistantship/fellowship only: 70%
Both full tuition waiver & assistantship/fellowship: 5%

Approximate percentage of incoming students with a B.A./B.S. only: 88% **Master's:** 12%

Approximate percentage of students who are Women: 88% **Ethnic Minority:** 12% **International:** 7%

Deaf or Hard of Hearing: 33% **Hearing:** 67%

Average years to complete the doctoral program (including internship): 6.25 years

Personal interview
Preferred in person but telephone acceptable

Attrition rate in past 7 years: not reported

Percentage of students applying for internship last year accepted into APPIC or APA internships: 75%

Formal tracks/concentrations: none

Research areas	# Faculty	# Grants
adult development of deaf lesbians and gay men	1	0
attachment in deaf persons	2	1
attention in deaf children	1	1
depression in deaf clients	1	0
cognitive processing and memory in deaf persons	1	0
ethics in mental health and deafness	1	0

neuropsychological assessment	1	0
parental involvement with education of deaf children	1	1

Clinical opportunities
Assessment and therapy with deaf and hard-of-hearing clients through our multidisciplinary mental health clinic. More than 60 externship programs available in Washington, D.C. metropolitan area.

George Fox University (Psy.D.)
Graduate Department of Clinical Psychology
School of Behavioral and Health Sciences
414 N Meridian Street
Newberg, OR 97132-2697
phone#: 800-631-0921 x2263
e-mail: psyd@georgefox.edu
Web address: psyd.georgefox.edu

1	2	**3**	4	5	6	7
Practice oriented		Equal emphasis			Research oriented	

Percentage of faculty subscribing to each of the following orientations:
Psychodynamic/Psychoanalytic	10%
Applied behavioral analysis/Radical behavioral	10%
Family systems/Systems	10%
Existential/Phenomenological/Humanistic	10%
Cognitive/Cognitive-behavioral	50%

Courses required for incoming students prior to enrolling:
18 semester hours or the equivalent (no specific courses required)

Courses recommended but not mandatory:
Abnormal, developmental, statistics, social, experimental, personality, psychobiology

GRE mean
Verbal + Quantitative 1180
Analytical Writing not used

GPA mean
Overall GPA 3.69

Number of applications/admission offers/incoming students in 2007
75 applied/33 admission offers/22 incoming

% of students receiving:
Full tuition waiver only: 0%
Partial tuition waiver only: 20%
Assistantship/fellowship only: 25%
Both full tuition waiver & assistantship/fellowship: 0%

Approximate percentage of incoming students with a B.A./B.S. only: 75%   Master's: 25%

Approximate percentage of students who are
Women: 55%   Ethnic Minority: 9%   International: 0%

Average years to complete the doctoral program (including internship): 5.2 years

Personal interview
Preferred in person but telephone acceptable in special circumstances.

Attrition rate in past 7 years: 5%

Percentage of students applying for internship last year accepted into APPIC or APA internships: 100%

Formal tracks/concentrations: None

Research areas	# Faculty	# Grants
adjudicated youth/adults	1	0
child and geriatric memory	1	0
clinical supervision	1	0
coping skills in students	1	1
marriage relationships	1	1
memory assessment	1	1
school consultation	1	1
pain management	1	1
shame	1	0
spirituality and mental health	1	1
Stroop effect	1	1
values and psychologist training	1	0

Clinical opportunities
addictions	inpatient hospital consultation
adolescent residential assessment	Native American setting
child psychopathology	neuropsychology
community mental health	hospital consultation
corrections	pain management
emergency room consultation	primary health care setting
geriatrics	public school setting
health psychology	rural psychology
	spirituality

George Mason University (Ph.D.)
Department of Psychology
4400 University Drive
Fairfax, VA 22030-4444
phone#: (703) 993-1342
e-mail: dwiggin3@gmu.edu
Web address:
www.gmu.edu/departments/psychology/clinical/

1	2	3	4	**5**	6	7
Practice oriented		Equal emphasis			Research oriented	

Percentage of faculty subscribing to each of the following orientations:
Psychodynamic/Psychoanalytic	25%
Applied behavioral analysis/Radical behavioral	0%
Family systems/Systems	15%
Existential/Phenomenological/Humanistic	25%
Cognitive/Cognitive-behavioral	80%
Community	25%

Courses required for incoming students to have completed prior to enrolling:
Statistics, abnormal, any laboratory science course

Recommended but not mandatory courses:
Tests and measurements, personality

GRE mean
Verbal 640   Quantitative 698
Analytical Writing not reported

GPA mean
Overall GPA 3.74

Number of applications/admission offers/incoming students in 2007
211 applied/15 admission offers/7 incoming

% of students receiving:
Full tuition waiver only: 0%
Assistantship/fellowship only: 0%
Both full tuition waiver & assistantship/fellowship: 100%

Approximate percentage of incoming students with a B.A./B.S. only: 100%   **Master's:** 0%

Approximate percentage of students who are Women: 78%   **Ethnic Minority:** 12%   **International:** 5%

Average years to complete the doctoral program (including internship): 6 years

Personal interview
Required in person (phone interview possible)

Attrition rate in past 7 years: 11.5%

Percentage of students applying for internship last year accepted into APPIC or APA internships: 80%

Formal tracks/concentrations: none

Research areas	# Faculty	# Grants
psychological adjustment	4	0
cognition and affect	4	0
domestic violence	1	0
criminal behavior	1	1
gay and lesbian issues	1	0
personality	1	1
positive human functioning	3	1
psychotherapy process	1	0
self-efficacy	1	0
social anxiety	1	0
stress and coping	2	0
program evaluation	1	1

Clinical opportunities
Child and adult assessment
cognitive-behavioral psychotherapy
community consultation/education
group/marriage/family psychotherapy
individual adult psychotherapy
program evaluation

George Washington University (Ph.D.)
Department of Psychology
2125 G Street, NW
Washington, DC 20052
phone#: (202) 994-6320
e-mail: ghowe@gwu.edu
Web address: www.gwu.edu/~clinpsyc

1	2	3	4	**5**	6	7
Practice oriented		Equal emphasis			Research oriented	

Percentage of faculty subscribing to each of the following orientations:

Psychodynamic/Psychoanalytic	0%
Applied behavioral analysis/Radical behavioral	10%
Family systems/Systems	30%
Existential/Phenomenological/Humanistic	10%
Cognitive/Cognitive-behavioral	60%

Courses required for incoming students to have completed prior to enrolling:
Equivalent of a major in psychology: statistics, research methods, basic psychology courses

Recommended but not mandatory courses:
None

GRE mean
Verbal 622   Quantitative 706
Analytical Writing Data not available

GPA mean
Overall GPA 3.56

Number of applications/admission offers/incoming students in 2007
299 applied/7 admission offers/5 incoming

% of students receiving:
Full tuition waiver only: 0%
Assistantship/fellowship only: 0%
Both full tuition waiver & assistantship/fellowship: 100%

Approximate percentage of incoming students with a B.A./B.S. only: 80%   **Master's:** 20%

Approximate percentage of students who are Women: 80%   **Ethnic Minority:** 40%   **International:** 0%

Average years to complete the doctoral program (including internship): 6.5 years

Personal interview
Preferred in person but telephone acceptable

Attrition rate in past 7 years: 7.5%

Percentage of students applying for internship last year accepted into APPIC or APA internships: 100%

Formal tracks/concentrations: none

Research areas	# Faculty	# Grants
adolescence	3	2
AIDS	1	2
anxiety disorders	1	0
behavioral medicine	1	0
child	2	1
community	6	1
depression	2	2
family	2	1
health	1	0
minority mental health	4	3
relaxation/biofeedback	1	0
stress	3	1

Clinical opportunities

adolescent problems	group therapy
AIDS	health
adolescent delinquency	hyperactivity
affective disorders	impulse control/aggression
anxiety disorders	marital/couples therapy
assessment	minority/cross-cultural
behavioral medicine	neuropsychology/
child	rehabilitation
conduct disorder	obsessive–compulsive
developmental disabilities/	disorder
autism	personality disorders
dissociative disorder	psychodynamic therapy
eating disorders	schizophrenia/psychoses
family therapy	substance abuse
forensic psychology	victim/battering abuse

George Washington University (Psy.D.)

Center for Professional Psychology
2300 M Street, NW, Suite 910
Washington, DC 20037
phone#: (202) 496-6260
e-mail: psyd@gwu.edu
Web address: www.gwu.edu/~psyd/index.htm

1	2	**3**	4	5	6	7
Practice oriented		Equal emphasis			Research oriented	

Percentage of faculty subscribing to each of the following orientations:

Psychodynamic/Psychoanalytic	90%
Applied behavioral analysis/Radical behavioral	0%
Family systems/Systems	0%
Existential/Phenomenological/Humanistic	0%
Cognitive/Cognitive-behavioral	10%

Courses required for incoming students to have completed prior to enrolling:
B.A./B.S.

Recommended but not mandatory courses:
Psychodynamicc theory, personality, development, psychodynamic therapy, cognitive development, statistics

GRE mean
Verbal 556   Quantitative 626   Analytical 641
Analytical Writing 5.2

GPA mean
Overall GPA 3.5

Number of applications/admission offers/incoming students in 2007
337 applied/admission offers/33 incoming

% of students receiving:
Full tuition waiver only: 0%
Assistantship/fellowship only: 33%
Both full tuition waiver & assistantship/fellowship: 0%

Approximate percentage of incoming students with a B.A./B.S. only: 63%   **Master's:** 17%

Approximate percentage of students who are Women: 76%   **Ethnic Minority:** 28%   **International:**

Average years to complete the doctoral program (including internship): 4.3 years

Personal interview
Required in person

Attrition rate in past 7 years: not reported

Percentage of students applying for internship last year accepted into APPIC or APA internships: 95%

Formal tracks/concentrations: adult, child, assessment

Research areas	# Faculty	# Grants
adult psychopathology	4	0
child clinical	2	1
child development	2	2
community intervention	3	1
group process	3	0
infant and childhood	1	1
intellectual assessment	3	0
personality assessment	3	0

Clinical opportunities

assessment	family therapy
children	learning disorders
clinical outcome studies	psychotherapy
developmental disorders	schizophrenia

University of Georgia (Ph.D.)

Department of Psychology
Athens, GA 30602
phone#: (706) 542-1787
e-mail: gradpsych@uga.edu
Web address:
www.uga.edu/psychology/graduate/clinical/index.html

1	2	3	4	5	**6**	7
Practice oriented		Equal emphasis			Research oriented	

Percentage of faculty subscribing to each of the following orientations:

Psychodynamic/Psychoanalytic	0%
Applied behavioral analysis/Radical behavioral	0%
Family systems/Systems	10%
Existential/Phenomenological/Humanistic	0%
Cognitive/Cognitive-behavioral	100%

Courses required for incoming students to have completed prior to enrolling:
None

Recommended but not mandatory courses:
Abnormal, statistics

GRE mean
1226

GPA mean
Overall GPA 3.56

Number of applications/admission offers/incoming students in 2007
184 applied/16 admission offers/5 incoming

% of students receiving:
Full tuition waiver only: 0%
Assistantship/fellowship only: 0%
Both full tuition waiver & assistantship/fellowship: 100%

Approximate percentage of incoming students with a B.A./B.S. only: 100%   **Master's:** 0%

Approximate percentage of students who are Women: 77%   **Ethnic Minority:** 13%   **International:** 3%

Average years to complete the doctoral program (including internship): 5.28 years

Personal interview
Preferred in person but telephone acceptable

Attrition rate in past 7 years: 5%

Percentage of students applying for internship last year accepted into APPIC or APA internships: 100%

Formal tracks/concentrations: child, neuropsychology

Research areas	# Faculty	# Grants
adolescence	3	0
adult psychopathology	3	1
affective disorder/depression	1	1
aggression	2	1
aging/gerontology	1	3
alcohol use and stress	1	0
anxiety disorders	2	1
battering	2	0
behavioral medicine	2	0
cardiovascular function	1	1
child clinical/child psychopathology	3	2
depression	1	0
developmental psychopathology	2	1
emotions	1	0
family systems	1	0
interpersonal processes	1	1
marriage/couples	1	1
neuropsychology	1	2
pain management	1	1
parent–child interaction	2	0
pediatric psychology	3	2
prevention	2	1
psychology of women	1	0
schizophrenia/psychoses	1	0
stress and coping	1	1
substance abuse	2	0
violence victim–offender	3	1
women's issues in therapy	1	0

Clinical opportunities

affective disorders	impulse control/aggression
anxiety disorders	marital/couples
assessment	neuropsychology
behavior therapy	pediatric psychology
behavioral medicine	personality disorders
developmental disorders	psychotherapy supervision
dissociative disorders	stress management
eating disorders	substance abuse
family therapy	victim/battering/abuse

Georgia State University (Ph.D.)

Department of Psychology
University Plaza
P.O. Box 5010
Atlanta, GA 30303
phone#: (404) 413-6200
e-mail: ffloyd@gsu.edu
Web address: www2.gsu.edu/~wwwpsy/ClinProg.htm

1	2	3	**4**	5	6	7
Practice oriented		Equal emphasis			Research oriented	

Percentage of faculty subscribing to each of the following orientations:

Psychodynamic/Psychoanalytic/Interpersonal	10%
Applied behavioral analysis/Radical behavioral	0%
Family systems/Systems	20%
Existential/Phenomenological/Humanistic	0%
Cognitive/Cognitive-behavioral	40%
Clinical Neuropsychology	30%

Courses required for incoming students to have completed prior to enrolling:
Research methods, psychological statistics, and two additional junior/senior-level psychology courses

Recommended but not mandatory courses:
Abnormal

GRE mean
Verbal 599 (Median)   Quantitative 634 (Median)

GPA mean
Overall GPA 3.74

Number of applications/admission offers/incoming students in 2007
339 applied/17 admission offers/7 incoming

% of students receiving:
Full tuition waiver only: 0%
Assistantship/fellowship only: 0%
Both full tuition waiver & assistantship/fellowship: 100%

Approximate percentage of incoming students with a B.A./B.S. only: 90%   **Master's:** 10%

Approximate percentage of students who are Women: 80%   **Ethnic Minority:** 40%   **International:** 11%

Average years to complete the doctoral program (including internship): 6 years

Personal interview
Preferred in person but telephone acceptable

Attrition rate in past 7 years: 8%

Percentage of students applying for internship last year accepted into APPIC or APA internships: 82%

Formal tracks/concentrations: general clinical, neuropsychology, clinical/community

Research areas	# Faculty	# Grants
ACT	1	0
alcohol and aggression	1	1
acquired brain injuries	3	1
couples therapy	1	0
crime and delinquency	2	1
brain injury	1	0
emotion and executive functioning	3	0
developmental neuropsychology	3	2
family traumatology	1	2
families and developmental disabilities	1	2
functional neuroimaging	3	1
HIV and families	1	1
HIV prevention	1	3
gender issues	1	1
multicultural issues	3	0
male parenting	1	1
pediatric psychology	1	1
reading/dyslexia	1	4
treatment of anxiety disorders	1	1

Clinical opportunities

adjustment problems
anxiety disorders
behavioral assessment
chronic health conditions
clinical-community
clinical neuropsychology
developmental disabilities
health psychology
HIV/AIDS
individual, couples, family, and group therapy
neuropsychological assessment
personality assessment
personality disorders
psychopathology of childhood
psychosocial rehabilitation
psychotherapy supervision
violence prevention

University of Hartford (Psy.D.)

Graduate Institute of Professional Psychology
200 Bloomfield Ave.
West Hartford, CT 06105
phone#: (860) 768-4778
e-mail for admissions questions: viereck@hartford.edu
Web address: www.hartford.edu/gipp

1	**2**	3	4	5	6	7
Practice oriented		Equal emphasis			Research oriented	

Percentage of faculty subscribing to each of the following orientations:

Psychodynamic/Psychoanalytic	25%
Applied behavioral analysis/Radical behavioral	6%
Family systems/Systems	25%
Existential/Phenomenological/Humanistic	13%
Cognitive/Cognitive-behavioral	63%

Courses required for incoming students prior to enrolling:
None specifically required

Courses recommended but not mandatory:
Psychology major, abnormal, social, research methods, personality, developmental, statistics

GRE mean
Verbal 518   Quantitative 572
Advanced Psychology not reported
Analytical Writing not reported

Number of applications/admission offers/incoming students in 2007
164 applied/56 admission offers/23 incoming

% of students receiving:
Full tuition waiver only: 0%
Assistantship/fellowship only: 43%
Both full tuition waiver & assistantship/fellowship: 0%

Approximate percentage of incoming students with a B.A./B.S. only: 87%   **Master's:** 13%

Approximate percentage of students who are Women: 87%   **Ethnic Minority:** 13%
International: not reported

Average years to complete the doctoral program (including internship): 5.5 years

Personal interview
Required in person (unless international students)

Attrition rate in past 7 years: 10%

Percentage of students applying for internship last year accepted into APPIC or APA internships: 100%

Formal tracks/concentrations: child & adolescent

Research areas	# Faculty	# Grants
child/adolescent	2	0
community treatment	1	0
intimate partner violence	1	0
clinical supervision/mentoring	1	0
psychological assessment	1	0
applied behavior analysis	1	0
substance abuse	1	0
stigma of mental illness	1	1

Clinical opportunities

acute psychiatry/mental health
anxiety disorders
depression
chronic mental illness
children, adolescents, and families
forensics
community mental health
hospital-based psychology departments
counseling centers
residential schools

University of Hawaii at Manoa (Ph.D.)

Clinical Studies Program
Department of Psychology
2430 Campus Road
Honolulu, HI 96822
phone#: (808) 956-7644
e-mail: cmueller@hawaii.edu or vkeough@hawaii.edu
Web address: www.psychology.hawaii.edu/pages/graduate_programs/clinical.html

1	2	3	4	5	6	7
Practice oriented			Equal emphasis			Research oriented

Percentage of faculty subscribing to each of the following orientations:

Psychodynamic/Psychoanalytic	0%
Behavioral	50%
Family systems/Systems	15%
Existential/Phenomenological/Humanistic	0%
Cognitive/Cognitive-behavioral	85%

Courses required for incoming students prior to enrolling:
Psychology major or 5–10 selected psychology courses

Courses recommended but not mandatory:
None

GRE mean
Verbal 620   Quantitative 730
Advanced Psychology not required
Analytical Writing 5.5

GPA mean
Overall GPA 3.48

Number of applications/admission offers/incoming students in 2007
117 applied/7 admission offers/6 incoming

% of students receiving:
Full tuition waiver only: 0%
Assistantship/fellowship only: 0%
Both full tuition waiver & assistantship/fellowship: 100%

Approximate percentage of incoming students with a B.A./B.S. only: 67%   **Master's:** 33%

Approximate percentage of students who are Women: 81%   **Ethnic Minority:** 41%
International: 6.6%

Average years to complete the doctoral program (including internship): 8 years

Personal interview
Telephone required

Attrition rate in past 7 years: 8%

Percentage of students applying for internship last year accepted into APPIC or APA internships: 67%

Formal tracks/concentrations: none

Research areas	# Faculty	# Grants
anxiety	1	1
assessment	7	2
behavioral medicine	1	0
childhood clinical	3	4
cross-cultural	2	1
data-based case management	2	0
depression	2	0
eating disorders	2	1
ethnic minority	2	2
health care compliance	2	0
mental health systems	5	6
neurocognitive assessment	1	0
schizophrenia	5	1
substance use prevention	1	3
treatment outcome	4	4

Clinical opportunities

assessment	dual diagnoses
behavioral medicine	eating disorders
case and system consultation	neuropsychology
child clinical	rehabilitation psychology
cross-cultural	severely mentally ill
developmental disabilities	substance use prevention

University of Houston (Ph.D.)
Department of Psychology
126 Heyne Building
Houston, TX 77204-5022
phone#: (713) 743-8600
e-mail: jvincent@uh.edu
Web address:
www.Psychology.uh.edu/GraduatePrograms/Clinical/

1	2	3	4	5	6	7
Practice oriented			Equal emphasis			Research oriented

Percentage of faculty subscribing to each of the following orientations:

Psychodynamic/Psychoanalytic	6%
Applied behavioral analysis/Radical behavioral	5%
Family systems/Systems	20%
Existential/Phenomenological/Humanistic	0%
Cognitive/Cognitive-behavioral	100%

Courses required for incoming students prior to enrolling:
None

Courses recommended but not mandatory:
Statistics, history and systems, physiological psychology, abnormal, experimental, social, developmental, research methods

GRE mean
Verbal 586   Quantitative 704   Analytical/Writing 615

GPA mean
Overall GPA 3.65

Number of applications/admission offers/incoming students in 2007
224 applied/21 admission offers/13 incoming

% of students receiving:
Full tuition waiver only: 0%
Assistantship/fellowship only: 10%
Both full tuition waiver & assistantship/fellowship: 100%

Approximate percentage of incoming students with a B.A./B.S. only: 80.8%   **Master's:** 19.2%

Approximate percentage of students who are Women: 67%   **Ethnic Minority:** 16.7%
International: 3%

Average years to complete the doctoral program (including internship): 5.5 years

Personal interview : Preferred in person but telephone acceptable

Attrition rate in past 7 years: 1.2%

Percentage of students applying for internship last year accepted into APPIC or APA internships: 100%

Formal tracks/concentrations: clinical neuropsychology, adult behavior disorders, child-family

Research areas	# Faculty	# Grants
adult psychopathology	6	3
affective disorder/depression	3	2
anxiety disorder	3	3
child clinical	3	2
chronic mental illness	3	1
cross-cultural	3	2
family research/therapy	3	2
forensic psychology	2	1
marriage/couples	2	1
neuropsychology	4	4
parent–child interaction	2	1
schizophrenia/psychoses	2	1
social skills	4	3

Clinical opportunities

adolescent suicide
Alzheimer's/dementia
anxiety disorders
child custody evaluation
child depression/anxiety
child victimization
clinical assessment
cognitive therapy
conduct disorder
couples therapy
domestic violence
family therapy

forensic psychology
health psychology
interpersonal psychotherapy
learning disabilities
multicultural
post traumatic stress
   disorder
rehabilitation
neuropsychology
schizophrenia/psychoses
traumatic brain injury
stroke

Howard University (Ph.D.)

Department of Psychology
520 Bryant Street, NW
Washington, DC 2005
phone#: (202) 806-6805
e-mail: dso@howard.edu
Web address: www.founders.howard.edu/
psychology-dept/Clinical%20Program%2020050412
.html & www.founders.howard.edu/psychology-dept/
index.htm

1	2	3	**4**	5	6	7
Practice oriented		Equal emphasis			Research oriented	

Percentage of faculty subscribing to each of the following orientations:

Psychodynamic/Psychoanalytic	20%
Applied behavioral analysis/Radical behavioral	0%
Family systems/Systems	20%
Existential/Phenomenological/Humanistic	20%
Cognitive/Cognitive-behavioral	40%

Courses required for incoming students to have completed prior to enrolling:
Psychology major, including: statistics, abnormal, experimental, developmental

Recommended but not mandatory courses:
Psychological testing or statistics II

GRE mean 2007 admission class
Verbal 575   Quantitative 633
Analytical Writing not reported

GPA mean
3.67

Number of applications/admission offers/incoming students in 2007
147 applied/6 admission offers/6 incoming

% of students receiving:
Full tuition waiver only: 0%
Assistantship/fellowship only: 0%
Both full tuition waiver & assistantship/fellowship: 0%

Approximate percentage of incoming students with a B.A./B.S. only: 60%   **Master's:** 40%

Approximate percentage of students who are Women: 67%   **Ethnic Minority:** 100%
International: 17%

Average years to complete the doctoral program (including internship): 6.5 years

Personal interview
required in person

Attrition rate in past 7 years: 5%

Percentage of students applying for internship last year accepted into APPIC or APA internships: 80%

Formal tracks/concentrations: adult, child

Research areas	# Faculty	# Grants
adolescent development	3	1
behavioral medicine	3	2
clinical training	4	2
family therapy	2	0
minority mental health	4	3
neuropsychology	2	1
psychophysiology	1	1
suicide prevention	1	0

Clinical opportunities

anxiety disorders
behavioral medicine
child violence prevention
community psychology
crisis intervention
substance use disorders

family
minority
neuropsychology
schizophrenia
victim/battering

Idaho State University (Ph.D.)

Psychology Department
Box 8112
Idaho State University
Pocatello ID 83209

phone#: (208) 282-2462
e-mail: robemark@isu.edu
Web address:
www.isu.edu/psych/clinicalprogram.shtml

1	2	3	**4**	5	6	7
Practice oriented			Equal emphasis			Research oriented

Percentage of faculty subscribing to each of the following orientations:

Psychodynamic/Psychoanalytic	15%
Applied behavioral analysis/Radical behavioral	33%
Family systems/Systems	33%
Existential/Phenomenological/Humanistic	100%
Cognitive/Cognitive-behavioral	100%

Courses required for incoming students to have completed prior to enrolling:
Psychology major or its equivalent. Methodology courses are mandatory.

Recommended but not mandatory courses:
None

GRE mean
Verbal 580   Quantitative 629
Analytical Writing 5.5
Advanced Psychology 665

GPA mean
Overall GPA 3.76

Number of applications/admission offers/incoming students in 2007
73 applied/12 admission offers/6 incoming

% of students receiving:
Full tuition waiver only: 0%
Assistantship/fellowship only: 58%
Both full tuition waiver & assistantship/fellowship: 35%

Approximate percentage of incoming students with a B.A./B.S. only: 90%   Master's: 10%

Approximate percentage of students who are
Women: 77%   Ethnic Minority: 4%   International: 4%

Average years to complete the doctoral program (including internship): 6.2 years

Personal interview
Preferred in person, but telephone acceptable

Attrition rate in past 7 years: 15%

Percentage of students applying for internship last year accepted into APPIC or APA internships: 100%

Formal tracks/concentrations: none

Research areas	# Faculty	# Grants
addictions	3	1
behavioral pharmocology	1	2
developmental psychopathology	1	1
mood and decision making	1	0
parent–child interaction therapy	1	0
sexual assault	1	2
trauma	2	1
working memory	1	2
person perception	1	0

Clinical opportunities
cognitive behavioral treatments
family systems therapy
parent–child interaction therapy
relapse prevention group therapy
neuropsychological evaluations
sexual dysfunction

University of Illinois at Chicago (Ph.D.)
Department of Psychology
1007 West Harrison
Chicago, IL 60680
phone#: (312) 996-1469
e-mail: jkassel@uic.edu
Web address: www.psch.uic.edu/clinicalprog.asp?sm
=clinical_program

1	2	3	4	5	**6**	7
Practice oriented			Equal emphasis			Research oriented

Percentage of faculty subscribing to each of the following orientations:

Psychodynamic/Psychoanalytic	0%
Applied behavioral analysis/Radical behavioral	5%
Family systems/Systems	15%
Existential/Phenomenological/Humanistic	20%
Cognitive/Cognitive-behavioral	80%
Community Psychology	10%

Courses required for incoming students prior to enrolling:
None

Courses recommended but not mandatory:
Statistics, science courses, independent research (for psychology majors), other research experience

GRE mean
Verbal 638   Quantitative 734
Advanced Psychology 710
Analytical Writing 5.4

GPA mean
Junior/Senior GPA 3.7

Number of applications/admission offers/incoming students in 2007
168 applied/10 admission offers/5 incoming

% of students receiving:
Full tuition waiver only: 0%
Assistantship/fellowship only: 0%
Both full tuition waiver & assistantship/fellowship: 100%

Approximate percentage of incoming students with a B.A./B.S. only: 100%   Master's: 0%

Approximate percentage of students who are
Women: 78%   Ethnic Minority: 14%   International: 5%

Average years to complete the doctoral program (including internship): 8 years

Personal interview
Preferred in person but telephone acceptable

Attrition rate in past 7 years: 15%

Percentage of students applying for internship last year accepted into APPIC or APA internships: 75%

Formal tracks/concentrations: none

Research areas	# Faculty	# Grants
AIDS	2	2
alcohol relapse	1	1
anxiety	3	1
cognitive deficits in schizophrenia	1	4
community psychology	1	1
depression	2	0
eating disorders and obesity	1	0
health behavior change	4	1
neurobehavioral and genetic aspects of autism	1	4
tobacco abuse	3	5

Clinical opportunities

adjustment reactions
anxiety and depression
health-related behaviors
HIV prevention
prevention
smoking cessation
weight reduction

University of Illinois at Urbana–Champaign (Ph.D.)

Department of Psychology
Psychology Building
603 East Daniel Street
Champaign, IL 61820
phone#: (217) 333-2169
e-mail: gradstdy@s.psych.uiuc.edu
Web address:
www.psych.uiuc.edu/divisions/clinicalcommunity.php

1	2	3	4	5	6	7
Practice oriented		Equal emphasis			Research oriented	

Percentage of faculty subscribing to each of the following orientations:

Psychodynamic/Psychoanalytic	100%
Applied behavioral analysis/Radical behavioral	0%
Family systems/Systems	100%
Existential/Phenomenological/Humanistic	0%
Cognitive/Cognitive-behavioral	100%

Courses required for incoming students to have completed prior to enrolling:
None

Recommended but not mandatory courses:
Psychology major, undergraduate statistics

GRE mean
Verbal 636   Quantitative 696
Advanced Psychology 716
Analytical Writing 5.0

GPA mean
Overall GPA 3.85

Number of applications/admission offers/incoming students in 2007
200 applied/18 admission offers/7 incoming

% of students receiving:
Full tuition waiver only: 0%
Assistantship/fellowship only: 0%
Both full tuition waiver & assistantship/fellowship: 100%

Approximate percentage of incoming students with a B.A./B.S. only: 100%   **Master's:** 0%

Approximate percentage of students who are Women: 75%   **Ethnic Minority:** 45%   **International:** 5%

Average years to complete the doctoral program (including internship): 7 years

Personal interview
Telephone required

Attrition rate in past 7 years: 12%

Percentage of students applying for internship last year accepted into APPIC or APA internships: 87.5%

Formal tracks/concentrations: none

Research areas	# Faculty	# Grants
behavior genetics	2	2
clinical neuropsychology	2	4
clinical psychophysiology	3	8
community psychology	5	4
research/program evaluation	4	3
cultural-community mental health	2	2
neuroimaging	3	8
intervention research	2	2
emotion and psychopathology	5	10
minority mental health	5	5
indigenous mental health	2	2
psychotherapy	1	1
schizophrenia	2	5
suicide	1	1
women's issues	3	2

Clinical opportunities

anxiety
child assessment
community development
community-based
   organizations consultation
community intervention
culturally-competent
   therapy
depression
diverse populations
family interventions
forensic evaluations
group therapy
health care systems
change assessment
individual adult
   psychotherapy
inpatient assessment
minority mental health
community organization
neuropsychological
   assessment
school consultation
educational settings and
   policy

Illinois Institute of Technology (Ph.D.)

Department of Psychology
IIT Center, LS252
Chicago, IL 60616
phone#: (312) 562-3503, 567-3500
e-mail: myoung@charlie.cns.iit.edu or
youngm@iit.edu
Web address:
www.iit.edu/colleges/psych/current/programs/clinical

1	2	3	4	5	6	7
Practice oriented			Equal emphasis			Research oriented

Percentage of faculty subscribing to each of the following orientations:

Psychodynamic/Psychoanalytic 0%
Applied behavioral analysis/Radical behavioral 0%
Family systems/Systems 10%
Existential/Phenomenological/Humanistic 0%
Cognitive/Cognitive-behavioral 90%

Courses required for incoming students to have completed prior to enrolling:

18 credits in psychology including experimental and statistics

Recommended but not mandatory courses:

None

GRE mean

Verbal 565   Quantitative 650
Analytical Writing

GPA mean

Overall GPA 3.51

Number of applications/admission offers/incoming students in 2007

110 applied/22 admission offers/13 incoming

% of students receiving:

Full tuition waiver only: 0%
Assistantship/fellowship only: 100%
Both full tuition waiver & assistantship/fellowship: 23%

Approximate percentage of incoming students with a B.A./B.S. only: 80% Master's: 20%

Approximate percentage of students who are Women: 80% Ethnic Minority: 17% International: 6%

Average years to complete the doctoral program (including internship): 5.5 years

Personal interview

Preferred in person but telephone acceptable

Attrition rate in past 7 years: 5%

Percentage of students applying for internship last year accepted into APPIC or APA internships: 67%

Formal tracks/concentrations: general clinical, combined rehab/clinical

Research areas	# Faculty	# Grants
ADHD	1	0
affective disorders	1	1
child behavior	2	1
family	1	0
health	1	1
marital	1	1
pediatric	2	1
severe mental illness	2	1
social support	1	0
rehabilitation	2	1
acceptance % commitment therapy	1	0

Clinical opportunities

affective disorders
child
family
health/behavioral medicine
marital/couples
minority/cross-cultural
neuropsychology
pain
severe mental illness

Immaculata University (Psy.D.)

Department of Graduate Psychology
Immaculata, PA 19345-0500
phone#: (610) 647-4400, ext. 3503
e-mail: jyalof@immaculata.edu
Web address: www.immaculata.edu/GraduateStudies/
Admission/Doctoral%20Clinical%20Psychology.htm

1	2	3	4	5	6	7
Practice oriented			Equal emphasis			Research oriented

Percentage of faculty subscribing to each of the following orientations:

Psychodynamic/Psychoanalytic 20%
Applied behavioral analysis/Radical behavioral 0%
Family systems/Systems 10%
Existential/Phenomenological/Humanistic 20%
Cognitive/Cognitive-behavioral 20%

Courses required for incoming students to have completed prior to enrolling:

Two tracks: MA or equivalent post baccalaureate, and bachelor's degree

Recommended but not mandatory courses:

None

GRE mean

A calculated mean is not used.

GPA mean

MA minimum of 3.0; BA minimum of 3.3

Number of applications/admission offers/incoming students in 2007

124 applied/53 admission offers/29 incoming

% of students receiving:

Full tuition waiver only: 0%
Assistantship/fellowship only: 0%
Both full tuition waiver & assistantship/fellowship: 0%

Approximate percentage of incoming students with a B.A./B.S. only: 51% Master's: 49%

179

Approximate percentage of students who are
Women: 93% **Ethnic Minority:** 7%
International: not reported

Average years to complete the doctoral program (including internship): 6 years

Personal interview
Required

Attrition rate in past 7 years: 15%

Percentage of students applying for internship last year accepted into APPIC or APA internships:
APPIC = 73%; APA = 20%

Formal tracks/concentrations: none

Research areas	# Faculty	# Grants
child, adolescent	2	0
development	3	0
existential-humanistic	2	0
diversity	3	0
psychotherapy process	2	0
family therapy	2	0
positive psychology	2	0
neuropsychology	2	0
personality assessment	2	0
school psychology	2	0
geriatric	1	0
ethics	2	0

Clinical opportunities

Indiana State University (Psy.D.)

Department of Psychology
Root Hall
Terre Haute, IN 47809
phone#: (812) 237-4314
e-mail: lizo@indstate.edu
Web address: www.indstate.edu/psych/36.html

1	2	**3**	4	5	6	7
Practice oriented		Equal emphasis			Research oriented	

Percentage of faculty subscribing to each of the following orientations:
Psychodynamic/Psychoanalytic   15%
Applied behavioral analysis/Radical behavioral   0%
Family systems/Systems   15%
Existential/Phenomenological/Humanistic   5%
Cognitive/Cognitive-behavioral   70%

Courses required for incoming students prior to enrolling:
Abnormal, personality, experimental, statistics, learning or cognition (24 credits in undergraduate psychology)

Courses recommended but not mandatory:
Physiological

GRE mean
1191

GPA mean
3.69

Number of applications/admission offers/incoming students in 2007
140 applied/9 admission offers/9 incoming

% of students receiving:
Full tuition waiver only: 0%
Assistantship/fellowship only: 0%
Both full tuition waiver & assistantship/fellowship: 100%

Approximate percentage of incoming students with a B.A./B.S. only: 80% **Master's:** 20%

Approximate percentage of students who are
Women: 67% **Ethnic Minority:** 0% **International:** 0%

Average years to complete the doctoral program (including internship): 5.5 years

Personal interview
Preferred in person but telephone acceptable

Attrition rate in past 7 years: 8%

Percentage of students applying for internship last year accepted into APPIC or APA internships: 86%

Formal tracks/concentrations: none

Research areas	# Faculty	# Grants
adult psychopathology	2	0
affective disorders	2	0
anxiety disorders	0	0
assessment	2	0
behavioral medicine	3	1
child psychopathology	1	0
clinical judgment	1	0
eating disorders	2	1
friendship/relationships/intimacy	1	0
gender roles	3	0
organizational/industrial	1	1
personality disorders	1	0
professional training	1	0
stress and coping	2	0
substance abuse	1	1
women's studies	2	0

Clinical opportunities
ADHD assessment   forensic psychology
behavioral medicine   rural psychology

Indiana University–Bloomington (Ph.D.)

Department of Psychological and Brain Sciences
1101 E. 10th Street
Bloomington, IN 47405
phone#: (812) 855-2311
e-mail: shiricha@indiana.edu
Web address: www.indiana.edu/%7Eclinpsy/

1	2	3	4	5	6	**7**
Practice oriented		Equal emphasis			Research oriented	

Percentage of faculty subscribing to each of the following orientations:

Psychodynamic/Psychoanalytic	0%
Applied behavioral analysis/Radical behavioral	0%
Family systems/Systems	100%
Existential/Phenomenological/Humanistic	0%
Cognitive/Cognitive-behavioral	100%

Courses required for incoming students to have completed prior to enrolling:
Psychology major

Recommended but not mandatory courses:
Basic sciences, math

GRE mean
Verbal 613   Quantitative 675

GPA mean
Overall GPA 3.75

Number of applications/admission offers/incoming students in 2007
91 applied/10 admission offers/5 incoming

% of students receiving:
Full tuition waiver only: 0%
Assistantship/fellowship only: 0%
Both full tuition waiver & assistantship/fellowship: 100%

Approximate percentage of incoming students with a B.A./B.S. only: 100%   **Master's:** 0%

Approximate percentage of students who are Women: 71%   **Ethnic Minority:** 35%   **International:** 7%

Average years to complete the doctoral program (including internship): 6 years

Personal interview
Preferred in person but telephone acceptable

Attrition rate in past 7 years: 10%

Percentage of students applying for internship last year accepted into APPIC or APA internships: 100%

Formal tracks/concentrations: none

Research areas	# Faculty	# Grants
antisocial behavior	3	2
behavioral genetics	3	4
childhood temperament	1	2
developmental psychopathology	4	4
eating disorders	1	0
health psychology	2	2
internalizing disorders	2	1
marital violence	1	1
mathematical models of causality	2	1
schizophrenia	2	4
sexuality and reproduction	1	3
social information processing	3	1
stress	1	1
substance abuse	4	4

Clinical opportunities

anxiety disorders
health-related family problems
child and family therapy
depression
marital violence/ therapy
neuropsychology
obsessive–compulsive disorder
schizophrenia
school/Head Start consultation
health psychology
smoking cessation

Indiana University of Pennsylvania (Psy.D.)

Department of Psychology
201 Uhler Hall
Indiana, PA 15705
phone#: (412) 357-4519
e-mail: goodwin@iup.edu
Web address:
www.iup.edu/natsciandmath/grad_psychology.html

1	2	**3**	4	5	6	7
Practice oriented		Equal emphasis			Research oriented	

Percentage of faculty subscribing to each of the following orientations:

Psychodynamic/Psychoanalytic	10%
Applied behavioral analysis/Radical behavioral	10%
Family systems/Systems	20%
Existential/Phenomenological/Humanistic	30%
Cognitive/Cognitive-behavioral	30%

Courses required for incoming students to have completed prior to enrolling:
personality, statistics or methods, abnormal, learning, social

Recommended but not mandatory courses:
6 credits in other areas of psychology

GRE mean
Verbal 550   Quantitative 650
Advanced Psychology 640

GPA mean
Overall GPA 3.5   Psychology GPA 3.6
Junior/Senior GPA 3.0

Number of applications/admission offers/incoming students in 2007
87 applied/22 admission offers/14 incoming

% of students receiving:
Full tuition waiver only: 0%
Assistantship/fellowship only: 0%
Both full tuition waiver & assistantship/fellowship: 100%

Approximate percentage of incoming students with a B.A./B.S. only: 72%   **Master's:** 28%

Approximate percentage of students who are Women: 81%   **Ethnic Minority:** 6%   **International:** 1%

Average years to complete the doctoral program (including internship): 5 years

Personal interview
Required in person

Attrition rate in past 7 years: 12%

What percentage of students applying for internship last year was accepted into APPIC or APA internships?
100%

Formal tracks/concentrations: child, family, behavioral medicine

Research areas	# Faculty	# Grants
abortion	0	0
aging	0	0
behavioral medicine	2	0
clinical judgment	1	0
cross-cultural	0	0
death and dying	1	0
ethical issues	2	0
family therapy	1	0
gender roles	1	0
minority mental health	3	0
parent–child	4	1
prevention	1	0
professional issues	5	1
psychopathology	3	0
psychopharmacology	0	0
women's studies	2	0
violence prevention	1	0
youth psychopathology	1	0

Clinical opportunities

assessment	intake interviews
behavioral medicine	stress and habit disorders
family therapy	

Indiana University–Purdue University Indianapolis (Ph.D.)

Clinical Rehabilitation Ph.D. Program
402 North Blackford Street, LD124
Indianapolis, IN 46202-3275
phone#: (317) 274-6945
e-mail: gradpsy@IUPUI.edu
Web address: www.psynt.iupui.edu/crp/index.aspx

1	2	3	4	5	6	7
Practice oriented		Equal emphasis			Research oriented	

Percentage of faculty subscribing to each of the following orientations:

Psychodynamic/Psychoanalytic	0%
Applied behavioral analysis/Radical behavioral	0%
Family systems/Systems	5%
Existential/Phenomenological/Humanistic	0%
Cognitive/Cognitive-behavioral	90%

Courses required for incoming students to have completed prior to enrolling:
Tests and measurements, statistics, physiology, abnormal

Recommended but not mandatory courses:
None

GRE mean
Verbal 515   Quantitative 635
Analytical Writing 5.28

GPA mean
Overall GPA greater than 3.2

Number of applications/admission offers/incoming students in 2007
45 applied/10 admission offers/5 incoming

% of students receiving:
Full tuition waiver only: 0%
Assistantship/fellowship only: 0%
Both full tuition waiver & assistantship/fellowship: 100%

Approximate percentage of incoming students with a B.A./B.S. only: 100%   **Master's:** 0%

Approximate percentage of students who are Women: 100%   **Ethnic Minority:** 17%
International: 0%

Average years to complete the doctoral program (including internship): 6 years

Personal interview
Required in person

Attrition rate in past 7 years: Not reported

Percentage of students applying for internship last year accepted into APPIC or APA internships: 100%

Formal tracks/concentrations: none

Research areas	# Faculty	# Grants
health psychology	3	1
neuropsychology	2	2–3
psychobiology	3	5–6
severe mental illness	2	3–4

Clinical opportunities

adaptive educational services	neurorehabilitation
adult behavioral medicine	intervention
crisis intervention unit	pediatric behavioral
hospice	medicine
neuropsychological	severe mental illness
assessment	women's prison

University of Indianapolis (Psy.D.)

School of Psychological Sciences
1400 East Hanna Avenue
Good Hall Room 109
Indianapolis, IN 46227-3697
phone#: (317) 788-3353
e-mail: ddowning@uindy.edu or
rholigrocki@uindy.edu
Web address: psych.uindy.edu/psyd/index.php

1	2	3	4	5	6	7
Practice oriented		Equal emphasis			Research oriented	

Percentage of faculty subscribing to each of the following orientations:

Psychodynamic/Psychoanalytic	17.5%
Applied behavioral analysis/Radical behavioral	17.5%
Family systems/Systems	17.5%
Existential/Phenomenological/Humanistic	17.5%
Cognitive/Cognitive-behavioral	35%

Courses required for incoming students prior to enrolling:
18 credit hours of psychology

Courses recommended but not mandatory:
Abnormal, child/development, statistics, personality, brain and behavior

GRE mean
Verbal 547   Quantitative 625
Advanced Psychology 638
Analytical Writing 4.8

GPA mean
Overall GPA 3.68

Number of applications/admission offers/incoming students in 2007
148 applied/49 admission offers/29 incoming

% of students receiving:
Full tuition waiver only: 7%
Assistantship/fellowship only: 24%
Both full tuition waiver & assistantship/fellowship: 0%

Approximate percentage of incoming students with a B.A./B.S. only: 79%   **Master's:** 21%

Approximate percentage of students who are Women: 88%   **Ethnic Minority:** 8%   **International:** 4%

Average years to complete the doctoral program (including internship): 5 years

Personal interview
Preferred in person but telephone acceptable

Attrition rate in past 7 years: 5%

Percentage of students applying for internship last year accepted into APPIC or APA internships: 93%

Formal tracks/concentrations: child and adolescent, health/behavioral medicine, adult and geropsychology

Research areas	# Faculty	# Grants
adult sibling relationships	1	1
child/family treatment outcome	1	1
eating disorders/obesity	1	0
forensics	1	0
geropsychology	2	1
multicultural mental health	2	1
neuro/health/stress//rehab	3	1
parent–child relationships	1	1
positive psychology	1	0
posttraumatic stress disorders	1	0
psychology of women	1	0
schizophrenia	1	1

Clinical opportunities
psychotherapy
assessment
behavioral medicine/health psychology
neuropsychological assessment
child psychology
medical centers
outpatient practices
schools
shelters
hospitals
community mental health centers
correctional facilities
university counseling centers

University of Iowa (Ph.D.)
Department of Psychology
E11 Seashore Hall
Iowa City, IA 52242-1407
phone#: (319) 335-2406
e-mail:la-clark@uiowa.edu
Web address:
www.psychology.uiowa.edu/training3.html

1	2	3	4	5	**6**	7

Practice oriented   Equal emphasis   Research oriented

Percentage of faculty subscribing to each of the following orientations:

Psychodynamic/Psychoanalytic	0%
Applied behavioral analysis/Radical behavioral	10%
Family systems/Systems	10%
Existential/Phenomenological/Humanistic	10%
Cognitive/Cognitive-behavioral/Third wave	100%

Courses required for incoming students prior to enrolling:
None

Courses recommended but not mandatory:
Undergraduate psychology major, statistics, abnormal, laboratory research, strong science background

GRE mean (accepted)
Verbal 600   Quantitative 700
Analytical Writing 5.0
Advanced Psychology not reported

GPA mean
Overall GPA 3.7

Number of applications/admission offers/incoming students in 2007
167 applied/8 admission offers/3 incoming

% of 2007 incoming students receiving:
Full tuition waiver only: 0%
Assistantship/fellowship and partial tuition waiver: 67%
Assistantship/fellowship and full tuition waiver: 33%

Approximate percentage of 2007 incoming students with a B.A./B.S. only: 100%   **Master's:** 0%

Approximate percentage of students who are: Women: 83%   **Ethnic Minority:** 11%   **International:** 6%

Average years to complete the doctoral program (including internship): 6.3 years

Personal interview
Preferred in person but telephone acceptable

Attrition rate in past 7 years: 8%

Percentage of students applying for internship last year accepted into APPIC or APA internships: 100%

Formal tracks/concentrations: adult psychopathology, child psychopathology, clinical health, neuropsychology

Research areas	# Faculty	# Grants
assessment	2	2
domestic violence/child abuse	2	1
depression	2	4
eating disorders	1	–
health psychology	3	4
couples therapy	1	0
personality disorders	1	1
quantitative models of psychopathology	1	0

Clinical opportunities

child abuse
adult psychiatry
child psychiatry/pediatrics
cognitive-behavioral therapy
couples therapy
depression
eating disorders
health psychology/behavioral medicine
infancy/postpartum
neuropsychology

Jackson State University (Ph.D.)

Department of Psychology
Clinical Psychology Ph.D. Program
P.O. Box 17550
Jackson, MS 39216-0350
phone#: (601) 979-5990
e-mail: psycdept@jswms.edu
Web address:
www.jsums.edu/~psycdept/grad/index.htm

1	2	3	4	**5**	6	7

Practice oriented — Equal emphasis — Research oriented

Percentage of faculty subscribing to each of the following orientations:

Psychodynamic/Psychoanalytic	10%
Applied behavioral analysis/Radical behavioral	0%
Family systems/Systems	0%
Existential/Phenomenological/Humanistic	0%
Cognitive/Cognitive-behavioral	90%

Courses required for incoming students to have completed prior to enrolling:
24 hours of coursework in psychology is required

Recommended but not mandatory courses:
Experimental, learning, statistics, physiological, abnormal

GRE mean
Verbal 496   Quantitative 560
Analytical Writing 4.0

GPA mean
Undergraduate GPA 2.28
Junior/Senior GPA 3.56
Master's GPA 3.86

Number of applications/admission offers/incoming students in 2007
27 applied/5 admission offers/5 incoming

% of students receiving:
Full tuition waiver only: 5%
Assistantship/fellowship only: 80%
Both full tuition waiver & assistantship/fellowship: 5%

Approximate percentage of incoming students with a B.A./B.S. only: 60%   **Master's:** 30%

Approximate percentage of students who are Women: 75%   **Ethnic Minority:** 60%
International: Not reported

Average years to complete the doctoral program (including internship): 6.5 years

Personal interview
Preferred in person but telephone acceptable

Attrition rate in past 7 years: 16.4%

Percentage of students applying for internship last year accepted into APPIC or APA internships: 86%

Formal tracks/concentrations: none

Research areas	# Faculty	# Grants
alcohol/substance abuse	2	0
childhood obesity	1	0
chronic pain/headache	3	1
depression	1	0
health care disparities	3	0
HIV/AIDS	3	3
posttraumatic stress disorder	1	0
psychological assessment	6	0
stigma	2	0

Clinical opportunities

behavioral medicine
campus counseling center
forensic
inpatient pediatric
inpatient psychiatric
neuropsychiatric rehab
outpatient pediatric
outpatient psychiatric

John F. Kennedy University (Psy.D.)

Graduate School of Professional Psychology
100 Ellinwood Way, Pleasant Hill, CA 94523
phone#: 925-969-3528
e-mail: proginfo@jfku.edu
Web address: www.jfku.edu/?a=gspp_psyd&cid=2&spid1=36&spid2=51

1	2	**3**	4	5	6	7

Practice oriented — Equal emphasis — Research oriented

Percentage of faculty subscribing to each of the following orientations:

Psychodynamic/Psychoanalytic	35%
Applied behavioral analysis/Radical behavioral	0%
Family systems/Systems	25%
Existential/Phenomenological/Humanistic	15%
Cognitive/Cognitive-behavioral	25%
Cultural Diversity	100%

Courses required for incoming students to have completed prior to enrolling:
Personality, statistics, and a diversity-related course

Recommended but not mandatory courses:
None

GRE mean
Not reported

GPA mean
Overall GPA 3,25

Number of applications/admission offers/incoming students in 2007
144 applied/86 admission offers/41 incoming

% of students receiving:
Full tuition waiver only: 0%
Assistantship/fellowship only: 0%
Both full tuition waiver & assistantship/fellowship: 0%

Approximate percentage of incoming students with a B.A./B.S. only: 88% **Master's:** 12%

Approximate percentage of students who are Women: 76% **Ethnic Minority:** 37% **International:** 3%

Average years to complete the doctoral program (including internship): 5 years

Personal interview
Required in person

Attrition rate in past 7 years: not reported

Percentage of students applying for internship last year accepted into APPIC or APA internships: 60%

Formal tracks/concentrations: none

Research areas	# Faculty	# Grants
LGBT policy	1	0
psychological games	1	0
psychology of immigration	1	0
disability psychology	1	0
community psychology	2	0

Clinical opportunities
We place our students in dozens of specialty clinics

University of Kansas (Ph.D.)
Clinical Child Psychology Program
2010 Dole Human Development Center
University of Kansas
100 Sunnyside Avenue
Lawrence, KS 66045
Phone #: (785) 864-4226

e-mail: clchild@ku.edu
Web address: www.ku.edu/~clchild

1	2	3	**4**	5	6	7

Practice oriented   Equal emphasis   Research oriented

Percentage of faculty subscribing to each of the following orientations:

Psychodynamic/Psychoanalytic	5%
Applied behavioral analysis/Radical behavioral	5%
Family systems/Systems	25%
Existential/Phenomenological/Humanistic	5%
Cognitive/Cognitive-behavioral	60%

Courses required for incoming students prior to enrolling:
Major in psychology or a minimum of 15–18 hours including: research methods, statistics, developmental, abnormal child psychology or Advanced Psychology GRE

Courses recommended but not mandatory:
None

GRE mean
Verbal 700   Quantitative 614
Analytical Writing Data not available

GPA mean
Overall GPA 3.86

Number of applications/admission offers/incoming students in 2007
96 applied/4 admission offers/4 incoming

% of students receiving:
Full tuition waiver only: 0%
Assistantship/fellowship only: 0%
Both full tuition waiver & assistantship/fellowship: 100%

Approximate percentage of incoming students with a B.A./B.S. only: 75% **Master's:** 25%

Approximate percentage of students who are Women: 58% **Ethnic Minority:** 33% **International:** 0%

Average years to complete the doctoral program (including internship): 6.5 years

Personal interview
Preferred in person but telephone acceptable; by invitation

Attrition rate in past 7 years: 3%

Percentage of students applying for internship last year accepted into APPIC or APA internships: 100%

Formal tracks/concentrations: child clinical, pediatrics

Research areas	# Faculty	# Grants
children with chronic illness	2	1
disasters and children	2	1
domestic violence	1	0
ethnicity/cultural issues	5	0
health promotion	2	1
school-based services	2	1
stress & coping	2	1
anxiety in children	1	
violence and children (bullying)	2	1

Clinical opportunities

community mental health
  center

early in-home intervention

serious emotional disorders

pediatric psychology

child abuse treatment

University of Kansas (Ph.D.)

Department of Psychology
Lawrence, KS 66045-7556
Phone #: (785) 864-4121
e-mail: rhiggins@ku.edu
Web address: www.psych.ku.edu/clinprog/

1	2	3	4	**5**	6	7
Practice oriented		Equal emphasis			Research oriented	

Percentage of faculty subscribing to each of the following orientations:

Psychodynamic/Psychoanalytic	10%
Applied behavioral analysis/Radical behavioral	10%
Family systems/Systems	10%
Existential/Phenomenological/Humanistic	30%
Cognitive/Cognitive-behavioral	70%

Courses required for incoming students to have completed prior to enrolling:

Bachelor's degree in psychology or minimum of 15 credit hours of psychology coursework

Recommended but not mandatory courses:

Psychological research, statistics, experimental design, abnormal, personality, brain & behavior, social psychology, cognitive psychology

GRE mean

Verbal 617   Quantitative 675
Analytical Writing 5.08
Advanced Psychology 740

GPA mean

Overall GPA 3.79

Number of applications/admission offers/incoming students in 2007

120 applied/8 admission offers/5 incoming

% of students receiving:

Full tuition waiver only: 0%
Assistantship/fellowship only: 0%
Both full tuition waiver & assistantship/fellowship: 90%

Approximate percentage of incoming students with a B.A./B.S. only: 75.5%   **Master's:** 24.5%

Approximate percentage of students who are Women: 68%   **Ethnic Minority:** 25%   **International:** 3%

Average years to complete the doctoral program (including internship): 6.5 years

Personal interview

Preferred in person but telephone acceptable

Attrition rate in past 7 years: 6%

Percentage of students applying for internship last year accepted into APPIC or APA internships: 100%

Formal tracks/concentrations: general adult, clinical health

Research areas	# Faculty	# Grants
pain & pain management		
stress & cardiovascular health	1	0
women's sexuality	1	0
outcome assessment	1	0
geriatric neuropsychology	1	0
anxiety disorders	2	1
multiple sclerosis	1	1
depression	3	1
adult psychopathology	1	0
health/pain management	1	0
marital & family	1	0

Clinical opportunities

dialectical behavior therapy

behavioral medicine—
  pediatrics

behavioral medicine—
  pain/oncology

anxiety disorders

forensic evaluation

neuropsychology/
  rehabilitation

cognitive-behavior therapy

weight loss

smoking cessation

general adult

Kent State University (Ph.D.)

Department of Psychology
Kent, OH 44242
phone#: (330) 672-2166
e-mail: jakamats@kent.edu
Web address:
dept.kent.edu/psychology/gradprograms/clinical.htm

1	2	3	4	5	**6**	7
Practice oriented		Equal emphasis			Research oriented	

Percentage of faculty subscribing to each of the following orientations:

Psychodynamic/Psychoanalytic	25%
Applied behavioral analysis/Radical behavioral	15%
Family systems/Systems	10%
Existential/Phenomenological/Humanistic	0%
Cognitive/Cognitive-behavioral	50%

Courses required for incoming students to have completed prior to enrolling:

None

Recommended but not mandatory courses:

Prefer 15–20 hours in psychology, including 1–2 statistics courses and at least 1 lab course

GRE mean

Verbal 613   Quantitative 702
Analytical Writing not used

GPA mean

Overall GPA 3.7

Number of applications/admission offers/incoming students in 2007

248 applied/25 admission offers/15 incoming

% of students receiving:
Full tuition waiver only: 0%
Assistantship/fellowship only: 0%
Both full tuition waiver & assistantship/fellowship: 100%

Approximate percentage of incoming students with a B.A./B.S. only: 89% **Master's:** 11%

Approximate percentage of students who are Women: 67% **Ethnic Minority:** 12% **International:** 10%

Average years to complete the doctoral program (including internship): 6 years

Personal interview
Preferred in person but telephone acceptable

Attrition rate in past 7 years: 8%

Percentage of students applying for internship last year accepted into APPIC or APA internships: 87%

Formal tracks/concentrations: assessment, child and family clinical, health, general

Research areas	# Faculty	# Grants
AIDS	2	1
aggression	1	1
anxiety and depression	2	0
eating disorders	1	0
family research	2	2
gerontology	1	0
MMPI	2	2
schizophrenia	1	1
stress and coping	4	2

Clinical opportunities

child/family therapy
eating disorders
forensic assessments
health psychology
marital therapy
neuropsychology
objective personality
   assessment
schizophrenia

University of Kentucky (Ph.D.)
Department of Psychology
Kastle Hall
Lexington, KY 40506-0044
phone#: (859) 257-8662
e-mail: mdiener@email.uky.edu
Web address:
www.uky.edu/AS/Psychology/graduate/clinical.html

1	2	3	4	**5**	6	7
Practice oriented		Equal emphasis			Research oriented	

Percentage of faculty subscribing to each of the following orientations:

Psychodynamic/Psychoanalytic	10%
Applied behavioral analysis/Radical behavioral	10%
Family systems/Systems	10%
Existential/Phenomenological/Humanistic	10%
Cognitive/Cognitive-behavioral	100%

Courses required for incoming students prior to enrolling:
Experimental methodology, statistics

Courses recommended but not mandatory:
Abnormal psychology, tests & measures, personality

GRE mean
Verbal 617   Quantitative 650
Analytical 5.0
Advanced Psychology not reported

GPA mean
Overall GPA 3.72

Number of applications/admission offers/incoming students in 2007
199 applied/9 admission offers/6 incoming

% of students receiving:
Full tuition waiver only: 0%
Assistantship/fellowship only: 0%
Both full tuition waiver & assistantship/fellowship: 100%

Approximate percentage of incoming students with a B.A./B.S. only: 78% **Master's:** 22%

Approximate percentage of students who are Women: 75% **Ethnic Minority:** 16% **International:** 5%

Average years to complete the doctoral program (including internship): 6.3 years

Personal interview
Preferred in person but telephone acceptable

Attrition rate in past 7 years: 16%

Percentage of students applying for internship last year accepted into APPIC or APA internships: 100%

Formal tracks/concentrations: neuropsychology, behavioral medicine

Research areas	# Faculty	# Grants
adolescent development	2	1
adult psychopathology	4	0
assessment/diagnosis/classification	3	0
behavioral medicine	2	1
child clinical	2	1
developmental psychopathology	1	1
eating disorders	1	1
neuropsychology	2	1
pain	1	1
personality assessment	3	1
personality disorders	2	0
psychoneuroimmunology	1	1
psychophysiology	2	1
substance abuse	4	2
violence/agression	1	2

Clinical opportunities

assessment
behavioral medicine
child
chronic mental illness
cognitive-behavioral therapies
community mental health
dialectical behavior therapy
neuropsychology
orofacial pain

La Salle University (Psy.D.)

Department of Psychology
Philadelphia, PA 19141
phone#: (215) 951-1350
e-mail: PsyD@lasalle.edu
Web address:
www.lasalle.edu/admiss/grad/doc_psych/index.php

1	2	3	**4**	5	6	7

Practice oriented   Equal emphasis   Research oriented

Percentage of faculty subscribing to each of the following orientations:

Psychodynamic/Psychoanalytic	0%
Applied behavioral analysis/Radical behavioral	10%
Family systems/Systems	10%
Existential/Phenomenological/Humanistic	0%
Cognitive/Cognitive-behavioral	80%

Courses required for incoming students to have completed prior to enrolling:

Developmental, personality, statistics, research methods, tests and measurements

Recommended but not mandatory courses:

Abnormal, physiological

GRE mean

Verbal 550   Quantitative 640
Advanced Psychology 620
Analytical Writing 5.0

GPA mean

Overall GPA 3.54

Number of applications/admission offers/incoming students in 2007

196 applied/72 admission offers/22 incoming

% of students receiving:

Full tuition waiver only: 0%
Assistantship/fellowship only: 27%
Both full tuition waiver & assistantship/fellowship: 0%

Approximate percentage of incoming students with a B.A./B.S. only: 70%   Master's: 30%

Approximate percentage of students who are Women: 73%   Ethnic Minority: 13% International: 1%

Average years to complete the doctoral program (including internship): 5 years

Personal interview

Required in person

Attrition rate in past 7 years: 14%

Percentage of students applying for internship last year accepted into APPIC or APA internships: 69%

Formal tracks/concentrations: general, clinical-child and family, clinical health, sport-performance

Research areas	# Faculty	# Grants
mindfulness interventions	2	1
adult assessment	1	1
anger and violence	1	1
sport psychology	1	0
anxiety/PTSD	1	0
post partum depression	1	1
psycho-oncology	1	1
child/adolescent disorders	1	0
emotion regulation	1	0

Clinical opportunities

anxiety disorders/PTSD
anger dyscontrol
sexual offenders
behavioral medicine/health promotion
mood disorders/post partum depression
child and adolescent services
adult assessment services

University of La Verne (Psy.D.)

Program in Clinical-Community Psychology
1950 Third Street
La Verne, CA 91750
phone#: (909) 593-3511 ext. 4181
email: rscott@ulv.edu
Web address: www.ulv.edu/psyd/

1	2	**3**	4	5	6	7

Practice oriented   Equal emphasis   Research oriented

Percentage of faculty subscribing to each of the following orientations:

Psychodynamic/Psychoanalytic	50%
Applied behavioral analysis/Radical behavioral	0%
Family systems/Systems	50%
Existential/Phenomenological/Humanistic	50%
Cognitive/Cognitive-behavioral	50%

Courses required for incoming students prior to enrolling:

Statistics, research methods, physiological, and abnormal. In addition, one course from: history & systems, social, personality, human development, and clinical or community.

Courses recommended but not mandatory:

None

GRE mean

Verbal   Quantitative Not reported
Analytical Writing not reported
Advanced Psychology not reported

GPA mean

Overall GPA 3.5

Number of applications/admission offers/incoming students in 2007

Not reported

% of students receiving:
Full tuition waiver only: 0%
Assistantship/fellowship only: 33%
Both full tuition waiver & assistantship/fellowship: 0%

Approximate percentage of incoming students with a B.A./B.S. only: 83%   **Master's:** 17%

Approximate percentage of students who are Women: 70%   **Ethnic Minority:** 35%
International: 10%

Average years to complete the doctoral program (including internship): 5 years

Personal interview
Required for admission

Attrition rate in past 7 years: not reported

Percentage of students applying for internship last year accepted into APPIC or APA internships: not reported

Formal tracks/concentrations: forensic, geropsychology, multicultural

Research areas	# Faculty	# Grants
multiculturalism	7	2
clinical forensics	2	0
community psychology	12	0
psychotherapy services	3	0
gender issues & sexuality	2	0
values and moral development	2	0

Clinical opportunities

children and adolescents	families
clinical forensics	HIV/AIDS
college counseling center	substance abuse

Loma Linda University (Ph.D.)

Department of Psychology
Loma Linda, CA 92350
phone#: (909) 558-8577 (Central Office)
e-mail: dvermeersch@llu.edu
Web address: www.llu.edu/llu/grad/psychology

1	2	3	4	**5**	6	7
Practice oriented		Equal emphasis			Research oriented	

Percentage of faculty subscribing to each of the following orientations:

Psychodynamic/Psychoanalytic	10%
Applied behavioral analysis/Radical behavioral	20%
Family systems/Systems	0%
Existential/Phenomenological/Humanistic	30%
Cognitive/Cognitive-behavioral	40%

Courses required for incoming students to have completed prior to enrolling:
Bachelors or masters degree in psychology or related field

Recommended but not mandatory courses:
computer literacy, math, research methods, sociology, biology, history and systems, learning, personality, statistics, social, developmental, psychobiology

GRE mean
Not reported

GPA mean
Not reported

Number of applications/admission offers/incoming students in 2007
Not reported

% of students receiving:
Full tuition waiver only: 0%
Assistantship/fellowship only: 0%
Both full tuition waiver & assistantship/fellowship: 0%

Approximate percentage of incoming students with a B.A./B.S. only: 70%   **Master's:** 30%

Approximate percentage of students who are Women: 70%   **Ethnic Minority:** 50%
International: Not reported

Average years to complete the doctoral program (including internship): 6 years

Personal interview
Preferred in person but telephone acceptable

Attrition rate in past 7 years: 10%

Percentage of students applying for internship last year accepted into APPIC or APA internships: 87.5%

Formal tracks/concentrations: clinical health psychology, pediatric health, neuropsychology, forensic

Research areas	# Faculty	# Grants
health psychology	6	3
clinical neuropsychology	2	0
pediatric health psychology	1	2
psychobiology	2	2
psychology and religion	2	0
psychotherapy outcome	1	0
statistics methods	3	0

Clinical opportunities

primary care	obesity treatment
medical/hospital	community outpatient
clinical neuropsychology	pediatric behavioral medicine
adult behavioral medicine	forensic

Loma Linda University (Psy.D.)

Department of Psychology
Loma Linda, CA 92350
phone#: (909) 558-8577 (central office)
e-mail: aarechiga@llu.edu
Web address: www.llu.edu/llu/grad/psychology

1	2	**3**	4	5	6	7
Practice oriented		Equal emphasis			Research oriented	

Percentage of faculty subscribing to each of the following orientations:

Psychodynamic/Psychoanalytic	10%
Applied behavioral analysis/Radical behavioral	20%
Family systems/Systems	0%
Existential/Phenomenological/Humanistic	30%
Cognitive/Cognitive-behavioral	40%

Courses required for incoming students to have completed prior to enrolling:
Bachelor's or master's degree in psychology or relevant field

Recommended but not mandatory courses:
computer literacy, math, sociology, biology, history and systems, learning, personality, statistics, social, developmental, psychobiology

GRE mean
Not reported

GPA mean
Not reported

Number of applications/admission offers/incoming students in 2007
Not reported

% of students receiving:
Full tuition waiver only: 0%
Assistantship/fellowship only: 0%
Both full tuition waiver & assistantship/fellowship: 0%

Approximate percentage of incoming students with a B.A./B.S. only: 70% **Master's:** 30%

Approximate percentage of students who are Women: 70% **Ethnic Minority:** 50% **International:** not reported

Average years to complete the doctoral program (including internship): 5 years

Personal interview
Preferred in person but telephone acceptable

Attrition rate in past 7 years: 10%

Percentage of students applying for internship last year accepted into APPIC or APA internships: 100%

Formal tracks/concentrations: clinical health, pediatric health, neuropsychology, forensic, family, culture psychology

Research areas	# Faculty	# Grants
health psychology	6	3
clinical neuropsychology	2	0
pediatric health psychology	1	2
psychobiology	2	2
psychology and religion	2	0
psychotherapy outcome	1	0
statistics	3	0

Clinical opportunities

primary care	community outpatient
medical/hospital	pediatric behavioral
clinical neuropsychology	medicine
adult behavioral medicine	forensic
obesity treatment	

Long Island University–C.W. Post Campus (Psy.D.) (2006 data)

Department of Psychology
College of Liberal Arts and Sciences
Brookville, NY 11548
phone#: (516) 299-2090
e-mail: doctoral.psychology@cwpost.liu.edu
Web address: http://www.cwpost.liu.edu/cwis/cwp/clas/psych/doctoral

1	2	3	4	5	6	7
Practice oriented		Equal emphasis			Research oriented	

Percentage of faculty subscribing to each of the following orientations:

Psychodynamic/Psychoanalytic	50%
Applied behavioral analysis/Radical behavioral	12%
Family systems/Systems	0%
Existential/Phenomenological/Humanistic	0%
Cognitive/Cognitive-behavioral	38%

Courses required for incoming students to have completed prior to enrolling:
18 credits of undergraduate psychology

Recommended but not mandatory courses:

GRE mean
Verbal 550   Quantitative 598
Advanced psychology 608
Analytical Writing

GPA mean
Not reported

Number of applications/admission offers/incoming students in 2005
204 applied/30 admission offers/12 incoming

% of students receiving:
Full tuition waiver only: 25%
Assistantship/fellowship only: 40%
Both full tuition waiver & assistantship/fellowship: 0%

Approximate percentage of incoming students with a B.A./B.S. only: 75% **Master's:** 25%

Approximate percentage of students who are Women: 67% **Ethnic Minority:** 20% **International:**

Average years to complete the doctoral program (including internship): 5.5 years

Personal interview
Required in person

Attrition rate in past 7 years:

Percentage of students applying for internship last year accepted into APPIC or APA internships:
not reported

Formal tracks/concentrations: none

Research areas	# Faculty	# Grants
anger management	1	0
attachment	1	1
developmental disabilities	1	0
marital violence	2	0
parent training	1	0
professional discipline	1	0
schizophrenia	1	0

Clinical opportunities

Adult behavior modification for habit control; depression, domestic violence; eating disorders; marital and relationship therapy; and phobias and anxiety disorders.
Child and family academic problems; aggressive behavior; family conflicts/family therapy; family violence; hyperactivity; parent/child conflicts; and socialization difficulties.
Group therapy anger management; assertiveness training; parent training; social skills; and stress management.
Psychological assessment achievement and intelligence testing; emotional and behavioral assessment; neuropsychological assessment; and personality assessment.

Long Island University (Ph.D.) (2006 data)

Department of Psychology
University Plaza
Brooklyn, NY 11201
phone#: (718) 488-1164
e-mail: nicholas.papouchis@liu.edu
Web address:
http://www.brooklyn.liu.edu/psych/psy_clin.html

1	2	3	**4**	5	6	7
Practice oriented		Equal emphasis			Research oriented	

Percentage of faculty subscribing to each of the following orientations:

Psychodynamic/Psychoanalytic	70%
Applied behavioral analysis/Radical behavioral	5%
Family systems/Systems	20%
Existential/Phenomenological/Humanistic	30%
Cognitive/Cognitive-behavioral	30%

Courses required for incoming students to have completed prior to enrolling:

Experimental, statistics, abnormal, developmental, personality

Recommended but not mandatory courses:

Social, history and systems, physiological, learning

GRE mean

Verbal 630   Quantitative 625   Analytical 635
Advanced Psychology 625   Analytical Writing 5.25

GPA mean

Overall GPA 3.59   Psychology GPA 3.65

Number of applications/admission offers/incoming students in 2005

187 applied/30 admission offers/15 incoming

% of students receiving:

Full tuition waiver only: 0%
Both full tuition waiver & assistantship/fellowship: 20%
Half tuition waiver & assistantship: 80%

Approximate percentage of incoming students with a B.A./B.S. only: 66%   Master's: 34%

Approximate percentage of students who are Women: 75%   Ethnic Minority: 20%   International: 5%

Average years to complete the doctoral program (including internship): 6.2 years

Personal interview
Required in person

Attrition rate in past 7 years:

Percentage of students applying for internship last year accepted into APPIC or APA internships:
not reported

Formal tracks/concentrations: none

Research areas	# Faculty	# Grants
aging and mental health	1	1
cultural/cross-cultural	4	0
developmental	4	1
developmental psychopathology	2	0
forensic	3	0
health psychology	1	1
neuropsychology	1	0
projective techniques	1	0
psychotherapy process	3	1
sociodevelopment	1	1
socioemotional development	1	0
trauma	1	1

Clinical opportunities

behavioral clinics	forensic units
child clinics and child	homeless shelters
hospital settings	hospital
college counseling	neuropsychology
community mental health	substance abuse
family therapy	

Louisiana State University (Ph.D.)

Department of Psychology
Audobon Hall, Room 236
Baton Rouge, LA 70803
phone#: (225) 578-8745
fax#: (225) 578-4125
e-mail: psrose@lsu.edu
Web address:
www.lsu.edu/psychology/graduate/Clinical.html

1	2	3	4	5	**6**	7
Practice oriented		Equal emphasis			Research oriented	

Percentage of faculty subscribing to each of the following orientations:

Psychodynamic/Psychoanalytic	0%
Applied behavioral analysis/Radical behavioral	100%
Family systems/Systems	0%
Existential/Phenomenological/Humanistic	0%
Cognitive/Cognitive-behavioral	50%

Courses required for incoming students to have completed prior to enrolling:
None

Are there courses you recommend that are not mandatory?
Statistics, experimental, physiological, learning

GRE mean
Not reported

GPA mean
Not reported

Number of applications/admission offers/incoming students in 2005
154 applied/8 admission offers/7 incoming

% of students receiving:
Full tuition waiver only: 0%
Assistantship/fellowship only: 0%
Both full tuition waiver & assistantship/fellowship: 100%

Approximate percentage of incoming students with a B.A./B.S. only: 50% **Master's:** 50%

Approximate percentage of students who are Women: 75% **Ethnic Minority:** 10%
International: not reported

Average years to complete the doctoral program (including internship): 5 years

Personal interview
No preference given

Attrition rate in past 7 years: not reported

Percentage of students applying for internship last year accepted into APPIC or APA internships:
not reported

Formal tracks/concentrations: none

Research areas	# Faculty	# Grants
anxiety disorders	1	1
autism	1	1
depression	1	1
eating disorders	1	1
mental retardation	1	1
neuropsychology	1	0
parent skills training	1	0
psychophysiology	1	0
social skills	2	1
stress and coping	1	0

Clinical opportunities

anxiety disorders	mental retardation
autism	neuropsychology
behavioral medicine	obsessive–compulsive
deafness disorder	schizophrenia
eating disorders	school/educational
family	

University of Louisville (Ph.D.)
Department of Psychological and Brain Sciences
Louisville, KY 40292
phone#: (502) 852-6775
e-mail: j.woodruff-borden@louisville.edu
Web address: www.louisville.edu/a-s/psychology/clinical/

1	2	3	4	**5**	6	7
Practice oriented		Equal emphasis				Research oriented

Percentage of faculty subscribing to each of the following orientations:

Psychodynamic/Psychoanalytic	10%
Applied behavioral analysis/Radical behavioral	0%
Family systems/Systems	0%
Existential/Phenomenological/Humanistic	0%
Cognitive/Cognitive-behavioral	80%
Interpersonal	10%

Courses required for incoming students to have completed prior to enrolling:
none

Recommended but not mandatory courses:
history, abnormal, personality, social, statistics, physiological, learning

GRE mean
Verbal 568   Quantitative 621
Analytical Writing Data not available

GPA mean
Junior/Senior GPA 3.6

Number of applications/admission offers/incoming students in 2007
99 applied/10 admission offers/9 incoming

% of students receiving:
Full tuition waiver only: 0%
Assistantship/fellowship only: 0%
Both full tuition waiver & assistantship/fellowship: 100%

Approximate percentage of incoming students with a B.A./B.S. only: 80% **Master's:** 20%

Approximate percentage of students who are Women: 62% **Ethnic Minority:** 12% **International:** 2%

Average years to complete the doctoral program (including internship): 6 years

Personal interview
Preferred in person but telephone acceptable

Attrition rate in past 7 years: 12%

Percentage of students applying for internship last year accepted into APPIC or APA internships: 84%

Formal tracks/concentrations: none

Research areas	# Faculty	# Grants
anxiety disorders	3	0
behavioral medicine	3	1
chronic mental illness	1	0
forensic psychology	1	0
gerontology/aging	2	1
stress and coping	2	0
substance abuse	1	0

Clinical opportunities

affective disorders	gerontology/aging
anxiety disorders	health psychology
child clinical psychology	interpersonal psychotherapy
developmental disabilities	psychosis
forensic psychology	

Loyola College in Maryland (Psy.D.)

Department of Psychology
Baltimore, MD 21210-2699
phone#: (410) 617-2696
e-mail: jlating@loyola.edu
Web address: www.loyola.edu/psychology

1	2	**3**	4	5	6	7

Practice oriented   Equal emphasis   Research oriented

Percentage of faculty subscribing to each of the following orientations:

Psychodynamic/Psychoanalytic	15%
Applied behavioral analysis/Radical behavioral	10%
Family systems/Systems	5%
Existential/Phenomenological/Humanistic	10%
Cognitive/Cognitive-behavioral	65%

Courses required for incoming students prior to enrolling:

Social, statistics or research methods, abnormal, personality, tests and measurements, learning or cognitive

Courses recommended but not mandatory:

None

GRE mean

Verbal 554   Quantitative 650   Analytical 650   Writing 5.0

GPA mean

Overall GPA 3.61

Number of applications/admission offers/incoming students in 2007

350 applied/25 admission offers/19 incoming

% of students receiving:

Full tuition waiver only: 0%
Assistantship/fellowship only: 40%
Both full tuition waiver & assistantship/fellowship: 0%

Approximate percentage of incoming students with a B.A./B.S. only: 84% Master's: 16%

Approximate percentage of students who are Women: 90% Ethnic Minority: 10% International: 0%

Average years to complete the doctoral program (including internship): 5.5 years

Personal interview

Required in person

Attrition rate in past 7 years: 6%

Percentage of students applying for internship last year accepted into APPIC or APA internships: 92%

Formal tracks/concentrations: none

Research areas	# Faculty	# Grants
child psychopathology	5	0
domestic violence	1	0
ethics and legal issues	2	0
gambling	1	0
gerontology	2	0
health psychology	3	0
homophobia	1	0
multicultural	3	0
neuropsychology	2	0
nonverbal communication	1	0
posttraumatic stress disorder	4	0
psychotherapy outcomes	1	0
sexuality	2	0
spirituality	2	0
social psychology	1	0
trichotillomania	1	0
women's issues	2	0

Clinical opportunities

adult inpatient	prison settings
behavioral medicine	stress and anxiety
child and family	Loyola Clinics:
eating disorders	multidisciplinary
juvenile forensics	assessment
private practice	

Loyola University of Chicago (Ph.D.)

Department of Psychology
Graduate Enrollment Services
820 North Michigan Avenue
Chicago, IL 60611
phone#: (312) 915-8900
e-mail: gradinfo@luc.edu
Web address: www.luc.edu/psychology/clinical.shtml

1	2	3	4	**5**	6	7

Practice oriented   Equal emphasis   Research oriented

Percentage of faculty subscribing to each of the following orientations:

Psychodynamic/Psychoanalytic	22%
Applied behavioral analysis/Radical behavioral	0%
Family systems/Systems	22%
Existential/Phenomenological/Humanistic	0%
Cognitive/Cognitive-behavioral	55%

Courses required for incoming students prior to enrolling:

Research methods, statistics, plus any 6 other psychology courses (24 hours total)

Courses recommended but not mandatory:

None

GRE mean
Verbal 563   Quantitative 682
Analytical Writing 5.17

GPA mean
Overall GPA 3.78

Number of applications/admission offers/incoming students in 2007
256 applied/10 admission offers/6 incoming

% of students receiving:
Full tuition waiver only: 0%
Assistantship/fellowship only: 0%
Both full tuition waiver & assistantship/fellowship: 100%

Approximate percentage of incoming students with a B.A./B.S. only: 90%   **Master's:** 10%

Approximate percentage of students who are Women: 76%   **Ethnic Minority:** 37%   **International:** 7%

Average years to complete the doctoral program (including internship): 6 years

Personal interview
Preferred in person but telephone acceptable

Attrition rate in past 7 years: 6%

Percentage of students applying for internship last year accepted into APPIC or APA internships: 100%

Formal tracks/concentrations: clinical child, neuropsychology

Research areas	# Faculty	# Grants
AIDS	2	1
adolescence	6	4
adult psychopathology	2	0
affective disorders	0	0
African American men	1	0
clinical-child/psychopathology	5	4
community psychology	3	0
death/bereavement	1	0
developmental psychopathology	4	3
disabilities	1	2
emerging adulthood	1	0
ethical issues	1	0
extracurricular activities	1	1
minority mental health	3	3
pediatric psychology	1	3
personality	2	0
prevention	3	2
psychotherapy	4	1
sexuality/dysfunctions	1	0
utilization of health services	1	0

Clinical opportunities
assessment (child and adult)
eating disorders
family psychology
health psychology
HIV/AIDS
neuropsychological
 assessment
personality disorders
psychotherapy (child and
 adult)
substance abuse
victims of abuse

University of Maine (Ph.D.)

Department of Psychology
5742 Little Hall
Orono, ME 04469-5742
phone#: (207) 581-2038
e-mail: Doug.Nangle@umit.maine.edu
Web address:
www.umaine.edu/psychology/dop/clinical.html

1	2	3	4	**5**	6	7
Practice oriented		Equal emphasis				Research oriented

Percentage of faculty subscribing to each of the following orientations:

Psychodynamic/Psychoanalytic	0%
Applied behavioral analysis/Radical behavioral	20%
Family systems/Systems	0%
Existential/Phenomenological/Humanistic	0%
Cognitive/Cognitive-behavioral	80%

Courses required for incoming students prior to enrolling:
3–4 advanced undergraduate psychology courses; background in natural sciences and mathematics

Courses recommended but not mandatory:
Learning, developmental, cognition

GRE mean
Verbal 608   Quantitative 690
Advanced Psychology 677
Analytical Writing not reported

GPA mean
Overall GPA 3.56

Number of applications/admission offers/incoming students in 2007
84 applied/9 admission offers/4 incoming

% of students receiving:
Full tuition waiver only: 0%
Assistantship/fellowship only: 0%
Both full tuition waiver & assistantship/fellowship: 100%

Approximate percentage of incoming students with a B.A./B.S. only: 80%   **Master's:** 20%

Approximate percentage of students who are Women: 70%   **Ethnic Minority:** 5%   **International:** 5%

Average years to complete the doctoral program (including internship): 6 years

Personal interview
Preferred in person but sometimes telephone interviews

Attrition rate in past 7 years: 17%

Percentage of students applying for internship last year accepted into APPIC or APA internships: 100%

Formal tracks/concentrations: general clinical, developmental

Research areas	# Faculty	# Grants
ADHD	1	0
anxiety disorders	2	1
behavioral medicine	1	1
depression	1	0
forensic psychology	2	1
psychotherapy outcome	3	0
social development	1	0
social skills	2	0
women's health	1	0

Clinical opportunities

ADHD clinic	community mental health
anxiety disorders clinic	crisis services—outpatient
autism spectrum disorders	health psychology
behavioral pediatrics	juvenile offenders
behavioral medicine	residential program for
body dysmorphic disorder	children

University of Manitoba (Ph.D.)

Psychology Graduate Office P514
Duff Roblin Building
Winnipeg, Manitoba R3T 2N2, Canada
phone#: (204) 474-6377
fax #: (204) 474-7917
e-mail: inglislf@ms.umanitoba.ca
Web address: www.umanitoba.ca/faculties/arts/
departments/psychology/media/GradBrochure.pdf

1	2	3	**4**	5	6	7
Practice oriented		Equal emphasis			Research oriented	

Percentage of faculty subscribing to each of the following orientations:

Psychodynamic/Psychoanalytic	10%
Applied behavioral analysis/Radical behavioral	20%
Clinical neuropsychology	14%
Family systems/Systems	20%
Existential/Phenomenological/Humanistic	10%
Cognitive/Cognitive-behavioral	30%

Courses required for incoming students prior to enrolling:
eight half (3 credit hour) courses in psychology, which include introductory psychology, research methods, and a second course in either research methods, statistics, or computer science

Courses recommended but not mandatory:
psychological measurement and assessment; psychological tests or design and analysis for psychological experiments; physiological psychology or sensory processes

GRE mean
Verbal 550   Quantitative 620
GPA mean 4.01 on a 4.50 scale

Number of applications/admission offers/incoming students in 2007
67 applied/9 admission offers/5 incoming

% of students receiving:
Full tuition waiver only: 0%
Assistantship/fellowship only: 25%
Both full tuition waiver & assistantship/fellowship: 0%

Approximate percentage of incoming students with a B.A./B.S. only: 25%   **B.A. Honors:** 50%   **Master's:** 25%

Approximate percentage of students who are Women: 67%   **Ethnic Minority:** 10%   **International:** 1%

Average years to complete the doctoral program (including internship): 7 years

Personal interview
Interview not required

Attrition rate in past 7 years: not reported

Percentage of students applying for internship last year accepted into APPIC or APA internships: 60%

Formal tracks/concentrations: none

Research areas	# Faculty	# Grants
anxiety disorders	4	0
applied behavioral analysis	3	2
childhood psychopathology	1	0
chronic illness	1	1
chronic pain	1	0
clinical supervision	1	0
community psychology	1	0
compliance issues	2	0
developmental disabilities	3	0
eating disorders	2	0
health psychology	2	1
hypnosis	1	0
neuropsychology	2	1
offender/abuse	2	0
psychoneuroimmunology	1	0
psychopathology	1	0
psychotherapy outcome	3	0
schizophrenia	1	0
sports psychology	1	1
trauma effects	3	0
victim/abuse	3	0

Clinical opportunities

anxiety disorders	developmental disabilities
behavioral medicine	family
child/play therapy	health psychology
clinical supervision	neuropsychology
cognitive behavioral	obsessive–compulsive
community psychology	disorders
couples	sports psychology
eating disorders	victim/battering/abuse

Marquette University (Ph.D.)

Psychology Department
P.O. Box 1881
Milwaukee, WI 53201-1881
phone#: (414) 288-7218
e-mail: Stephen.Saunders@mu.edu
Web address:
www.marquette.edu/psyc/doctoralprogram.html

1	2	3	**4**	5	6	7
Practice oriented		Equal emphasis			Research oriented	

Percentage of faculty subscribing to each of the following orientations:

Psychodynamic/Psychoanalytic	15%
Applied behavioral analysis/Radical behavioral	10%
Family systems/Systems	40%
Existential/Phenomenological/Humanistic	15%
Cognitive/Cognitive-behavioral	80%

Courses required for incoming students prior to enrolling:
Research methods, statistics, developmental, abnormal, personality, social, cognition, neuroscience

Courses recommended but not mandatory:
History and systems

GRE mean
Verbal 625   Quantitative 650   Analytical Writing

GPA mean
Overall GPA 3.5

Number of applications/admission offers/incoming students in 2007
95 applied/15 admission offers/6 incoming

% of students receiving:
Full tuition waiver only: 10%
Assistantship/fellowship only: 0%
Both full tuition waiver & assistantship/fellowship: 90%

Approximate percentage of incoming students with a B.A./B.S. only: 85%   Master's: 15%

Approximate percentage of students who are
Women: 70%   Ethnic Minority: 20%   International: 5%

Average years to complete the doctoral program (including internship): 6.5 years

Personal interview
Preferred in person but telephone acceptable

Attrition rate in past 7 years: 9%

Percentage of students applying for internship last year accepted into APPIC or APA internships: 80%

Formal tracks/concentrations: child/family, adult

Research areas	# Faculty	# Grants
adult development	1	0
ADHD	1	0
Alzheimer's disease	1	0
body esteem	1	0
child development	3	1
child–parent relationships	3	1
depression	1	0
family conflict	2	1
fear conditioning	1	0
friendships/relationships	1	0
group dynamics	1	0
help-seeking for mental illness	1	1
Latino mental health	1	0
memory problems	1	2
mental imagery	1	0
minority mental health	1	0
multicultural psychology	1	0
neuropsychology	2	0
organizational behavior	1	0
pediatric psychology	1	0
psychosocial aspects of illness	1	0
psychotherapy process	3	0
psychotherapy outcome	3	0
social stigmatization	1	1
treatment utilization	1	0

Clinical opportunities
ADHD
adult neuropsychology
child neuropsychology
pediatric neuropsychology
child and adolescent
  medical health
adult psychotherapy
child psychotherapy
trauma
family/couples therapy
pain clinic (pediatric)

Marshall University (Psy.D.)
Department of Psychology
Huntington, WV 25755
phone#: (304) 696-2774
e-mail: Marianna Linz—linz@marshall.edu, Okey Napier—okey.napier@marshall.edu
Web address: www.marshall.edu/psych/psyd.htm

1	2	**3**	4	5	6	7
Practice oriented		Equal emphasis			Research oriented	

Percentage of faculty subscribing to each of the following orientations:

Psychodynamic/Psychoanalytic	33%
Applied behavioral analysis/Radical behavioral	10%
Family systems/Systems	10%
Existential/Phenomenological/Humanistic	0%
Cognitive/Cognitive-behavioral	60%

Courses required for incoming students to have completed prior to enrolling:
Statistics, research methods, personality, psychometrics, abnormal

Recommended but not mandatory courses:
None

GRE mean
Verbal 525   Quantitative 547
Advanced Psychology not reported
Analytical Writing not reported

GPA mean
Overall GPA 3.86

Number of applications/admission offers/incoming students in 2007
50 applied/15 admission offers/10 incoming

% of students receiving:
Full tuition waiver only: 0%
Assistantship/fellowship only: 0%
Both full tuition waiver & assistantship/fellowship: 75%

Approximate percentage of incoming students with a B.A./B.S. only: 70% **Master's:** 30%

Approximate percentage of students who are Women: 85% **Ethnic Minority:** 15% **International:** 2%

Average years to complete the doctoral program (including internship): 5 years

Personal interview
Preferred in person but telephone acceptable

Attrition rate in past 7 years: <1%

Percentage of students applying for internship last year accepted into APPIC or APA internships: 50%

Formal tracks/concentrations: none

Research areas	# Faculty	# Grants
depression/suicide	1	0
common factors in psychotherapy	1	0
rural mental health	2	1
women's health	1	0
GLBT issues	1	0
learning disabilities	1	0
animal behavior	1	0
poverty	1	0
meta analysis	1	0
racial identity development	1	0

Clinical opportunities

school-based health centers
university training clinic
juvenile correctional facility
adult correctional facility
inpatient psychiatric—adult
medical school practice
community mental health
rural community

University of Maryland, Baltimore County (Ph.D.)

Department of Psychology
1000 Hilltop Circle
Baltimore, MD 21250
phone#: (410) 455-2567
e-mail: psycdept@umbc.edu
Web address: www.umbc.edu/psyc/grad/hsp.html

1	2	3	4	**5**	6	7
Practice oriented		Equal emphasis				Research oriented

Percentage of faculty subscribing to each of the following orientations:

Psychodynamic/Psychoanalytic	10%
Applied behavioral analysis/Radical behavioral	10%
Family systems/Systems	40%
Existential/Phenomenological/Humanistic	0%
Cognitive/Cognitive-behavioral	80%

Courses required for incoming students to have completed prior to enrolling:
Psychological statistics, abnormal, experimental

Recommended but not mandatory courses:
Personality, physiological, developmental

GRE mean
Verbal 600   Quantitative 676
Advanced Psychology 655
Analytical Writing 4.92

GPA mean
Overall GPA 3.66

Number of applications/admission offers/incoming students in 2007
122 applied/13 admission offers/6 incoming

% of students receiving:
Full tuition waiver only: 0%
Assistantship/fellowship only: 0%
Both full tuition waiver & assistantship/fellowship: 100%

Approximate percentage of incoming students with a B.A./B.S. only: 84% **Master's:** 16%

Approximate percentage of students who are Women: 84% **Ethnic Minority:** 33% **International:** 16%

Average years to complete the doctoral program (including internship): 7 years

Personal interview
Preferred in person but telephone acceptable

Attrition rate in past 7 years: 8%

Percentage of students applying for internship last year accepted into APPIC or APA internships: 83%

Formal tracks/concentrations: behavioral medicine, community

Research areas	# Faculty	# Grants
addictive disorders	2	2
behavioral medicine	4	3
cardiovascular disease	1	1
community psychology	4	2
delinquency	1	1
domestic violence	1	1
family therapy	1	1
HIV/AIDS	2	1
interpersonal processes	1	0
psychology of religion	1	0
psychoneuroimmunology	1	0
suicide	1	0

Clinical opportunities

addictive disorders
applied behavior analysis
domestic abuse
emergency mental health
family therapy
forensic psychology
medical liaison
neuropsychology
pediatric psychology
prevention
rehabilitation psychology
school-based mental health
severe and chronic mental illness

University of Maryland College Park (Ph.D.)

Department of Psychology
Biology–Psychology Building
College Park, MD 20742-4411
phone#: (301) 405-5890

e-mail: jcoldren@psyc.umd.edu
Web address:
www.bsos.umd.edu/psyc/clinicalpsyc/index.htm

1	2	3	4	5	**6**	7
Practice oriented		Equal emphasis			Research oriented	

Percentage of faculty subscribing to each of the following orientations:
Psychodynamic/Psychoanalytic   0%
Applied behavioral analysis/Radical behavioral   0%
Family systems/Systems   0%
Existential/Phenomenological/Humanistic   0%
Cognitive/Cognitive-behavioral   100%

Courses required for incoming students to have completed prior to enrolling:
B.A. or B.S. in psychology or related areas

Recommended but not mandatory courses:
Statistics, abnormal, laboratory courses in psychology

GRE mean
Verbal 628   Quantitative 668
Analytical Writing not reported

GPA mean
Overall GPA 3.6

Number of applications/admission offers/incoming students in 2007
227 applied/10 admission offers/5 incoming

% of students receiving:
Full tuition waiver only: 0%
Assistantship/fellowship only: 0%
Both full tuition waiver & assistantship/fellowship: 100%

Approximate percentage of incoming students with a B.A./B.S. only: 90%   **Master's:** 10%

Approximate percentage of students who are Women: 90%   **Ethnic Minority:** 30%   **International:** 0%

Average years to complete the doctoral program (including internship): 6 years

Personal interview
Required in person

Attrition rate in past 7 years: 10%

Percentage of students applying for internship last year accepted into APPIC or APA internships: 100%

Formal tracks/concentrations: none

Research areas	# Faculty	# Grants
addictive behaviors	3	4
anxiety disorder	0	0
behavioral undercontrol	2	1
personality and physiology	1	0
psychotherapy outcome	2	2
serious mental illnesses	1	2

Clinical opportunities
Multiple opportunities in training clinic, extern, and intern levels in inpatient, outpatient, and specialized settings

Marywood University (Psy.D.)

Department of Psychology and Counseling
Scranton, PA 18509
phone #: (416) 736-5115
e-mail: cannonb@marywood.edu
Web address: www.marywood.edu/departments/psyd/

1	2	**3**	4	5	6	7
Practice oriented		Equal emphasis			Research oriented	

Percentage of faculty subscribing to each of the following orientations:
Psychodynamic/Psychoanalytic   40%
Applied behavioral analysis/Radical behavioral   0%
Family systems/Systems   0%
Existential/Phenomenological/Humanistic   0%
Cognitive/Cognitive-behavioral   90%

Courses required for incoming students to have completed prior to enrolling:
Statistics, research methods, abnormal; at least 18 credits in psychology

Recommended but not mandatory courses:
none

GRE mean
Verbal 548   Quantitative 630
Advanced Psychology 666
Analytical Writing 5.1

GPA mean
Overall GPA 3.8

Number of applications/admission offers/incoming students in 2007
55 applied/9 admission offers/9 incoming

% of students receiving:
Full tuition waiver only: 0%
Full assistantship/fellowship only: 0%
Both full tuition waiver & assistantship/fellowship: 4%
(96% of students receive a $3,600 scholarship)

Percentage of incoming students with a B.A./B.S. only: 78%   **Master's:** 22%

Percentage of students who are Women: 80%   **Ethnic Minority:** 5%   **International:** 0%

Average years to complete (including internship):
5 years (3 years for post-master's admission)

Personal interview
Preferred in person but telephone acceptable

Attrition rate in past 7 years: 4%

Percentage of students applying for internship last year accepted into APPIC or APA internships: 100%

Formal tracks/concentrations: none

Research areas	# Faculty	# Grants
malingering	1	0
psychology and media	2	0
clinical training and supervision	4	0
positive psychology	1	0
multicultural issues	2	0
stress, anxiety and coping	3	0
aggression in boys	1	0
outcome assessment in mental health	1	0
self-esteem change	1	0
technology and education	3	0

Clinical opportunities

outpatient mental health
inpatient psychiatry
inpatient behavioral medicine
outpatient childhood disorders
university counseling center
community mental health
inpatient geriatric

University of Massachusetts at Amherst (Ph.D.)

Department of Psychology
135 Hicks Way-Tobin Hall
Amherst, MA 01003
phone#: (413) 545-0662
e-mail: mpj@psych.umass.edu
Web address: www.umass.edu/psychology/div4

1	2	3	4	**5**	6	7

Practice oriented   Equal emphasis   Research oriented

Percentage of faculty subscribing to each of the following orientations:

Psychodynamic/Psychoanalytic	21%
Applied behavioral analysis/Radical behavioral	0%
Family systems/Systems	5%
Existential/Phenomenological/Humanistic	0%
Cognitive/Cognitive-behavioral	37%

Courses required for incoming students to have completed prior to enrolling:
Undergraduate background in psychology which, at a minimum, consists of statistics, methods, and 3 advanced subjects

Recommended but not mandatory courses:
none

GRE mean
Verbal 598   Quantitative 667
Analytical Writing

GPA mean
Overall GPA 3.65

Number of applications/admission offers/incoming students in 2007
156 applied/7 admission offers/4 incoming

% of students receiving:
Full tuition waiver only: 0%
Assistantship/fellowship only: 0%
Both full tuition waiver & assistantship/fellowship: 100%

Approximate percentage of incoming students who a B.A./B.S. only: 66%   **Master's:** 33%

Approximate percentage of students who are Women: 79.5%   **Ethnic Minority:** 33% **International:** 12.8%

Average years to complete the doctoral program (including internship): 6 years

Personal interview
Preferred in person but telephone acceptable

Attrition rate in past 7 years: 0%

Percentage of students applying for internship last year accepted into APPIC or APA internships: 90%

Formal tracks/concentrations: child/family concentration, adult

Research areas	# Faculty	# Grants
child, adolescent, family	4	3
aging/gerontology	2	0
developmental psychopathology	1	1
stress/coping	1	1
psychotherapy process	3	1
psychotherapist's development	3	0
psychological assessment	1	1
psychotherapy research	3	1
substance abuse	1	0

Clinical opportunities

child and adolescent therapy
cognitive-behavior therapy
cultural diversity experience
gerontology
psychoanalytic therapy
psychotherapy supervision
psychological/neuro-psychological assessment
college counseling
outpatient medical settings
inpatient medical settings
residential treatment

University of Massachusetts at Boston (Ph.D.)

Department of Psychology
Boston, MA 02125-3393
phone#: (617) 287-6340
e-mail: clinical.Psych@umb.edu
Web address: www.umb.edu/academics/cla/dept/psychology/graduate.html

1	2	3	**4**	5	6	7

Practice oriented   Equal emphasis   Research oriented

Percentage of faculty subscribing to each of the following orientations:

Psychodynamic/Psychoanalytic	30%
Applied behavioral analysis/Radical behavioral	0%
Family systems/Systems	30%
Existential/Phenomenological/Humanistic	0%
Cognitive/Cognitive-behavioral	40%

Courses required for incoming students to have completed prior to enrolling:
statistics; 6 courses total in psychology

199

Recommended but not mandatory courses:
development, abnormal, personality, research methods

GRE mean
Verbal 613   Quantitative 667
Advanced Psychology 670
Analytical Writing 5.18

GPA mean
Overall GPA 3.5   Psychology GPA 3.8
Junior/Senior GPA 3.7

Number of applications/admission offers/incoming students in 2007
256 applied/12 admission offers/8 incoming

% of students receiving:
Full tuition waiver only: 0%
Assistantship/fellowship only: 0%
Both full tuition waiver & assistantship/fellowship: 100%

Approximate percentage of incoming students with a B.A./B.S. only: 87.5%   **Master's:** 12.5%

Approximate percentage of students who are Women: 79%   **Ethnic Minority:** 34%
International: 2%

Average years to complete the doctoral program (including internship): 6.5 years

Personal interview
Required in person

Attrition rate in past 7 years: 0%

Percentage of students applying for internship last year accepted into APPIC or APA internships: 75%

Formal tracks/concentrations: none

Research areas	# Faculty	# Grants
cross-cultural	3	1
family	3	1
media and psychology	1	0
severe psychopathology	1	1
social stereotypes	0	0
trauma	3	1

Clinical opportunities
Students are placed at the major teaching hospitals and mental health centers in the greater Boston area.

Massachusetts School of Professional Psychology (Psy.D.)

221 Rivermoor Street
Boston, MA 02132
phone#: (617) 327-6777
toll free (888) 664-MSPP
e-mail: admissions@mspp.edu
Web address: www.mspp.edu

1	2	**3**	4	5	6	7
Practice oriented		Equal emphasis			Research oriented	

Percentage of faculty subscribing to each of the following orientations:

Psychodynamic/Psychoanalytic	50%
Applied behavioral analysis/Radical behavioral	0%
Family systems/Systems	19%
Existential/Phenomenological/Humanistic	12%
Cognitive/Cognitive-behavioral	19%

Courses required for incoming students prior to enrolling:
Abnormal and two out of the following six courses: developmenta, social, personality, behavioral statistics, tests and measurements, physiological

Courses recommended but not mandatory:
All psychology related

GRE mean
Verbal 540   Quantitative 603
Analytical Writing 4.5

GPA mean
Overall GPA 3.0

Number of applications/admission offers/incoming students in 2007
333 applied/121 admission offers/55 incoming

% of students receiving:
Full tuition waiver only: 0%
Assistantship/fellowship only: 45%
Both full tuition waiver & assistantship/fellowship: 0%

Approximate percentage of incoming students with a B.A./B.S. only: 60%   **Master's:** 40%

Approximate percentage of students who are Women: 75%   **Ethnic Minority:** 12%
International: 12%

Average years to complete the doctoral program (including internship): 4.5 years

Personal interview
Required in person

Attrition rate in past 7 years: 2.2%

Percentage of students applying for internship last year accepted into APPIC or APA internships: 100%

Formal tracks/concentrations: health, forensic, childhood, adolescence and family

Research areas: a wide variety

Clinical opportunities
We have 190 sites per year in diverse areas.

McGill University (Ph.D.)

Department of Psychology
1205 Avenue Docteur Penfield
Montreal, Quebec H3A 1B1, Canada
phone#: (514) 398-6124
e-mail: gradsec@psych.mcgill.ca
Web address: www.psych.mcgill.ca/grad/clnprg.htm

1	2	3	4	5	**6**	7
Clinically oriented		Equal emphasis			Research oriented	

Percentage of faculty subscribing to each of the following orientations:

Psychodynamic/Psychoanalytic	20%
Applied behavioral analysis/Radical behavioral	0%
Family systems/Systems	0%
Existential/Phenomenological/Humanistic	0%
Cognitive/Cognitive-behavioral	80%

Courses required for incoming students to have completed prior to enrolling:
Courses in the biological, cognitive, and social bases of behavior as well as statistics.

Recommended but not mandatory courses:
none

GRE mean
Verbal 660   Quantitative 660
Analytical Writing Data not available

GPA mean
Overall GPA 3.7

Number of applications/admission offers/incoming students in 2007
180 applied/5 admission offers/4 incoming

% of students receiving:
Full tuition waiver only: 0%
Assistantship/fellowship only: 100%
Both full tuition waiver & assistantship/fellowship: 0%

Approximate percentage of incoming students with a B.A./B.S. only: 95%   Master's: 5%

Approximate percentage of students who are Women: 66%   Ethnic Minority: 10% International: 20%

Average years to complete the doctoral program (including internship): 6 years

Personal interview
Telephone required

Attrition rate in past 7 years:

Percentage of students applying for internship last year accepted into APPIC or APA internships: 100%

Formal tracks/concentrations: none

Research areas	# Faculty	# Grants
aggression	1	1
aging (including Alzheimer's)	2	1
assessment/diagnosis	2	0
attention-deficit disorder	1	1
behavior therapy	1	0
behavioral genetics	1	1
behavioral medicine	2	2
child	1	1
child psychopathology	1	1
cognitive information processing	1	0
depression	2	2
developmental	1	1
eating disorders	1	1
emotion	1	1
family	2	1
gender	1	1
health psychology	2	2
interpersonal relations	2	2
memory	2	1
neuropsychology	1	1
olfaction	1	1
personality	1	1
personality assessment	2	0
psychopathology	2	2
psychopharmacology	2	1
psychophysiology	2	1
psychotherapy process/outcome	1	1
sexual dysfunction	1	1
stress	1	1
substance abuse	1	1

Clinical opportunities
The McGill University Psychology Internship Consortium is closely associated with our graduate program in clinical psychology. The Consortium consists of psychology departments in 3 university teaching hospitals, a children's hospital, and a psychiatric hospital.

The University of Memphis (Ph.D.)
Department of Psychology
Memphis, TN 38152
phone#: (901) 678-3015
e-mail: hlevitt@memphis.edu
Web address: www.psyc.memphis.edu/programs/grad/clinical/clinicalhome.shtml

1	2	3	4	**5**	6	7
Practice oriented		Equal emphasis			Research oriented	

Percentage of faculty subscribing to each of the following orientations:

Psychodynamic/Psychoanalytic	0%
Applied behavioral analysis/Radical behavioral	0%
Family systems/Systems	30%
Existential/Phenomenological/Humanistic	20%
Cognitive/Cognitive-behavioral	50%

Courses required for incoming students to have completed prior to enrolling:
A minimum of 18 semester hours in undergraduate psychology courses, including courses in research and statistics methods.

Recommended but not mandatory courses:
none

GRE mean
Verbal 560   Quantitative 670
Analytical Writing not reported

GPA mean
Overall GPA 3.63

Number of applications/admission offers/incoming students in 2007
153 applied/11 admission offers/10 incoming

% of students receiving:
Full tuition waiver only: 0%
Assistantship/fellowship only: 0%
Both full tuition waiver & assistantship/fellowship: 100%

Approximate percentage of incoming students with a B.A./B.S. only: 89%   **Master's:** 11%

Approximate percentage of students who are Women: 72%   **Ethnic Minority:** 23%   **International:** 5%

Average years to complete the doctoral program (including internship): 6.5 years

Personal interview
Interview required

Attrition rate in past 7 years: 11.6%

Percentage of students applying for internship last year accepted into APPIC or APA internships: 66%

Formal tracks/concentrations: behavioral medicine, psychotherapy research, child clinical

Research areas	# Faculty	# Grants
behavioral medicine	4	1
child clinical	2	0
psychotherapy research	3	0

Clinical opportunities

addiction	eating disorders
affective disorders	family therapy
anxiety disorders	gambling
behavioral medicine	inpatient psychology
cancer and emotional	minority/cross-cultural
adjustment	school/educational
developmental disabilities	

University of Miami (Ph.D.)

Department of Psychology
P.O. Box 249229
Coral Gables, FL 33124
phone#: (305) 284-2814
e-mail: inquire@psy.miami.edu
Web address: www.psy.miami.edu/

1	2	3	4	5	6	7

Practice oriented   Equal emphasis   Research oriented

Percentage of faculty subscribing to each of the following orientations:

Psychodynamic/Psychoanalytic	10%
Applied behavioral analysis/Radical behavioral	0%
Family systems/Systems	30%
Existential/Phenomenological/Humanistic	10%
Cognitive/Cognitive-behavioral	80%

Courses required for incoming students to have completed prior to enrolling:
statistics, experimental

Recommended but not mandatory courses:
strong science background, especially biology and mathematics

GRE mean
Verbal 610   Quantitative 700
Analytical Writing

GPA mean
Overall GPA 3.6

Number of applications/admission offers/incoming students in 2007
340 applied/21 admission offers/14 incoming

% of students receiving:
Full tuition waiver only: 0%
Assistantship/fellowship only: 0%
Both full tuition waiver & assistantship/fellowship: 100%

Approximate percentage of incoming students with a B.A./B.S. only: 90%   **Master's:** 10%

Approximate percentage of students who are Women: 70%   **Ethnic Minority:** 30%   **International:** 1%

Average years to complete the doctoral program (including internship): 6 years

Personal interview
Required in person

Attrition rate in past 7 years: 12%

Percentage of students applying for internship last year accepted into APPIC or APA internships: 100%

Formal tracks/concentrations: adult clinical, child clinical, health clinical, pediatric health

Research areas	# Faculty	# Grants
AIDS	6	2
adult psychopathology	6	2
affective disorders	3	1
cancer	4	1
cardiovascular disease	4	2
child clinical psychology	6	2
child psychopathology	5	2
diabetes	3	2
family therapy	2	1
health psychology	14	2
hypertension	3	1
pediatric psychology	3	2
psychoneuroimmunology	6	2
stress and coping	9	2
trauma	4	2

Clinical opportunities

abuse	group therapy
AIDS	long-term care
behavioral medicine	marital therapy
conduct disorder	minority/cross-cultural
developmental disabilities	neuropsychology
diabetes	pediatrics
eating disorders	substance abuse
family therapy	

Miami University (Ph.D.)

Department of Psychology
Oxford, OH 45056
phone#: (513) 529-2400

e-mail: kerigpk@muohio.edu
Web address:
www.units.muohio.edu/psychology/clinical/index.html

1	2	3	4	**5**	6	7
Practice oriented		Equal emphasis			Research oriented	

Percentage of faculty subscribing to each of the following orientations:
Psychodynamic/Psychoanalytic 8%
Applied behavioral analysis/Radical behavioral 0%
Family systems/Systems 17%
Existential/Phenomenological/Humanistic 25%
Cognitive/Cognitive-behavioral 17%
Developmental 33%

Courses required for incoming students prior to enrolling:
statistics

Courses recommended but not mandatory:
None

GRE mean
Verbal 600   Quantitative 660   Analytical 670
Analytical Writing 5.5/6

GPA mean
Overall GPA 3.7

Number of applications/admission offers/incoming students in 2007
198 applied/7 admission offers/6 incoming

% of students receiving:
Full tuition waiver only: 0%
Assistantship/fellowship only: 0%
Both full tuition waiver & assistantship/fellowship: 100%

Approximate percentage of incoming students with a B.A./B.S. only: 71%   Master's: 28%

Approximate percentage of students who are Women: 70%   Ethnic Minority: 29% International: 14%

Average years to complete the doctoral program (including internship): 6 years

Personal interview
Preferred in person but telephone acceptable

Attrition rate in past 7 years: .075%

Percentage of students applying for internship last year accepted into APPIC or APA internships: 78%

Formal tracks/concentrations: trauma and resilience, child, family, and school-based mental health, adult psychotherapy research

Research areas	# Faculty	# Grants
action research	2	1
anxiety disorders	3	1
bullying youth	3	2
child psychopathology	6	4
consultation/school improvement	3	2
dating violence	3	1
dating violence prevention	1	1
dreams	1	0
early childhood mental health	1	1
eating disorders	1	0
family research	3	1
fetal alcohol spectrum disorders	1	0
immigration/acculturation	2	0
interparental conflict & violence	3	2
narrative methodologies	2	0
parent–child boundary dissolution	1	1
personality disorders	3	0
program development/evaluation	2	2
psychotherapy process	3	0
PTSD and juvenile delinquency	1	1
school-based mental health	4	3
school–family community partnership	4	3
training/technical assistance	2	1
trauma recovery	4	1

Clinical opportunities
adult psychotherapy
anxiety disorders
assessment with adults
assessment with children
attachment disorders
ADHD
child psychotherapy
college student counseling
community mental health
conduct disorder
consultation
cross-cultural psychology
depression
developmental disabilities
family therapy
group psychotherapy
juvenile delinquency
inpatient mental health
parent-child therapy
posttraumatic stress
   disorder
prevention
rural mental health
school-based mental health

University of Michigan (Ph.D.)
Department of Psychology
530 Church Street
Ann Arbor, MI 48109-1109
phone#: (734) 764-6332
e-mail: psych2sect@umich.edu
Web address: www.lsa.umich.edu/psych/areas/clinical/

1	2	3	4	**5**	6	7
Practice oriented		Equal emphasis			Research oriented	

Percentage of faculty subscribing to each of the following orientations:
Psychodynamic/Psychoanalytic 33%
Applied behavioral analysis/Radical behavioral 0%
Family systems/Systems 33%
Existential/Phenomenological/Humanistic 0%
Cognitive/Cognitive-behavioral 33%

What percentage of students applying for internship last year was accepted into APPIC or APA internships?
100%

Courses required for incoming students to have completed prior to enrolling:
none

Recommended but not mandatory courses:
Basic course work in psychology

GRE mean
Verbal 700   Quantitative 705
Analytical Writing not reported

GPA mean
Overall GPA 3.75   Psychology GPA 3.9

Number of applications/admission offers/incoming students in 2007
320 applied/9 admission offers/7 incoming

% of students receiving:
Full tuition waiver only: 0%
Assistantship/fellowship only: 0%
Both full tuition waiver & assistantship/fellowship: 100%

Approximate percentage of incoming students with a B.A./B.S. only: 90%   **Master's:** 10%

Approximate percentage of students who are Women: 100%   **Ethnic Minority:** 50%
International: 20%

Average years to complete the doctoral program (including internship): 5 years

Personal interview
Preferred in person but telephone acceptable

Attrition rate in past 7 years: 0%

Percentage of students applying for internship last year accepted into APPIC or APA internships: 90%

Formal tracks/concentrations: none

Research areas	# Faculty	# Grants
child abuse/neglect	1	0
childhood illness/family coping	1	1
childhood loss	2	2
chronic illness and coping	1	0
conscious/unconscious processes	1	0
divorce	1	1
family systems	4	1
family violence	2	2
health psychology	2	0
homeless families	1	0
inner city children	4	2
low birthweight children	1	0
neuropsychology	6	0
peer relations/social skills	2	2
personality disorders	2	0
psychotherapy research	5	0
schizophrenia	1	0
social competence in children	2	0
substance abuse	2	2
television violence	1	1

Clinical opportunities
adult
child and family

Michigan State University (Ph.D.)
Department of Psychology
East Lansing, MI 48824
phone#: (517) 432-9953

e-mail: mcvay@msu.edu
Web address:
psychology.msu.edu/academic/clinical/index.htm

1	2	3	4	**5**	6	7

Practice oriented   Equal emphasis   Research oriented

Percentage of faculty subscribing to each of the following orientations:

Psychodynamic/Psychoanalytic	40%
Applied behavioral analysis/Radical behavioral	0%
Family systems/Systems	40%
Existential/Phenomenological/Humanistic	0%
Cognitive/Cognitive-behavioral	40%
Feminist	10%

Courses required for incoming students prior to enrolling:
12 hours of psychology courses at the bachelor's level

Courses recommended but not mandatory:
Statistics, research design, competence with computer programs (SPSS, SYSTAT, etc.)

GRE mean
Verbal 553   Quantitative 631
Advanced Psychology 629
Analytical Writing 5.0

GPA mean
Overall GPA 3.55

Number of applications/admission offers/incoming students in 2007
200 applied/7 admission offers/5 incoming

% of incoming students receiving:
Full tuition waiver only: 0%
Assistantship/fellowship only: 0%
Both full tuition waiver & assistantship/fellowship: 100%

Approximate percentage of incoming students who entered with a B.A./B.S. only: 100%   **Master's:** 0%

Approximate percentage of students who are Women: 93%   **Ethnic Minority:** 40%   **International:** 9%

Average years to complete the doctoral program (including internship): 6.7 years

Personal interview
Preferred in person but telephone acceptable

Attrition rate in past 7 years: 11%

Percentage of students applying for internship last year accepted into APPIC or APA internships: 100%

Formal tracks/concentrations: none

Research areas	# Faculty	# Grants
ADHD	1	3
aging/gerontology	1	0
antisocial behavior	1	1
eating disorders	1	2
family research/systems	3	1
family violence	2	1
intimate partner violence	2	1

neuropsychology of alchoholism	1	1
neuroscience of anxiety	1	2
racial harassment/gendered bullying	1	2

Clinical opportunities

assessment
couples therapy
depression and anxiety
eating disorders
family therapy
gerontology/aging

intimate partner violence
loss and trauma group therapy
minority/cross-cultural
play therapy

University of Minnesota (Ph.D.)

Department of Psychology
N218 Elliot Hall, 75 East River Road
Minneapolis, MN 55455
phone#: (612) 625-2546
e-mail: cspr@umn.edu
Web address:
www.psych.umn.edu/areas/clinical/index.htm

1	2	3	4	5	**6**	7

Practice oriented   Equal emphasis   Research oriented

Percentage of faculty subscribing to each of the following orientations:

Psychodynamic/Psychoanalytic	17%
Applied behavioral analysis/Radical behavioral	17%
Family systems/Systems	0%
Existential/Phenomenological/Humanistic	0%
Cognitive/Cognitive-behavioral	83%

Courses required for incoming students to have completed prior to enrolling:
statistics, abnormal

Recommended but not mandatory courses:
none

GRE mean
Verbal 600   Quantitative 695
Analytical Writing 5.5

GPA mean
Overall GPA 3.74

Number of applications/admission offers/incoming students in 2007
181 applied/9 admission offers/6 incoming

% of students receiving:
Full tuition waiver only: 0%
Assistantship/fellowship only: 0%
Both full tuition waiver & assistantship/fellowship: 100%

Approximate percentage of incoming students with a B.A./B.S. only: 100%   Master's: 0%

Approximate percentage of students who are Women: 70%   Ethnic Minority: 24% International: 10.8%

Average years to complete the doctoral program (including internship): 6 years

Personal interview
Interview not required

Attrition rate in past 7 years: 2%

Percentage of students applying for internship last year accepted into APPIC or APA internships: 89%

Formal tracks/concentrations: adult psychopathology, developmental psychopathology

Research areas

affective disorders
antisocial personality
anxiety disorders
behavioral genetics
cross-cultural psychology
developmental psychopathology
eating disorders
molecular genetics

personality assessment
personality disorders
psychopharmacology
psychophysiology/ neuroimaging
response to extreme stress
schizophrenia
substance abuse

Clinical opportunities

ADHD
affective disorders
antisocial disorders
anxiety disorders
behavior therapy
childhood disorders
cognitive therapy
community psychology
conduct disorder
crisis intervention
eating disorders
family therapy

forensic psychology
psychodynamic therapy
neuropsychology
obsessive–compulsive disorder
panic disorder
post-traumatic stress disorder
psychopathic personality
psychotic disorders
schizophrenia
substance abuse

University of Mississippi (Ph.D.)

Department of Psychology
University, MS 38677
phone#: (662) 915-7383
e-mail: pygross@olemiss.edu
Web address: www.olemiss.edu/depts/psychology/Clinical/index.html

1	2	3	4	**5**	6	7

Practice oriented   Equal emphasis   Research oriented

Percentage of faculty subscribing to each of the following orientations:

Psychodynamic/Psychoanalytic	0%
Applied behavioral analysis/Radical behavioral	29%
Family systems/Systems	14%
Existential/Phenomenological/Humanistic	14%
Cognitive/Cognitive-behavioral	71%

Courses required for incoming students prior to enrolling:
statistics, lab course

Courses recommended but not mandatory:
physiological, abnormal, developmental, and some grounding in biology/physiology/chemistry

GRE mean
Verbal 554   Quantitative 674
Verbal + Quantitative 1228
Advanced Psychology 635
Analytical Writing N/A

GPA mean
Overall GPA 3.72   Psychology GPA 3.5
Junior/Senior GPA 3.5

Number of applications/admission offers/incoming students in 2007
applied not reported/15 admission offers/8 incoming

% of students receiving:
Full tuition waiver only: 0%
Assistantship/fellowship only: 0%
Both full tuition waiver & assistantship/fellowship: 100%

Approximate percentage of incoming students with a B.A./B.S. only: 87.5%   Master's: 12.5%

Approximate percentage of students who are
Women: 84%   Ethnic Minority: 20%   International: 0%

Average years to complete the doctoral program (including internship): 6 years

Personal interview
Preferred in person but telephone acceptable

Attrition rate in past 7 years: 8%

Percentage of students applying for internship last year accepted into APPIC or APA internships: 100%

Formal tracks/concentrations: none

Research areas	# Faculty	# Grants
behavior problems in children	3	0
community psychology	2	0
compliance	1	0
computer-based research	1	1
emotion	2	1
posttraumatic stress disorder	1	0
psychological assessment	2	0
race relations	1	0
rape	2	0
rural mental health	2	0
smoking cessation/addiction	1	1
social skills/competence	2	0

Clinical opportunities
child/adolescent
children's social skills
chronic mental illness
clinical assessment
community mental health
consultation
eating disorders
family/marital therapy
health psychology
mental retardation
posttraumatic stress
  disorder
sexual aggression
smoking cessation
substance abuse

University of Missouri–Columbia (Ph.D.)
Department of Psychology
210 McAlester Hall
Columbia, MO 65211

phone#: (573) 882-6860
e-mail: belldeb@missouri.edu
Web address: psychology.missouri.edu/clinical.php

1	2	3	4	5	**6**	7
Practice oriented		Equal emphasis			Research oriented	

Percentage of faculty subscribing to each of the following orientations:
Psychodynamic/Psychoanalytic	5%
Applied behavioral analysis/Radical behavioral	5%
Family systems/Systems	15%
Existential/Phenomenological/Humanistic	0%
Cognitive/Cognitive-behavioral	75%

Courses required for incoming students to have completed prior to enrolling:
None

Recommended but not mandatory courses:
Other sciences, statistics/mathematics

GRE mean
Verbal + Quantitative 1375
Analytical Writing 5.5
Advanced Psychology not reported

GPA mean
Overall GPA 3.7   Psychology GPA 3.95
Junior/Senior GPA 3.9

Number of applications/admission offers/incoming students in 2007
121 applied/10 admission offers/2 incoming

Percent of students receiving:
Full tuition waiver only: 0%
Assistantship/fellowship only: 0%
Both full tuition waiver & assistantship/fellowship: 100%

Approximate percentage of incoming students with a B.A./B.S. only: 94%   Master's: 6%

Approximate percentage of students who are
Women: 74%   Ethnic Minority: 11%   International: 6%

Average years to complete the doctoral program (including internship): 7.9 years

Personal interview
Preferred in person but telephone acceptable

Attrition rate in past 7 years: 12.8%

Percentage of students applying for internship last year accepted into APPIC or APA internships: 100%

Formal tracks/concentrations: clinical adult, clinical child

Research areas	# Faculty	# Grants
addictions	5	~10
anxiety disorders (child)	2	1
autism/devel. disorders	1	0
eating disorders	1	1
multisystemic therapy	1	1
personality disorders	1	2
schizophrenia	1	1
treatment dissemination	1	1

Clinical opportunities

adult, outpatient and inpatient

child, outpatient and inpatient

health psychology

medical center

rehabilitation psychology

prevention

state hospital

VA hospital

University of Missouri–Kansas City (Ph.D.)

Department of Psychology
5100 Rockhill Road
Kansas City, MO 64110
phone#: (816)-235-1073
e-mail: catleyd@umkc.edu
Web address: cas.umkc.edu/psyc/grad/clinical.htm

1	2	3	4	5	6	**7**

Practice oriented | Equal emphasis | Research oriented

Percentage of faculty subscribing to each of the following orientations:

Psychodynamic/Psychoanalytic	0%
Applied behavioral analysis/Radical behavioral	0%
Family systems/Systems	0%
Existential/Phenomenological/Humanistic	0%
Cognitive/Cognitive-behavioral	100%

Courses required for incoming students to have completed prior to enrolling:
A B.A./B.S. in psychology is preferred but not required.
At least 9 credits of psychology, including research methods and statistics

Recommended but not mandatory courses:
At least two of the following: abnormal, biopsychology, child, cognitive, learning, motivation, personality, sensation and perception, social

GRE mean
Verbal 535   Quantitative 660
Advanced Psychology not reported
Analytical Writing 5.0

GPA mean
Overall GPA 3.69

Number of applications/admission offers/incoming students in 2007
46 applied/6 admission offers/4 incoming

% of students receiving:
Full tuition waiver only: 0%
Assistantship/fellowship only: 0%
Both full tuition waiver & assistantship/fellowship: 100%

Approximate percentage of incoming students with a B.A./B.S. only: 78%   **Master's:** 22%

Approximate percentage of students who are Women: 77%   **Ethnic Minority:** 5%   **International:** 0%

Average years to complete the doctoral program (including internship): 5.5 years

Personal interview
Telephone required

Attrition rate in past 7 years: 7%

Percentage of students applying for internship last year accepted into APPIC or APA internships: 0%

Formal tracks/concentrations: health and life sciences

Research areas	# Faculty	# Grants
emotional social development	2	1
eating disorders/obesity	1	0
smoking cessation/Cardiovascular disease	2	2
HIV	1	3
serious mental illness	1	1
social attitudes and ideology	1	0
health and gender	1	0
attention and emotion	1	0
sensory and cognitive neuroscience	1	1

Clinical Opportunities
chronic pain
psychiatry

University of Missouri–St. Louis (Ph.D.)

Department of Psychology
One University Blvd.
St. Louis, MO 63121
phone#: (314) 516-5391
e-mail: ann_steffen@umsl.edu
Web address: www.umsl.edu/divisions/artscience/psychology/clinical/index.html

1	2	3	**4**	5	6	7

Practice oriented | Equal emphasis | Research oriented

Percentage of faculty subscribing to each of the following orientations:

Psychodynamic/Psychoanalytic	12%
Applied behavioral analysis/Radical behavioral	0%
Family systems/Systems	0%
Existential/Phenomenological/Humanistic	12%
Cognitive/Cognitive-behavioral	75%

Courses required for incoming students to have completed prior to enrolling:
A total of 24 undergraduate credits, including statistics and research methods

Recommended but not mandatory courses:
Personality, social, learning and motivation, history and systems, physiological, developmental

GRE mean
Verbal 643   Quantitative 689
Advanced Psychology 736
Analytical Writing 4.8

GPA mean
Overall GPA 3.74 Psychology GPA 3.86

Number of applications/admission offers/incoming students in 2007
115 applied/16 admission offers/7 incoming

% of students receiving:
Full tuition waiver only: 0%
Assistantship/fellowship only: 0%
Both full tuition waiver & assistantship/fellowship: 100%

Approximate percentage of incoming students with a B.A./B.S. only: 85%   **Master's:** 15%

Approximate percentage of students who are Women: 75%   **Ethnic Minority:** 17%
International: 9.4%

Average years to complete the doctoral program (including internship): 6.0 years

Personal interview
Preferred in person but telephone acceptable

Attrition rate in past 7 years: 11%

Percentage of students applying for internship last year accepted into APPIC or APA internships: 75%

Formal tracks/concentrations: behavioral medicine, child clinical, trauma studies, women and gender studies

Research areas	# Faculty	# Grants
behavioral medicine	1	1
child & adolescents	2	1
clinical geropsychology	1	2
multicultural issues	1	0
women & sexuality	1	0
trauma studies	2	2

Clinical opportunities
adults
children/adolescents & families
older adults
anxiety disorders
behavioral medicine
PTSD/trauma
neuropsychological assessment

University of Montana (Ph.D.)
Department of Psychology
Missoula, MT 59812-1584
phone#: (406) 243-4521
e-mail: david.schuldberg@umontana.edu
Web address: psychweb.psy.umt.edu/www/graduate_clinical_about.asp

1	2	3	**4**	5	6	7
Practice oriented		Equal emphasis			Research oriented	

Percentage of faculty subscribing to each of the following orientations:

Psychodynamic/Psychoanalytic	64%
Applied behavioral analysis/Radical behavioral	9%
Family systems/Systems	45%
Existential/Phenomenological/Humanistic	27%
Cognitive/Cognitive-behavioral	73%

Courses required for incoming students to have completed prior to enrolling:
None

Recommended but not mandatory courses:
Research methods, statistics, abnormal, personality, physiological

GRE mean (for current entering class)
Verbal 510   Quantitative 625
Advanced Psychology 596
Analytical Writing not reported

GPA mean
Overall GPA 3.24   Graduate GPA for students entering with M.A.: 3.87

Number of applications/admission offers/incoming students in 2007
142 applied/11 admission offers/7 incoming

% of students receiving:
Full tuition waiver only: 0%
Assistantship/fellowship only: 0%
Both full tuition waiver & assistantship/fellowship: 57%

Approximate percentage of incoming students with a B.A./B.S. only: 57%   **Master's:** 42%

Approximate percentage of students who are Women: 85%   **Ethnic Minority:** 28%   **International:** 3%

Average years to complete the doctoral program (including internship): 6 years

Personal interview
Preferred in person but telephone acceptable

Attrition rate in past 7 years: 8.9%

Percentage of students applying for internship last year accepted into APPIC or APA internships: 100%

Formal tracks/concentrations: child, adolescent, family clinical emphasis, neuropsychology emphasis

Research areas	# Faculty	# Grants
assessment	2	1
attention-deficit disorder	0	0
behavioral medicine/health psychology	3	0
child psychopathology	2	1
closed-head injury	1	0
cross-cultural (Native American)	2	1
depression	1	0
emotion regulation	0	0
gender issues	1	1
malingering	1	0
neuropsychology	1	0
nonlinear dynamic systems	1	0
psychotherapy process/outcome	3	0
schizophrenia	1	0
sexuality	0	0
substance abuse	2	1
health care systems	1	0
LGBT health	1	0
elderly	1	1

intimate partner violence	2	1
resilience	2	0
PTSD	3	1
mindfulness	1	0

Clinical opportunities

adolescent and child	functional analytic therapy
anxiety disorders	motivational interviewing
assessment	neuropsychology
attachment disorder	pain management
borderline personality	prison populations
disorder	rural psychology
community health	schizophrenia/psychoses
couples/family	substance abuse
depression	trauma
domestic violence	

University of Nebraska–Lincoln (Ph.D.)

Department of Psychology
209 Burnett Hall
Lincoln, NE 68588-0311
phone#: (402) 472-3229
e-mail: rbarnes1@unl.edu
Web address: psycweb.unl.edu

1	2	3	**4**	5	6	7

Practice oriented   Equal emphasis   Research oriented

Percentage of faculty subscribing to each of the following orientations:

Psychodynamic/Psychoanalytic	0%
Applied behavioral analysis/Radical behavioral	10%
Family systems/Systems	25%
Existential/Phenomenological/Humanistic	10%
Cognitive/Cognitive-behavioral	85%

Courses required for incoming students to have completed prior to enrolling:

Psychology major preferred

Recommended but not mandatory courses:

Methodology and quantitative courses

GRE mean

Verbal 610   Quantitative 660
Analytical Writing
Advanced Psychology not reported

GPA mean

Overall GPA 3.68

Number of applications/admission offers/incoming students in 2007

214 applied/12 admission offers/10 incoming

% of students receiving:

Full tuition waiver only: 0%
Assistantship/fellowship only: 0%
Both full tuition waiver & assistantship/fellowship: 100%

Approximate percentage of incoming students with a B.A./B.S. only: 80% Master's: 20%

Approximate percentage of students who are
Women: 65% **Ethnic Minority:** 20% **International:** 5%

Average years to complete the doctoral program (including internship): 6.0 years

Personal interview

Preferred in person but telephone acceptable

Attrition rate in past 7 years: 5%

Percentage of students applying for internship last year accepted into APPIC or APA internships: 100%

Formal tracks/concentrations: adult/general, child and family, forensic

Research areas	# Faculty	# Grants
anxiety disorders	2	2
child abuse/family violence	2	2
child/adolescence	2	1
serious mental illness	1	1
forensic	2	2
psychology and law	3	2
psychopathology	3	2
trauma/PTSD	2	2

Clinical opportunities

anxiety disorders	minority issues
child abuse/family violence	neuropsychology
serious mental illness	substance abuse
forensic	

University of Nevada–Las Vegas (Ph.D.)

Department of Psychology
Las Vegas, NV 89154
phone#: (702) 895-0183
e-mail: chris.kearney@unlv.edu
Web address: psychology.unlv.edu

1	2	3	4	**5**	6	7

Practice oriented   Equal emphasis   Research oriented

Percentage of faculty subscribing to each of the following orientations:

Psychodynamic/Psychoanalytic	5%
Applied behavioral analysis/Radical behavioral	5%
Family systems/Systems	5%
Existential/Phenomenological/Humanistic	5%
Cognitive/Cognitive-behavioral	80%

Courses required for incoming students to have completed prior to enrolling:

Statistics, abnormal, experimental

Recommended but not mandatory courses:

Standardized testing, child behavior disorders, motivation and learning, history of psychology

GRE mean

Verbal 566   Quantitative 604
Analytical Writing not reported
Advanced Psychology 620

GPA mean

Overall GPA 3.74

Number of applications/admission offers/incoming students in 2007
105 applied/10 admission offers/6 incoming

% of students receiving:
Full tuition waiver only: 0%
Assistantship/fellowship only: 0%
Both full tuition waiver & assistantship/fellowship: 100%

Approximate percentage of incoming students with a B.A./B.S. only: 82%   **Master's:** 18%

Approximate percentage of students who are Women: 84%   **Ethnic Minority:** 22%   **International:** 0%

Average years to complete the doctoral program (including internship): 6 years

Personal interview
Preferred in person but telephone acceptable

Attrition rate in past 7 years: 2%

Percentage of students applying for internship last year accepted into APPIC or APA internships: 85%

Formal tracks/concentrations: none

Research areas	# Faculty	# Grants
child externalizing disorders	1	1
child internalizing disorders	1	0
descriptive experience sampling	2	0
women's health/sexuality	1	0
eating disorders	1	0
social skills	1	0
psychopharmacology	1	0
neuropsychology	1	1
statistics	1	0

Clinical opportunities
Achievement Center (childhood externalizing disorders)
School Refusal and Anxiety Disorders Clinic
university-based counseling
Student counseling and psychological services

University of Nevada–Reno (Ph.D.)
Department of Psychology
MSS 298
Reno, NV 89557
e-mail: follette@unr.edu
Web address: www.psyc.unr.edu

1	2	3	4	**5**	6	7
Practice oriented		Equal emphasis			Research oriented	

Percentage of faculty subscribing to each of the following orientations:

Psychodynamic/Psychoanalytic	0%
Applied behavioral analysis/Radical behavioral	40%
Family systems/Systems	15%
Existential/Phenomenological/Humanistic	0%
Cognitive/Cognitive-behavioral	45%

Courses required for incoming students to have completed prior to enrolling:
not reported

Recommended but not mandatory courses:
personality, abnormal, statistics, experimental design, history of psychology, behavior principles, behavior analysis

GRE mean
Verbal 645   Quantitative 660
Advanced Psychology 700
Analytical Writing not reported

GPA mean
Overall GPA 3.6   Psychology GPA 3.85

Number of applications/admission offers/incoming students in 2007
122 applied/8 admission offers/6 incoming

% of students receiving:
Full tuition waiver only: 0%
Assistantship/fellowship only: 0%
Both full tuition waiver & assistantship/fellowship: 100%

Approximate percentage of incoming students with a B.A./B.S. only: 67%   **Master's:** 33%

Approximate percentage of students who are Women: 70%   **Ethnic Minority:** 10%   **International:** 2%

Average years to complete the doctoral program (including internship): 7.5 years

Personal interview
Preferred in person but telephone acceptable

Attrition rate in past 7 years: 7%

Percentage of students applying for internship last year accepted into APPIC or APA internships: 100%

Formal tracks/concentrations: none

Research areas	# Faculty	# Grants
aging	1	2
anxiety disorders	2	0
behavior analysis	3	0
behavioral assessment	3	0
behavioral health	2	0
couples	2	0
drug and alcohol abuse	2	1
gerontology	1	2
health care administration	1	1
incest survivors	2	0
minority mental health	1	0
mood disorders	1	0
prevention	4	2
sexual offenders	1	1
social skills	3	0
suicide	1	0
treatment development	3	1
verbal behavior	4	0

Clinical opportunities

AIDS	gerontology
anxiety disorders	health care administration
behavioral health care	incest survivors
couples	personality disorders
depression	posttraumatic stress
drug and alcohol abuse	disorder

University of New Brunswick (Ph.D.)

Department of Psychology
Fredericton, New Brunswick E3B 6E4 Canada
phone#: (506) 453-4707
e-mail: psyc@unb.ca
Web address:
www.unbf.ca/arts//psychology/graduate.html

1	2	3	**4**	5	6	7

Practice oriented	Equal emphasis	Research oriented

Percentage of faculty subscribing to each of the following orientations:

Psychodynamic/Psychoanalytic	0%
Applied behavioral analysis/Radical behavioral	40%
Family systems/Systems	20%
Existential/Phenomenological/Humanistic	0%
Cognitive/Cognitive behavioral	100%
Feminist	20%

Courses required for incoming students to have completed prior to enrolling:
Honor's degree or equivalent in psychology, honor's thesis, history and systems, biological psychology, cognitive-affective bases of behavior, developmental, social

Recommended but not mandatory courses:
none

GRE mean
Verbal 537   Quantitative 570
Advanced Psychology 693
Analytical Writing 5.5

GPA mean
Overall GPA 3.9

Number of applications/admission offers/incoming students in 2007
66 applied/9 admission offers/5 incoming

% of students receiving:
Full tuition waiver only: 0%
Assistantship/fellowship only: 47%
Both full tuition waiver & assistantship/fellowship: 0%

Approximate percentage of incoming students with a B.A./B.S. only: 80%   **Master's:** 20%

Approximate percentage of students who are Women: 91%   **Ethnic Minority:** 15%
International: 0%

Average years to complete the doctoral program (including internship): 8 years

Personal interview
Telephone required

Attrition rate in past 7 years: 3%

Percentage of students applying for internship last year accepted into APPIC or APA internships: 100%

Formal tracks/concentrations: none

Research areas	# Faculty	# Grants
health & rehabilitation	1	1
human sexuality	3	2
anxiety/depression	3	1
infant development	1	1
cognitive neuroscience	3	3
feminist approaches	2	1
adolescent help seeking	1	0
neuropsychology	1	0
addiction	1	1
forensic psychology	1	1
adult attachment	1	0

Clinical opportunities

health psychology	inpatient mental health
rehabilitation psychology	First Nations community
neuropsychology	mental health
community mental health	student counseling

University of New Mexico (Ph.D.)

Department of Psychology
MSCO3 2220
Albuquerque, NM 87131-0001
phone#: (505) 277-4121
e-mail: janellen@unm.edu (director),
advising@unm.edu (graduate office) or
trishara@unm.edu (coordinator)
Web address: psych.unm.edu/clinical.html

1	2	3	4	**5**	6	7

Practice oriented	Equal emphasis	Research oriented

Percentage of faculty subscribing to each of the following orientations:

Psychodynamic/Psychoanalytic	0%
Applied behavioral analysis/Radical behavioral	20%
Family systems/Systems	38%
Existential/Phenomenological/Humanistic	25%
Cognitive/Cognitive-behavioral	50%

Courses required for incoming students to have completed prior to enrolling:
Statistics, research methods, psychology major or equivalent course work

Recommended but not mandatory courses:
Basic science courses, laboratory courses, supervised research

GRE mean
Verbal + Quantitative 1281
Analytical Writing note reported
Advanced Psychology not reported

GPA mean
Overall GPA 3.64

Number of applications/admission offers/incoming students in 2007
114 applied/9 admission offers/5 incoming

% of students receiving:
Full tuition waiver only: 0%
Assistantship/fellowship only: 0%
Both full tuition waiver & assistantship/fellowship: 100%

Approximate percentage of incoming students with a B.A./B.S. only: 100%   Master's: 0%

Approximate percentage of students who are Women: 80%   Ethnic Minority: 20% International: 2%

Average years to complete the doctoral program (including internship): 7 years

Personal interview
Preferred in person but telephone acceptable

Attrition rate in past 7 years: not reported

Percentage of students applying for internship last year accepted into APPIC or APA internships: 80%

Formal tracks/concentrations: none

Research areas	# Faculty	# Grants
eating disorders	1	1
family interactions	2	3
minority/cultural issues	3	1
health psychology	3	0
human learning/language	1	0
neuropsychology	2	4
pediatric psychology	1	0
substance abuse	6	8

Clinical opportunities

behavioral medicine	neuropsychological
forensic settings	assessment
inpatient and outpatient	pediatrics
psychotherapy	personality assessment
multicultural	school setting
neuroimaging	substance abuse

The New School (Ph.D.)

(formerly listed as New School University)
New School for Social Research, Department of Psychology
65 Fifth Avenue, F 330
New York, NY 10003
phone#: (212) 229-5727
e-mail: SafranJ@newschool.edu
Web address:
www.socialresearch.newschool.edu/psy/index.htm

1	2	3	**4**	5	6	7
Practice oriented			Equal emphasis			Research oriented

Percentage of faculty subscribing to each of the following orientations:

Psychodynamic/Psychoanalytic	90%
Applied behavioral analysis/Radical behavioral	0%
Family systems/Systems	0%
Existential/Phenomenological/Humanistic	0%
Cognitive/Cognitive-behavioral	10%

Courses required for incoming students to have completed prior to enrolling:
1 course in each of the following: personality, social, developmental; psychopathology; 1 course in assessment of individual differences; 1 course in statistics; 1 research methods course

Recommended but not mandatory courses:
Undergraduate major in psychology

GRE mean
Verbal 525   Quantitative 590
Advanced Psychology 595
Analytical Writing not reported

GPA mean
GPA 3.63

Number of applications/admission offers/incoming students in 2007
21 applied/16 admission offers/15 incoming
Note: Only applications from New School University master's students in psychology are considered for enrollment.

% of students receiving:
Full tuition waiver only: 7%
Assistantship/fellowship only: 6%
Both full tuition waiver & assistantship/fellowship: 2%
(33% of students receive a partial tuition waiver)

Approximate percentage of incoming students with a B.A./B.S. only: 0%   Master's: 100%

Approximate percentage of students who are Women: 77%   Ethnic Minority: 13% International: 14%

Average years to complete the doctoral program (including internship): 5.5 years

Personal interview
Required in person

Attrition rate in past 7 years: 5.8%

Percentage of students applying for internship last year accepted into APPIC or APA internships: 100%

Formal tracks/concentrations: none

Research areas	# Faculty	# Grants
assessment/diagnosis	2	1
child clinical	1	1
developmental	1	0
emotions	1	0
memory	2	1
moral development	1	0
narrative methodologies	2	0

personality assessment	1	0
prevention	2	1
psychoanalysis	2	0
psychopathology	2	0
psychotherapy process & outcome	3	1

Clinical opportunities
New School–Beth Israel Center
variety of clinical settings

University of North Carolina at Chapel Hill (Ph.D.)

Department of Psychology
Davie Hall 013A
Chapel Hill, NC 27514
phone#: (919) 962-5082
fax#: (919) 962-2537
e-mail: mitch.prinstein@unc.edu
Web address: www.unc.edu/depts/clinpsy/

1	2	3	4	5	**6**	7
Practice oriented		Equal emphasis			Research oriented	

Percentage of faculty subscribing to each of the following orientations:

Psychodynamic/Psychoanalytic	0%
Applied behavioral analysis/Radical behavioral	0%
Family systems/Systems	0%
Existential/Phenomenological/Humanistic	0%
Cognitive/Cognitive-behavioral	100%

Courses required for incoming students to have completed prior to enrolling:
A psychology major or its equivalent (8 or more courses).

Recommended but not mandatory courses:
None

GRE mean
Verbal + Quantitative 1350
Analytical Writing not reported
Advanced Psychology not reported

GPA mean
Psychology GPA 3.5   Junior/Senior GPA 3.5

Number of applications/admission offers/incoming students in 2007
450 applied/12 admission offers/9 incoming

% of students receiving:
Full tuition waiver only: 0%
Assistantship/fellowship only: 0
Both full tuition waiver & assistantship/fellowship: 100%

Approximate percentage of incoming students with a B.A./B.S. only: 85%   Master's: 15%

Approximate percentage of students who are
Women: 71%   **Ethnic Minority:** 28%
International: not reported

Average years to complete the doctoral program (including internship): 6 years

Personal interview
Preferred in person but telephone acceptable

Attrition rate in past 7 years: 7%

Percentage of students applying for internship last year accepted into APPIC or APA internships: 100%

Formal tracks/concentrations: adult clinical, clinical child and adolescent

Research areas	# Faculty	# Grants
schizophrenia	1	2
anxiety disorders	1	0
couples therapy/research	1	2
behavioral medicine	1	2
pediatric bipolar disorder	1	2
adolescent substance use	1	1
adolescent peer relationships	1	1
adolescent depression	1	1
ethnic minority youth; health disparities	2	0
family functioning and health	1	0

Clinical opportunities

couples therapy	child bipolar treatment
anxiety disorders	child assessment
adult therapy and assessment	health/pediatric psychology
child behavior therapy	developmental disabilities

University of North Carolina at Greensboro (Ph.D.)

Department of Psychology
296 Eberhart Building
Greensboro, NC 27402-6170
phone#: (336) 256-0006
e-mail: ada@uncg.edu
Web address: www.uncg.edu/psy/areas_clinical.htm

1	2	3	**4**	5	6	7
Practice oriented		Equal emphasis			Research oriented	

Percentage of faculty subscribing to each of the following orientations:

Psychodynamic/Psychoanalytic	0%
Applied behavioral analysis/Radical behavioral	12%
Family systems/Systems	62%
Existential/Phenomenological/Humanistic	0%
Cognitive/Cognitive-behavioral	100%

Courses required for incoming students to have completed prior to enrolling:
Equivalent of undergraduate major in psychology, which should include statistics and 4 other courses in psychology

Recommended but not mandatory courses:
Physiological, abnormal, learning, cognitive

GRE mean
Verbal 580   Quantitative 710
Advanced Psychology not required
Analytical Writing 5.0

GPA mean
Overall GPA 3.8

Number of applications/admission offers/incoming students in 2007
256 applied/10 admission offers/6 incoming

% of students receiving:
Full tuition waiver only: 0%
Assistantship/fellowship only: 0%
Both full tuition waiver & assistantship/fellowship: 100%

Approximate percentage of incoming students with a B.A./B.S. only: 84%   **Master's:** 16%

Approximate percentage of students who are Women: 84%   **Ethnic Minority:** 33%
International: not reported

Average years to complete the doctoral program (including internship): 6 years

Personal interview
Required in person

Attrition rate in past 7 years: 8.8%

Percentage of students applying for internship last year accepted into APPIC or APA internships: 67%

Formal tracks/concentrations: clinical child specialization, ADHD specialization

Research areas	# Faculty	# Grants
ADHD	1	2
adolescents' externalizing disorder	0	0
behavioral analysis	1	0
behavioral assessment	1	0
children's internalizing disorder	1	0
children's social relationships	2	2
depression	1	0
personality disorders	1	0
schizophrenia	1	1

Clinical opportunities
preschool intervention program
university-based community clinic
university counseling center

University of North Dakota (Ph.D.)
Department of Psychology
Box 8380
Grand Forks, ND 58202
phone#: (701) 777-3451
e-mail: alan_king@UND.nodak.edu
Web address:
ndwild.psych.und.nodak.edu/dept/clinical.html

1	2	3	4	**5**	6	7
Practice oriented		Equal emphasis			Research oriented	

Percentage of faculty subscribing to each of the following orientations:

Psychodynamic/Psychoanalytic	5%
Applied behavioral analysis/Radical behavioral	15%
Family systems/Systems	0%
Existential/Phenomenological/Humanistic	5%
Cognitive/Cognitive-behavioral	75%

Courses required for incoming students to have completed prior to enrolling:
Psychology courses (at least 18 hours) in developmental, abnormal, statistics, research methods. One semester of college algebra and a year of biological science.

Recommended but not mandatory courses:
A background in social and natural sciences

GRE mean
Verbal + Quantitative 1074
Analytical Writing 4.9
Advanced Psychology not reported

GPA mean
Overall GPA 3.64

Number of applications/admission offers/incoming students in 2007
90 applied/11 admission offers/8 incoming

% of students receiving:
Full tuition waiver only: 0%
Assistantship/fellowship only: 0%
Both full tuition waiver & assistantship/fellowship: 100%

Approximate percentage of incoming students with a B.A./B.S. only: 100%   **Master's:** 0%

Approximate percentage of students who are Women: 75%   **Ethnic Minority:** 36%
International: <1%

Average years to complete the doctoral program (including internship): 5.0 years

Personal interview
Preferred in person but telephone acceptable

Attrition rate in past 7 years: 7%

Percentage of students applying for internship last year accepted into APPIC or APA internships: 64%

Formal tracks/concentrations: none

Research areas	# Faculty	# Grants
adult psychopathology	6	0
self-harm behavior	1	1
suicidality	1	1
anxiety disorders	1	0
applied behavioral analysis	2	0
behavioral medicine	2	0
community psychology	2	0
cross-cultural psychology	2	1
friendship/relationships	2	0
gender roles	2	0
minority mental health	2	0
pain management/control	1	0
personality assessment	2	0

personality disorders	3	0
psychophysiology	1	0
relaxation/biofeedback	1	0
rural psychology	2	2
stress and coping	6	0
substance abuse	1	0
women's studies	2	0

Clinical opportunities

affective disorders	minority/cross-cultural
anxiety disorders	obsessive–compulsive
assessment	personality disorders
behavioral medicine	rural psychology
community psychology	substance abuse
interpersonal psychotherapy	victim/battering abuse
marital/couples therapy	

University of North Texas (Ph.D.)

Clinical Psychology Program
Department of Psychology
Box 311280
Denton, TX 76203-1280
phone#: (940) 565-2652
e-mail: amym@unt.edu
Web address: www.psyc.unt.edu/gradclinical.shtml

1	2	3	**4**	5	6	7
Practice oriented			Equal emphasis			Research oriented

Percentage of faculty subscribing to each of the following orientations:

Psychodynamic/Psychoanalytic	25%
Applied behavioral analysis/Radical behavioral	0%
Family systems/Systems	25%
Existential/Phenomenological/Humanistic	37%
Cognitive/Cognitive-behavioral	37%

Courses required for incoming students to have completed prior to enrolling:

Statistics, plus three of the following: research methods, learning, perception, motivation, cognition, psychological measurement, physiological, research thesis

Are there courses you recommend that are not mandatory?

See above

GRE mean

Verbal 590   Quantitative 703
Analytical Writing not reported
Advanced Psychology not reported

GPA mean

3.83

Number of applications/admission offers/incoming students in 2007

157 applied/11 admission offers/8 incoming

% of students receiving:

Full tuition waiver only: 0%
Assistantship/fellowship only: 0%
Both full tuition waiver & assistantship/fellowship: 100%

Approximate percentage of incoming students with a B.A./B.S. only: 88%   **Master's:** 12%

Approximate percentage of students who are Women: 88%   **Ethnic Minority:** 25%   **International:** 8%

Average years to complete the doctoral program (including internship): 6 years

Personal interview

Required in person

Attrition rate in past 7 years: 13.6%

Percentage of students applying for internship last year accepted into APPIC or APA internships: 88%

Formal tracks/concentrations: none

Research areas	# Faculty	# Grants
abuse	2	0
AIDS	2	0
affect management	1	0
aging	1	1
children	1	1
disaster intervention	2	0
forensics	3	1
malingering	2	0
neuropsychology	1	0
posttraumatic stress disorder	2	0
schizophrenia	2	0
stress	2	1

Clinical opportunities

children	psychopathy
depression	posttraumatic stress
forensic psychology	disorder

Northern Illinois University (Ph.D.)

Department of Psychology
DeKalb, IL 60115
phone#: (815) 753-0772
e-mail: mlovejoy@niu.edu
Web address:
www.niu.edu/psyc/grad_clinical/clinical_index.shtml

1	2	3	4	**5**	6	7
Practice oriented			Equal emphasis			Research oriented

Percentage of faculty subscribing to each of the following orientations:

Psychodynamic/Psychoanalytic	17%
Applied behavioral analysis/Radical behavioral	67%
Family systems/Systems	67%
Existential/Phenomenological/Humanistic	33%
Cognitive/Cognitive-behavioral	100%

Courses required for incoming students prior to enrolling:

None

Courses recommended but not mandatory:

Statistics, research methods, laboratory course, history

GRE mean
Verbal 556   Quantitative 683
Analytical Writing 5.0

GPA mean
Overall GPA 3.86

Number of applications/admission offers/incoming students in 2007
191 applied/16 admission offers/8 incoming

% of students receiving:
Full tuition waiver only: 0%
Assistantship/fellowship only: 0%
Both full tuition waiver & assistantship/fellowship: 100%

Approximate percentage of incoming students with a B.A./B.S. only: 88%   **Master's:** 12%

Approximate percentage of students who are Women: 75%   **Ethnic Minority:** 25%   **International:** 4%

Average years to complete the doctoral program (including internship): 7.0 years

Personal interview
Preferred in person but telephone acceptable

Attrition rate in past 7 years: 12%

Percentage of students applying for internship last year accepted into APPIC or APA internships: 89%

Formal tracks/concentrations: none

Research areas	# Faculty	# Grants
adolescents	3	0
adult psychopathology	3	0
anxiety disorders	3	0
child sexual abuse	1	1
couples	1	0
developmental psychopathology	3	1
diversity	1	1
eating disorders	1	0
mood disorders	3	0
parenting	3	1
personality disorders	1	0
physical abuse	1	0
prevention	1	0
psychometrics	3	0
sexual aggression	1	0

Clinical opportunities

ADHD clinic	forensic evaluations
anxiety disorders	individual psychotherapy
assessment	parent training
child psychotherapy	personality and cognitive
developmental disabilities	assessment
family therapy	victim/battering/abuse

Northwestern University (Ph.D.)

Department of Psychology
102 Swift Hall, 2029 Sheridan Road
Evanston, IL 60208-2710
phone#: (847) 491-5190
e-mail: rzinbarg@northwestern.edu

Web address: www.wcas.northwestern.edu/psych/programs/clinical.html

1	2	3	4	5	6	7
Practice oriented		Equal emphasis			Research oriented	

Percentage of faculty subscribing to each of the following orientations:

Psychodynamic/Psychoanalytic	10%
Applied behavioral analysis/Radical behavioral	0%
Family systems/Systems	10%
Existential/Phenomenological/Humanistic	0%
Cognitive/Cognitive-behavioral	80%

Courses required for incoming students to have completed prior to enrolling:
None

Recommended but not mandatory courses:
Psychology major, undergraduate statistics

GRE mean
Verbal 680   Quantitative 750
Advanced Psychology 750
Analytical Writing not reported

GPA mean
Overall GPA 3.83   Junior/Senior GPA 3.88

Number of applications/admission offers/incoming students in 2007
Not reported

% of students receiving:
Full tuition waiver only: 0%
Assistantship/fellowship only: 0%
Both full tuition waiver & assistantship/fellowship: 100%

Approximate percentage of incoming students with a B.A./B.S. only: 90%   **Master's:** 10%

Approximate percentage of students who are Women: 60%   **Ethnic Minority:** 10%
International: not reported

Average years to complete the doctoral program (including internship): 6 years

Personal interview
not reported

Attrition rate in past 7 years: 10%

Percentage of students applying for internship last year accepted into APPIC or APA internships: 50%
(74% in past 7 years)

Formal tracks/concentrations: none

Research areas	# Faculty	# Grants
anxiety	2	1
behavioral genetics	1	0
cognitive functioning	2	1
depression	2	0
personality	4	2
psychotherapy	1	0

Clinical opportunities

anxiety disorders	depression
behavioral medicine	family
couples	neuropsychology
crisis intervention	psychosis

Northwestern University, Feinberg School of Medicine (Ph.D.)

Department of Psychiatry and Behavioral Sciences
Division of Psychology
Abbott Hall, Suite 1205
710 North Lakeshore Drive
Chicago, IL 60611
phone#: (312) 908-8262
e-mail: clinpsych@northwestern.edu
Web address:
www.clinpsych.northwestern.edu/doc_prog.htm

1	2	3	**4**	5	6	7
Practice oriented		Equal emphasis			Research oriented	

Percentage of faculty subscribing to each of the following orientations:

Psychodynamic/Psychoanalytic	30%
Applied behavioral analysis/Radical behavioral	10%
Family systems/Systems	10%
Existential/Phenomenological/Humanistic	10%
Cognitive/Cognitive-behavioral	40%

Courses required for incoming students to have completed prior to enrolling:
Statistics, research designs, abnormal

Recommended but not mandatory courses:
None

GRE mean
Verbal 650   Quantitative 640
Advanced Psychology 650
Analytical Writing not reported

GPA mean
Not reported

Number of applications/admission offers/incoming students in 2007
229 applied/8 admission offers/5 incoming

% of students receiving:
Full tuition waiver only: 0%
Assistantship/fellowship only: 0%
Both full tuition waiver & assistantship/fellowship: 0%
(Note: Half or 3/4 tuition: 100%)

Approximate percentage of incoming students with a B.A./B.S. only: 80%   **Master's:** 20%

Approximate percentage of students who are Women: 88%   **Ethnic Minority:** 12%   **International:** 6%

Average years to complete the doctoral program (including internship): 6 years

Personal interview
Required in person

Attrition rate in past 7 years: 3%

Percentage of students applying for internship last year accepted into APPIC or APA internships: 62%

Formal tracks/concentrations: neuropsychology, general adult clinical, child clinical

Research areas	# Faculty	# Grants
adolescent/adult depression	3	2
child mental health	3	1
mental health services and policy	2	1
neuropsychology	3	1
psycholegal studies (youth in criminal justice system)	2	1

Clinical opportunities

adult, adolescent, and child outpatient clinics	neuropsychology
chronic mental illness	student mental health

Nova Southeastern University (Ph.D.)

Dean, Center for Psychological Studies
3301 College Avenue
Fort Lauderdale, FL 33314
phone#: (954) 262-5790
e-mail: cpsinfo@nova.edu
Web address: www.cps.nova.edu

1	2	3	4	5	**6**	7
Practice oriented		Equal emphasis			Research oriented	

Percentage of faculty subscribing to each of the following orientations:

Psychodynamic/Psychoanalytic	8%
Applied behavioral analysis/Radical behavioral	22%
Family systems/Systems	9%
Existential/Phenomenological/Humanistic	8%
Cognitive/Cognitive-behavioral	53%

Courses required for incoming students to have completed prior to enrolling:
18 credits in psychology and 3 credits in statistics

Recommended but not mandatory courses:
Courses in statistics, psychology, biology

GRE mean
Verbal 489   Quantitative 562
Advanced Psychology not reported
Analytical Writing 4.4

GPA mean
3.51

Number of applications/admission offers/incoming students in 2007
211 applied/37 admission offers/16 incoming

% of students receiving:
Full tuition waiver only: 0%
Assistantship/fellowship only: 27%
Both full tuition waiver & assistantship/fellowship: 0%

Approximate percentage of incoming students with a B.A./B.S. only: 100%   **Master's:** 0%

217

Approximate percentage of students who are
Women: 99% **Ethnic Minority:** 25% **International:** 1%

Average years to complete the doctoral program (including internship): 5.6 years

Personal interview
Required in person

Attrition rate in past 7 years: 7.5%

Percentage of students applying for internship last year accepted into APPIC or APA internships: 100%

Formal tracks/concentrations: forensic, health, neuropsychology, psychodynamic psychotherapy, child, adolescent, and family psychology, multicultural/diversity, trauma

Research areas	# Faculty	# Grants
ADHD	3	1
alcohol/substance abuse	3	5
anxiety disorders	2	0
behavior therapy	12	0
biofeedback	1	0
child/adolescent depression	4	0
child/adolescent psychotherapy	8	1
child neuropsychology	4	0
community mental health	3	0
cross-cultural counseling	2	0
domestic/interpersonal violence	2	1
forensic psychology	3	2
gerontology	1	0
health psychology	7	2
long-term mental illness	2	0
MMPI-2	1	0
neuropsychology	5	2
posttraumatic stress disorder	5	0
psychoanalysis	3	0
survivors of sexual abuse/assault	2	0
trauma and victimization	7	0

Clinical opportunities

anxiety disorders
behavioral modification
biofeedback
child/adolescent
child/adolescent depression
community support services
crisis assessment and
   intervention
depression
family therapy
forensic
group therapy
interpersonal violence

multilingual services
neuropsychological
   assessment
pain management
parenting skills training
psychodynamic
   psychotherapy
psychological consultation
psychological testing
serious emotional
disturbance
stress management
substance abuse

Nova Southeastern University (Psy.D.)

Dean, Center for Psychological Studies
3301 College Avenue
Fort Lauderdale, FL 33314
phone#: (954) 262-5790
e-mail: cpsinfo@cps.acast.nova.edu
Web address: www.cps.nova.edu

1	2	3	4	5	6	7
Practice oriented		Equal emphasis			Research oriented	

Percentage of faculty subscribing to each of the following orientations:

Psychodynamic/Psychoanalytic	8%
Applied behavioral analysis/Radical behavioral	22%
Family systems/Systems	9%
Existential/Phenomenological/Humanistic	8%
Cognitive/Cognitive-behavioral	53%

Courses required for incoming students to have completed prior to enrolling:
18 credits in psychology and 3 credits in statistics

Recommended but not mandatory courses:
Courses in statistics, psychology, biology

GRE mean
Verbal 462   Quantitative 535
Advanced Psychology not reported
Analytical Writing 4.3

GPA mean
Overall GPA 3.41

Number of applications/admission offers/incoming students in 2007
321 applied/143 admission offers/97 incoming

% of students receiving:
Full tuition waiver only: 0%
Assistantship/fellowship only: 77%
Both full tuition waiver & assistantship/fellowship: 0%

Approximate percentage of incoming students with a B.A./B.S. only: 95% **Master's:** 5%

Approximate percentage of students who are
Women: 95% **Ethnic Minority:** 33% **International:** 4%

Average years to complete the doctoral program (including internship): 5 years

Personal interview
Required in person

Attrition rate in past 7 years: 7.5%

Percentage of students applying for internship last year accepted into APPIC or APA internships: 100%

Formal tracks/concentrations: forensic, health, neuropsychology, psychodynamic psychotherapy, child, adolescent, and family psychology, multicultural/diversity, trauma

Research areas	# Faculty	# Grants
ADHD	3	1
alcohol/substance abuse	3	5
anxiety disorders	2	0
behavior therapy	12	0
biofeedback	1	0
child/adolescent depression	4	0
child/adolescent psychotherapy	8	1
child neuropsychology	4	0
community mental health	3	0
cross-cultural counseling	2	0

domestic/interpersonal violence	2	1
forensic psychology	3	2
gerontology	1	0
health psychology	7	2
long-term mental illness	2	0
MMPI-2	1	0
neuropsychology	5	2
posttraumatic stress disorder	5	0
psychoanalysis	3	0
survivors of sexual abuse/assault	2	0
trauma and victimization	7	0

Clinical opportunities

anxiety disorders
behavioral modification
biofeedback
child/adolescent
child/adolescent traumatic stress and depression
community support services
crisis assessment and intervention
depression
family treatment
forensic
group therapy
interpersonal violence
multilingual services
neuropsychological assessment
pain management
parenting skills and training
psychodynamic psychotherapy
psychological consultation
psychological testing
serious emotional disturbance
stress management
substance abuse

Ohio State University (Ph.D.)

Department of Psychology
108 Psychology Building
1835 Neil Avenue Mall
Columbus, OH 43210
phone#: (614) 292-4112
e-mail: emery.33@osu.edu
Web address: www2.psy.ohio-state.edu/programs/clinical/

1	2	3	4	5	**6**	7
Practice oriented		Equal emphasis			Research oriented	

Percentage of faculty subscribing to each of the following orientations:

Psychodynamic/Psychoanalytic	0%
Applied behavioral analysis/Radical behavioral	0%
Family systems/Systems	0%
Existential/Phenomenological/Humanistic	0%
Cognitive/Cognitive-behavioral	100%

Courses required for incoming students prior to enrolling:

Experimental, abnormal, statistics, personality

Courses recommended but not mandatory:

None

GRE mean

Verbal 640   Quantitative 683
Analytical Writing 5.1

GPA mean

Psychology GPA 3.65

Number of applications/admission offers/incoming students in 2007

252 applied/24 admission offers/14 incoming

% of students receiving:

Full tuition waiver only: 0%
Assistantship/fellowship only: 0%
Both full tuition waiver & assistantship/fellowship: 100%

Approximate percentage of incoming students with a B.A./B.S. only: 100%   Master's: 0%

Approximate percentage of students who are Women: 86%   Ethnic Minority: 20%   International: 14%

Average years to complete the doctoral program (including internship): 5.5 years

Personal interview

Preferred in person but telephone acceptable

Attrition rate in past 7 years: 11%

Percentage of students applying for internship last year accepted into APPIC or APA internships: 100%

Formal tracks/concentrations: adult clinical, child clinical, health

Research areas	# Faculty	# Grants
anxiety disorders	2	1
cardiovascular health	3	4
child psychopathology	3	4
childhood mood disorders	2	4
depression	3	1
oncology	1	3
pediatric neuropsychology	2	3
personality	1	0
psychoneuroimmunology	2	5
psychosocial aspects of pediatric oncology	2	3

Clinical opportunities

anxiety disorder
child and adolescent psychopathology
childhood mood disorders
crisis intervention
depressive disorders
eating disorders
family
gerontology
health psychology
neuropsychology
oncology
psycho-education evaluations
sex therapy

Ohio University (Ph.D.)

Department of Psychology
Athens, OH 45701-2979
phone#: (740) 593-1707
e-mail: psychology@ohio.edu
Web address: www.psych.ohiou.edu/academics/grad_studies/clinical.html

1	2	3	**4**	5	6	7
Practice oriented		Equal emphasis			Research oriented	

Percentage of faculty subscribing to each of the following orientations:

Psychodynamic/Psychoanalytic	40%
Applied behavioral analysis/Radical behavioral	0%
Family systems/Systems	30%
Existential/Phenomenological/Humanistic	30%
Cognitive/Cognitive-behavioral	60%

Courses required for incoming students to have completed prior to enrolling:
27 quarter hours of undergraduate psychology, including experimental psychology and statistics

Recommended but not mandatory courses:
Computer science, abnormal, personality

GRE mean:
Verbal 556   Quantitative 639   Psychology 637

GPA mean
3.60

Number of applications/admission offers/incoming students in 2007
143 applied/13 admission offers/10 incoming

% of students receiving:
Full tuition waiver only: 0%
Assistantship/fellowship only: 0
Both full tuition waiver & assistantship/fellowship: 100%

Approximate percentage of incoming students with a B.A./B.S. only: 80%   **Master's:** 20%

Approximate percentage of students who are Women: 69%   **Ethnic Minority:** 20%   **International:** 9%

Average years to complete the doctoral program (including internship): 5.9 years

Personal interview
Preferred in person but telephone acceptable

Attrition rate in past 7 years: 10.8%

Percentage of students applying for internship last year accepted into APPIC or APA internships: 90%

Formal tracks/concentrations: child clinical, clinical health

Research areas	# Faculty	# Grants
adult psychopathology and psychotherapy	2	0
family and child	2	2
health psychology	4	6
sexual assault	1	1
neuropsychology	1	1

Clinical opportunities

adult inpatient and outpatient	pain management and cardiac rehabilitation
child and family	substance abuse
neuropsychological assessment	primary care patients pediatric

Oklahoma State University (Ph.D.)

Department of Psychology
116 North Murray Hall
Stillwater, OK 74078
phone#: (405) 744-7494
e-mail: thad.leffingwell@okstate.edu
Web address: psychology.okstate.edu/grad/index.html

1	2	3	4	**5**	6	7
Practice oriented		Equal emphasis			Research oriented	

Percentage of faculty subscribing to each of the following orientations:

Psychodynamic/Psychoanalytic	0%
Applied behavioral analysis/Radical behavioral	0%
Family systems/Systems	20%
Existential/Phenomenological/Humanistic	0%
Cognitive/Cognitive-behavioral	80%

Courses required for incoming students to have completed prior to enrolling:
Statistics, experimental psychology

Recommended but not mandatory courses:
Abnormal psychology, history and systems

GRE mean
Verbal 516   Quantitative 622
Advanced Psychology not reported
Analytical Writing 4.8

GPA mean
Overall GPA 3.84

Number of applications/admission offers/incoming students in 2007
119 applied/7 admission offers/5 incoming

% of students receiving:
Full tuition waiver only: 0%
Assistantship/fellowship only: 0%
Both full tuition waiver & assistantship/fellowship: 100%

Approximate percentage of incoming students with a B.A./B.S. only: 100%   **Master's:** 0%

Approximate percentage of students who are Women: 100%   **Ethnic Minority:** 40%
International: not reported

Average years to complete the doctoral program (including internship): 5 years

Personal interview
No preference given

Attrition rate in past 7 years: 10%

What percentage of students applying for internship last year was accepted into APPIC or APA internships?
50% (92% in last six years)

Formal tracks/concentrations: child clinical, behavioral medicine/health psychology

Research areas	# Faculty	# Grants
anxiety disorders	1	0
health psychology	2	0
pediatric psychology	0	0
sexual abuse	0	0
substance abuse	1	0
depression	1	0

Clinical opportunities

anxiety disorder	marital therapy
behavioral medicine	pediatric psychology
family therapy	substance abuse

University of Oregon (Ph.D.)

Department of Psychology
Eugene, OR 97403
phone#: (541) 346-5060
e-mail: gradsec@psych.uoregon.edu
Web address: psychweb.uoregon.edu/

1	2	3	4	**5**	6	7

Practice oriented   Equal emphasis   Research oriented

Percentage of faculty subscribing to each of the following orientations:

Psychodynamic/Psychoanalytic	0%
Applied behavioral analysis/Radical behavioral	20%
Family systems/Systems	20%
Existential/Phenomenological/Humanistic	0%
Cognitive/Cognitive-behavioral	55%

Courses required for incoming students to have completed prior to enrolling:
Good background in psychology

Recommended but not mandatory courses:
Research, statistics or math background

GRE mean
high 600 range or higher
Analytical Writing 5.23
Advanced Psychology not reported

GPA mean
Cumulative undergraduate GPA should be above 3.0

Number of applications/admission offers/incoming students in 2007
200 applied/6 admission offers/4 incoming

% of students receiving:
Full tuition waiver only: 0%
Assistantship/fellowship only: 0%
Both full tuition waiver & assistantship/fellowship: 100%

Approximate percentage of incoming students with a B.A./B.S. only: 75% Master's: 25%

Approximate percentage of students who are Women: 87% Ethnic Minority: 43% International: 1%

Average years to complete the doctoral program (including internship): 5 years

Personal interview
Preferred in person but telephone acceptable under special circumstances

Attrition rate in past 7 years: 0%

Percentage of students applying for internship last year accepted into APPIC or APA internships: 100%

Formal tracks/concentrations: please visit departmental website at http://psychweb.uoregon.edu

Research areas	# Faculty	# Grants
affective disorders	3	2
anxiety disorders	2	2
cultural psychology	1	1
developmental psychopathology	2	1
life stress	1	0
neuropsychology	2	2

Clinical opportunities

anxiety disorders	cognitive therapy
behavioral genetics	depression
child, family, and adult assessment	marital
	neuropsychology

University of Ottawa (Ph.D.)

School of Psychology
Lamoureux Hall
145 Jean-Jacques Lussier
Ottawa, Ontario K1N 6N5, Canada
phone#: (613) 562-5801
e-mail: psycgrad@uottawa.ca
Web address: www.grad.uottawa.ca/programs/doctorates/psychology/program_objective.html

1	2	3	**4**	5	6	7

Practice oriented   Equal emphasis   Research oriented

Percentage of faculty subscribing to each of the following orientations:

Psychodynamic/Psychoanalytic	6%
Applied behavioral analysis/Radical behavioral	0%
Family systems/Systems	6%
Existential/Phenomenological/Humanistic	12%
Cognitive/Cognitive-behavioral	82%

Courses required for incoming students to have completed prior to enrolling:
Canadian Honors B.A. or its equivalent (60 credits in psychology, plus research experience similar to honors thesis)

Recommended but not mandatory courses:
History and systems

GRE mean
GRE is not required for admission

GPA mean
Overall GPA 8 on a scale of 10

Number of applications/admission offers/incoming students in 2007
193 applied/23 admission offers/17 incoming

% of students receiving:
Full tuition waiver only: 0%
Assistantship/fellowship only: 0%
Both full tuition waiver & assistantship/fellowship: 100%

Approximate percentage of incoming students with a B.A./B.S. only: 70%   **Master's:** 30%

Approximate percentage of students who are Women: 90%   **Ethnic Minority:** not reported **International:** 2%

Average years to complete the doctoral program (including internship): 6.6 years after BA; 6.1 years after MA

Personal interview
Interview not required

Attrition rate in past 7 years: 4%

Percentage of students applying for internship last year accepted into APPIC or APA internships: 92%

Formal tracks/concentrations: neuroscience

Research areas	# Faculty	# Grants
aging	1	1
child psychopathology	4	1
community psychology	2	3
evaluation of psychotherapy	1	0
family functioning	1	1
forensic psychology	1	0
health psychology	2	1
immigrants' adaptation	1	0
marital therapy	2	1
sexual functioning	1	1
social development of children	2	2

Clinical opportunities

anxiety	groups
community psychology	pain management
couples therapy	parent training
depression	posttraumatic stress
family therapy	disorders
geropsychology	sex therapy

Pacific Graduate School of Psychology (Ph.D.)

Department of Clinical Psychology
935 East Meadow
Palo Alto, CA 94303
phone#: (650) 843-3419
e-mail: admissions@pgsp.edu
Web address: www.pgsp.edu/

1	2	3	4	5	6	7
Practice oriented		Equal emphasis			Research oriented	

Percentage of faculty subscribing to each of the following orientations:

Psychodynamic/Psychoanalytic	40%
Applied behavioral analysis/Radical behavioral	0%
Family systems/Systems	20%
Existential/Phenomenological/Humanistic	0%
Cognitive/Cognitive-behavioral	40%

Courses required for incoming students to have completed prior to enrolling:
None

Recommended but not mandatory courses:
Statistics, personality or abnormal, developmental, physiological; a solid academic background

GRE mean
Verbal + Quantitative 1120
Analytical Writing 4.5

GPA mean
Undergraduate GPA 3.43

Number of applications/admission offers/incoming students in 2007
Not reported

% of students receiving:
Full tuition waiver only: 0%
Assistantship/fellowship only: 35%
Both full tuition waiver & assistantship/fellowship: 0%

Approximate percentage of incoming students with a B.A./B.S. only: 75%   **Master's:** 25%

Approximate percentage of students who are Women: 80%   **Ethnic Minority:** 33%   **International:** 6%

Average years to complete the doctoral program (including internship): 6.5 years

Personal interview
Interview not required

Attrition rate in past 7 years: 4%

Percentage of students applying for internship last year accepted into APPIC or APA internships: 79%

Formal tracks/concentrations: neuropsychology, forensics, child and family, LGBTQ, health, psychology and the Law (J.D./Ph.D.), meditation, joint MBA/Ph.D.

Research areas	# Faculty	# Grants
adult psychopathology	1	1
aging	1	1
assessment	3	0
bereavement	2	0
children	3	0
culture	5	0
forensics	2	0
health psychology	4	1
LGBT	1	1
minority aging	2	0
neuropsychology	3	1
neuropsychology & aging	1	0
psychology & law	2	0
psychotherapy	5	2
substance abuse	2	0

Clinical opportunities

AIDS	neuropsychology
assessment	forensics
child psychology	inpatient services
family	older adults program
health psychology	shyness program
minority	LGBTQ

Pacific Graduate School of Psychology/ Stanford University Medical School Consortium (Psy.D.)

935 E. Meadow Dr.,
Palo Alto, CA, 94303
phone#: (800)-818-6136 or (650) 843-3536
e-mail: Bruce Arnow, Ph.D. (arnow@stanford.edu) or
Jim Breckenridge, Ph.D. (jbreckenridge@pgsp.edu)
Web address:
www.pgsp.edu/program_stanford_psyd_home.php

1	**2**	3	4	5	6	7
Practice oriented		Equal emphasis			Research oriented	

Percentage of faculty subscribing to each of the following orientations:

Psychodynamic/Psychoanalytic	15%
Applied behavioral analysis/Radical behavioral	0%
Family systems/Systems	15%
Existential/Phenomenological/Humanistic	10%
Cognitive/Cognitive-behavioral	60%

Courses required for incoming students to have completed prior to enrolling:
Abnormal, statistics, biopsychology, developmental

Recommended but not mandatory courses: None

GRE mean
Verbal 574   Quantitative 667
Advanced Psychology not reported
Analytical Writing 5.12

GPA mean
Overall GPA 3.44

Number of applications/admission offers/incoming students in 2007
173 applied/48 admission offers/30 incoming

% of students receiving:
Full tuition waiver only: 0%
Assistantship/fellowship only: 60%
Both full tuition waiver & assistantship/fellowship: 0%

Approximate percentage of incoming students with a B.A./B.S. only: 87%   Master's: 13%

Approximate percentage of students who are Women: 79%   Ethnic Minority: 29%   International: 4%

Average years to complete the doctoral program (including internship): 5 years

Personal interview
Preferred in person but telephone acceptable

Attrition rate in past 7 years: 12%

Percentage of students applying for internship last year accepted into APPIC or APA internships: 68%

Formal tracks/concentrations: none

Research areas	# Faculty	# Grants
anxiety disorders	6	4
depression	2	2
eating disorders	2	1
terrorism	2	2
medical illness/comorbidity	2	1
substance abuse	2	0
trauma & abused children	2	0
cultural diversity	2	1

Clinical opportunities

anxiety clinic	cross-cultural counseling
behavioral medicine	borderline personality
spinal cord rehab inpatient	disorders (DBT)
child psychotherapy	neuropsychological
college counseling	assessment
post traumatic stress	geropsychology
disorder	substance abuse
HIV	pain management
domestic violence	depression
LGBT	community mental health
veterans (VA Palo Alto	homeless
healthcare system)	family

Pacific University (Psy.D.)

Department of Clinical Psychology
School of Professional Psychology
2004 Pacific Avenue
Forest Grove, OR 97116
phone#: (503) 352-2240
e-mail: waldronk@pacificu.edu (Admissions)
Web address: www.pacificu.edu/spp/clinical/index.cfm

1	2	**3**	4	5	6	7
Practice oriented		Equal emphasis			Research oriented	

Percentage of faculty subscribing to each of the following orientations:

Psychodynamic/Psychoanalytic	18%
Applied behavioral analysis	0%
Family systems/Systems	6%
Existential/Phenomenological/Humanistic	11%
Cognitive/Cognitive-behavioral	65%

Courses required for incoming students to have completed prior to enrolling:
A strong undergraduate background in psychology

Recommended but not mandatory courses:
4 of the 7 following courses: introduction, personality, abnormal, experimental, physiological, social, statistics

GRE mean
Verbal 536   Quantitative 605
Analytical Writing 4.6
Psychology Subject Test not reported

GPA mean
Overall GPA 3.47

Number of applications/admission offers/incoming students in 2005
125 applied/95 admission offers/55 incoming

% of students receiving:
Full tuition waiver only: 0%
Assistantship/fellowship only: 25%
Both full tuition waiver & assistantship/fellowship: 0%

Approximate percentage of incoming students with a B.A./B.S. only: 90% **Master's:** 10%

Approximate percentage of students who are Women: 70% **Ethnic Minority:** 14% **International:** 3%

Average years to complete the doctoral program (including internship): 5.5 years

Personal interview
Required in person

Attrition rate in past 7 years: 5%

Percentage of students applying for internship last year accepted into APPIC or APA internships:

Formal tracks/concentrations: Latina/bilingual; forensic; neuropsychology; child/adolescent; organizational/consulting

Research areas	# Faculty	# Grants
anxiety disorders	2	0
behavioral health	1	0
behavior therapy	7	0
child psychopathology	4	6
dynamic psychotherapy	2	0
forensic psychology	2	0
gestalt therapy	1	0
integrative approaches	2	0
neuropsychology	1	1
organizational behavior	4	0
posttraumatic stress disorders	1	0
psychology of women	2	0
psychotherapy with minorities	4	0
single case research	1	0
training, supervision and consultation	3	2

Clinical opportunities
Psychological service center in downtown Portland
38 community sites

University of Pennsylvania (Ph.D.)

Department of Psychology
3720 Walnut Street
Philadelphia, PA 19104-6241
phone#: (215) 898-4712
e-mail: cingulli@psych.upenn.edu
Web address: www.psych.upenn.edu/grad/clinprog.htm

1	2	3	4	5	6	7
Practice oriented		Equal emphasis			Research oriented	

Percentage of faculty subscribing to each of the following orientations:

Psychodynamic/Psychoanalytic	5%
Applied behavioral analysis/Radical behavioral	10%
Family systems/Systems	0%
Existential/Phenomenological/Humanistic	10%
Cognitive/Cognitive-behavioral	85%

Courses required for incoming students to have completed prior to enrolling:
None

Recommended but not mandatory courses:
Statistics

GRE mean
Verbal 698   Quantitative 754
Advanced Psychology 793
Analytical Writing 5.4

GPA mean
Overall GPA 3.77

Number of applications/admission offers/incoming students in 2007
345 applied/10 admission offers/5 incoming

% of students receiving:
Full tuition waiver only: 0%
Assistantship/fellowship only: 0%
Both full tuition waiver & assistantship/fellowship: 100%

Approximate percentage of incoming students with a B.A./B.S. only: 100% **Master's:** 0%

Approximate percentage of students who are Women: 50% **Ethnic Minority:** 12% **International:** 19%

Average years to complete the doctoral program (including internship): 6 years

Personal interview
Required in person

Attrition rate in past 7 years: 15%

Percentage of students applying for internship last year accepted into APPIC or APA internships: 75%

Formal tracks/concentrations: none

Research areas	# Faculty	# Grants
anxiety disorders	2	5
depression	3	4
family/community	1	0
psychodynamic treatment	2	2
psychopharmacology	3	3
substance abuse	1	1

Clinical opportunities
assessment and diagnostic interviewing
behavioral therapy
cognitive-behavioral therapy
psychodynamic therapy

Pennsylvania State University (Ph.D.)

Department of Psychology
417 Bruce V. Moore Building
University Park, PA 16802
phone#: (814) 863-1751
e-mail: mgn1@psu.edu
Web address: psych.la.psu.edu/Clinical/index.html

1	2	3	**4**	5	6	7
Practice oriented		Equal emphasis			Research oriented	

Percentage of faculty subscribing to each of the following orientations:

Psychodynamic/Psychoanalytic	20%
Applied behavioral analysis/Radical behavioral	0%
Family systems/Systems	20%
Existential/Phenomenological/Humanistic	10%
Cognitive/Cognitive-behavioral	50%

Courses required for incoming students prior to enrolling:

No course requirements. Broad psychology background.

Courses recommended but not mandatory:

Statistics and methodology

GRE mean

Verbal 670   Quantitative 680
Analytical Writing not reported

GPA mean

Overall GPA 3.88

Number of applications/admission offers/incoming students in 2007

Not reported

% of students receiving:

Full tuition waiver only: 0%
Assistantship/fellowship only: 0%
Both full tuition waiver & assistantship/fellowship: 100%

Approximate percentage of incoming students with a B.A./B.S. only: 100%   Master's: 0%

Approximate percentage of students who are Women: 72%   Ethnic Minority: 21%   International:

Average years to complete the doctoral program (including internship): 7.6 years

Personal interview

Preferred in person but telephone acceptable

Attrition rate in past 7 years: not reported

Percentage of students applying for internship last year accepted into APPIC or APA internships:

Formal tracks/concentrations: none

Research areas	# Faculty	# Grants
adult psychopathology	5	1
affective disorders	2	0
anxiety disorders	7	3
behavioral medicine	2	0
child clinical	3	2
cognition/information processing	2	0
cross-cultural psychology	1	1
childhood and adolescence	2	1
developmental disabilities	3	1
emotions	5	1
family research/therapy	2	1
hypnosis	1	0
neuropsychology	2	1
parent–child interactions	3	2
personality assessment	3	1
personality development	1	0
personality disorders	2	0
psychoanalysis/psychodynamics	2	0
psychophysiology	2	0
psychotherapy process/outcome	4	3
relaxation/biofeedback	2	1
rural psychology	1	1
violence/abuse	2	0

Clinical opportunities

We offer a broad range of clinical experiences involving a variety of psychopathologies.

Pepperdine University (Psy.D.)

Department of Psychology
Graduate School of Education and Psychology
6100 Center Drive
Los Angeles, CA 90045
phone#: (310) 568-5600
e-mail: cheryl.saunders@pepperdine.edu
Web address: gsep.pepperdine.edu/psychology/
psyd-clinical-psychology/

1	2	**3**	4	5	6	7
Practice oriented		Equal emphasis			Research oriented	

Percentage of faculty subscribing to each of the following orientations:

Psychodynamic/Psychoanalytic	42%
Applied behavioral analysis/Radical behavioral	0%
Family systems/Systems	27%
Existential/Phenomenological/Humanistic	12%
Cognitive/Cognitive-behavioral	65%

Courses required for incoming students prior to enrolling:

A master's degree in psychology or closely related field that reflectsknowledge in the following domains: biological aspects of behavior; cognitive and affective aspects of behavior; social aspects of behavior; psychological measurement; research methodology; and techniques of data analysis.

Courses recommended but not mandatory:

None

GRE mean

Verbal 565   Quantitative 601
Advanced Psychology 655
Analytical Writing 4.87

GPA mean

Overall GPA 3.37   Master's GPA 3.91

Number of applications/admission offers/incoming students in 2007
150 applied/42 admission offers/26 incoming

% of students receiving:
Full tuition waiver only:
Partial scholarship: 70%
Assistantship/fellowship only: 10%
Both tuition waiver & assistantship/fellowship: 0%

Approximate percentage of incoming students with a B.A./B.S. only: 0%   **Master's:** 100%

Approximate percentage of students who are Women: 92%   **Ethnic Minority:** 20%   **International:** 0

Average years to complete the doctoral program (including internship): 5.1 years

Personal interview
Preferred in person but telephone acceptable

Attrition rate in past 7 years: < 3%

Percentage of students applying for internship last year accepted into APPIC or APA internships: 86%

Formal tracks/concentrations: psychodynamic psychotherapy, family systems, cultural-ecological and community-clinical, forensic assessment

Research areas	# Faculty	# Grants
ADHD	1	2
clinical supervision	1	0
clinical application of neuroscience (theoretical scholarship)	2	0
ethnic minority trauma recovery	1	1
forensic psychology	1	0
positive psychology	2	1
posttraumatic stress disorder	1	2
program evaluation	1	1
psychiatric diagnosis	1	1
psychology, religion& spirituality	4	0
psychotherapy training, process, outcome	6	1
psychotherapy effectiveness with Latinos	1	0

Clinical opportunities

adolescence
ADHD
AIDS
adoption
aging
assessment
behavior therapy
behavioral medicine
child clinical
cognitive behavioral therapy
community psychology
chronically mentally ill
eating disorders
existential-humanistic psychotherapy

forensic
group
inpatient
marital/family/systemic psychothrapy
multicultural psychology
neuropsychology
posttraumatic stress disorder
psychodynamic psychotherapy
rehabilitation
religion and spirituality
schizophrenia
school psychology
substance abuse
veteran population

Philadelphia College of Osteopathic Medicine (Psy.D.)

Department of Psychology
4190 City Avenue
Philadelphia, PA 19131-1695
phone#: 215-871-6442
e-mail: StephanieF@pcom.edu
Web address: www.pcom.edu/Academic_Programs/
aca_psych/PsyD_in_Clinical_Psychology/
psyd_in_clinical_psychology.html

1	2	3	4	5	6	7
Practice oriented		Equal emphasis			Research oriented	

Percentage of faculty subscribing to each of the following orientations:

Psychodynamic/Psychoanalytic	0%
Applied behavioral analysis/Radical behavioral	0%
Family systems/Systems	0%
Existential/Phenomenological/Humanistic	0%
Cognitive/Cognitive-behavioral	100%

Courses required for incoming students to have completed prior to enrolling:
personality, abnormal, statistics/research, and developmental psychology

Recommended but not mandatory courses:
none

GRE mean
GRE not required for admission

GPA mean
Overall GPA 3.8

Number of applications/admission offers/incoming students in 2007
154 applied/42 admission offers/29 incoming

% of students receiving:
Full tuition waiver only: 0%
Assistantship/fellowship only: 2%
Both full tuition waiver & assistantship/fellowship: 0%

Approximate percentage of incoming students with a B.A./B.S. only: 0%   **Master's:** 100%

Approximate percentage of students who are Women: 76%   **Ethnic Minority:** 18%   **International:** 0.5%

Average years to complete the doctoral program (including internship): 6.9 years

Personal interview
Required in person

Attrition rate in past 7 years: 4%

Percentage of students applying for internship last year accepted into APPIC or APA internships: 57%

Formal tracks/concentrations: none

Research areas	# Faculty	# Grants
anxiety disorders	7	0
cognitive distortions	1	0
critical incident stress management	1	0
cognitive behavioral treatment of stress-related medical disorders	3	0
patient non-adherence	1	0
anger	1	0
coping with chronic illnesses	2	1
personality disorders	1	0
pain management	1	0
somatization disorder	1	0
child and adolescent anxiety disorders	1	0
psychotherapy outcome/process	1	0
memory and aging	1	0
psychological assessment	3	0
cognitive behavioral therapy for adult ADHD	1	0
substance use disorders	1	0
addictions	1	0
personality assessment	3	0
children's aggressive behavior	1	0
impact of parental psychopathology on children	1	1
CBT treatment of mood & anxiety	7	0
multicultural issues	4	0
crisis/trauma	1	0
childhood sexual abuse	1	0
supervision/clinical training	1	0
eating disorders	1	0

Clinical opportunities

culturally diverse, underserved primary care

outpatient cognitive-behavior therapy clinic

internal medicine

family medicine

geriatric medicine

University of Pittsburgh (Ph.D.)

Department of Psychology
Psychology Graduate Office
Sennott Square, 3rd Floor
210 South Bouquet Street
Pittsburgh, PA 15260
phone#: (412) 624-4502
e-mail: psygrad@pitt.edu
Web address:
www.psychology.pitt.edu/graduate/clinical/index.php

1	2	3	4	5	**6**	7
Practice oriented		Equal emphasis				Research oriented

Percentage of faculty subscribing to each of the following orientations:

Psychodynamic/Psychoanalytic	0%
Applied behavioral analysis/Radical behavioral	0%
Family systems/Systems	30%
Existential/Phenomenological/Humanistic	0%
Cognitive/Cognitive-behavioral	70%

Courses required for incoming students to have completed prior to enrolling:
None

Recommended but not mandatory courses:
Basic psychology courses, including research methods and statistics; background in biology, math, & computer science

GRE mean
Verbal 641   Quantitative 726
Advanced Psychology 726
Analytical Writing 5.56

GPA mean
Overall GPA 3.72

Number of applications/admission offers/incoming students in 2007
280 applied/12 admission offers/4 incoming

% of students receiving:
Full tuition waiver only: 0%
Assistantship/fellowship only: 0%
Both full tuition waiver & assistantship/fellowship: 100%

Approximate percentage of incoming students with a B.A./B.S. only: 95%   **Master's:** 5%

Approximate percentage of students who are Women: 80%   **Ethnic Minority:** 13%   **International:** 4%

Average years to complete the doctoral program (including internship): 7 years

Personal interview
Preferred in person but telephone acceptable

Attrition rate in past 7 years: 4%

Percentage of students applying for internship last year accepted into APPIC or APA internships: 100%

Formal tracks/concentrations: adult psychopathology, developmental psychopathology, health psychology

Research areas	# Faculty	# Grants
adult psychopathology	7	19
mood disorders/depression	6	22
at-risk adolescents	8	28
attention-deficit disorder	1	2
autism	3	16
behavioral genetics	4	11
behavioral medicine/health psychology	14	38
cancer/behavioral oncology	1	3
cardiovascular behavioral medicine	4	13
child & family psychopathology	14	45
chronic disease	2	6
emotion	5	19
eating disorders	1	4
neuroimaging	7	27
neuropsychology	7	27
prevention	3	9
program evaluation	2	3
psychoneuroimmunology	3	9
psychopharmacology	3	8
psychophysiology	5	16

schizophrenia	1	1
social cognition/cognition	4	10
social support	1	4
statistics	2	2
stress and coping	4	15
substance abuse/addictions	8	21
weight management	1	4

Clinical opportunities

adolescent treatment
affective disorders
anxiety disorders
assessment
attention-deficit disorder
autism
behavioral medicine
child treatment
cognitive-behavioral
  therapy
conduct disorder
chronic mental illness
eating disorders
emergency room
  assessment
family therapy
gay/lesbian
group therapy
inpatient
minority populations
neuropsychological
  assessment
obsessive-compulsive
pain management
parent training
pediatric
personality disorders
schizophrenia
smoking cessation
substance abuse
suicide prevention
veterans medical center
victim/sexual abuse
weight management

Ponce School of Medicine (Psy.D.)

Clinical Psychology Doctoral Program
P.O. Box 7004
Ponce, PR 00732
phone#: (787) 813-5700
e-mail: jpons@psm.edu
Web address: www.psm.edu/Academic%20Affair%20
&%20Programs/programs/PsyD/index.htm

1	2	**3**	4	5	6	7

Practice oriented · · · Equal emphasis · · · Research oriented

Percentage of faculty subscribing to each of the following orientations:

Psychodynamic/Psychoanalytic	33%
Applied behavioral analysis/Radical behavioral	0%
Family systems/Systems	33%
Existential/Phenomenological/Humanistic	0%
Cognitive/Cognitive-behavioral	33%

Courses required for incoming students to have completed prior to enrolling:

developmental, statistics, research methods, abnormal

Recommended but not mandatory courses:

personality, physiological

GRE mean

Most of our students take the Spanish version of the GRE—
EXADEP

GPA mean

Overall GPA 3.49

Number of applications/admission offers/incoming students in 2007

91 applied/33 mission offers/30 incoming

% of students receiving:

Full tuition waiver only: 0%
Assistantship/fellowship only: 5%
Both full tuition waiver & assistantship/fellowship: 5%

Approximate percentage of incoming students with a B.A./B.S. only: 85% Master's: 15%

Approximate percentage of students who are Women: 74% Ethnic Minority: 100% International: 3%

Average years to complete the doctoral program (including internship): not reported

Personal interview

Required in person

Attrition rate in past 7 years: 8%

Percentage of students applying for internship last year accepted into APPIC or APA internships: 26%

Formal tracks/concentrations: health psychology, neuropsychology

Research areas	# Faculty	# Grants
adaptation of tests	4	1
HIV stigma and health disparities	3	2
fear conditioning and extinction	1	1

Clinical opportunities

general community hospital
community mental health clinics

Purdue University (Ph.D.)

Department of Psychological Sciences
703 Third Street
West Lafayette, IN 47907-2081
phone#: (765) 494-6977
e-mail: (secretary) dlbatta@psych.purdue.edu,
(director) rollock@psych.purdue.edu
Web address: www.psych.purdue.edu/ [Use pull-down menu under "Areas" to click on "Clinical"]

1	2	3	4	5	**6**	7

Practice oriented · · · Equal emphasis · · · Research oriented

Percentage of faculty subscribing to each of the following orientations:

Psychodynamic/Psychoanalytic	10%
Applied behavioral analysis/Radical behavioral	10%
Family systems/Systems	10%
Existential/Phenomenological/Humanistic	0%
Cognitive/Cognitive-behavioral	70%

Courses required for incoming students to have completed prior to enrolling:

The most competitive students have solid, broad coursework in psychology, especially methodology and statistics, as well as undergraduate research experience.

Recommended but not mandatory courses:

Strong record of coursework in mathematics (calculus preferable), natural sciences, other social sciences

GRE mean
Verbal: 593
Quantitative: 666

GPA mean
Overall 3.47

Number of applications/admission offers/incoming students in 2007
127 applied/5 admission offers/3 incoming

% of incoming students receiving:
Full tuition waiver only: 0%
Assistantship/fellowship only: 0%
Both full tuition waiver & assistantship/fellowship: 100%

Approximate percentage of incoming students with a B.A./B.S. only: 100%   **Master's:** 0%

Approximate percentage of students who are:
Women: 70.6%   **Ethnic Minority:** 26.5%
International: 2.9%

Average years to complete the doctoral program (including internship): 7.3 years

Personal interview
Personal interviews; telephone interviews are acceptable under extenuating circumstances.

Attrition rate in past 7 years: 26.3%

Percentage of students applying for internship last year accepted into APPIC or APA internships: 100%

Formal tracks/concentrations: adult, child

Research areas	# Faculty	# Grants
adolescence	1	0
anger & antisocial behavior	3	1
anxiety disorders	1	0
ethnicity minority/cultural issues	2	0
family processes & child/adolescent development	2	2
marital/intimate partner violence	2	0
personality and psychopathology	3	0
personality assessment	1	0
social skills deficits and pathology	2	0

Clinical opportunities
childhood disorders
anxiety (adult & child)
assessment (neuropsychological; adult & child)
assessment (general clinical; child & adult)
depression (adult & child)
family and adolescence
HeadStart consultations
personality disorders (adult)

Regent University (Ph.D.)
Doctoral Program in Clinical Psychology
CRB 154
1000 Regent University Drive
Virginia Beach, VA 23464
phone#: (800) 373-5504 ext. 4498
e-mail: stepbru@regent.edu
Web address: www.regent.edu/psyd

1	2	**3**	4	5	6	7
Practice oriented		Equal emphasis			Research oriented	

Percentage of faculty subscribing to each of the following orientations:
Psychodynamic/Psychoanalytic   30%
Applied behavioral analysis/Radical behavioral   20%
Family systems/Systems   40%
Existential/Phenomenological/Humanistic   30%
Cognitive/Cognitive-behavioral   60%

Courses required for incoming students to have completed prior to enrolling:
18 hours of psychology (undergraduate)

Recommended but not mandatory courses:
Statistics, research methods, personality, human development, abnormaly, social, physiological

GRE mean
Verbal and Quantitative: 1080
Analytical Writing 3.5

GPA mean
3.69

Number of applications/admission offers/incoming students in 2007
87 applied/33 admission offers/18 incoming

% of students receiving:
Full tuition waiver only: 0%
(100% of incoming students received Partial tuition waiver)
Assistantship/fellowship only: 13%
Both full tuition waiver & assistantship/fellowship: 13%

Approximate percentage of incoming students with a B.A./B.S. (Honors) only: 79%   **Master's:** 21%

Approximate percentage of students who are
Women: 68%   **Ethnic Minority:** 18%   **International:** 4%

Average years to complete the doctoral program (including internship): 5.4 years

Personal interview
Required in person

Attrition rate in past 7 years: 11.6%

Percentage of students applying for internship last year accepted into APPIC or APA internships: 85%

Formal tracks/concentrations: marital & family, clinical child, health, religion

Research areas	# Faculty	# Grants
ADHD	1	1
consultation to religious and community organizations	4	3
diversity in the military	1	0
personality and religion	1	1
marital functioning and spirituality	2	1
sexual and religious identity	1	3
God image & adjustment	1	1

Clinical opportunities

behavioral medicine
child mental health settings
Christian counseling centers
forensic settings

military mental health
neuropsychology
psychiatric hospitals

University of Rhode Island (Ph.D.)

Department of Psychology
Chafee Center
Kingston, RI 02881
phone#: (401) 874-2193
e-mail: alberman@uri.edu
Web address:
www.uri.edu/artsci/psy/clinical/index.html

1	2	3	**4**	5	6	7
Practice oriented			Equal emphasis			Research oriented

Percentage of faculty subscribing to each of the following orientations:

Psychodynamic/Psychoanalytic   10%
Applied behavioral analysis/Radical behavioral   0%
Family systems/Systems   40%
Existential/Phenomenological/Humanistic   30%
Cognitive/Cognitive-behavioral   50%
Feminist   10%

Courses required for incoming students to have completed prior to enrolling:
Background in undergraduate psychology

Recommended but not mandatory courses:
Tests and measurements

GRE mean
Verbal 560   Quantitative 620
Analytical Writing not reported
Advanced Psychology not reported

GPA mean
Undergraduate GPA 3.4

Number of applications/admission offers/incoming students in 2007
248 applied/9 admission offers/6 incoming

% of students receiving:
Full tuition waiver only: 22%
Assistantship/fellowship only: 78%
Both full tuition waiver & assistantship/fellowship: 0%

Approximate percentage of incoming students with a B.A./B.S. only: 50%   **Master's:** 50%

Approximate percentage of students who are Women: 74%   **Ethnic Minority:** 37%   **International:** 10%

Average years to complete the doctoral program (including internship): 6.8 years

Personal interview
Required in person

Attrition rate in past 7 years: 14%

Percentage of students applying for internship last year accepted into APPIC or APA internships: 100%

Formal tracks/concentrations: neuropsychology, child/family, applied methodology

Research areas	# Faculty	# Grants
behavioral medicine/health psychology	3	10
child clinical	1	0
clinical judgment	1	0
community psychology	1	4
family research	1	0
multicultural issues	1	0

Clinical opportunities

child therapy
community psychology
family therapy
health psychology

individual psychotherapy
marriage and couples
  therapy
sex therapy

University of Rochester (Ph.D.)

Department of Psychology
Meliora Hall
Rochester, NY 14627-0266
phone#: (585) 275-8704
e-mail: gilbert@psych.rochester.edu
Web address:
www.psych.rochester.edu/graduate/clinical/

1	2	3	4	**5**	6	7
Practice oriented			Equal emphasis			Research oriented

Percentage of faculty subscribing to each of the following orientations:

Psychodynamic/Psychoanalytic   24%
Applied behavioral analysis/Radical behavioral   12%
Family systems/Systems   1%
Existential/Phenomenological/Humanistic   6%
Cognitive/Cognitive-behavioral   57%

Courses required for incoming students to have completed prior to enrolling:
Equivalent of psychology major

Recommended but not mandatory courses:
None

GRE mean
Verbal 618   Quantitative 690   Analytical Writing 5.5

GPA mean
Overall GPA 3.8

Number of applications/admission offers/incoming students in 2007
190 applied/4 admission offers/4 incoming

% of students receiving:
Full tuition waiver only: 0%
Assistantship/fellowship only: 0%
Both full tuition waiver & assistantship/fellowship: 100%

Approximate percentage of students who are Women: 81%   **Ethnic Minority:** 16%   **International:** 13%

Average years to complete the doctoral program (including internship): 7 years

Personal interview
Required in person

Attrition rate in past 7 years: 7%

Percentage of students applying for internship last year accepted into APPIC or APA internships: 100%

Formal tracks/concentrations: developmental psychopathology

Research areas	# Faculty	# Grants
attention-deficit disorder	1	1
autism	2	2
child abuse	1	2
depression	1	1
marriage	1	0
motivation	1	3

Clinical opportunities

attention-deficit disorder
autism
child maltreatment/abuse

neuropsychology
psychodynamic therapy
smoking prevention

Roosevelt University (Psy.D.)

School of Psychology
Chicago, IL 60605
phone#: (312)-341-3760
e-mail: skvaal@roosevelt.edu
Web address: www.roosevelt.edu/cas/sp/psyd.htm

1	2	3	4	5	6	7

Practice oriented   Equal emphasis   Research oriented

Percentage of faculty subscribing to each of the following orientations:

Psychodynamic/Psychoanalytic	42%
Applied behavioral analysis/Radical behavioral	1%
Family systems/Systems	17%
Existential/Phenomenological/Humanistic	17%
Cognitive/Cognitive-behavioral	42%

Courses required for incoming students to have completed prior to enrolling:
Abnormal, research methods, statistics

Recommended but not mandatory courses:
Personality, tests and measurement

GRE mean
Verbal 544   Quantitative 626
Advanced Psychology not reported
Analytical Writing 5.0

GPA mean
Overall GPA 3.5

Number of applications/admission offers/incoming students in 2007
130 applied/30 admission offers/17 incoming

% of students receiving:
Full tuition waiver only: 0%
Assistantship/fellowship only: 0%
Both full tuition waiver & assistantship/fellowship: 3%

Approximate percentage of incoming students with a B.A./B.S. only: 95%   **Master's:** 5%

Approximate percentage of students who are Women: 75%   **Ethnic Minority:** 21%
International: 2%

Average years to complete the doctoral program (including internship): 6 years

Personal interview
Required in person

Attrition rate in past 7 years: 8%

Percentage of students applying for internship last year accepted into APPIC or APA internships: 60%

Formal tracks/concentrations: none

Research areas	# Faculty	# Grants
assessment	3	0
children and adolescents	4	1
health psychology	4	1
neuropsychology	3	0
group psychotherapy/psychodrama	1	0
social cognition	1	0
learning theory	1	0
college teaching	1	0

Clinical opportunities

children and families
adult chronic psychiatric
behavioral medicine
torture survivors
neuropsychology (child, adolescent, adult)

therapeutic day schools
veteran's administration hospitals
jail/prison populations
anxiety disorders
eating disorders

Rosalind Franklin University of Medicine and Science (Ph.D.)

Department of Psychology
3333 Green Bay Road
North Chicago, IL 60064
phone#: (847) 578-3305
e-mail: chinni.chilamkurti@rosalindfranklin.edu
Web address:
www.rosalindfranklin.edu/srhs/psychology/

1	2	3	4	5	6	7

Practice oriented   Equal emphasis   Research oriented

Percentage of faculty subscribing to each of the following orientations:

Psychodynamic/Psychoanalytic	5%
Applied behavioral analysis/Radical behavioral	5%
Family systems/Systems	15%
Existential/Phenomenological/Humanistic	5%
Cognitive/Cognitive-behavioral	70%

Courses required for incoming students to have completed prior to enrolling:
Statistics and biological/physiological psychology

Recommended but not mandatory courses:
abnormal, developmental, social

GRE mean
Verbal 513   Quantitative 600
Advanced Psychology 668
Analytical Writing 4.2

GPA mean
Overall GPA 3.42

Number of applications/admission offers/incoming students in 2007
68 applied/21 admission offers/12 incoming

% of students receiving:
Full tuition waiver only: 0%
Assistantship/fellowship only: 0%
Both full tuition waiver & assistantship/fellowship: 55%

Approximate percentage of incoming students with a B.A./B.S. only: 50%   **Master's:** 50%

Approximate percentage of students who are Women: 71%   **Ethnic Minority:** 14%   **International:** 0%

Average years to complete the doctoral program (including internship): 7 years

Personal interview
Preferred in person but telephone acceptable

Attrition rate in past 7 years: not reported

Percentage of students applying for internship last year accepted into APPIC or APA internships: 82%

Formal tracks/concentrations: neuropsychology, health psychology, psychopathology

Research areas	# Faculty	# Grants
aging	1	1
anxiety disorders	1	1
cancer	1	0
diabetes	1	0
epilepsy/neuropsychology	1	2
pain	1	1
psychopathy	1	0
risk behaviors in adolescents	1	0
schizophrenia	1	0
sports concussion	1	0

Clinical opportunities

anxiety disorders	neuropsychiatric
behavioral medicine	neuropsychological

Rutgers, The State University of New Jersey (Ph.D.)

Department of Psychology
Graduate School of Arts and Sciences
New Brunswick, NJ 08903

e-mail: tewilson@rci.rutgers.edu
Web address:
psych.rutgers.edu/program_areas/clin/clin.html

1	2	3	4	**5**	6	7
Practice oriented			Equal emphasis			Research oriented

Percentage of faculty subscribing to each of the following orientations:

Psychodynamic/Psychoanalytic	0%
Applied behavioral analysis/Radical behavioral	14%
Family systems/Systems	6%
Existential/Phenomenological/Humanistic	0%
Cognitive/Cognitive-behavioral	80%

Courses required for incoming students to have completed prior to enrolling:
A major in psychology or equivalent courses

Recommended but not mandatory courses:
None

GRE mean
Verbal 690   Quantitative 750
Advanced Psychology 750
Analytical Writing not reported

GPA mean
Overall GPA 3.77

Number of applications/admission offers/incoming students in 2007
244 applied/8 admission offers/4 incoming

% of students receiving:
Full tuition waiver only: 0%
Assistantship/fellowship only: 0%
Both full tuition waiver & assistantship/fellowship: 100%

Approximate percentage of incoming students with a B.A./B.S. only: 100%   **Master's:** 0%

Approximate percentage of students who are Women: 75%   **Ethnic Minority:** 29%   **International:** 6%

Average years to complete the doctoral program (including internship): 6 years

Personal interview
Preferred in person but telephone acceptable

Attrition rate in past 7 years: 0.3%

Percentage of students applying for internship last year accepted into APPIC or APA internships: 100%

Formal tracks/concentrations: none

Research areas	# Faculty	# Grants
applied behavioral analysis	2	0
autism	1	1
behavioral medicine	5	1
depression	0	0
developmental psychopathology	1	1
eating disorders	1	1
ethical issues	0	0
marriage/couples	2	1

philosophical issues	1	0
prevention	2	1
program design and evaluation	1	1
psychopathology	1	1
psychotherapy process/outcome	5	3
somatization disorders	1	1
substance abuse	3	2

Clinical opportunities

adolescent delinquency
affective disorders
alcohol use disorders
anxiety disorders
assessment
behavioral medicine
community psychology
conduct disorder
depression
developmental disabilities

eating disorders
family therapy
minority
obsessive–compulsive
    disorder
personality disorders
sex therapy
somatization disorders
substance abuse

Rutgers, The State University of New Jersey (Psy.D.)

Graduate School of Applied and Professional Psychology
152 Frelinghuysen Road
Piscataway, NJ 08854-8085
phone#: (732) 445-2000 x 117
e-mail: clinpsyd@rci.rutgers.edu
Web address: gsappweb.rutgers.edu

1	2	3	4	5	6	7

Practice oriented   Equal emphasis   Research oriented

Percentage of faculty subscribing to each of the following orientations:

Psychodynamic/Psychoanalytic	30%
Applied behavioral analysis/Radical behavioral	10%
Family systems/Systems	20%
Existential/Phenomenological/Humanistic	10%
Cognitive/Cognitive-behavioral	30%

Courses required for incoming students to have completed prior to enrolling:
Statistics, abnormal, and the biological bases of psychology

Recommended but not mandatory courses:
Students also should have taken 1 and preferably 2 courses of the following: cognitive, perception, conditioning and learning, developmental, personality, social. We also prefer that 1 of the above has a laboratory component.

GRE mean
Verbal 630
Quantitative 690
Advanced Psychology 700

GPA mean
Overall GPA 3.71

Number of applications/admission offers/incoming students in 2007
470 applied/27 admission offers/15 incoming

% of students receiving:
Full tuition waiver only: 0%
Scholarships only: 47%
Both full tuition waiver & assistantship/fellowship: 53%

Approximate percentage of incoming students with a B.A./B.S. only: 87.5% **Master's:** 12.5%

Approximate percentage of students who are Women: 67% **Ethnic Minority:** 27% **International:** 7%

Average years to complete the doctoral program (including internship) 5.8 years

Personal interview
Preferred in person but telephone acceptable

Attrition rate in past 7 years: 4%

Percentage of students applying for internship last year accepted into APPIC or APA internships: 94%

Formal tracks/concentrations: community, sports

Research areas	# Faculty	# Grants
adolescence	3	1
adoption	1	1
anxiety disorders	3	1
applied behavioral analysis	1	1
autism	1	1
community	2	1
developmental disabilities	3	2
diagnosis and classification	2	0
dissociative disorders	1	0
eating disorders	1	1
empirically supported treatment	2	1
ethical issues	1	0
family/marriage/couples	3	1
feminist theory and psychology	1	0
mental health policy	2	1
mind/body/health	1	1
multicultural issues	2	0
organizational psychology	1	0
personality disorders	2	0
philosophy and psychology	2	0
program design and evaluation	1	0
psychiatric disabilities	1	1
psychoanalytic theory	4	1
psychology and the arts	1	0
psychophysiological disorders	1	0
psychotherapy process/outcome	3	1
severe mental illness	2	1
social learning theory	1	1
substance abuse	4	2

Clinical opportunities (see website for listing of practicum sites)

AIDS
adolescent delinquency
affective disorders
anxiety disorders
assessment
behavioral medicine
community psychology
conduct disorder
developmental disabilities
dissociative disorder

infancy/postpartum
interpersonal psychotherapy
marital/couples therapy
minority
neuropsychology
obsessive–compulsive
    disorder
organizational psychology
personality disorders
psychodynamic therapy

eating disorders
family therapy
forensic psychology
gerontology
group therapy
hyperactivity
hypnosis
impulse control

rational-emotive
 psychotherapy
schizophrenia
school psychology
sex therapy
substance abuse
victim/abuse

St. John's University (Ph.D.)

Department of Psychology
8000 Utopia Parkway
Jamaica, NY 11439
phone#: (718) 990-6369
e-mail: nevidj@stjohns.edu
Web address:
www.stjohns.edu/academics/graduate/liberalarts/
departments/psychology/programs/phd_cp

1	2	3	**4**	5	6	7

Practice oriented   Equal emphasis   Research oriented

Percentage of faculty subscribing to each of the following orientations:

Psychodynamic/Psychoanalytic   30%
Applied behavioral analysis/Radical behavioral   0%
Family systems/Systems   10%
Existential/Phenomenological/Humanistic   0%
Cognitive/Cognitive-behavioral   60%

Courses required for incoming students to have completed prior to enrolling:

Statistics, experimental laboratory

Recommended but not mandatory courses:

None

GRE mean

Verbal 638   Quantitative 677
Advanced Psychology 688.8
Analytical Writing 4.9

GPA mean

Overall GPA 3.60   Psychology GPA 3.65

Number of applications/admission offers/incoming students in 2007

255 applied/30 admission offers/12 incoming

% of incoming students receiving:

Full tuition waiver only: 8%
Assistantship/fellowship only: 0%
Both full tuition waiver & assistantship/fellowship: 0%
(92% of students are given partial support)

Approximate percentage of incoming students with a B.A./B.S. only: 83%   Master's: 17%

Approximate percentage of students who are Women: 79.7%   Ethnic Minority: 29.7% International: 0%

Average years to complete the doctoral program (including internship): 6.2 years

Personal interview

Preferred in person but telephone acceptable

Attrition rate in past 7 years: 10%

Percentage of students applying for internship last year accepted into APPIC or APA internships: 100%

Formal tracks/concentrations: child clinical

Research areas	# Faculty	# Grants
anxiety disorders	2	0
autism	1	1
bilingualism	2	0
bullying behavior/victimization	1	0
child abuse	1	2
gender issues	2	0
health psychology	2	1
minority mental health	5	1
moral development	3	0
intervention	1	1
schizophrenia	1	0
smoking cessation	1	0
stress management	1	1

Clinical opportunities

clinical child psychology
cognitive-behavioral
 therapy
group therapy
neuropsychological
 assessment

psychodynamic therapy
medical centers
municipal hospitals
outpatient clinics
research institutes

Saint Louis University (Ph.D.)

Department of Psychology
221 North Grand Boulevard
St. Louis, MO 63103
phone#: (314) 977-2284
e-mail: psyclini@slu.edu
Web address: www.slu.edu/graduate/

1	2	3	**4**	5	6	7

Practice oriented   Equal emphasis   Research oriented

Percentage of faculty subscribing to each of the following orientations:

Psychodynamic/Psychoanalytic   15%
Applied behavioral analysis/Radical behavioral   0%
Family systems/Systems   25%
Existential/Phenomenological/Humanistic   15%
Cognitive/Cognitive-behavioral   70%

Courses required for incoming students to have completed prior to enrolling:

Statistics, abnormal, and 6 upper-division psychology courses

Recommended but not mandatory courses:

Personality, learning, social, physiological, developmental, tests and measurement

GRE mean

Verbal 550   Quantitative 550
Analytical Writing 4.0

GPA mean
Overall GPA 3.5

Number of applications/admission offers/incoming students in 2007
165 applied/14 admission offers/8 incoming

% of students receiving:
Full tuition waiver only: 0%
Assistantship/fellowship only: 0%
Tuition full waiver & assistantship/fellowship: 100% for first year

Approximate percentage of incoming students with a B.A./B.S. only: 85% Master's: 15%

Approximate percentage of students who are
Women: 70% Ethnic Minority: 20% International: 10%

Average years to complete the doctoral program (including internship): 6 years

Personal interview
Preferred in person but telephone acceptable

Attrition rate in past 7 years: 5%

Percentage of students applying for internship last year accepted into APPIC or APA internships: 70%

Formal tracks/concentrations: none

Research areas	# Faculty	# Grants
abuse/violence	2	1
adjustment	2	0
anxiety	2	0
assessment	2	0
child/adolescent	2	1
community	1	0
depression	2	0
eating disorders	1	1
ethical issues	2	0
family	3	0
minority issues	1	0
neuropsychology	1	0
personality disorders	2	0
professional issues	2	0
sport psychology	1	0
stress and coping	2	0

Clinical opportunities

anxiety	hyperactivity
assessment	learning disabilities
clinical neuropsychology	marital
eating disorders and obesity	parent skills training
ethnic diversity	personality disorders
family therapy	psychodynamic therapy
health psychology	victims of abuse and assault

Sam Houston State University (Ph.D.)
Department of Psychology and Philosophy
Huntsville, TX 77341-2210
phone#: (936) 294-1210
e-mail: maconroy@shsu.edu
Web address: www.shsu.edu/clinpsy

1	2	3	**4**	5	6	7
Practice oriented		Equal emphasis			Research oriented	

Percentage of faculty subscribing to each of the following orientations:
Psychodynamic/Psychoanalytic	0%
Applied behavioral analysis/Radical behavioral	0%
Family systems/Systems	33%
Existential/Phenomenological/Humanistic	0%
Cognitive/Cognitive-behavioral	67%

Courses required for incoming students to have completed prior to enrolling:
none

Recommended but not mandatory courses:
none

GRE mean
Verbal 561 Quantitative 644
Advanced Psychology 654
Analytical Writing not reported

GPA mean
Overall GPA 3.65

Number of applications/admission offers/incoming students in 2007
92 applied/12 admission offers/7 incoming

% of students receiving:
Full tuition waiver only: 0%
Assistantship/fellowship only: 100%
Both full tuition waiver & assistantship/fellowship: 0%

Approximate percentage of incoming students with a B.A./B.S. only: 73% Master's: 27%

Approximate percentage of students who are
Women: 84% Ethnic Minority: 18%
International: 0%

Average years to complete the doctoral program (including internship): 6 years

Personal interview
Preferred in person but telephone acceptable

Attrition rate in past 7 years: 12%

Percentage of students applying for internship last year accepted into APPIC or APA internships: 100%

Formal tracks/concentrations: forensic

Research areas	# Faculty	# Grants
juvenile justice	2	2
violence risk	2	1
witness preparation/testimony	1	1
family psychology	1	1
criminal justice system	1	1
addictive behavior	1	1
advanced data analysis	1	0
trauma	1	2
body image/eating disorders	1	0
mental health and pregnancy	1	0
behavioral medicine	1	0

health psychology: chronic pain, fatigue	1	1
neurobehavioral functioning	1	1
person perception	1	0
jury decision making	1	0
social influences	1	0
group dynamics	1	0
relationship commitment	1	0

Clinical opportunities
not reported

San Diego State University/University of California–San Diego (Ph.D.)

Joint doctoral program in clinical psychology
San Diego, CA 92182
phone#: (619) 594-2246
e-mail: eklonoff@sunstroke.sdsu.edu
Web address: www.psychology.sdsu.edu/doctoral/

1	2	3	4	5	**6**	7

Practice oriented   Equal emphasis   Research oriented

Percentage of faculty subscribing to each of the following orientations:

Psychodynamic/Psychoanalytic	5%
Applied behavioral analysis/Radical behavioral	30%
Family systems/Systems	10%
Existential/Phenomenological/Humanistic	5%
Cognitive/Cognitive-behavioral	50%

Courses required for incoming students to have completed prior to enrolling:
psychology major or 18 semester hours in psychology including: personality, abnormal, social, statistics, testing, experimental with lab, physiological.

Recommended but not mandatory courses:
Perception, learning, biology, mathematics, linguistics, computer science, medical physics

GRE mean
Verbal 637   Quantitative 671
Advanced Psychology 3.73
Analytical Writing not reported

GPA mean
Overall GPA 3.67   Psychology GPA 3.80

Number of applications/admission offers/incoming students in 2007
309 applied/18 admission offers/10 incoming

% of students receiving:
Full tuition waiver only: 0%
Assistantship/fellowship only: 0%
Tuition full waiver & assistantship/fellowship: 100%

Approximate percentage of incoming students with a B.A./B.S. only: 73%   **Master's:** 27%

Approximate percentage of students who are Women: 78%   **Ethnic Minority:** 22%
International: not reported

Average years to complete the doctoral program (including internship): 6 years

Personal interview
Preferred in person but telephone acceptable

Attrition rate in past 7 years: 2%

Percentage of students applying for internship last year accepted into APPIC or APA internships: 100%

Formal tracks/concentrations: behavioral medicine/health psychology, experimental psychopathology, neuropsychology

Research areas	# Faculty	# Grants
AIDS	7	1
aging	8	1
Alzheimer's/dementia	6	0
anxiety	4	1
applied behavioral analysis	4	0
autism	2	0
bereavement	2	0
biofeedback	1	0
cancer disparities	4	0
cancer prevention	2	2
cardiovascular disease	4	1
child, marriage, and family	5	0
childhood brain damage	2	0
chronic disease	4	1
cognition and memory	13	0
cognitive psychology/therapy	2	0
community psychology	1	0
cross-cultural psychology	10	0
decision making	1	0
depression	3	2
developmental neuropsychology	7	0
developmental psychopathology	3	0
ethnicity and health	2	0
exercise	2	1
gender and health	2	0
gender issues	2	0
information processing	4	0
interpersonal psychology	1	0
neuropsychological testing	2	1
nutrition	3	0
pain	2	0
posttraumatic stress disorder	1	0
problem solving	1	0
psychological testing	4	0
psychology of humor	1	0
psychopathology	3	0
psychopharmacology	6	2
psychophysiology	5	0
psychotherapy process and outcome	4	0
schizophrenia/psychosis	7	2
sexuality	1	0
sleep	4	0
smoking	7	1
social skills training	1	0
social support	2	0
statistics	4	0
stress and coping	13	0

substance abuse	12	5
women's health	3	0

Clinical opportunities

anxiety disorders
behavioral medicine
child and family therapy

cognitive therapy
neuropsychology
school psychology

University of Saskatchewan (Ph.D.)

Department of Psychology
Doctoral Program in Clinical Psychology
Saskatoon, Saskatchewan S7N 5A5, Canada
e-mail: psychology@usask.ca
Web address: www.usask.ca/psychology/programs/
clinprog/welcome/index.html

1	2	3	**4**	5	6	7

Practice oriented Equal emphasis Research oriented

Percentage of faculty subscribing to each of the following orientations:

Psychodynamic/Psychoanalytic	12.5%
Applied behavioral analysis/Radical behavioral	12.5%
Family systems/Systems	12.5%
Existential/Phenomenological/Humanistic	25%
Cognitive/Cognitive-behavioral	50%

Courses required for incoming students prior to enrolling:

An honors B.A. or B.Sc. degree in psychology or its equivalent, including statistics, research methods, and an honors thesis

Courses recommended but not mandatory:

Basic area courses, for example, biological, cognitive, and social bases of behavior

GRE mean

Verbal   Quantitative   Advanced Psychology
Analytical Writing

GPA mean

Overall GPA 86%

Number of applications/admission offers/incoming students in 2007

54 applied/8 admission offers/5 incoming

% of students receiving:

Full tuition waiver only: 0%
Assistantship/fellowship only: 100%
Both full tuition waiver & assistantship/fellowship: 0%

Approximate percentage of incoming students with a B.A./B.S. only: 80%   Master's: 20%

Approximate percentage of students who are Women: 80%   Ethnic Minority: 25%   International: 0%

Average years to complete the doctoral program (including internship): 7 years

Personal interview

Preferred in person but telephone acceptable

Attrition rate in past 7 years: 5%

Percentage of students applying for internship last year accepted into APPIC or APA internships: 80%

Formal tracks/concentrations: none

Research areas	# Faculty	# Grants
bereavement	1	0
child trauma and violence	1	1
forensic/psychopathy	4	2
health psychology	3	2
metaphor/narrative	1	1
neuropsychology	1	1
psychotherapy process	2	1

Clinical opportunities

adult psychotherapy
child clinical psychology
behavioral medicine
developmental disabilities

inpatient forensic
neuropsychology
young offenders

Seattle Pacific University (Ph.D.)

Department of Graduate Psychology
3307 Third Avenue West, Suite 107
Seattle, WA 98119
phone#: (206) 281-2987
e-mail: mbbaldwin@spu.edu
Web address: www.spu.edu/clinpsych

1	2	3	**4**	5	6	7

Practice oriented Equal emphasis Research oriented

Percentage of faculty subscribing to each of the following orientations:

Psychodynamic/Psychoanalytic	33%
Applied behavioral analysis/Radical behavioral	33%
Family systems/Systems	50%
Existential/Phenomenological/Humanistic	16%
Cognitive/Cognitive-behavioral	83%

Courses required for incoming students to have completed prior to enrolling:

Statistics and 5 from among: abnormal, developmental, experimental, physiological, social, learning, motivation, personality, cognitive, tests and measurement

Recommended but not mandatory courses:

See above

GRE mean

Verbal 553   Quantitative 627
Advanced Psychology not reported
Analytical Writing not reported

GPA mean

Overall GPA 3.58

Number of applications/admission offers/incoming students in 2007

48 applied/23 admission offers/12 incoming

% of students receiving:

Full tuition waiver only: 0%
Assistantship/fellowship only: 40%
Both full tuition waiver & assistantship/fellowship: 0%

Approximate percentage of incoming students with a B.A./B.S. only: 83%   **Master's:** 17%

Approximate percentage of students who are Women: 80%   **Ethnic Minority:** 14%
International: 0%

Average years to complete the doctoral program (including internship): 6 years

Personal interview
Preferred in person but telephone acceptable

Attrition rate in past 7 years: 0%

Percentage of students applying for internship last year accepted into APPIC or APA internships: 44%

Formal tracks/concentrations: none

Research areas	# Faculty	# Grants
gender and psychology	3	1
developmental psychopathology	3	3
psychology of religion	3	1
child and adolescent development	3	1
health psychology	2	0
family psychology	2	0
ethnicity and psychology	2	0
career and life development	2	0
treatment program evaluation	2	1
mental disorder in women	2	1
program and policy development	2	1
hypnosis	2	0
biofeedback	1	1
child development	1	1
conduct problems in young children	1	1
attention and self-regulation	1	1
severe mental disorders	1	1
cognitive models of psychopathology	1	1
addictive behavior	1	1
evaluation of career interventions	1	0
counseling process and outcome	1	0
relationships in ministry	1	0
disaster psychology	1	0
relationship between couples	1	0
multisystemic interventions	1	0
interventions for chronic pain	1	0
gender differences in health	2	0
psychodynamic psychotherapy	1	0
supervision/ethics	1	0
psychophysiology of stress	1	0
exercise and quality of life	1	0
self-psychology and self-esteem	1	0
prejudice and intergroup relations	1	0
leadership development	1	0
developmental disabilities	1	0
psychologies of peace and war	1	0
ethnic identity, ethnic memories	1	0
Pacific Native American communities	1	0

Clinical opportunities
behavioral medicine
neuropsychology
rehabilitation medicine
juvenile rehabilitation
serious mental illness
Latino/a mental health
child and adolescent mental health
university counseling center
cancer care
corrections
autism/autism spectrum
Christian counseling
foster care
family therapy
community mental health

Simon Fraser University (Ph.D.)
Department of Psychology
Burnaby, British Columbia V5A 1S6, Canada
Phone#: (778) 782-3354
e-mail: turner@sfu.ca
Web address:
www.psyc.sfu.ca/grad/index.php?topic=clin_overview

1	2	3	**4**	5	6	7
Practice oriented		Equal emphasis			Research oriented	

Percentage of faculty subscribing to each of the following orientations:
Psychodynamic/Psychoanalytic 15%
Applied behavioral analysis/Radical behavioral 0%
Family systems/Systems 35%
Existential/Phenomenological/Humanistic 0%
Cognitive/Cognitive-Behavioral 85%

Courses required for incoming students to have completed prior to enrolling:
Undergraduate degree (BA, BSc or equivalent) with an honor's or major in psychology

Recommended but not mandatory courses:
Psychology honors program; advanced undergraduate courses across all substantive areas of psychology

GRE mean
Verbal 609   Quantitative 700
Advanced Psychology 753
Analytical Writing not reported

GPA mean
Overall GPA 4.04
Psychology GPA 4.07

Number of applications/admission offers/incoming students in 2007
163 applied/9 admission offers/8 incoming

% of students receiving:
Full tuition waiver only: 0%
Assistantship/fellowship only: 100%
Both full tuition waiver & assistantship/fellowship: 0%

Approximate percentage of incoming students with a B.A./B.S. only: 87.5%   **Master's:** 12.5%

Approximate percentage of students who are Women: 81%   **Ethnic Minority:** not reported
International: not reported

Average years to complete the doctoral program (including internship): 7 years

Personal interview
Preferred in person but telephone acceptable

Attrition rate in past 7 years: 5%

Percentage of students applying for internship last year accepted into APPIC or APA internships:

Formal tracks/concentrations: general, child clinical, clinical forensic, clinical neuropsychology

Research areas	# Faculty	# Grants
behavioral medicine	1	1
child clinical	3	6
child psychopathology	3	5
cognition	5	6
depression	2	1
developmental	6	6
family	3	3
forensic	3	8
gender	0	0
neuropsychology	3	5
psychopathology	8	8
sex offenders	2	2
stress and coping	1	1
violence and abuse	5	5

University of South Carolina (Ph.D.)

Department of Psychology
Columbia, SC 29208
Phone#: (803) 777-2312
E-mail: marthab@gwm.sc.edu
Web address:
www.cas.sc.edu/psyc/grad_psyccc/ccprog.html

1	2	3	**4**	5	6	7
Practice oriented		Equal emphasis			Research oriented	

Percentage of faculty subscribing to each of the following orientations:

Psychodynamic/Psychoanalytic	30%
Applied behavioral analysis/Radical behavioral	20%
Family systems/Systems	10%
Existential/Phenomenological/Humanistic	0%
Cognitive/Cognitive-behavioral	40%

Courses required for incoming students to have completed prior to enrolling:
18 hours in psychology, including statistics

Recommended but not mandatory courses:
Research methods, learning, biopsychology, abnormal, social, developmental, personality

GRE mean
Verbal 667   Quantitative 691
Advanced Psychology 710
Analytical Writing not reported

GPA mean
Overall GPA 3.68   Psychology GPA 3.82
Junior/Senior GPA 3.85

Number of applications/admission offers/incoming students in 2007
130 applied/11 admission offers/9 incoming

% of students receiving:
Full tuition waiver only: 0%
Assistantship/fellowship only: 0%
Both full tuition waiver & assistantship/fellowship: 100%

Approximate percentage of incoming students with a B.A./B.S. only: 80%   **Master's:** 20%

Approximate percentage of students who are Women: 65%   **Ethnic Minority:** 25%
International: not reported

Average years to complete the doctoral program (including internship): 6 years

Personal interview
Preferred in person but telephone acceptable

Attrition rate in past 7 years: 6%

Percentage of students applying for internship last year accepted into APPIC or APA internships: 86%

Formal tracks/concentrations: children, adolescents, and families

Research areas	# Faculty	# Grants
citizen participation	1	0
community coalition development	1	1
conduct disorders	1	1
marital relationships	4	0
neuropsychology	2	1
prevention (racism/cross-cultural)	5	3
self-perception in minority youth	1	1
violence/rape/battering	2	1

Clinical opportunities
community psychology
family therapy
neuropsychology

University of South Dakota (Ph.D.)

Department of Psychology
Vermillion, SD 57069
phone#: (605) 677-5353
e-mail: byutrzen@usd.edu
Web address: www.usd.edu/psyc/ctp

1	2	3	**4**	5	6	7
Practice oriented		Equal emphasis			Research oriented	

Percentage of faculty subscribing to each of the following orientations:

Psychodynamic/Psychoanalytic	30%
Applied behavioral analysis/Radical behavioral	0%
Family systems/Systems	30%
Existential/Phenomenological/Humanistic	0%
Cognitive/Cognitive-behavioral	100%

Courses required for incoming students to have completed prior to enrolling:
18 semester hours in psychology distributed among standard coursework

Recommended but not mandatory courses:
Research design, statistics, history/systems, learning, abnormal, physiological

GRE mean
Verbal 547   Quantitative 628
Advanced Psychology 668
Analytical Writing not reported

GPA mean
3.86

Number of applications/admission offers/incoming students in 2007
95 applied/11 admission offers/6 incoming

% of students receiving:
Full tuition waiver only: 0%
Assistantship/fellowship only: 100%
Both full tuition waiver & assistantship/fellowship: 0%
(all students on assistantships also receive tuition reduction to 1/3 of in-state tuition costs)

Approximate percentage of incoming students with a B.A./B.S. only: 84%   **Master's:** 16%

Approximate percentage of students who are Women: 67%   **Ethnic Minority:** 4%   **International:** 1%

Average years to complete the doctoral program (including internship): 6 years

Personal interview
Interviews are by invitation and are required.

Attrition rate in past 7 years: 8%

Percentage of students applying for internship last year accepted into APPIC or APA internships: 89%

Formal tracks/concentrations: clinical disaster psychology

Research areas	# Faculty	# Grants
child clinical	3	0
cross-cultural	7	2
depression	2	0
disaster mental health	4	1
ethics	1	0
family violence	2	0
health psychology	2	0
psychosis/serious mental illness	2	0
rural community psychology	6	0
substance abuse	2	1

Clinical opportunities
crisis intervention/disaster mental health
minority/cross-cultural (American Indian mental health)
rural/community mental health
substance abuse
severe and persistent mental illness
forensic/sex offenders

University of South Florida (Ph.D.)
Department of Psychology
4202 Fowler Avenue, PCP 4118G
Tampa, FL 33620
phone#: (813) 974-2492

e-mail: phares@cas.usf.edu
Web address:
www.cas.usf.edu/psychology/gra_cli_stud_index.htm

1	2	3	4	5	6	7
Practice oriented		Equal emphasis			Research oriented	

Percentage of faculty subscribing to each of the following orientations:
Psychodynamic/Psychoanalytic — 0%
Applied behavioral analysis/Radical behavioral — 9%
Family systems/Systems — 9%
Existential/Phenomenological/Humanistic — 9%
Cognitive/Cognitive-behavioral — 73%

Courses required for incoming students prior to enrolling: None

Courses recommended but not mandatory:
Research design, statistics, abnormal

GRE mean
Verbal 619   Quantitative 680
Advanced Psychology not reported
Analytical Writing 5.3

GPA mean
Junior/Senior GPA 3.79

Number of applications/admission offers/incoming students in 2007
237 applied/13 admission offers/7 incoming

% of students receiving:
Full tuition waiver only: 0%
Assistantship/fellowship only: 0%
Both full tuition waiver & assistantship/fellowship: 100%

Approximate percentage of incoming students with a B.A./B.S. only: 100%   **Master's:** 0%

Approximate percentage of students who are Women: 81%   **Ethnic Minority:** 17%
International: 6%

Average years to complete the doctoral program (including internship): 6.7 years

Personal interview
Preferred in person but telephone acceptable

Attrition rate in past 7 years: 5%

Percentage of students applying for internship last year accepted into APPIC or APA internships: 78%

Specializations: health psychology, personality/ psychopathology, clinical neuropsychology, addictive behaviors, clinical child psychology

Research areas	# Faculty	# Grants
child/adolescent	4	2
depression	1	0
eating disorders	2	1
emotions	2	0
family dysfunction	1	0
health psychology	5	5
neuropsychology	1	0

personality assessment	1	0
psychosocial oncology	2	5
substance abuse/addictions	2	5
suicidality	1	2

Clinical opportunities

ADHD	intellectual assessment
clinical assessment	learning disorders
adult neuropsychology	oppositional defiant
anxiety—child and adult	disorder
child and adolescent	psychosocial oncology
disorders	selective mutism
depression/anxiety	substance abuse
eating disorders	survivors of torture
family dysfunction	weight management
health psychology	

University of Southern California (Ph.D.)

Doctoral Program in Psychological Clinical Science
Department of Psychology
3620 McClintock, SGM 501
Los Angeles, CA 90089-1061
phone#: (213) 821-2407
e-mail: lgore@usc.edu
Web address: www.usc.edu/schools/college/psyc/
graduate/clinical_program_ove.shtml

1	2	3	4	5	**6**	7
Practice oriented		Equal emphasis			Research oriented	

Percentage of faculty subscribing to each of the following orientations:

Psychodynamic/Psychoanalytic	0%
Applied behavioral analysis/Radical behavioral	10%
Family systems/Systems	50%
Existential/Phenomenological/Humanistic	10%
Cognitive/Cognitive-behavioral	100%

Courses required for incoming students to have completed prior to enrolling:
None

Recommended but not mandatory courses:
Statistics, research methods or experimental psychology, and courses in biology, physical sciences, social sciences, mathematics

GRE mean
Verbal 625   Quantitative 721
Analytical Writing 5.1

GPA mean
Overall GPA 3.56

Number of applications/admission offers/incoming students in 2007
285 applied/14 admission offers/8 incoming

% of students receiving:
Full tuition waiver only: 0%
Assistantship/fellowship only: 0%
Both full tuition waiver & assistantship/fellowship: 100%

Approximate percentage of incoming students with a B.A./B.S. only: 75%   **Master's:** 25%

Approximate percentage of students who are Women: 84%   **Ethnic Minority:** 42%
International: 12%

Average years to complete the doctoral program (including internship): 5.0 years

Personal interview
Strongly preferred

Attrition rate in past 7 years: 9%

Percentage of students applying for internship last year accepted into APPIC or APA internships: 100%

Formal tracks/concentrations: child and family, aging

Research areas	# Faculty	# Grants
adolescent substance abuse	2	0
alcohol use/abuse	2	2
behavioral medicine	3	5
child psychopathology	3	3
childhood victimization	3	2
clinical neuroscience/experimental	1	0
cognitive behavioral therapy	3	1
gerontology	4	13
marital and family research/abuse	4	3

Clinical opportunities

community	marital/family
gerontology	minority mental health
individual adult	

Southern Illinois University (Ph.D.)

Department of Psychology
Life Science Building II, Room 281
Carbondale, IL 62901
phone#: (618) 453-3564 (graduate program secretary)
e-mail: dollngr@siu.edu
Web address: www.psychology.siu.edu/clinical.htm

1	2	3	**4**	5	6	7
Practice oriented		Equal emphasis			Research oriented	

Percentage of faculty subscribing to each of the following orientations:

Psychodynamic/Psychoanalytic	0%
Applied behavioral analysis/Radical behavioral	0%
Family systems	10%
Existential/Phenomenological/Humanistic	0%
Cognitive/Cognitive-behavioral	90%

Courses required for incoming students prior to enrolling: None

Courses recommended but not mandatory:
History and systems, tests and measurements, abnormal, personality, learning, developmental, physiological, statistics, social

GRE mean
Verbal 567   Quantitative 638

GPA mean
3.89

Number of applications/admission offers/incoming students in 2007
123 applied/9 admission offers/6 incoming

% of students receiving:
Full tuition waiver only: 0%
Assistantship/fellowship only: 0%
Both full tuition waiver & assistantship/fellowship: 100%

Approximate percentage of incoming students with a B.A./B.S. only: 85% **Master's:** 15%

Approximate percentage of students who are Women: 70% **Ethnic Minority:** 20% **International:** 15%

Average years to complete the doctoral program (including internship): 7.5 years

Personal interview
Preferred in person but telephone acceptable

Attrition rate in past 7 years: 11%

Percentage of students applying for internship last year accepted into APPIC or APA internships: 90%

Formal tracks/concentrations: child and adult

Research areas	# Faculty	# Grants
abortion	1	0
abuse	1	0
AIDS attitudes	1	0
adolescent issues	2	0
anxiety disorders	3	0
assessment	8	0
behavioral genetics	1	0
behavioral medicine	2	0
child clinical	3	0
child sexual abuse	1	0
clinical judgment	1	0
community psychology	1	0
delinquency	1	1
depression	2	0
family systems	1	0
gender roles	1	0
learning disabilities	2	1
marital	1	0
pediatric psychology	1	0
personality (five-factor model)	3	0
personality assessment	4	0
psychology of religion	1	0
relationships	2	0
sleep (child)	1	0
smoking	1	many
stress, coping, and social support	1	0

Clinical opportunities

family therapy	severe psychopathology
forensic psychology	sexual abuse
juvenile corrections	substance abuse
neuropsychology	

University of Southern Mississippi (Ph.D.)

Department of Psychology
Box 5025 Southern Station
Hattiesburg, MS 39406-5025
phone#: (601) 266-4588
e-mail: mitchell.berman@usm.edu
Web address: www.usm.edu/psy/clinical/home.htm

1	2	3	4	**5**	6	7
Clinically oriented			Equal emphasis			Research oriented

Percentage of faculty subscribing to each of the following orientations:

Psychodynamic/Psychoanalytic	12%
Applied behavioral analysis/Radical behavioral	13%
Family systems/Systems	0%
Existential/Phenomenological/Humanistic	0%
Cognitive/Cognitive-behavioral	75%

Courses required for incoming students to have completed prior to enrolling: None

Recommended but not mandatory courses:
Research methods, statistics, history and systems

GRE mean
Verbal 561 Quantitative 660
Analytical Writing not reported

GPA mean
Overall GPA 3.70

Number of applications/admission offers/incoming students in 2007
87 applied/16 admission offers/8 incoming

% of students receiving:
Full tuition waiver only: 0%
Assistantship/fellowship only: 0%
Both full tuition waiver & assistantship/fellowship: 100%

Approximate percentage of incoming students with a B.A./B.S. only: 80% **Master's:** 20%

Approximate percentage of students who are Women: 70% **Ethnic Minority:** 20%
International: 8%

Average years to complete the doctoral program (including internship): 5 years

Personal interview
Required in person or phone interviews

Attrition rate in past 7 years: 24%

Percentage of students applying for internship last year accepted into APPIC or APA internships: 100%

Formal tracks/concentrations: adult, child

Research areas	# Faculty	# Grants
adult clinical	5	1
child clinical	3	0

Clinical opportunities
adult clinical
child clinical

Spalding University (Psy.D.)

School of Professional Psychology
851 South Fourth Street
Louisville, KY 40203
phone#: (502) 585-7127
e-mail: esimpson@spalding.edu
Web address:
www.spalding.edu/content.aspx?id=1938&cid=1086

1	2	3	4	5	6	7

Practice oriented   Equal emphasis   Research oriented

Percentage of faculty subscribing to each of the following orientations:
Psychodynamic/Psychoanalytic   10%
Applied behavioral analysis/Radical behavioral 10%
Family systems/Systems   10%
Existential/Phenomenological/Humanistic   20%
Cognitive/Cognitive-behavioral   50%

Courses required for incoming students to have completed prior to enrolling:
18 hours of undergraduate work.

Recommended but not mandatory courses:
Undergraduate research, physiological

GRE mean
Verbal 550   Quantitative 590
Advanced Psychology not reported

GPA mean
Overall GPA 3.5

Number of applications/admission offers/incoming students in 2007
Not reported

% of students receiving:
Full tuition waiver only: 0%
Assistantship/fellowship only: 17%
Both full tuition waiver & assistantship/fellowship: 0%

Approximate percentage of incoming students with a B.A./B.S. only: 67%   **Master's:** 33%

Approximate percentage of students who are Women: 74%   **Ethnic Minority:** 12%   **International:** 7%

Average years to complete the doctoral program (including internship): 5.5 years

Personal interview
Preferred in person but telephone acceptable

Attrition rate in past 7 years: 11%

Percentage of students applying for internship last year accepted into APPIC or APA internships: 85%

Formal tracks/concentrations: forensic, health, adult, child, adolescent, and family

Research areas	# Faculty	# Grants
child development	1	0
clinical supervision	1	0
health psychology	2	1
program evaluation	1	0
sports psychology	1	0

Clinical opportunities
family/systems psychology
health psychology

Stony Brook University/State University of New York (Ph.D.)

Department of Psychology
Stony Brook, NY 11794-2500
phone#: (631) 632-7830
e-mail: k.d.oleary@sunysb.edu
Web address: www.psychology.sunysb.edu/
psychology/graduate/areasofstudy/clinical

1	2	3	4	5	6	7

Practice oriented   Equal emphasis   Research oriented

Percentage of faculty subscribing to each of the following orientations:
Psychodynamic/Psychoanalytic   45%
Applied behavioral analysis/Radical behavioral 82%
Family systems/Systems   64%
Existential/Phenomenological/Humanistic   36%
Cognitive/Cognitive-behavioral   91%

Courses required for incoming students to have completed prior to enrolling: None

Recommended but not mandatory courses:
Statistics, experimental with lab, abnormal, research methods

GRE mean Applicants Accepted for Academic Year 2006–2007
Verbal 640   Quantitative 737
Analytical Writing 5.8

GPA mean
Overall GPA 3.68

Number of applications/admission offers/incoming students in 2006–2007
305 applied/13 admission offers/6 incoming

% of students receiving:
Full tuition waiver only: 0%
Assistantship/fellowship only: 0%
Both full tuition waiver & assistantship/fellowship: 100%

Approximate percentage of incoming students with a B.A./B.S. only: 100%   **Master's:** 16.6%

Approximate percentage of students who are Women: 83%   **Ethnic Minority:** 33%
International: not reported

Average years to complete the doctoral program (including internship): 6.8 years

Personal interview
Prefer in person but telephone acceptable

Attrition rate in past 7 years: 17%

Percentage of students applying for internship last year accepted into APPIC or APA internships: 100%

Formal tracks/concentrations: close relationship concentration

Research areas	# Faculty	# Grants
affective disorders	1	4
attachment/close relationships	1	3
psychopathology/self mutilation	1	1
developmental disabilities	1	2
marriage/spousal abuse	3	5
parent–child interactions	1	1
problem solving	1	0
psychotherapy outcome/integration	2	2

Clinical opportunities
psychological center
marital clinic
university hospital
student counseling center
various community agencies

Suffolk University (Ph.D.)
Department of Psychology
41 Temple St., 6th Floor
Boston, MA 02114-4280
phone#: (617) 573-8293
e-mail: phd@suffolk.edu
Web address: www.suffolk.edu/college/7093.html

1	2	3	**4**	5	6	7
Practice oriented		Equal emphasis			Research oriented	

Percentage of faculty subscribing to each of the following orientations:

Psychodynamic/Psychoanalytic	5%
Applied behavioral analysis/Radical behavioral	0%
Family systems/Systems	30%
Existential/Phenomenological/Humanistic	5%
Cognitive/Cognitive-behavioral	60%

Courses required for incoming students to have completed prior to enrolling:
5 courses in psychology, including statistics and research methods

Recommended but not mandatory courses:
Not reported

GRE mean
Verbal 582   Quantitative 665
Analytical Writing 5.1
Advanced Psychology 637

GPA mean
Overall GPA 3.56

Number of applications/admission offers/incoming students in 2007
313 applied/29 admission offers/13 incoming

% of students receiving:
Full tuition waiver only: 15%
Assistantship/fellowship only: 85%
Both full tuition waiver & assistantship/fellowship: 0%

Approximate percentage of incoming students with a B.A./B.S. only: 69%   **Master's:** 31%

Approximate percentage of students who are Women: 80%   **Ethnic Minority:** 15%   **International:** 4%

Average years to complete the doctoral program (including internship): 6.3 years

Personal interview
Required; may occur in person or by telephone

Attrition rate in past 7 years: 2%

Percentage of students applying for internship last year accepted into APPIC or APA internships: 91%

Formal tracks/concentrations: child, neuropsychology, general

Research areas
See web site for specific research areas

Clinical opportunities
adult inpatient and outpatient
child and adolescent inpatient and outpatient
college/university counseling center
forensic
neuropsychological assessment
schools

Syracuse University (Ph.D.)
Department of Psychology
430 Huntington Hall
Syracuse, NY 13244-2340
phone#: (315) 443-2760
e-mail: kemaster@syr.edu
Web address: psychweb.syr.edu/GPClinical.htm

1	2	3	4	**5**	6	7
Practice oriented		Equal emphasis			Research oriented	

Percentage of faculty subscribing to each of the following orientations:

Psychodynamic/Psychoanalytic	0%
Applied behavioral analysis/Radical behavioral	0%
Family systems/Systems	11%
Existential/Phenomenological/Humanistic	0%
Cognitive/Cognitive-behavioral	89%

Courses required for incoming students prior to enrolling:
15 credits of psychology courses, statistics, laboratory course

Courses recommended but not mandatory:
Numerous laboratory, research experience, science courses

GRE mean
Verbal 570   Quantitative 660
Analytical Writing not reported

GPA mean
Overall GPA 3.7 Psychology GPA 3.7

Number of applications/admission offers/incoming students in 2007
105 applied/10 admission offers/6 incoming

% of students receiving:
Full tuition waiver only: 0%
Assistantship/fellowship only: 0%
Both full tuition waiver & assistantship/fellowship: 100%

Approximate percentage of incoming students with a B.A./B.S. only: 80%   Master's: 20%

Approximate percentage of students who are Women: 75%   Ethnic Minority: 10% International: 25%

Average years to complete the doctoral program (including internship): 6 years

Personal interview
Preferred in person but telephone acceptable

Attrition rate in past 7 years: 28%

Percentage of students applying for internship last year accepted into APPIC or APA internships: 100%

Formal tracks/concentrations: health, HIV/AIDS, addictions

Research areas	# Faculty	# Grants
family	1	2
psychophysiology	3	2
sexual health, AIDS prevention	2	4
substance abuse	3	6

Clinical opportunities
addictions	crisis intervention
anxiety disorders	family
behavioral medicine	neuropsychology
community psychology	school/educational
couples	

Teachers College–Columbia University (Ph.D.)
Department of Clinical Psychology
525 West 120th Street
New York, NY 10027
phone#: (212) 678-3267
fax#: (212) 678-4048
e-mail: farber@tc.edu
Web address:
www.tc.columbia.edu/academic/ccp/clinical/

1	2	3	**4**	5	6	7
Practice oriented		Equal emphasis			Research oriented	

Percentage of faculty subscribing to each of the following orientations:
Psychodynamic/Psychoanalytic	60%
Applied behavioral analysis/Radical behavioral	0%
Family systems/Systems	0%
Existential/Phenomenological/Humanistic	0%
Cognitive/Cognitive-behavioral	40%

Courses required for incoming students prior to enrolling:
Statistics and 9 credits from among: experimental, personality, history and systems, developmental, or social

Courses recommended but not mandatory:
Abnormal psychology

GRE mean
Verbal 623   Quantitative 644
Analytical Writing 4.9
Advanced Psychology 680

GPA mean
Overall GPA 3.7

Number of applications/admission offers/incoming students in 2007
310 applied/10 admission offers/10 incoming

% of students receiving:
Full tuition waiver only: 0%
Assistantship/fellowship only: 0%
Both full tuition waiver & assistantship/fellowship: 10%
(87.5% of students receive a partial tuition wavier)

Approximate percentage of incoming students with a B.A./B.S. only: 25%   Master's: 75%

Approximate percentage of students who are Women: 70%   Ethnic Minority: 20% International: 20%

Average years to complete the doctoral program (including internship): 7 years

Personal interview
Required in person

Attrition rate in past 7 years: 1.4%

Percentage of students applying for internship last year accepted into APPIC or APA internships: 90%

Formal tracks/concentrations: child clinical

Research areas	# Faculty	# Grants
altruism	1	0
child abuse	1	1
geriatrics	1	1
psychotherapy research	3	1
risk and resilience	2	2
spirituality	1	1
trauma, stress and coping	2	1

Clinical opportunities
child therapy
psychodynamic therapy

Temple University (Ph.D.)
Department of Psychology
Broad and Montgomery Streets
Philadelphia, PA 19122-6085
phone#: (215) 204-7326
e-mail: lalloy@temple.edu
Web address:
www.temple.edu/psychology/Clinical/index.html

1	2	3	4	5	**6**	7
Practice oriented			Equal emphasis			Research oriented

Percentage of faculty subscribing to each of the following orientations:

Psychodynamic/Psychoanalytic	0%
Applied behavioral analysis/Radical behavioral	29%
Family systems/Systems	42%
Existential/Phenomenological/Humanistic	14%
Cognitive/Cognitive-behavioral	100%

Courses required for incoming students prior to enrolling:
B.A. or B.S. and at least 4 courses in psychology (including 1 laboratory course), a natural sciences lab, statistics

Courses recommended but not mandatory:
None

GRE mean
Verbal + Quantitative 1400
Analytical Writing not reported

GPA mean
GPA 3.73

Number of applications/admission offers/incoming students in 2007
423 applied/15 admission offers/10 incoming

% of students receiving:
Full tuition waiver only: 0%
Assistantship/fellowship only: 0%
Both full tuition waiver & assistantship/fellowship: 100%

Approximate percentage of incoming students with a B.A./B.S. only: 80%   **Master's:** 20%

Approximate percentage of students who are Women: 100%   **Ethnic Minority:** 10%   **International:** 0%

Average years to complete the doctoral program (including internship): 6 years

Personal interview
Required in person

Attrition rate in past 7 years: 7.1%

Percentage of students applying for internship last year accepted into APPIC or APA internships: 89%

Formal tracks/concentrations: none

Research areas	# Faculty	# Grants
adult anxiety disorders/treatment	1	2
child anxiety disorders/treatment	1	3
childhood externalizing problems	1	3
vulnerability to mood disorders	1	1
resilience among minority children	1	1
neuropsychology of	1	2
relationship difficulties/couples therapy	1	0

Clinical opportunities
anxiety disorders in children
adult anxiety disorders
bipolar spectrum disorders
conduct disorder and depression
clinical neuropsychology
specialty clinics in a large urban area

University of Tennessee (Ph.D.)
Department of Psychology
Austin Peay Psychology Building
Knoxville, TN 37996-0900
phone#: (865) 974-3328
e-mail: cjogle@utk.edu
Web address: web.utk.edu/~welsh/clinical/

1	2	3	**4**	5	6	7
Practice oriented			Equal emphasis			Research oriented

Percentage of faculty subscribing to each of the following orientations:

Psychodynamic/Psychoanalytic	25%
Applied behavioral analysis/Radical behavioral	0%
Family systems/Systems	15%
Existential/Phenomenological/Humanistic	0%
Cognitive/Cognitive-behavioral	60%

Courses required for incoming students to have completed prior to enrolling: None

Recommended but not mandatory courses:
None

GRE mean
Verbal 577   Quantitative 678
Analytical Writing not reported
Advanced Psychology 599

GPA mean
Overall GPA 3.76

Number of applications/admission offers/incoming students in 2007
113 applied/14 admission offers/7 incoming

% of students receiving:
Full tuition waiver only: 100%
Assistantship/fellowship only: 0%
Both full tuition waiver & assistantship/fellowship: 0%

Approximate percentage of incoming students with a B.A./B.S. only: 67%   **Master's:** 33%

Approximate percentage of students who are Women: 67%   **Ethnic Minority:** 9%   **International:** 4%

Average years to complete the doctoral program (including internship): 5.5 years

Personal interview
Preferred in person but telephone acceptable

Attrition rate in past 7 years: 5%

Percentage of students applying for internship last year accepted into APPIC or APA internships: 100%

Formal tracks/concentrations: none

Research areas	# Faculty	# Grants
family/relationship	6	2
adult psychopathology	4	1
developmental psychopathology	3	1
psychotherapy	4	1
health	3	1

Clinical opportunities

romantic relationships

hypnosis

borderline personality
    disorder

therapy with cancer patients

substance abuse

conduct disorder

Texas A&M University (Ph.D.)

Department of Psychology
College Station, TX 77843-4235
phone#: (979) 845-2581
e-mail: d-snyder@tamu.edu
Web address: psychology.tamu.edu/AOS.php?ID=1

1	2	3	4	**5**	6	7
Practice oriented		Equal emphasis			Research oriented	

Percentage of faculty subscribing to each of the following orientations:

Psychodynamic/Psychoanalytic	20%
Applied behavioral analysis/Radical behavioral	0%
Family systems/Systems	15%
Existential/Phenomenological/Humanistic	15%
Cognitive/Cognitive-behavioral	50%

Courses required for incoming students prior to enrolling:
Abnormal and at least 3 other psychology courses including experimental

Courses recommended but not mandatory:
Advanced research-based seminars

GRE mean
Verbal 600   Quantitative 650
Analytical Writing not required

GPA mean
Overall GPA 3.5

Number of applications/admission offers/incoming students in 2007
180 applied/10 admission offers/7 incoming

% of students receiving:
Full tuition waiver only: 0%
Assistantship/fellowship only: 0%
Both full tuition waiver & assistantship/fellowship: 100%

Approximate percentage of incoming students with a B.A./B.S. only: 70%   **Master's:** 30%

Approximate percentage of students who are Women: 60%   **Ethnic Minority:** 30%   **International:** 10%

Average years to complete the doctoral program (including internship): 5 years

Personal interview
Preferred in person but telephone acceptable

Attrition rate in past 7 years: 12%

Percentage of students applying for internship last year accepted into APPIC or APA internships: 100%

Formal tracks/concentrations: none

Research areas	# Faculty	# Grants
addictive disorders	1	1
aging	2	1
anxiety disorders	3	1
assessment	3	0
child behavior disorders	4	3
health psychology	2	1
marital/family studies	5	3
psychopathology	2	1
psychotherapy	7	2

Clinical opportunities

community

family

forensic

neuropsychology

rural psychology

substance abuse

University of Texas at Austin (Ph.D.)

Department of Psychology
1 University Station A8000
Austin, TX 78712
phone#: (512) 471-3393
e-mail: gradoffice@psy.utexas.edu
Web address:
www.psy.utexas.edu/psy/clinical/index.html

1	2	3	4	5	**6**	7
Practice oriented		Equal emphasis			Research oriented	

Percentage of faculty subscribing to each of the following orientations:

Psychodynamic/Psychoanalytic	0%
Applied behavioral analysis/Radical behavioral	0%
Family systems/Systems	0%
Existential/Phenomenological/Humanistic	25%
Cognitive/Cognitive-behavioral	75%

Courses required for incoming students to have completed prior to enrolling:
None

Recommended but not mandatory courses:
Abnormal, biopsychology, research methods, statistics

GRE mean
Verbal + Quantitative 1344
Analytical Writing not reported

GPA mean
Psychology GPA 3.75

Number of applications/admission offers/incoming students in 2007
Not reported

% of students receiving:
Full tuition waiver only: 0%
Assistantship/fellowship only: 0%
Both full tuition waiver & assistantship/fellowship: 100%

Approximate percentage of incoming students with a B.A./B.S. only: 80% **Master's:** 20%

Approximate percentage of students who are Women: 60% **Ethnic Minority:** 40% **International:** 9%

Average years to complete the doctoral program (including internship): 6.6 years

Personal interview
Telephone required

Attrition rate in past 7 years: 6%

Percentage of students applying for internship last year accepted into APPIC or APA internships: 100%

Formal tracks/concentrations: none

Research areas	# Faculty	# Grants
addictions	1	1
ADHD	1	1
anxiety	1	0
depression	1	1
developmental disabilities	1	1
epidemiology	1	0
health psychology	1	1
neurological disorders	1	1
neuropsychology	1	0
sexual dysfunction	1	1
stress and coping	1	1

Clinical opportunities

anxiety disorders
behavioral medicine
child/family
child/adolescent severe
   mental illness
community
crisis intervention
depression
student populations

marital
neuropsychology
obsessive–compulsive
   disorder
personality disorders
sleep psychology
student counseling center
survivors of torture

University of Texas Southwestern Medical Center at Dallas (Ph.D.)

Division of Psychology
5323 Harry Hines Boulevard
Dallas, Texas 75390-9044
phone#: (214) 648-5277
e-mail:
ClinicalPsychologyProgram@UTSouthwestern.edu
Web address:
www.utsouthwestern.edu/graduateschool/
clinicalpsychology.html

1	2	3	**4**	5	6	7
Practice oriented		Equal emphasis			Research oriented	

Percentage of faculty subscribing to each of the following orientations:

Psychodynamic/Psychoanalytic	35%
Applied behavioral analysis/Radical behavioral	5%
Family systems/Systems	20%
Existential/Phenomenological/Humanistic	5%
Cognitive/Cognitive-behavioral	35%

Courses required for incoming students to have completed prior to enrolling:
Learning, statistics

Recommended but not mandatory courses:
Developmental, physiological, experimental

GRE mean
Verbal + Quantitative 1250
Analytical Writing not reported
Advanced Psychology not reported

GPA mean
Overall GPA 3.6

Number of applications/admission offers/incoming students in 2007
150 applied/10 admission offers/10 incoming

% of students receiving:
Full tuition waiver only: 0%
Assistantship/fellowship: 100% (in 1st semester of 2nd year through end of 4th year)
Both full tuition waiver & assistantship/fellowship: 0%

Approximate percentage of incoming students with a B.A./B.S. only: 50% **Master's:** 50%

Approximate percentage of students who are Women: 70% **Ethnic Minority:** 20% **International:** 10%

Average years to complete the doctoral program (including internship): 4.5 years

Personal interview
Required in person

Attrition rate in past 7 years: 10%

Percentage of students applying for internship last year accepted into APPIC or APA internships: 100%

Formal tracks/concentrations: health psychology, child, neuropsychology

Research areas	# Faculty	# Grants
Alzheimer's	1	1
child depression	2	1
community mental health	1	0
cultural issues	2	0
depression	3	3
developmental psychology	1	1
health psychology	3	3
health services research	1	1
learning disabilities	1	0
neurobiological aspects of psychological disorders	2	2

neuropsychology	2	2
pain management	1	1
pediatric psychology	1	0
rehabilitation psychology	1	1
sleep disorders	1	1

Clinical opportunities

affective disorders	inpatient psychiatry
behavioral psychology	neuropsychology
clinical child	outpatient psychotherapy
community mental health	personality disorders
deafness	primary care consultation
developmental disabilities	psychiatric emergency care
family therapy	rehabilitation psychology
forensic psychology	sleep disorders
health/medical psychology	vocational assessment

Texas Tech University (Ph.D.)

Department of Psychology
P.O. Box 42501
Lubbock, TX 79409
phone#: (806) 742-3711
fax#: (806) 742-0818
e-mail: kay.hill@ttu.edu or lee.cohen@ttu.edu
Web address: http://www.depts.ttu.edu/psy/
psy.php?page=graduate/clinical/clinical

1	2	3	**4**	5	6	7
Practice oriented		Equal emphasis			Research oriented	

Percentage of faculty subscribing to each of the following orientations:

Behavioral	87.5%
Cognitive-Behavioral	100%
Existential/Humanistic/Phenomenological	25%
Family systems/Systems	37.5%
Interpersonal	25%
Personal Construct/Narrative	12.5%
Psychodynamic/Psychoanalytic	12.5%

Courses required for incoming students prior to enrolling:

18 semester hours of psychology

Courses recommended but not mandatory:

Statistics, abnormal, developmental, physiological, and a research course such as experimental design or independent research

GRE mean

Verbal 535   Quantitative 594   Analytical Writing 4.9

GPA mean

Overall GPA 3.75

Number of applications/admission offers/incoming students in 2007

126 applied/8 admission offers/7 incoming

% of students receiving:

Full tuition waiver only: 0%
Assistantship/fellowship only: 0%
Both full tuition waiver & assistantship/fellowship: 100%

Approximate percentage of incoming students with a B.A./B.S. only: 71%   **Master's:** 29%

Approximate percentage of students who are Women: 71%   **Ethnic Minority:** 9%   **International:** 0%

Average years to complete the doctoral program (including internship): 6 years

Personal interview
In person interviews strongly encouraged but telephone interviews acceptable

Attrition rate in past 7 years: 9%

Percentage of students applying for internship last year accepted into APPIC or APA internships: 88%

Formal tracks/concentrations: none

Research areas	# Faculty	# Grants
addictions	1	1
behavioral assessment	1	0
behavioral medicine	1	1
behavioral parent training	1	0
child depression and anxiety	1	0
child maltreatment and abuse	1	0
cognitive-behavioral therapies	3	0
community interventions	1	0
eating disorders	1	0
ethics/regulatory issues	1	0
ethnic minority/cultural	1	2
health psychology	2	0
high-risk patients/suicide	2	3
high-risk youth	1	0
child assessment	1	0
MMPI/MMPI-2	1	0
neuropsychological assessment	1	0
nicotine dependence/withdrawal	1	1
personal meaning-making	1	0
methodology factor	2	0
Spanish-speaking families	1	1
suicide	2	0
teachers' evaluations of children's problems	2	0
trauma	2	0

Clinical opportunities

Extensive opportunities with diverse populations are available

University of Toledo (Ph.D.)

Department of Psychology
2801 West Bancroft Street
Toledo, OH 43606-3390
phone#: (419) 530-2721
e-mail: jmihura@pop3.utoledo.edu
Web address: www.psychology.utoledo.edu/

1	2	3	**4**	5	6	7
Practice oriented		Equal emphasis			Research oriented	

Percentage of faculty subscribing to each of the following orientations:

Psychodynamic/Psychoanalytic	67%
Applied behavioral analysis/Radical behavioral	0%
Family systems/Systems	17%
Existential/Phenomenological/Humanistic	0%
Cognitive/Cognitive-behavioral	67%

Courses required for incoming students to have completed prior to enrolling:
Psychology major including statistics and research methods

Recommended but not mandatory courses:
None

GRE mean
Verbal 559   Quantitative 645
Analytic Writing 5.1
Advanced Psychology not reported

GPA mean
Psychology GPA 3.7

Number of applications/admission offers/incoming students in 2007
106 applied/10 admission offers/5 incoming

% of students receiving:
Full tuition waiver only: 0%
Assistantship/fellowship only: 0%
Both full tuition waiver & assistantship/fellowship: 100%

Approximate percentage of incoming students with a B.A./B.S. only: 90%   **Master's:** 10%

Approximate percentage of students who are Women: 69%   **Ethnic Minority:** 11%   **International:** 3%

Average years to complete the doctoral program (including internship): 5.3 years

Personal interview
In person (although international students can interview by telephone)

Attrition rate in past 7 years: 19%

Percentage of students applying for internship last year accepted into APPIC or APA internships: 100%

Formal tracks/concentrations: cognitive-behavioral, psychodynamic, family and systems, child and adolescent

Research areas	# Faculty	# Grants
child/adolescent psychopathology	3	0
public mental health	2	1
program evaluation	2	1
psychotherapy research	3	1
anxiety and depression	2	0
cognitive behavioral therapy	2	0
psychological assessment	2	0
media violence	1	0
children and violence	1	0
diversity & Multicultural Issues	2	0

Clinical opportunities

cognitive behavioral therapy	psychological assessment
	chronic mental illness
child & adolescent therapy	anxiety and depression
psychodynamic therapy	in-house clinic
family & couple therapy	

University of Tulsa (Ph.D.)

Department of Psychology
Tulsa, OK 74104
phone#: (918) 631-2248
e-mail: sandra-barney@utulsa.edu
Web address: www.cas.utulsa.edu/psych/

1	2	3	4	5	6	7
Practice oriented		Equal emphasis				Research oriented

Percentage of faculty subscribing to each of the following orientations:

Psychodynamic/Psychoanalytic	10%
Applied behavioral analysis/Radical behavioral	0%
Family systems/Systems	0%
Existential/Phenomenological/Humanistic	0%
Cognitive/Cognitive-behavioral	90%

Courses required for incoming students prior to enrolling:
18 hours of psychology including abnormal, statistics or research methods, and core psychology courses

Courses recommended but not mandatory:
Advanced courses in psychology

GRE mean
Verbal 590   Quantitative 670
Analytical Writing 5.0

GPA mean
GPA 3.81

Number of applications/admission offers/incoming students in 2007
49 applied/10 admission offers/5 incoming

% of students receiving:
Full tuition waiver only: 0%
Assistantship/fellowship only: 0%
Both full tuition waiver & assistantship/fellowship 50%

Approximate percentage of incoming students with a B.A./B.S. only: 83%   **Master's:** 17%

Approximate percentage of students who are Women: 100%   **Ethnic Minority:** 0%   **International:** 0%

Average years to complete the doctoral program (including internship): 5 years

Personal interview
Held on interview day for all candidates

Attrition rate in past 7 years: 17%

Percentage of students applying for internship last year accepted into APPIC or APA internships: 78%

Formal tracks/concentrations: clinical

Research areas	# Faculty	# Grants
clinical gerontology	0	0
life-span development	2	1
neuropsychology	1	1
personality disorders	2	0
posttraumatic stress disorder	2	0
stress	3	0

Clinical opportunities

Practicum program is community-based with access to over 22 general and specialty clinics

Uniformed Services University of Health Sciences (Ph.D.)

4301 Jones Bridge Road
Bethesda, MD 20814-4799
phone#: (301) 295-3270
e-mail: mfeuerstein@usuhs.edu
Web address: www.usuhs.mil/mps/clinindex.html

1	2	3	**4**	5	6	7

Practice oriented   Equal emphasis   Research oriented

Percentage of faculty subscribing to each of the following orientations:

Psychodynamic/Psychoanalytic	10%
Applied behavioral analysis/Radical behavioral	0%
Family systems/Systems	10%
Existential/Phenomenological/Humanistic	20%
Cognitive/Cognitive-behavioral	70%

Courses required for incoming students prior to enrolling:
experimental, abnormal, statistics

Courses recommended but not mandatory:
Biological psychology and care courses in psychology; some course work in the biological sciences and research design

GRE mean
Verbal 600   Quantitative 600
Analytical Writing not reported

GPA mean
GPA 3.5

Number of applications/admission offers/incoming students in 2007
50 applied/5 admission offers/5 incoming

% of students receiving:
Full tuition waiver only: 0%
Assistantship/fellowship only: 0%
Both full tuition waiver & assistantship/fellowship: 100%

Approximate percentage of incoming students with a B.A./B.S. only: 50%   **Master's:** 50%

Approximate percentage of students who are Women: 54%   **Ethnic Minority:** 27%
International: none—must be a United States citizen

Average years to complete the doctoral program (including internship): 5 years

Personal interview
Preferred in person but telephone acceptable

Attrition rate in past 7 years: 5%

Percentage of students applying for internship last year accepted into APPIC or APA internships: 100%

Formal tracks/concentrations: military clinical psychology, medical clinical psychology

Research areas	# Faculty	# Grants
cancer survivorship	1	0
drug abuse and behavioral toxicology	1	3
mood disorders	1	2
neuropsychology	1	1
obesity and eating disorders	1	1
occupational health psychology	1	3
stress and pain in the workplace	–	–
sexual dysfunction	1	0
stress and animal models	1	3
stress and cardiovascular disease	2	4

Clinical opportunities

children and adolescent medical centers
military teaching hospitals
substance abuse
VA hospitals
unique military settings

University of Utah (Ph.D.)

Department of Psychology
380 S 1530 E, Room 502
Salt Lake City, UT 84112
phone#: (801) 581-6126
e-mail: mary.looser@psych.utah.edu
Web address:
www.psych.utah.edu/researchareas/clinical/

1	2	3	**4**	5	6	7

Practice oriented   Equal emphasis   Research oriented

Percentage of faculty subscribing to each of the following orientations:

Psychodynamic/Psychoanalytic	30%
Applied behavioral analysis/Radical behavioral	0%
Family systems/Systems	50%
Existential/Phenomenological/Humanistic	0%
Cognitive/Cognitive-behavioral	50%

Courses required for incoming students to have completed prior to enrolling:
Undergraduate degree in psychology or its equivalent, including statistics, research design and abnormal

Recommended but not mandatory courses:
Advanced statistics and research design

GRE mean
Verbal 592   Quantitative 652
Analytical Writing 5.25
Advanced Psychology 663

GPA mean
Junior/Senior GPA 3.57

Number of applications/admission offers/incoming students in 2007
141 applied/10 admission offers/5 incoming

% of students receiving:
Full tuition waiver only: 0%
Assistantship/fellowship only: 0%
Both full tuition waiver & assistantship/fellowship: 100%

Approximate percentage of incoming students with a B.A./B.S. only: 80% **Master's:** 20%

Approximate percentage of students who are Women: 75% **Ethnic Minority:** 12%
International: not reported

Average years to complete the doctoral program (including internship): 7 years

Personal interview
Required in person

Attrition rate in past 7 years: 21%

Percentage of students applying for internship last year accepted into APPIC or APA internships: 95%

Formal tracks/concentrations: adult, child/adolescent/family, health, clinical neuropsychology

Research areas	# Faculty	# Grants
adolescent/child psychology	1	0
adult psychopathology	4	0
health psychology	2	1
developmental	1	0
family/couple research	4	1
forensic	1	1
minority mental health	1	1
neuropsychology	1	2
personality assessment	3	0
personality disorders	1	0
sexuality	1	0
stress and coping	2	0

Clinical opportunities

adolescent/child	inpatient psychiatry
health psychology	interpersonal psychotherapy
anxiety disorders	minority mental health
CBT	pediatric psychology
clinical neuropsychology	personality disorders
depression	rational-emotive therapy
family therapy	sex therapy/sexuality
forensic psychology	substance abuse treatment
homeless/disadvantaged population	

Vanderbilt University—Departments of Psychology and Psychology and Human Development (Ph.D.)

111 21st Avenue South
Nashville, TN 37203
phone#: (615) 322-0080
e-mail: vay.welch@vanderbilt.edu or
sharone.hall@vanderbilt.edu

Web address: www.vanderbilt.edu/psychological
_sciences/doctoral/clinical

1	2	3	4	5	6	7

Practice oriented   Equal emphasis   Research oriented

Percentage of faculty subscribing to each of the following orientations:

Psychodynamic/Psychoanalytic	0%
Applied behavioral analysis/Radical behavioral	5%
Family systems/Systems	5%
Existential/Phenomenological/Humanistic	0%
Cognitive/Cognitive-behavioral	90%

Courses required for incoming students to have completed prior to enrolling: None

Recommended but not mandatory courses:
Abnormal; biological bases of behavior; research methods; statistics

GRE mean
Verbal 630   Quantitative 720
Analytical Writing not reported

GPA mean
Overall GPA 3.5   Psychology GPA 3.8

Number of applications/admission offers/incoming students in 2007
321 applied/9 admission offers/6 incoming

% of students receiving:
Full tuition waiver only: 0%
Assistantship/fellowship only: 0%
Both full tuition waiver & assistantship/fellowship: 100%

Approximate percentage of incoming students with a B.A./B.S. only: 95% **Master's:** 5%

Approximate percentage of students who are Women: 75% **Ethnic Minority:** 19%
International: 3%

Average years to complete the doctoral program (including internship): 6 years

Personal interview
On invitation only

Attrition rate in past 7 years: 10%

Percentage of students applying for internship last year accepted into APPIC or APA internships: 100%

Formal tracks/concentrations: child, adolescent, and family, adult psychopathology

Research areas	# Faculty	# Grants
anxiety	7	2
autism	2	1
depression	8	5
eating	3	2
emotion	9	2
ethics and professional practice	1	0
gender issues	2	0

health disparities	2	2
health psychology	5	3
imaging	5	5
intervention	4	3
neuropsychology	3	3
personality	1	1
prevention	3	2
psychopathology	12	5
psychopathy	1	0
psychopharmacology	2	2
psychophysiology	6	2
schizophrenia	2	2
statistics	2	1
substance abuse	3	0
vocal communication	1	0

Clinical opportunities

affective disorders
aggression/conduct
anxiety disorders
behavioral medicine
child and family
developmental disabilities
neuropsychology
pediatric psychology
personality disorders
schizophrenia
substance abuse

University of Vermont (Ph.D.)

Department of Psychology
John Dewey Hall
Burlington, VT 05405
phone#: (802) 656-2670
e-mail: rex.forehand@uvm.edu
Web address: www.uvm.edu/~psych/?Page=programs/
graduate/clinical/clinical_overview.html&SM
=gradmenu.html

1	2	3	**4**	5	6	7

Practice oriented   Equal emphasis   Research oriented

Percentage of faculty subscribing to each of the following orientations:

Psychodynamic/Psychoanalytic	0%
Applied behavioral analysis/Radical behavioral	0%
Family systems/Systems	10%
Existential/Phenomenological/Humanistic	0%
Cognitive/Cognitive-behavioral	90%

Courses required for incoming students to have completed prior to enrolling:

Psychology major or equivalent including statistics, research design, and at least 3 other psychology courses

Recommended but not mandatory courses:

None

GRE mean

Verbal 600   Quantitative 650
Analytical Writing not reported
Advanced Psychology 635

GPA mean

Overall GPA 3.53

Number of applications/admission offers/incoming students in 2007

190 applied/6 admission offers/6 incoming

% of students receiving:

Full tuition waiver only: 0%
Assistantship/fellowship only: 80%
Both full tuition waiver & assistantship/fellowship: 20%

Approximate percentage of incoming students with a B.A./B.S. only: 100%   Master's: 0%

Approximate percentage of students who are Women: 85%   Ethnic Minority: 10%   International: 8%

Average years to complete the doctoral program (including internship): 5 years

Personal interview

In person interview required

Attrition rate in past 7 years: 5%

Percentage of students applying for internship last year accepted into APPIC or APA internships: 100%

Formal tracks/concentrations: none

Research areas	# Faculty	# Grants
adolescent treatment	2	1
anxiety disorders	1	3
child psychopathology	4	2
health psychology	3	2
lesbian/gay issues	1	1
prevention	2	1
sex offenders/abuse	2	0

Clinical opportunities

adolescent psychotherapy
anxiety disorders
behavioral medicine
childhood disorders
chronically mentally ill
depression
eating disorders
family therapy
HIV/AIDS
mental retardation
neuropsychology
prevention
substance abuse

University of Victoria (Ph.D.)

Department of Psychology
Victoria, British Columbia V8W 3P5, Canada
phone#: (250) 721-7525
e-mail: ptaylor@uvic.ca
Web address: www.uvic.ca/psyc/clinical/

1	2	3	**4**	5	6	7

Practice oriented   Equal emphasis   Research oriented

Percentage of faculty subscribing to each of the following orientations:

Psychodynamic/Psychoanalytic	12%
Applied behavioral analysis/Radical behavioral	0%
Family systems/Systems	25%
Existential/Phenomenological/Humanistic	12%
Cognitive/Cognitive-behavioral	100%
Interpersonal	25%

Courses required for incoming students to have completed prior to enrolling:

"A"-level grades for 1 full year of course work in at least 4 areas: social, biological, cognitive, developmental, cultural, abnormal

Recommended but not mandatory courses:

Additional clinical psychology selections

GRE mean

Verbal 630   Quantitative 630
Analytical Writing 4.8

GPA mean

Overall GPA 8.0   Psychology GPA 8.3

Number of applications/admission offers/incoming students in 2007

101 applied/8 admission offers/4 incoming

% of students receiving:

Full tuition waiver only: 0%
Assistantship/fellowship only: 100%
Both full tuition waiver & assistantship/fellowship: 0%

Approximate percentage of incoming students with a B.A./B.S. only: 100%   Master's: 0

Approximate percentage of students who are Women: 75%   Ethnic Minority: 25%   International: 15%

Average years to complete the doctoral program (including internship): 7 years

Personal interview

Preferred in person but telephone acceptable

Attrition rate in past 7 years: 8%

Percentage of students applying for internship last year accepted into APPIC or APA internships: 90%

Formal tracks/concentrations: clinical life span emphasis, clinical neuropsychology emphasis

Research areas	# Faculty	# Grants
addictions	1	1
attention-deficit disorder	1	1
couples treatment	1	1
childhood sexual abuse	1	1
cognitive disorders in the elderly	1	1
cross-cultural psych	1	1
epilepsy	1	1
families and disabilities	1	1
families and divorce	1	1
fetal alcohol syndrome	1	1
traumatic brain injury	2	2

Clinical opportunities

forensic
adult psychiatric
adult rehabilitation
mental health

child and adult inpatient
neuropsychology
young adult counselling
couples, family and group

University of Virginia–Department of Human Services (Ph.D.)

Curry School of Education
P.O. Box 400270
Charlottesville, VA 22904-4270
phone#: (434) 924-7472
e-mail: clin-psych@virginia.edu
Web address: curry.edschool.virginia.edu/clinpsych/

1	2	3	**4**	5	6	7

Practice oriented   Equal emphasis   Research oriented

Percentage of faculty subscribing to each of the following orientations:

Psychodynamic/Psychoanalytic	0%
Applied behavioral analysis/Radical behavioral	0%
Family systems/Systems	63%
Existential/Phenomenological/Humanistic	0%
Cognitive/Cognitive-behavioral	63%

Courses required for incoming students to have completed prior to enrolling:

None

Recommended but not mandatory courses:

Undergraduate statistics, child development, learning, abnormal, physiological/biopsychology, social

GRE mean

Verbal 613   Quantitative 659
Analytical Writing 5.3
Advanced Psychology 687

GPA mean

Overall GPA 3.5   Psychology GPA 3.6
Junior/Senior GPA 3.6

Number of applications/admission offers/incoming students in 2007

145 applied/10 admission offers/7 incoming

% of students receiving:

Full tuition waiver only: 0%
Assistantship/fellowship only: 0%
Both full tuition waiver & assistantship/fellowship: 100%

Approximate percentage of incoming student with a B.A./B.S. only: 88%   Master's: 12%

Approximate percentage of students who are Women: 83%   Ethnic Minority: 17%   International: 5%

Average years to complete the doctoral program (including internship): 5.3 years

Personal interview

Preferred in person but telephone acceptable

Attrition rate in past 7 years: 3%

Percentage of students applying for internship last year accepted into APPIC or APA internships: 93%

Formal tracks/concentrations: forensic, family therapy, child clinical

Research areas

Research areas	# Faculty	# Grants
adolescent suicide	2	0
child clinical	1	0
cognitive/learning disorders	1	0
forensic psychology	2	2
incarcerated populations	2	1
multicultural	3	1
multiproblem families	1	0
parenting behavior	3	1
school interventions	4	1
test development	3	0
youth mentoring	4	6
youth violence	2	1

Clinical opportunities

adult psychotherapy
child and family
couples therapy
crisis intervention
developmental
  psychopathology
family therapy
forensic psychology
medical consultation

neuropsychology
parenting/parent–child
  interaction
school interventions
school psychology
systems consultation
correctional facilities
inpatient facilities

University of Virginia–Department of Psychology

College of Arts and Sciences
P.O. Box 400400
Charlottesville, VA 22904-4477
phone#: (434) 982-4750
e-mail: psy-dept@virginia.edu
Web address: www.virginia.edu/psychology/research/
areas.php#clinical

1	2	3	4	5	**6**	7

Practice oriented   Equal emphasis   Research oriented

Percentage of faculty subscribing to each of the following orientations:

Psychodynamic/Psychoanalytic	25%
Applied behavioral analysis/Radical behavioral	0%
Family systems/Systems	25%
Existential/Phenomenological/Humanistic	0%
Cognitive/Cognitive-behavioral	50%

Courses required for incoming students prior to enrolling: B.A. in psychology or equivalent

Courses recommended but not mandatory:
Abnormal, statistics

GRE mean
Verbal 620   Quantitative 620   Analytical 620
Advanced Psychology 620
Analytical Writing not reported

GPA mean
Overall GPA 3.5

Number of applications/admission offers/incoming students in 2007
493 applied/26 admission offers/13 incoming

% of students receiving:
Full tuition waiver only: 0%
Assistantship/fellowship only: 0%
Both full tuition waiver & assistantship/fellowship: 100%

Approximate percentage of incoming students with a B.A./B.S. only: 62%   **Master's:** 38%

Approximate percentage of students who are Women: 60%   **Ethnic Minority:** 8%
International: 9%

Average years to complete the doctoral program (including internship): 6 years

Personal interview
Preferred in person but telephone acceptable

Attrition rate in past 7 years: 17%

Percentage of students applying for internship last year accepted into APPIC or APA internships: 100%

Formal tracks/concentrations: none

Research areas	# Faculty	# Grants
adult psychopathology	3	3
anxiety disorders	1	0
behavioral genetics	2	1
child clinical/psychopathology	5	5
community psychology	3	3
developmental adolescence	3	3
epidemiology	2	1
family research/systems	2	2
minority mental health	2	2
neuropsychology	1	0
personality disorders	2	1
prevention	3	2
schizophrenia/psychosis	2	0
violence/abuse/victim–offender	4	2

Clinical opportunities

anxiety disorders
behavioral medicine
community psychology
depression
family therapy
forensic psychology
marital/couples therapy

neuropsychology
obsessive–compulsive
  disorder
pediatric psychology
psychology & law
schizophrenia/psychosis
victim/battering/abuse

Virginia Commonwealth University (Ph.D.)

Department of Psychology
806 West Franklin Street
Richmond, VA 23284-2018
phone#: (804) 828-1158 (admissions)
e-mail: clin-psy@vcu.edu
Web address:
http://www.has.vcu.edu/psy/clinical/index.html

1	2	3	4	**5**	6	7

Practice oriented   Equal emphasis   Research oriented

Percentage of faculty subscribing to each of the following orientations:

Psychodynamic/Psychoanalytic	15%
Applied behavioral analysis/Radical behavioral	0%
Family systems/Systems	30%
Existential/Phenomenological/Humanistic	0%
Cognitive/Cognitive-behavioral	100%
Interpersonal	20%

Courses required for incoming students to have completed prior to enrolling:
18 hours of psychology including experimental and statistics

Recommended but not mandatory courses:
Additional courses in psychology, statistics, and science, as well as substantial research experience

GRE mean
Verbal 615   Quantitative 672
Analytical Writing not reported
Advanced Psychology not required

GPA mean
Overall GPA 3.5

Number of applications/admission offers/incoming students in 2007
200 applied/15 admission offers/13 incoming

% of students receiving:
Full tuition waiver only: 0%
Assistantship/fellowship only: 0%
Both full tuition waiver & assistantship/fellowship: 100%

Approximate percentage of incoming students with a B.A./B.S. only: 65%   **Master's:** 35%

Approximate percentage of students who are Women: 70%   **Ethnic Minority:** 25%   **International:** 8%

Average years to complete the doctoral program (including internship): 6 years

Personal interview
In person interview strongly recommended, telephone interview may be acceptable in extenuating circumstances

Attrition rate in past 7 years: 6%

Percentage of students applying for internship last year accepted into APPIC or APA internships: 100%

Formal tracks/concentrations: child/adolescent, behavioral medicine

Research areas	# Faculty	# Grants
adolescent	5	4
anxiety	2	1
behavioral medicine	5	3
child clinical/pediatric	5	4
community	5	3
divorce	1	0
forensic psychology	1	1
minority/cross-cultural	2	1
pregnancy issues	1	1
psychopathology	1	1
psychophysiology	2	0

psychotherapy	3	3
stress and coping	2	0
substance abuse	1	1

Clinical opportunities

assessment and testing	inpatient
behavioral medicine	neuropsychological
child and adult anxiety	assessments
child pediatric	poly-trauma treatment
children of divorce	pain management
child custody evaluations	school
chronic mental illness	substance abuse
community psychology	mood disorder
correctional psychology	

Virginia Consortium Program in Clinical Psychology (Psy.D.)

(College of William & Mary, Eastern Virginia Medical School, Norfolk State University, & Old Dominion University)
Higher Education Center
1881 University Drive, Suite 239
Virginia Beach, VA 23453
phone#: (757) 368-1820
e-mail: rlewis@odu.edu
Web address: www.sci.odu.edu/vcpcp

1	2	**3**	4	5	6	7
Practice oriented		Equal emphasis			Research oriented	

Percentage of faculty subscribing to each of the following orientations:

Psychodynamic/Psychoanalytic	31%
Applied behavioral analysis/Radical behavioral	13%
Family systems/Systems	28%
Existential/Phenomenological/Humanistic	7%
Cognitive/Cognitive-behavioral	31%

Courses required for incoming students prior to enrolling:
B.A. in psychology or equivalent

Courses recommended but not mandatory:
Strong background in psychology

GRE mean
Verbal 603   Quantitative 639
Advanced Psychology not required
Analytical Writing 5.0

GPA mean
Undergraduate GPA 3.93

Number of applications/admission offers/incoming students in 2007
207 applied/17 admission offers/10 incoming

% of students receiving:
Full tuition waiver only: 0%
Assistantship/fellowship only: 0%
Both tuition waiver & assistantship/fellowship: 100%
(significant tuition reduction but not a complete waiver)

Approximate percentage of incoming students with a B.A./B.S. only: 71% **Master's:** 19%

Approximate percentage of students who are:
Women: 79% **Ethnic Minority:** 29% **International:** 2%

Average years to complete the doctoral program (including internship): 5 years

Personal interview:
Required in person

Attrition rate in past 7 years: 6%

Percentage of students applying for internship last year accepted into APPIC or APA internships: 78%

Formal tracks/concentrations: neuropsychology

Research areas	# Faculty	# Grants
ADHD	1	0
attribution	1	0
behavioral pharmacology	1	0
biofeedback	1	0
body image	2	0
cardiovascular behavioral medicine	1	1
child/adolescent psychotherapy	2	0
chronic illness	1	0
clinical neuropsychology	2	0
cognitive-behavioral therapy	4	0
community psychology	1	0
depression	4	0
developmental psychopathology	1	0
drug abuse and prevention	1	1
eating disorders	3	1
emotional regulation in children	1	0
family systems and therapy	4	0
feminism	1	0
gender issues	4	0
GL issues	1	0
health-risk behaviors	1	0
high risk infants	1	0
HIV	1	0
humor in therapy	1	0
interpersonal therapy	2	0
judgment and decision-making	1	0
learning disabilities	1	0
MMPI-2	2	2
moral development	2	0
multicultural	6	0
multimodal behavior therapy	1	0
parent-child interactions	3	1
pediatric psychology	3	0
personal relationships	5	0
personality constructs	1	0
professional issues	1	0
rehabilitation	1	0
schizophrenia	1	0
sleep disorders	1	1
special education	1	0
trauma	2	0
women's issues	4	0

Clinical opportunities
Over 30 public and private agencies that serve adults, adolescents, and children

Virginia Polytechnic Institute and State University (Ph.D.)

Department of Psychology
5088 Derring Hall
Blacksburg, VA 24061-0436
phone#: (540) 231-6275
e-mail: rswinett@vt.edu
Web address: www.psyc.vt.edu/graduate/clinical

1	2	3	4	5	6	7
Practice oriented		Equal emphasis			Research oriented	

Percentage of faculty subscribing to each of the following orientations:

Psychodynamic/Psychoanalytic	0%
Applied behavioral analysis/Radical behavioral	5%
Family systems/Systems	20%
Existential/Phenomenological/Humanistic	0%
Cognitive/Cognitive-behavioral	100%

Courses required for incoming students to have completed prior to enrolling:
Research methods, statistics, learning, electives

Recommended but not mandatory courses:
Abnormal, social, developmental, personality

GRE mean
Verbal 600   Quantitative 650
Analytical Writing not reported
Advanced Psychology not reported

GPA mean
Overall GPA 3.6

Number of applications/admission offers/incoming students in 2007
157 applied/9 admission offers/9 incoming

% of students receiving:
Full tuition waiver only: 0%
Assistantship/fellowship only: 0%
Both full tuition waiver & assistantship/fellowship: 100%

Approximate percentage of incoming students with a B.A./B.S. only: 80% **Master's:** 20%

Approximate percentage of students who are Women: 75% **Ethnic Minority:** 15%
International: not reported

Average years to complete the doctoral program (including internship): 6 years

Personal interview
Preferred in person but telephone acceptable

Attrition rate in past 7 years: 15%

Percentage of students applying for internship last year accepted into APPIC or APA internships: 100%

Formal tracks/concentrations: none

Research areas	# Faculty	# Grants
AIDS	2	0
affective disorders/depression	2	0
anxiety disorders	3	1
attention-deficit disorder	1	0
autism	1	0
behavioral medicine	3	2
child clinical	3	2
eating disorders	1	0
gender roles	1	0
hypnosis	1	1
marriage/couples	1	0
minority mental health	2	1
neuropsychology	2	0
pain management	2	0
parent–child interaction	2	1
pediatric psychology	1	1
prevention	4	3
psychotherapy outcome	2	1
shyness	1	0
social skills	3	0
stress and coping	1	0
substance abuse	2	3

Clinical opportunities

ADHD	data management systems
AIDS	gerontology
affective disorders	marital/couples therapy
anxiety disorders	neuropsychology
behavioral medicine	prevention
child clinical	substance abuse
conduct disorder	systems management
consultation	

University of Washington (Ph.D.)

Department of Psychology
Seattle, WA 98195
e-mail: resmith@u.washington.edu
Web address:
web.psych.washington.edu/graduate/apply.html

1	2	3	4	5	**6**	7
Practice oriented		Equal emphasis			Research oriented	

Percentage of faculty subscribing to each of the following orientations:

Psychodynamic/Psychoanalytic	0%
Applied behavioral analysis/Radical behavioral	10%
Family systems/Systems	20%
Existential/Phenomenological/Humanistic	0%
Cognitive/Cognitive-behavioral	70%

Courses required for incoming students to have completed prior to enrolling: None

Recommended but not mandatory courses:
Abnormal, biological, developmental, statistics, learning & motivation, social

GRE median
Verbal 645   Quantitative 620
Analytical Writing not reported
Advanced Psychology not reported

GPA mean
Overall GPA 3.68

Number of applications/admission offers/incoming students in 2007
312 applied/10 admission offers/9 incoming

% of students receiving:
Full tuition waiver only: 0%
Assistantship/fellowship only: 0%
Both full tuition waiver & assistantship/fellowship: 100%

Approximate percentage of incoming students with a B.A./B.S. only: 100%   **Master's:** 0%

Approximate percentage of students who are Women: 82%   **Ethnic Minority:** 21%
International: 0.1%

Average years to complete the doctoral program (including internship): 6 years

Personal interview
Interview not required

Attrition rate in past 7 years: 3%

Percentage of students applying for internship last year accepted into APPIC or APA internships: 90%

Formal tracks/concentrations: adult clinical, child clinical

Research areas	# Faculty	# Grants
anxiety disorders	3	1
autism	1	1
child emotional development	3	3
cognitive therapy	4	2
depression	3	1
minority	5	4
psychology process	1	1
spouse abuse	2	1
substance abuse	3	3
suicide	1	1

Clinical opportunities

anxiety disorders	neuropsychology
autism	pediatric psychology
community psychology	personality disorders
couples	psychoeducational
family	rehabilitation medicine
minority	substance abuse

Washington State University (Ph.D.)

Department of Psychology
P.O. Box 644820
Pullman, WA 99164-4820
phone#: (509) 335-2631
e-mail: psychhelpdesk@wsu.edu
Web address:
www.wsu.edu/psychology/graduateprograms/clinical

1	2	3	**4**	5	6	7
Practice oriented		Equal emphasis			Research oriented	

Percentage of faculty subscribing to each of the following orientations:

Psychodynamic/Psychoanalytic	23%
Applied behavioral analysis/Radical behavioral	0%
Family systems/Systems	23%
Existential/Phenomenological/Humanistic	8%
Cognitive/Cognitive-behavioral	100%

Courses required for incoming students to have completed prior to enrolling: None

Recommended but not mandatory courses:
Abnormal, social, developmental, personality, statistics, research methods

GRE mean
Verbal + Quantitative 1159
Analytical Writing not required

GPA mean
Overall GPA 3.66

Number of applications/admission offers/incoming students in 2007
181 applied/8 admission offers/6 incoming

% of students receiving:
Full tuition waiver only: 0%
Assistantship/fellowship only: 0%
Both full tuition waiver & assistantship/fellowship: 100%

Approximate percentage of incoming students with a B.A./B.S. only: 67% **Master's:** 33%

Approximate percentage of students who are Women: 80% **Ethnic Minority:** 25% **International:** 10%

Average years to complete the doctoral program (including internship): 6 years

Personal interview
Preferred in person but telephone acceptable

Attrition rate in past 7 years: 12%

Percentage of students applying for internship last year accepted into APPIC or APA internships: 80%

Formal tracks/concentrations: none

Research areas	# Faculty	# Grants
adult psychopathology	5	6
health psychology	5	8
child clinical	4	4
neuropsychology	1	1

Clinical opportunities

adult and child inpatient	psychotherapy
neuropsychological assessment	health psychology

Washington University in St. Louis (Ph.D.)

Department of Psychology
Campus Box 1125
One Brookings Drive
St. Louis, MO 63130-4899
phone#: (314) 935-6520
e-mail: toltmann@artsci.wustl.edu
Web address: www.psych.wustl.edu/clinical/

1	2	3	4	5	**6**	7
Practice oriented		Equal emphasis			Research oriented	

Percentage of faculty subscribing to each of the following orientations:

Psychodynamic/Psychoanalytic	0%
Applied behavioral analysis/Radical behavioral	0%
Family systems/Systems	10%
Existential/Phenomenological/Humanistic	10%
Cognitive/Cognitive-behavioral	80%

Courses required for incoming students to have completed prior to enrolling:
24 credits of psychology and 30 credits in the physical, biological, and social sciences; experimental (with laboratory); quantitative methods

Recommended but not mandatory courses:
History and systems

GRE mean
Verbal 650   Quantitative 680
Advanced Psychology 700
Analytical Writing 5.0

GPA mean
Overall GPA 3.77   Psychology GPA 3.8
Junior/Senior GPA 3.8

Number of applications/admission offers/incoming students in 2007
131 applied/10 admission offers/2 incoming

% of students receiving:
Full tuition waiver only: 0%
Assistantship/fellowship only: 0%
Both full tuition waiver & assistantship/fellowship: 100%

Approximate percentage of incoming students with a B.A./B.S. only: 80% **Master's:** 20%

Approximate percentage of students who are Women: 70% **Ethnic Minority:** 33% **International:** 17%

Average years to complete the doctoral program (including internship): 6 years

Personal interview
Required in person

Attrition rate in past 7 years: 15%

Percentage of students applying for internship last year accepted into APPIC or APA internships: 100%

Formal tracks/concentrations: none

Research areas	# Faculty	# Grants
aging/gerontology	3	3
neuropsychology	4	5
psychopathology	4	3
psychological treatment	4	2

Clinical opportunities
psychological services center
practicum agencies in St. Louis area

University of Waterloo (Ph.D.)

Department of Psychology
Waterloo, Ontario N2L 3G1 Canada
phone#: (519) 888-4567, ext. #33659
e-mail: jmoakman@uwaterloo.ca
Web address: www.psychology.uwaterloo.ca/
gradprog/programs/phd/clinical/index.html

1	2	3	4	**5**	6	7
Practice oriented		Equal emphasis			Research oriented	

Percentage of faculty subscribing to each of the following orientations:
Psychodynamic/Psychoanalytic 33%
Applied behavioral analysis/Radical behavioral 22%
Family systems/Systems 33%
Existential/Phenomenological/Humanistic 44%
Cognitive/Cognitive-behavioral 100%

Courses required for incoming students prior to enrolling:
Statistics, research design, research courses, undergraduate thesis or equivalent

Courses recommended but not mandatory:
History of psychology

GRE mean
Verbal 655   Quantitative 679
Advanced Psychology 704
Analytical Writing not reported

GPA mean
3.51

Number of applications/admission offers/incoming students in 2007
137 applied/9 admission offers/6 incoming

% of students receiving:
Full tuition waiver only: 0%
Assistantship/fellowship only: 100%
Both full tuition waiver & assistantship/fellowship: 0%

Approximate percentage of incoming students with a B.A./B.S. only: 66%   **Master's:** 33%

Approximate percentage of students who are Women: 76%   **Ethnic Minority:** 28%   **International:** 4%

Average years to complete the doctoral program (including internship): 6.5 years

Personal interview
Preferred in person, but telephone acceptable

Attrition rate in past 7 years: 18.5%

Percentage of students applying for internship last year accepted into APPIC or APA internships: 50%

Formal tracks/concentrations: none

Research areas	# Faculty	# Grants
social anxiety	2	2
human sexuality	1	1
obsessive–compulsive disorder	3	2
self-determination theory	1	1
depression	1	1
interpersonal circumplex	2	1
anxiety disorders	3	1
reading	3	1
cognitive development	1	1
culture	1	1

Clinical opportunities
child/adolescent/adult   neuropsychology
hypnosis   school/educational

Wayne State University (Ph.D.)

Department of Psychology
5057 Woodward Avenue, 7th Floor
Detroit, MI 48202
phone#: (313) 577-2800
e-mail: aallen@wayne.edu
Web address: www.psych.wayne.edu

1	2	3	4	**5**	6	7
Practice oriented		Equal emphasis			Research oriented	

Percentage of faculty subscribing to each of the following orientations:
Psychodynamic/Psychoanalytic 10%
Applied behavioral analysis/Radical behavioral 0%
Family systems/Systems 20%
Existential/Phenomenological/Humanistic 0%
Cognitive/Cognitive-behavioral 60%

Courses required for incoming students to have completed prior to enrolling:
12 semester hours in psychology, including experimental (with laboratory) and statistics

Recommended but not mandatory courses:
Undergraduate courses in mathematics and life sciences

GRE mean
Verbal 620   Quantitative 680
Analytical Writing 5.0

GPA mean
Overall GPA 3.8

Number of applications/admission offers/incoming students in 2007
150 applied/15 admission offers/9 incoming

% of students receiving:
Full tuition waiver only: 10%
Assistantship/fellowship only: 30%
Both full tuition waiver & assistantship/fellowship: 50%

Approximate percentage of incoming students with a B.A./B.S. only: 90%   **Master's:** 10%

Approximate percentage of students who are Women: 70%   **Ethnic Minority:** 10%   **International:** 10%

Average years to complete the doctoral program (including internship): 6.5 years

Personal interview
Required in person

Attrition rate in past 7 years: 0%

Percentage of students applying for internship last year accepted into APPIC or APA internships: 90%

Formal tracks/concentrations: health, child clinical, clinical neuropsychology, community

Research areas	# Faculty	# Grants
	not reported	not reported

Clinical opportunities

behavioral medicine	early intervention
community psychology	gerontology
neuropsychology	substance abuse
cross-cultural mental health	rehabilitation

West Virginia University (Ph.D.)

Department of Psychology
1124 Life Sciences Building
Morgantown, WV 26506-6040
phone#: (304) 293-2001, ext. # 31628
e-mail: debra.swinney@mail.wvu.edu
Web address: www.wvu.edu/~psychology/
graduateprogram/index.htm

1	2	3	4	**5**	6	7
Practice oriented		Equal emphasis			Research oriented	

Percentage of faculty subscribing to each of the following orientations:

Psychodynamic/Psychoanalytic	0%
Applied behavioral analysis/Radical behavioral	50%
Family systems/Systems	0%
Existential/Phenomenological/Humanistic	0%
Cognitive/Cognitive-behavioral	50%

Courses required for incoming students to have completed prior to enrolling: None

Recommended but not mandatory courses:
Psychology major or related field, research

GRE mean
Verbal + Quantitative 1169
Analytical Writing 4.6
Advanced Psychology 634

GPA mean
Overall GPA 3.72

Number of applications/admission offers/incoming students in 2007
107 applied/11 admission offers/9 incoming

% of students receiving:
Full tuition waiver only: 0%
Assistantship/fellowship only: 0%
Both full tuition waiver & assistantship/fellowship: 100%

Approximate percentage of incoming students with a B.A./B.S. only: 66.7% **Master's:** 33.3%

Approximate percentage of students who are Women: 67% **Ethnic Minority:** 11% **International:** 0%

Average years to complete the doctoral program (including internship): 5 years

Personal interview
Preferred in person but telephone acceptable

Attrition rate in past 7 years: 11%

Percentage of students applying for internship last year accepted into APPIC or APA internships: 100%

Formal tracks/concentrations: clinical, clinical child, clinical health, developmental, behavior analysis

Research areas	# Faculty	# Grants
anxiety disorders	2	0
behavioral dentistry	1	1
behavioral medicine	3	0
cardiovascular reactivity	1	0
child behavior disorders	1	0
developmental psychopathology	1	0
ethnic minority	1	0
forensics	2	0
gerontology	2	0
pain	1	0
posttraumatic stress disorder	1	0
suicide	1	1

Clinical opportunities

anxiety disorders	gerontology
behavioral dentistry	parent training
behavioral medicine	primary care service
forensic psychology	school interventions

Western Michigan University (Ph.D.)

Department of Psychology
Kalamazoo, MI 49008
phone#: (269) 387-4330
e-mail: donna.areaux@wmich.edu
Web address:
www.wmich.edu/psychology/grad/clinical.html

1	2	3	**4**	5	6	7
Practice oriented		Equal emphasis			Research oriented	

Percentage of faculty subscribing to each of the following orientations:

Psychodynamic/Psychoanalytic	0%
Applied behavioral analysis/Radical behavioral	71%
Family systems/Systems	14%
Existential/Phenomenological/Humanistic	0%
Cognitive/Cognitive-behavioral	43%

Courses required for incoming students to have completed prior to enrolling:
Psychology major at an accredited institution

Recommended but not mandatory courses:
Basic course in behavioral principles/theory

GRE mean
Verbal + Quantitative 1126
Analytical Writing not reported
Advanced Psychology not reported

GPA mean
Undergraduate GPA not reported
Psychology GPA 3.69

Number of applications/admission offers/incoming students in 2007
99 applied/6 admission offers/5 incoming

% of students receiving:
Full tuition waiver only: 0%
Assistantship/fellowship only: 0%
Both full tuition waiver & assistantship/fellowship: 100%

Approximate percentage of incoming students with a B.A./B.S. only: 100%   **Master's:** 0%

Approximate percentage of students who are Women: 71%   **Ethnic Minority:** 11%   **International:** 7%

Average years to complete the doctoral program (including internship): 6 years

Personal interview
Preferred in person but telephone acceptable

Attrition rate in past 7 years: 10%

Percentage of students applying for internship last year accepted into APPIC or APA internships: 80%

Formal tracks/concentrations: none

Research areas	# Faculty	# Grants
aging	1	1
AIDS prevention/education	1	1
anxiety disorders/PTSD	1	0
autism/developmental disabilities	1	1
behavioral medicine	1	1
behavioral neuroscience	1	0
behavior therapy	2	0
depression	2	1
habit behaviors	1	0
interpersonal victimization	1	0
program evaluation	1	0
psychotherapy outcome	4	0
sexual dysfunctions	1	1

Clinical opportunities

forensic mental health	refugee mental health
function-based treatment	school refusal
posttraumatic stress disorder	

Wheaton College (Psy.D.)

Department of Psychology
Wheaton, IL 60187-5593
phone#: (630) 752-7053
e-mail: Robert.J.Gregory@wheaton.edu
Web address: www.wheaton.edu/psychology/
graduate/overview/index.html

1	2	**3**	4	5	6	7
Practice oriented			Equal emphasis			Research oriented

Percentage of faculty subscribing to each of the following orientations:

Psychodynamic/Psychoanalytic	28%
Applied behavioral analysis/Radical behavioral	0%
Family systems/Systems	33%
Existential/Phenomenological/Humanistic	0%
Cognitive/Cognitive-behavioral	39%

Courses required for incoming students to have completed prior to enrolling:
personality, physiological, abnormal, research methods, statistics

Recommended but not mandatory courses
developmental, cognition, social

GRE mean
Verbal 530   Quantitative 580
Advanced Psychology not reported
Analytical Writing 4.7

GPA mean
Overall GPA 3.45

Number of applications/admission offers/incoming students in 2007
65 applied/31 admission offers/19 incoming

% of students receiving:
Full tuition waiver only: 0%
Assistantship/fellowship only: 100%
Both full tuition waiver & assistantship/fellowship: 0%

Approximate percentage of incoming students with a B.A./B.S. only: 78%   **Master's:** 22%

Approximate percentage of students who are Women: 70%   **Ethnic Minority:** 20%
International: not reported

Average years to complete the doctoral program (including internship): 5 years

Personal interview
Required in person

Attrition rate in past 7 years: 1.5%

Percentage of students applying for internship last year accepted into APPIC or APA internships: 67%

Formal tracks/concentrations: none

Research areas	# Faculty	# Grants
spirituality/psychology integration	4	0
marriage & family	4	0
gender & sexuality	2	0
older adult and aging	1	1
meta-analysis	1	0
parent training (multicultural)	3	0
rural psychology	2	0
child & adolescent	3	0

Clinical opportunities

Chicago area has a great variety of offerings including hospitals, public and private agencies, community-based services, school-based services, and private practice.

Wichita State University (Ph.D.)

Department of Psychology
Wichita, KS 67260-0034
phone#: (316) 978-3170
e-mail: ddorr@cox.net
Web address: psychology.wichita.edu/cc/default.htm

1	2	3	**4**	5	6	7

Practice oriented · Equal emphasis · Research oriented

Percentage of faculty subscribing to each of the following orientations:

Psychodynamic/Psychoanalytic	20%
Applied behavioral analysis/Radical behavioral	10%
Family systems/Systems	25%
Existential/Phenomenological/Humanistic	10%
Cognitive/Cognitive-behavioral	35%

Courses required for incoming students to have completed prior to enrolling:

Most successful applicants have an undergraduate degree in psychology with course work in statistics, research methods, and history and systems

Recommended but not mandatory courses:
See above

GRE mean
Verbal 594   Quantitative 552
Analytical Writing 4.3
Advanced Psychology not reported

GPA mean
Overall GPA 3.7

Number of applications/admission offers/incoming students in 2007
40 applied/6 admission offers/5 incoming

% of students receiving:
Full tuition waiver only: 0%
Assistantship/fellowship only: 0%
Both full tuition waiver & assistantship/fellowship: 0%
(All students receive a Teaching Assistantship and partial tuition remission)

Approximate percentage of incoming students with a B.A./B.S. only: 80%   Master's: 20%

Approximate percentage of students who are
Women: 93%   Ethnic Minority: 11%   International: 0%

Average years to complete the doctoral program (including internship): 5 years

Personal interview
Required in person

Attrition rate in past 7 years: 6%

Percentage of students applying for internship last year accepted into APPIC or APA internships: 100%

Formal tracks/concentrations: none

Research areas	# Faculty	# Grants
antisocial behavior in children	1	2
personal relationships	1	0
teen pregnancy prevention	1	2
acceptance commitment therapy	1	0
MMPI-2	1	0
self help	1	5
teaching excellence	1	1

Clinical opportunities
anxiety disorders
depression

Widener University (Psy.D.)

Institute for Graduate Clinical Psychology
One University Place
Graduate Clinical Psychology
Chester, PA 19013
phone#: (610) 499-1208
e-mail: graduate.psychology@widener.edu
Web address: www3.widener.edu/Academics/
Schools_amp_Colleges/School_of_Human_Service
Professions/Institute_for_Graduate_Clinical
_Psychology/Welcome/391/

1	2	3	4	5	6	7

Practice oriented · Equal emphasis · Research oriented

Percentage of faculty subscribing to each of the following orientations:

Psychodynamic/Psychoanalytic	35%
Applied behavioral analysis/Radical behavioral	0%
Family systems/Systems	15%
Existential/Phenomenological/Humanistic	15%
Cognitive/Cognitive-behavioral	15%

Courses required for incoming students to have completed prior to enrolling:
abnormal, developmental, research methods, statistics

Recommended but not mandatory courses: Personality

GRE mean
Verbal 567   Quantitative 654
Analytical Writing 4.7
Advanced Psychology not reported

GPA mean
Overall GPA 3.57

Number of applications/admission offers/incoming students in 2007
362 applied/56 admission offers/30 incoming

% of students receiving:
Full tuition waiver only: 0%
Assistantship/fellowship only: 0%
Both full tuition waiver & assistantship/fellowship: 0%

Approximate percentage of incoming students with a B.A./B.S. only: 65% **Master's:** 35%

Approximate percentage of students who are Women: 75% **Ethnic Minority:** 16% **International:** 4%

Average years to complete the doctoral program (including internship): 5 years

Personal interview
Required in person

Attrition rate in past 7 years: 10%

Percentage of students applying for internship last year accepted into APPIC or APA internships: 100%

Formal tracks/concentrations: cross cultural/diversity, family therapy, forensic, group, health, neuropsychology, organizational, psychoanalytic

Research areas	# Faculty	# Grants
assessment/diagnosis	5	0
early childhood	4	1
learning disabilities	3	0
problem solving	2	0
stress and coping	2	2

Clinical opportunities

assessment
biofeedback
brief intervention
cognitive behavioral
couples therapy
cross-cultural & diversity
family therapy

forensic psychology
health psychology
group therapy
neuropsychology
psychoanalytic psychology
sex therapy

University of Windsor (Ph.D.)

Department of Psychology
Windsor, Ontario N9B 3P4, Canada
phone#: (519) 253-3000
fax#: (519) 973-7021
e-mail: bzakoor@uwindsor.ca
Web address: web4.uwindsor.ca/units/psychology/
clinical.nsf/831fc2c71873e46285256d6e006c367a/
76637c78d4470b818525691a0063cdfc!OpenDocument

1	2	**3**	4	5	6	7
Practice oriented		Equal emphasis			Research oriented	

Percentage of faculty subscribing to each of the following orientations:

Psychodynamic/Psychoanalytic	30%
Applied behavioral analysis/Radical behavioral	5%
Family systems/Systems	15%
Existential/Phenomenological/Humanistic	25%
Cognitive/Cognitive-behavioral	35%

Courses required for incoming students to have completed prior to enrolling:
Honor's B.A. in psychology or its equivalent

Recommended but not mandatory courses: None

GRE mean
Verbal 72nd percentile
Quantitative 60th percentile
Analytical Writing 72nd percentile
Advanced Psychology 86th percentile

GPA mean
Overall 3.5

Number of applications/admission offers/incoming students in 2007
158 applied/25 admission offers/11 incoming

% of students receiving:
Full tuition waiver only: 20%
Assistantship/fellowship only: 10%
Both full tuition waiver & assistantship/fellowship: 70%

Approximate percentage of incoming students with a B.A./B.S. only: 93% **Master's:** 7%

Approximate percentage of students who are Women: 86% **Ethnic Minority:** not reported **International:** 0%

Average years to complete the doctoral program (including internship): 6 years

Personal interview
Telephone interview required

Attrition rate in past 7 years: 8%

Percentage of students applying for internship last year accepted into APPIC or APA internships: 86%

Formal tracks/concentrations: adult clinical, child clinical, clinical neruopsychology

Research areas	# Faculty	# Grants
addiction	2	1
child research	4	3
community psychology	2	2
eating disorders	2	1
gambling behavior	1	3
health psychology	3	5
neuropsychological	4	4
psychotherapy research	3	2

Clinical opportunities
Psychological Service Center
Student Counseling Centre
practica and internships in the Detroit area

University of Wisconsin–Madison (Ph.D.)

Department of Psychology
W. J. Brogden Psychology Building
1202 West Johnson Street
Madison, WI 53706
phone#: (608) 262-2079
e-mail: dgooding@.wisc.edu
Web address: psych.wisc.edu/gradstudies/
clinical.html

1	2	3	4	5	6	**7**

Practice oriented   Equal emphasis   Research oriented

Percentage of faculty subscribing to each of the following orientations:

Psychodynamic/Psychoanalytic	20%
Applied behavioral analysis/Radical behavioral	0%
Family systems/Systems	8%
Existential/Phenomenological/Humanistic	8%
Cognitive/Cognitive-behavioral	92%
Motivational Interviewing	25%

Courses required for incoming students prior to enrolling:
Psychology major or related field training

Courses recommended but not mandatory: None

GRE mean
Verbal + Quantitative 1300
Analytical Writing not reported
Advanced Psychology not reported

GPA mean
GPA 3.73

Number of applications/admission offers/incoming students in 2007
180 applied/12 admission offers/4 incoming

% of students receiving:
Full tuition waiver only: 0%
Assistantship/fellowship only: 0%
Both full tuition remission (out of state portion only) & assistantship/fellowship: 100%

Approximate percentage of incoming students with a B.A./B.S. only: 100%   **Master's:** 0%

Approximate percentage of students who are Women: 75%   **Ethnic Minority:** 25%   **International:** 25%

Average years to complete the doctoral program (including internship): 7 years

Personal interview
Preferred in person but telephone acceptable

Attrition rate in past 7 years: not reported

Percentage of students applying for internship last year accepted into APPIC or APA internships: 80%

Formal tracks/concentrations: adult psychopathology

Research areas	# Faculty	# Grants
affective disorders	4	
developmental psychopathology	4	
health	3	
personality disorders: psychopathy	1	
schizophrenia and psychoses	2	
substance abuse	2	

Clinical opportunities
addictive disorders
assessment
assessment of forensic populations
assessment of schizophrenia and at-risk populations
childhood psychopathology

affective neuroscience
cognitive therapy
families/couples therapy
brief dynamic psychotherapy
therapy with criminal offenders

University of Wisconsin–Milwaukee (Ph.D.)

Department of Psychology
P.O. Box 413
Milwaukee, WI 53201
phone#: (414) 224-5521
e-mail: makovsky@uwm.edu
Web address:
www.uwm.edu/Dept/Psychology/clinical/index.html

1	2	3	**4**	5	6	7

Practice oriented   Equal emphasis   Research oriented

Percentage of faculty subscribing to each of the following orientations:

Psychodynamic/Psychoanalytic	0%
Applied behavioral analysis/Radical behavioral	30%
Family systems/Systems	20%
Existential/Phenomenological/Humanistic	0%
Cognitive/Cognitive-behavioral	50%

Courses required for incoming students to have completed prior to enrolling:
B.A.or B.S. in psychology or equivalent

Recommended but not mandatory courses:
Statistics, research methodology, advanced laboratory course in psychology

GRE mean
Verbal 585   Quantitative 669
Advanced Psychology 661
Analytical Writing not reported

GPA mean
Overall GPA 3.55   Psychology GPA 3.69
Junior/Senior GPA 3.68

Number of applications/admission offers/incoming students in 2007
117 applied/8 admission offers/6 incoming

% of students receiving:
Full tuition waiver only: 0%
Assistantship/fellowship only: 0%
Both full tuition waiver & assistantship/fellowship: 100%

Approximate percentage of incoming students with a B.A./B.S. only: 79%   **Master's:** 21%

Approximate percentage of students who are Women: 55%   **Ethnic Minority:** 17.2%
International: 0%

Average years to complete the doctoral program (including internship): 6.5 years

Personal interview
Preferred in person but telephone acceptable

Attrition rate in past 7 years: <5%

Percentage of students applying for internship last year accepted into APPIC or APA internships: 86%

Formal tracks/concentrations: none

Research areas	# Faculty	# Grants
alcohol and substance abuse	1	0
anxiety/impulse control disorders	3	3
attachment	2	0
child psychology	4	3
developmental disabilities	1	1
emotion regulation	2	0
health psychology	2	0
learning disabilities	1	0
mood disorders	1	2
multicultural issues	1	0
neuropsychology	2	1
psychotherapy research	2	4

Clinical opportunities

acceptance and commitment therapy
behavior therapy
behavioral medicine
neuropsychology
child development
couples therapy
developmental disabilities
family violence
functional analytic psychotherapy
inpatient psychiatric
learning disability
OC spectrum disorders
premature infants

The Wright Institute (Psy.D.)

2728 Durant Avenue
Berkeley, CA 94704
phone#: (510) 841-9230
e-mail: info@wrightinst.edu
Web address:
www.wrightinst.edu/program_program.html

1	2	3	4	5	6	7
Practice oriented		Equal emphasis			Research oriented	

Percentage of faculty subscribing to each of the following orientations:

Psychodynamic/Psychoanalytic	40%
Applied behavioral analysis/Radical behavioral	0%
Family systems/Systems	20%
Existential/Phenomenological/Humanistic	10%
Cognitive/Cognitive-behavioral	30%

Courses required for incoming students to have completed prior to enrolling:
None

Recommended but not mandatory courses:
Development, personality, abnormal, statistics

GRE mean
GRE scores not used in admission decisions

GPA mean
Overall GPA 3.3   Psychology GPA 3.3

Number of applications/admission offers/incoming students in 2007
Not reported

% of students receiving:
Full tuition waiver only: 0%
Assistantship/fellowship only: 18%
Both full tuition waiver & assistantship/fellowship: 0%

Approximate percentage of incoming students with a B.A./B.S. only: 60%   **Master's:** 40%

Approximate percentage of students who are Women: 75%   **Ethnic Minority:** 20%
International: not reported

Average years to complete the doctoral program (including internship): 5.5 years

Personal interview
Preferred in person but telephone acceptable

Attrition rate in past 7 years: not reported

Percentage of students applying for internship last year accepted into APPIC or APA internships: not reported

Formal tracks/concentrations: none

Research areas	# Faculty	# Grants
chronic illness	1	0
cross-cultural psychology	3	0
evolutionary psychology	1	1
gender studies	3	0
infant/parent psychotherapy	3	0
jail and prison facilities	1	0
neurogerontology	1	0
parenting	3	0
step-families	1	0
stress-related somatic difficulties	1	0
substance abuse	2	0

Clinical opportunities

AIDS/HIV
affect disorders
assessment
brief and long-term therapy
child/adolescent assessment
child/adolescent psychopathology
couples therapy
crisis intervention
empirically supported treatments
ethnic minority
family therapy
forensic populations
geropsychology
GLBT
group therapy
men's issues
neuropsychology
pediatric/developmental
personality disorders
program development/ evaluation
psychodynamic
public policy/advocacy
rehabilitation psychology
schizophrenia
substance abuse
university counseling
women's issues

Wright State University (Psy.D.)

School of Professional Psychology
3640 Colonel Glenn Highway
Dayton, OH 45435
phone#: (937) 775-3492

e-mail: sopp1@wright.edu
Web address: www.wright.edu/sopp/

1	2	3	4	5	6	7
Practice oriented		Equal emphasis			Research oriented	

Percentage of faculty subscribing to each of the following orientations:
Psychodynamic/Psychoanalytic	40%
Applied behavioral analysis/Radical behavioral	0%
Family systems/Systems	20%
Existential/Phenomenological/Humanistic	10%
Cognitive/Cognitive-behavioral	30%

Courses required for incoming students to have completed prior to enrolling: Statistics

Recommended but not mandatory courses:
Development, personality, abnormal

GRE mean
not used in admissions decisions

GPA mean
Overall GPA 3.3
Psychology GPA 3.3

Number of applications/admission offers/incoming students in 2007
290 applied/115 admission offers/68 incoming

% of students receiving:
Full tuition waiver only: 0%
Assistantship/fellowship only: 18%
Both full tuition waiver & assistantship/fellowship: 0%

Approximate percentage of incoming students with a B.A./B.S. only: 60%   Master's: 40%

Approximate percentage of students who are
Women: 75%   Ethnic Minority: 25%   International: 7%

Average years to complete the doctoral program (including internship): 5.5 years

Personal interview
Preferred in person but telephone acceptable

Attrition rate in past 7 years: 8.8%

Percentage of students applying for internship last year accepted into APPIC or APA internships: 45%

Formal tracks/concentrations: none

Research areas	# Faculty	# Grants
chronic illness	1	0
cross-cultural psychology	3	0
evolutionary psychology	1	1
gender studies	3	0
infant/parent psychotherapy outcome	3	0
jail and prison facilities	1	0
neurogerontology	1	0
parenting	3	0
step-families	1	0
stress-related somatic difficulties	1	0
substance abuse	2	0

Clinical opportunities
AIDS/HIV	GLBT
affect disorders	group therapy
assessment	men's issues
brief and long-term therapy	neuropsychology
child/adolescent assessment	pediatric/developmental
child/adolescent psychopathology	personality disorders
	program evaluation
couples therapy	psychodynamic
crisis intervention	public policy/advocacy
empirically supported treatments	rehabilitation psychology
	schizophrenia
ethnic minority	substance abuse
family therapy	university counseling
forensic populations	women's issues
geropsychology	

University of Wyoming (Ph.D.)
Department of Psychology
Box 3415 University Station
Laramie, WY 82071
phone#: (307) 766-6303
e-mail: psyc.uw@uwyo.edu
Web address: uwadmnweb.uwyo.edu/psychology/
clinicalpsychology.asp

1	2	3	4	5	6	7
Practice oriented		Equal emphasis			Research oriented	

Percentage of faculty subscribing to each of the following orientations:
Psychodynamic/Psychoanalytic	0%
Applied behavioral analysis/Radical behavioral	40%
Family systems/Systems	0%
Existential/Phenomenological/Humanistic	0%
Cognitive/Cognitive-behavioral	60%

Courses required for incoming students to have completed prior to enrolling:
None

Recommended but not mandatory courses:
Statistics, 30–45 psychology credits, research experience

GRE mean
Verbal + Quantitative 1250
Advanced Psychology 655
Analytical Writing 5.2

GPA mean
Overall GPA 3.74   Psychology GPA 3.9
Junior/Senior GPA 3.8

Number of applications/admission offers/incoming students in 2007
63 applied/6 admission offers/5 incoming

% of students receiving:
Full tuition waiver only: 0%
Assistantship/fellowship only: 0%
Both full tuition waiver & assistantship/fellowship: 100%

Approximate percentage of incoming students with a B.A./B.S. only: 75%   Master's: 25%

Approximate percentage of students who are
Women: 70%   **Ethnic Minority:** 10%   **International:** 0%

Average years to complete the doctoral program (including internship): 7 years

Personal interview
Preferred in person but telephone acceptable

Attrition rate in past 7 years: 5%

What percentage of students applying for internship last year was accepted into APPIC or APA internships? 75%

Formal tracks/concentrations: integrated behavioral health

Research areas	# Faculty	# Grants
anxiety	2	1
depression	3	2
HIV/AIDS prevention	1	1
mental retardation	2	1
Native American mental health	2	1
primary care	4	1
psychology and the law	2	1
substance abuse	1	1
trauma/posttraumatic stress disorder	1	1
ADHD	1	0
schizophrenia	1	0

Clinical opportunities
inpatient and residential
bereavement
developmental disabilities
empirically supported psychotherapies
mood/anxiety disorders
primary/interdisciplinary care
rural/community health care

Xavier University (Psy.D.)

Department of Psychology
3800 Victory Parkway
Cincinnati, OH 45207-6511
phone#: (513) 745-3533
e-mail: maybury@xavier.edu
Web address: www.xavier.edu/psychology_doctorate/

1	2	**3**	4	5	6	7
Practice oriented		Equal emphasis			Research oriented	

Percentage of faculty subscribing to each of the following orientations:
Psychodynamic/Psychoanalytic 40%
Applied behavioral analysis/Radical behavioral 0%
Family systems/Systems 20%
Existential/Phenomenological/Humanistic 0%
Cognitive/Cognitive-behavioral 60%

Courses required for incoming students prior to enrolling:
Minimum 18 semester hours includingstatistics, research methods, abnormal, testing, and social

Courses recommended but not mandatory:
Anatomy and physical science, calculus

GRE mean
Not reported

GPA mean
Not reported

Number of applications/admission offers/incoming students in 2007
218 applied/49 offers/17 incoming

% of students receiving:
Full tuition waiver only: 0%
Assistantship/fellowship only: 42% (includes partial tuition remission)
Both full tuition waiver & assistantship/fellowship: 0%

Approximate percentage of incoming students with a B.A./B.S. only: 99%   **Master's:** 1%

Approximate percentage of students who are
Women: 76%   **Ethnic Minority:** 12%
International: not reported

Average years to complete the doctoral program (including internship): 5.5 years

Personal interview
Interview not required

Attrition rate in past 7 years: 8%

Percentage of students applying for internship last year accepted into APPIC or APA internships: 69%

Formal tracks/concentrations: children/adolescents & their families, older adults, severe mental illness

Research areas	# Faculty	# Grants
cognitive/behavioral	5	0
geropsychology	2	0
psychoanalytic	4	0
social/experimental	1	0
statistician	2	0

Clinical opportunities
college-related concerns
Xavier University Psychology Services Center

Yale University (Ph.D.)

Department of Psychology
P.O. Box 208205
New Haven, CT 06520-8205
Phone #: (203) 432-4505
E-mail: william.corbin@yale.edu
Web address: www.yale.edu/psychology/clinical.html

1	2	3	4	5	6	**7**
Practice oriented		Equal emphasis			Research oriented	

Percentage of faculty subscribing to each of the following orientations:

Psychodynamic/Psychoanalytic	0%
Applied Behavioral Analysis/Radical Behavioral	0%
Family Systems/Systems	0%
Existential/Phenomenological/Humanistic	14%
Cognitive/Cognitive-behavioral	100%

Courses required for incoming students prior to enrolling: none

Courses recommended but not mandatory:
broad psychology background, undergraduate psychology

GRE Mean:
Verbal: 653   Quantitative: 707
Analytical Writing 5.6
Advanced Psychology not reported

GPA Mean:
Overall GPA: 3.82

Number of applications/admission offers/incoming students in 2007
316 applied/3 admission offers/1 incoming

% of students receiving:
Full tuition waiver only: 0%
Assistantship/fellowship only: 0%
Both full tuition waiver & assistantship/fellowship: 100%

Approximate percentage of incoming students with a B.A./B.S. only: 100%   **Master's:** 0%

Approximate percentage of students who are:
Women: 86%   **Ethnic minority:** 18%
International: not reported

Average years to complete the doctoral program (including internship): 6 years

Personal interview: No preference given

Attrition rate in past 7 years: 14%

Percentage of students applying for internship last year accepted into APPIC or APA internships: 100%

Formal tracks/concentrations: none

Research areas	# Faculty	# Grants
adult psychopathology	5	0
alcohol use/dependence	1	2
anxiety disorders	2	0
behavior genetics	1	0
cognitive processes	3	0
depression/suicidality	3	0
disruptive behavior disorders	1	0
developmental psychopathology	2	0
eating disorders	2	0
health psychology	2	2
longitudinal epidemiology	1	0
public health/social policy	1	0

Clinical Opportunities

adolescents	eating and weight disorders
anxiety and mood disorders	health psychology
child psychotherapy	substance abuse
conduct disorders	

Yeshiva University (Ph.D.)

Ferkauf Graduate School of Psychology
Jack and Pearl Resnick Campus
1300 Morris Park Ave
Bronx, NY 10461
phone#: (718) 430-3856
e-mail: ssuchday@aecom.yu.edu
Web address: www.yu.edu/Ferkauf/page.aspx?id=705
&ekmensel=242_submenu_282_btnlink

1	2	3	4	**5**	6	7
Practice oriented		Equal emphasis			Research oriented	

Percentage of faculty subscribing to each of the following orientations:

Psychodynamic/Psychoanalytic	0%
Applied behavioral analysis/Radical behavioral	0%
Family systems/Systems	0%
Existential/Phenomenological/Humanistic	0%
Cognitive/Cognitive-behavioral	100%

Courses required for incoming students to have completed prior to enrolling:
Minimum of 15 credits in psych, statistics, abnormal, experimental, personality, or physiological

Recommended but not mandatory courses:
Courses in mathematics, natural sciences, and social sciences

GRE mean
Verbal 560   Quantitative 630
Advanced Psychology 650
Analytical Writing 4.9

GPA mean
Overall GPA 3.5

Number of applications/admission offers/incoming students in 2007
115 applied/45 admission offers/14 incoming

% of students receiving:
Full tuition waiver only: 1%
Assistantship/fellowship only: 33%
Both full tuition waiver & assistantship/fellowship: 0%

Approximate percentage of incoming students with a B.A./B.S. only: 82%   **Master's:** 18%

Approximate percentage of students who are
Women: 80%   **Ethnic Minority:** 14%   **International:** 4%

Average years to complete the doctoral program (including internship): 5.5 years

Personal interview
Required in person

Attrition rate in past 7 years: 2%

Percentage of students applying for internship last year accepted into APPIC or APA internships: 78%

Formal tracks/concentrations: none

Research areas	# Faculty	# Grants
cardiovascular psychology	1	0
acculturation and global health	2	3
neuropsychology	2	2
multiple sclerosis	1	3
obesity	1	0
asthma	1	1
psychosocial oncology	1	2
migraines	1	3
diabetes	1	1

Clinical opportunities

behavioral medicine	asthma and anxiety
cardiovascular psychology	neuropsychology
weight management	geropsychology

Yeshiva University (Psy.D.)

Department of Psychology
Ferkauf Graduate School of Psychology
1300 Morris Park Avenue
Bronx, NY 10461
phone#: (718) 430-3850
e-mail: gill@aecom.yu.edu
Web address: www.yu.edu/ferkauf/index_sub.asp?504

1	2	3	4	5	6	7
Practice oriented		Equal emphasis			Research oriented	

Percentage of faculty subscribing to each of the following orientations:

Psychodynamic/Psychoanalytic	40%
Applied behavioral analysis/Radical behavioral	5%
Family systems/Systems	10%
Existential/Phenomenological/Humanistic	5%
Cognitive/Cognitive-behavioral	40%

Courses required for incoming students to have completed prior to enrolling:
Statistics, abnormal, experimental, physiological, personality

Recommended but not mandatory courses:
None

GRE mean
Verbal 550   Quantitative 600
Analytical Writing not reported
Advanced Psychology not reported

GPA mean
Overall GPA 3.5   Psychology GPA 3.5

Number of applications/admission offers/incoming students in 2007
Not reported

% of students receiving:
Full tuition waiver only: 0%
Assistantship/fellowship only: 70%
Both full tuition waiver & assistantship/fellowship: 0%

Approximate percentage of incoming students with a B.A./B.S. only: 85%   **Master's:** 15%

Approximate percentage of students who are Women: 73%   **Ethnic Minority:** 15%
International: not reported

Average years to complete the doctoral program (including internship): 5 years

Personal interview
Required in person

Attrition rate in past 7 years: 2%

Percentage of students applying for internship last year accepted into APPIC or APA internships: 98%

Formal tracks/concentrations: geropsychology, psychodynamics, CBT, mental health counseling

Research areas	# Faculty	# Grants
anxiety disorders	1	0
depression	2	0
early childhood intervention	1	0
ethnicity and identity	2	0
family therapy	1	0
forensics	1	0
geropsychology	1	1
parenting styles	1	0
psychoanalytic therapy	5	0
psychotherapy process/outcome	3	0
sleep disorders/nightmares	1	0
stress and coping	4	1
trauma	2	0

Clinical opportunities

anxiety disorders	marital/couples
cognitive behavior therapy	parent training
depression	psychodynamic therapy
family therapy	psychoeducational
geriatrics	assessment
interpersonal therapy	

York University–Adult Clinical Program (Ph.D.)

Department of Psychology
Toronto, Ontario M3J 1P3, Canada
phone#: (416) 736-5115
e-mail: clindir@yorku.ca
Web address:
www.yorku.ca/health/psyc/graduate/clinical.htm

1	2	3	4	5	6	7
Practice oriented		Equal emphasis			Research oriented	

Percentage of faculty subscribing to each of the following orientations:

Psychodynamic/Psychoanalytic	25%
Applied behavioral analysis/Radical behavioral	0%
Family systems/Systems	6%
Existential/Phenomenological/Humanistic	38%
Cognitive/Cognitive-behavioral	31%

Courses required for incoming students to have completed prior to enrolling:
Psychological/neuropsychology, organizational/social/groups, research design, statistics, learning/perception, personality/abnormal/individual differences

Recommended but not mandatory courses:
Multicultural psychology, sex-roles, tests and measurements, health psychology

GRE mean
Verbal 563   Quantitative 559
Advanced Psychology 664
Analytical Writing not reported

GPA mean
Overall GPA A

Number of applications/admission offers/incoming students in 2007
133 applied/8 admission offers/8 incoming

% of students receiving:
Full tuition waiver only: 0%
Assistantship/fellowship only: 100% incoming students; 36% all other
Both full tuition waiver & assistantship/fellowship: 0%

Approximate percentage of incoming students with a B.A./B.S. only: 92%   **Master's:** 8%

Approximate percentage of students who are Women: 90%   **Ethnic Minority:** not reported
International: not reported

Average years to complete the doctoral program (including internship): 7 years

Personal interview
Preferred in person but telephone acceptable

Attrition rate in past 7 years: not reported

Percentage of students applying for internship last year accepted into APPIC or APA internships: 78%

Formal tracks/concentrations: adult clinical, health

Research areas	# Faculty	# Grants
alcohol and substance abuse	1	0
anxiety/stress/coping	1	1
major depression	1	1
eating disorders & body image	1	1
grief and trauma	1	0
psychopathology/psychotherapy	1	2
health—cardiovascular disease	1	2
relationship research	1	1
neuropsychology of memory and aging	2	1
narrative processes	1	1
clinical neuropsychology	1	1
cognitive rehabilitation	1	1
motivation & psychotherapy	1	1
pain	1	1
personality factors	1	0
psychotherapy process/outcome	3	3
schizophrenia	2	1

Clinical opportunities

substance abuse	forensic
anxiety disorders	geriatric
depression	health psychology
eating disorders	neuropsychology

York University—Clinical-Developmental Program (Ph.D.)
Department of Psychology
Toronto, Ontario M3J 1P3, Canada
phone#: (416) 736-5290
e-mail: cldevdir@yorku.ca
Web address: www.yorku.ca/health/psyc/graduate/clinical_development.htm

1	2	3	**4**	5	6	7
Practice oriented		Equal emphasis			Research oriented	

Percentage of faculty subscribing to each of the following orientations:

Psychodynamic/Psychoanalytic	10%
Applied behavioral analysis/Radical behavioral	25%
Family systems/Systems	75%
Existential/Phenomenological/Humanistic	0%
Cognitive/Cognitive-behavioral	75%

Courses required for incoming students to have completed prior to enrolling:
Honors degree in psychology

Recommended but not mandatory courses:
developmental, atypical development

GRE mean
Verbal 600   Quantitative 735
Advanced Psychology 670
Analytical Writing not reported

GPA mean
Not reported

Number of applications/admission offers/incoming students in 2007
109 applied/13 admission offers/11 incoming

% of students receiving:
Full tuition waiver only: 0%
Assistantship/fellowship only: 100%
Both full tuition waiver & assistantship/fellowship: 0%

Approximate percentage of incoming students with a B.A./B.S. only: 90%   **Master's:** 10%

Approximate percentage of students who are Women: 80%   **Ethnic Minority:** 20%
International: not reported

Average years to complete the doctoral program (including internship): 6.5 years

Personal interview
Preferred in person but telephone acceptable

Attrition rate in past 7 years: 10%

Percentage of students applying for internship last year accepted into APPIC or APA internships: 90%

Formal tracks/concentrations: clinical-developmental

Research areas	# Faculty	# Grants
adolescent peer relations	3	3
aggression	3	3
autism, developmental disability	2	3
bullying and victimization	2	1
child abuse	3	2
child testimony	1	2
cognitive and language development	2	1
interpersonal support	1	0
pediatric/child health	2	2
problem-solving/emotion	1	0
stress and coping	1	0
teen violence	2	2

Clinical opportunities

children's rehabilitation
developmental disabilities
dual diagnosis clinic
gender disorder clinic
learning disability/ADHD

mental health centers
psychiatric clinics
regional hospital clinics
school boards

Clinical Psychology Program That Has Been Discontinued

New York University (accredited, inactive)

Clinical Psychology Programs Withdrawing from APA Accreditation

Dalhousie University

University of Western Ontario

Clinical Psychology Programs Not Reporting Information

Argosy University–Tampa Campus

University of North Texas and University of North Texas Health Sciences Center

REPORTS ON INDIVIDUAL COUNSELING PSYCHOLOGY PROGRAMS

University of Akron (Ph.D.)

Department of Counseling and Department of
Psychology
Akron, OH 44325-4301
phone#: (330) 972-7280 or (330) 972-7777
e-mail: shardin@uakron.edu
Web address:
www3.uakron.edu/psychology/counseling

1	2	3	4	5	6	7
Practice oriented			Equal emphasis			Research oriented

Percentage of faculty subscribing to each of the following orientations:

Psychodynamic/Psychoanalytic	10%
Applied behavioral analysis/Radical behavioral	0%
Family systems/Systems	10%
Existential/Phenomenological/Humanistic	20%
Cognitive/Cognitive-behavioral	60%

Courses required for incoming students to have completed prior to enrolling:

The program has 2 tracks: 1 track (Department of Psychology) admits students with a bachelor's degree in psychology; the other track (Department of Counseling) admits students with a master's degree in counseling.

Recommended but not mandatory courses:

Psychology research, quantitative methods, personality

GRE mean

1100 recommended
Analytical Writing not reported

GPA mean

Overall GPA 3.25

Number of applications/admission offers/incoming students in 2007

80 applied/15 admission offers/7 incoming

% of students receiving:

Full tuition waiver only: 0%
Assistantship/fellowship only: 0%
Both full tuition waiver & assistantship/fellowship: 100%

Approximate percentage of incoming students with a B.A./B.S. only: 50%   Master's: 50%

Approximate percentage of students who are

Women: 75%   Ethnic Minority: 10%
International: not reported

Average years to complete the doctoral program (including internship): 6 years

Personal interview

No preference given

Attrition rate in past 7 years: 10%

Percentage of students applying for internship last year accepted into APPIC or APA internships: 100%

Formal tracks/concentrations: none

Research areas	# Faculty	# Grants
multicultural	2	0
personality assessment	2	0
suicide	2	0
vocational counseling	2	0
women's issues	3	0

Clinical opportunities

child study and family therapy
community mental health center
college counseling center

University at Albany/State University of New York (Ph.D.)

Department of Educational and Counseling
Psychology
ED 220
Albany, NY 12222
phone#: (518) 442-5040
e-mail: mfriedlander@uamail.albany.edu
Web address: www.albany.edu/counseling_psych

1	2	3	4	5	6	7
Practice oriented			Equal emphasis			Research oriented

Percentage of faculty subscribing to each of the following orientations:

Psychodynamic/Psychoanalytic	15%
Family systems/Systems	15%
Existential/Phenomenological/Humanistic	20%
Cognitive/Cognitive-behavioral	50%

Courses required for incoming students to have completed prior to enrolling:

Preparation in basic psychology (18 credits minimum, including statistics)

Recommended but not mandatory courses: abnormal, developmental, personality

GRE mean

Verbal + Quantitative 1150
Analytical Writing not reported
Advanced Psychology not considered

GPA mean

Overall GPA 3.6   Psychology GPA 3.8

Number of applications/admission offers/incoming students in 2007

120 applied/10 admission offers/7 incoming

% of students receiving:

Full tuition waiver only: 0%
Assistantship/fellowship only: 0%
Both full tuition waiver & assistantship/fellowship: 95%

Approximate percentage of incoming students who entered with a B.A./B.S. only: 45%   Master's: 55%

Approximate percentage of students who are

Women: 75%   Ethnic Minority: 22%   International: 15%

Average years to complete the doctoral program (including internship): 6.5 years

Personal interview
Preferred in person but telephone acceptable

Attrition rate in past 7 years: 2%

Percentage of students applying for internship last year accepted into APPIC or APA internships: 91%

Formal tracks/concentrations: none

Research areas	# Faculty	# Grants
career development	2	1
cross-cultural	3	2
family dynamics	1	0
family therapy	1	1
methodology	2	2
prevention	1	0
psychotherapy process	1	1
social justice	1	0
spirituality	1	0
supervision	2	0
women's issues	2	0

Clinical opportunities
adolescent residential treatment centers
college and university counseling centers
community agencies
county mental health clinics
neuropsychology rehabilitation center
various units at VA hospitals, including neuropsychology, outpatient, day treatment, substance abuse

Arizona State University (Ph.D.)

Division of Psychology and Education
Arizona State University
Tempe, AZ 85287-0611
phone#: (480) 965-6339
e-mail: dpe@asu.edu
Web address: coe.asu.edu/psyched/

1	2	3	4	**5**	6	7
Practice oriented		Equal emphasis			Research oriented	

Percentage of faculty subscribing to each of the following orientations:
Psychodynamic/Psychoanalytic 20%
Applied behavioral analysis/Radical behavioral 0%
Family systems/Systems 10%
Existential/Phenomenological/Humanistic 30%
Cognitive/Cognitive-behavioral 40%

Courses required for incoming students to have completed prior to enrolling:
None

Recommended but not mandatory courses:
Psychology or related background

GRE mean
Verbal 540 Quantitative 570
Analytical Writing not reported

GPA mean
Overall GPA 3.26 Junior/Senior GPA 3.67

Number of applications/admission offers/incoming students in 2007
159 applied/10 admission offers/8 incoming

% of students receiving:
Full tuition waiver only: 0%
Assistantship/fellowship only: 12%
Both full tuition waiver & assistantship/fellowship: 88%

Approximate percentage of incoming students with a B.A./B.S. only: 40% **Master's:** 60%

Approximate percentage of students who are Women: 75% **Ethnic Minority:** 50% **International:** 5%

Average years to complete the doctoral program (including internship): 5 years

Personal interview
Required in person

Attrition rate in past 7 years: 6%

Percentage of students applying for internship last year accepted into APPIC or APA internships: 93%

Formal tracks/concentrations: none

Research areas	# Faculty	# Grants
career development	3	1
cognitive appraisal	1	0
cognitive-behavioral interventions	1	1
consultation	2	0
counseling process	4	0
counseling the gifted and talented	2	1
counseling women and minorities	5	1
culture sensitivity training	4	0
experimental methodology	2	0
family enrichment	1	0
gender issues in counseling	2	0
group counseling	1	0
health psychology	1	0
HIV	1	0
international issues	1	0
interpersonal therapy	3	0
psychology of women	2	0
retention	4	1
social psychological counseling	2	0
training and supervision	4	0
values and decision making	1	0

Clinical opportunities
varied

Auburn University (Ph.D.)

Department of Counselor Education, Counseling Psychology, and School Psychology
Auburn, AL 36849-5218
phone#: (334) 844-5160
e-mail: ccp@mail.auburn.edu
Web address: www.auburn.edu/coun

1	2	3	**4**	5	6	7
Practice oriented		Equal emphasis			Research oriented	

Percentage of faculty subscribing to each of the following orientations:

Psychodynamic/Psychoanalytic	33%
Applied behavioral analysis/Radical behavioral	0%
Family systems/Systems	0%
Existential/Phenomenological/Humanistic	33%
Cognitive/Cognitive-behavioral	33%

Courses required for incoming students to have completed prior to enrolling: None

Recommended but not mandatory courses: None

GRE mean
Verbal not reported
Quantitative not reported
Advanced Psychology not required
Analytical Writing not reported

GPA mean
Overall GPA 3.6

Number of applications/admission offers/incoming students in 2007
84 applied/6 admission offers/5 incoming

% of students receiving:
Full tuition waiver only: 0%
Assistantship/fellowship only: 20%
Both full tuition waiver & assistantship/fellowship: 80%

Approximate percentage of incoming students with a B.A./B.S. only: 40%   **Master's:** 60%

Approximate percentage of students who are Women: 80%   **Ethnic Minority:** 0%   **International:** 20%

Average years to complete the doctoral program (including internship): 5.5 years

Personal interview
Preferred in person but telephone acceptable

Attrition rate in past 7 years: 8%

Percentage of students applying for internship last year accepted into APPIC or APA internships: 100%

Formal tracks/concentrations: none

Research areas	# Faculty	# Grants
alternative methods	1	0
gay/lesbian/bisexual	2	0
professional issues/ethics	3	0
psychometrics	2	0
substance abuse prevention	3	1

Clinical opportunities
mental health center (outpatient)
substance abuse unit (inpatient and outpatient)
university counseling center
rehabilitation

Ball State University (Ph.D.)

Department of Counseling Psychology
Muncie, IN 47306
phone#: (765) 285-8040

fax#: (765) 285-2067
e-mail: SBOWMAN@BSU.EDU
Web address: www.bsu.edu/counselingpsychology

1	2	3	**4**	5	6	7
Practice oriented		Equal emphasis			Research oriented	

Percentage of faculty subscribing to each of the following orientations:

Psychodynamic/Psychoanalytic	15%
Applied behavioral analysis/Radical behavioral	0%
Family systems/Systems	35%
Existential/Phenomenological/Humanistic	20%
Cognitive/Cognitive-behavioral	30%

Courses required for incoming students to have completed prior to enrolling:
Counseling theories, counseling techniques, practicum, one other counseling course

Recommended but not mandatory courses: None

GRE mean
Verbal + Quantitative 1123
Analytical Writing not reported

GPA mean
Overall master's GPA 3.8

Number of applications/admission offers/incoming students in 2007
70 applied/13 admission offers/10 incoming

% of students receiving:
Full tuition waiver only: 0%
Assistantship/fellowship only: 0%
Both full tuition waiver & assistantship/fellowship: 100%

Approximate percentage of incoming students with a B.A./B.S. only: 0%   **Master's:** 100%

Approximate percentage of students who are Women: 69%   **Ethnic Minority:** 20%   **International:** 18%

Average years to complete the doctoral program (including internship): 4.6 years

Personal interview
Preferred in person but telephone acceptable

Attrition rate in past 7 years: 9%

Percentage of students applying for internship last year accepted into APPIC or APA internships: 66%

Formal tracks/concentrations: marriage and family, multicultural/social justice

Research areas	# Faculty	# Grants
behavioral medicine	2	0
career/vocational	4	0
child/adolescent	2	0
clinical judgment	1	0
multicultural	4	1
organizational/EAP	1	0
social psychology applications	3	0
rehabilitation	1	1
women's identity	2	0

Clinical opportunities
BSU Practicum Clinic
Cancer Center
university counseling center

Boston College (Ph.D.)

Department of Counseling, Developmental and
Educational Psychology
School of Education
Chestnut Hill, MA 02167
phone#: (617) 552-4710 or (617) 552-4214
e-mail: gsoe@bc.edu
Web address: www.bc.edu/schools/lsoe/academics/
graduate/phd/counsel.html

1	2	3	4	**5**	6	7
Practice oriented			Equal emphasis			Research oriented

Percentage of faculty subscribing to each of the following orientations:

Psychodynamic/Psychoanalytic	35%
Applied behavioral analysis/Radical behavioral	0%
Family systems/Systems	2%
Existential/Phenomenological/Humanistic	10%
Cognitive/Cognitive-behavioral	20%

Courses required for incoming students to have completed prior to enrolling:
For applicants without a master's degree, we require at least 18 credit hours of undergraduate psychology

Recommended but not mandatory courses:
Statistics, abnormal, developmental, personality

GRE mean
Verbal 613   Quantitative 608
Analytical Writing 5.5

GPA mean
Overall GPA 3.43

Number of applications/admission offers/incoming students in 2007
243 applied/8 admission offers/6 incoming

% of students receiving:
Full tuition waiver only: 0%
Assistantship/fellowship only: 0%
Both full tuition waiver & assistantship/fellowship: 100%

Approximate percentage of incoming students with a B.A./B.S. only: 0%   **Master's:** 100%
Note. We are now expanding our applicant pool to include students without a master's degree as well as students with Master's degrees in counseling or related areas. Therefore, the statistics represented above will change in subsequent years.

Approximate percentage of students who are Women: 85%   **Ethnic Minority:** 43%
International: 14%

Average years to complete the doctoral program (including internship): 5.5 years

Personal interview
Preferred in person but telephone acceptable

Attrition rate in past 7 years: 8%

Percentage of students applying for internship last year accepted into APPIC or APA internships: 100%

Formal tracks/concentrations: none

Research areas	# Faculty	# Grants
adolescent development	2	2
career development	1	3
gender roles	2	0
schools and agencies	4	6
mentoring in adolescence	1	1
multicultural	3	3
risk and resilience	4	2
violence prevention	3	2

Clinical opportunities
acute psychiatric
college counseling center
community mental health
inpatient adult unit
inpatient child
school based mental health clinic
violence prevention/ intervention

Brigham Young University (Ph.D.)

Department of Counseling Psychology and
Special Education
Provo, UT 84602-5093
phone#: (801) 422-3859
e-mail: aaron_jackson@byu.edu
Web address: education.byu.edu/cpse/index.html

1	2	3	**4**	5	6	7
Practice oriented			Equal emphasis			Research oriented

Percentage of faculty subscribing to each of the following orientations:

Psychodynamic/Psychoanalytic	30%
Applied behavioral analysis/Radical behavioral	0%
Family systems/Systems	0%
Existential/Phenomenological/Humanistic	35%
Cognitive/Cognitive-behavioral	35%

Courses required for incoming students to have completed prior to enrolling:
Abnormal, personality, developmental, research methods

Recommended but not mandatory courses:
Statistics

GRE mean
Verbal 616   Quantitative 560
Analytical Writing 4.7

GPA mean
Overall GPA 3.69

Number of applications/admission offers/incoming students in 2007
38 applied/6 admission offers/6 incoming

% of students receiving:
Full tuition waiver only: 0%
Assistantship/fellowship only: 100%
Both full tuition waiver & assistantship/fellowship: 0%

Approximate percentage of incoming students with a B.A./B.S. only: 83% **Master's:** 17%

Approximate percentage of students who are Women: 66% **Ethnic Minority:** 27% **International:** 6%

Average years to complete the doctoral program (including internship): 5 years

Personal interview
Preferred in person but telephone acceptable

Attrition rate in past 7 years: 4%

Percentage of students applying for internship last year accepted into APPIC or APA internships: 89%

Formal tracks/concentrations: none

Research areas	# Faculty	# Grants
crisis intervention	1	1
mental health and spirituality	6	3
mental health in schools	3	2
multicultural counseling	2	2
Native American vocational development	1	1
outcome research	3	3
women's issues	2	1

Clinical opportunities
eating disorders
family clinic

University of British Columbia (Ph.D.)
Department of Educational and Counseling Psychology,
and Special Education
2125 Main Mall
Vancouver, British Columbia V6T 1Z4, Canada
phone#: (604) 822-8539
e-mail: lynn.miller@ubc.edu
Web address: ecps.educ.ubc.ca/

1	2	3	**4**	5	6	7
Practice oriented		Equal emphasis			Research oriented	

Percentage of faculty subscribing to each of the following orientations:
Psychodynamic/Psychoanalytic 5%
Applied behavioral analysis/Radical behavioral 0%
Family systems/Systems 60%
Existential/Phenomenological/Humanistic 60%
Cognitive/Cognitive-behavioral 50%

Courses required for incoming students to have completed prior to enrolling:
Ph.D. applicants are required to have completed courses equivalent to the M.A. in Counseling offered by the department. Please check the Web site.

Recommended but not mandatory courses:
Yes. We encourage more methods courses (a methods certificate can be additionally earned).

GRE mean
Verbal 500   Quantitative 570

GPA mean
Overall 3.5

Number of applications/admission offers/incoming students in 2007
20 applied/6 admission offers/6 incoming

% of students receiving:
Full tuition waiver only: 100%
Assistantship/fellowship only: 0%
Both full tuition waiver & assistantship/fellowship: 80%

Approximate percentage of incoming students with a B.A./B.S. only: 0% **Master's:** 100%

Approximate percentage of students who are Women: 70% **Ethnic Minority:** 50% **International:** 15%

Average years to complete the doctoral program (including internship): 4.8 years

Personal interview
Preferred in person but telephone acceptable; telephone required

Attrition rate in past 7 years: 2%

What percentage of students applying for internship last year was accepted into APPIC or APA internships? 25%

Formal tracks/concentrations: not reported

Research areas	# Faculty	# Grants
aboriginal approaches to healing	3	7
anxiety in other cultures	2	2
Asian approaches to counseling	1	2
assessment in rehabilitation	1	1
counseling process	1	0
ethics	1	0
career development	4	4
infertility	1	0
stress and coping	1	2
trauma	3	3
women's sexuality	2	1

Clinical opportunities
Not reported

Colorado State University (Ph.D.)
Department of Psychology
Fort Collins, CO 80523
phone#: (970) 491-6363
e-mail: jmoran@lamar.colostate.edu
Web address:
www.colostate.edu/Depts/Psychology/counseling/

1	2	**3**	4	5	6	7
Practice oriented		Equal emphasis			Research oriented	

Percentage of faculty subscribing to each of the following orientations:

Psychodynamic/Psychoanalytic	0%
Applied behavioral analysis/Radical behavioral	0%
Family systems/Systems	0%
Existential/Phenomenological/Humanistic	0%
Cognitive/Cognitive-behavioral	70%

Courses required for incoming students to have completed prior to enrolling: none

Recommended but not mandatory courses:
learning, personality, history and systems, developmental, abnormal, statistics

GRE mean
Verbal 592   Quantitative 692
Advanced Psychology not required
Analytical Writing 4.8

GPA mean
Overall GPA 3.87

Number of applications/admission offers/incoming students in 2007
211 applied/20 admission offers/10 incoming

% of students receiving:
Full tuition waiver only: 0%
Assistantship/fellowship only: 0%
Both full tuition waiver & assistantship/fellowship: 0%
Both half tuition waiver & assistantship/fellowship: 100%

Approximate percentage of incoming students with a B.A./B.S. only: 90%   Master's: 10%

Approximate percentage of students who are Women: 90%   Ethnic Minority: 10% International: 0%

Average years to complete the doctoral program (including internship): 5 years

Personal interview
No interview required

Attrition rate in past 7 years: 0%

Percentage of students applying for internship last year accepted into APPIC or APA internships: 100%

Formal tracks/concentrations: none

Research areas	# Faculty	# Grants
ADHD	1	0
adolescents	3	5
aggression (anger research and reduction)	1	0
aging/geriatrics	3	0
anxiety (reduction)	1	0
assessment (including multicultural)	3	0
body image beating disturbances	1	0
child		
cognitive	5	1
college teaching	1	0
educational outcomes	1	1
emotional disorders	1	0
ethics	1	0

health psychology	8	4
interpersonal relationships	1	0
learning disabilities	1	0
men	1	0
multicultural	6	3
parent–child interaction	1	0
psychopathology	3	0
psychotherapy process	1	0
stress and coping processes	2	0
substance abuse	4	3
supervision and training	2	0
violence/abuse	2	0
vocational psychology	2	0
women	3	1

Clinical opportunities

family stress center	juvenile detention facility
inpatient psychiatry	neuropsychology practice
university counseling center	community college counseling
primary care	

Teacher's College–Columbia University (Ph.D.)

Department of Counseling and Clinical Psychology
New York, NY 10027
phone#: (212) 678-3257
e-mail: miville@exchange.tc.columbia.edu
Web address:
devweb.tc.columbia.edu/academic/CCP/CounPsych/
proginfo.asp?Id=programinfo=Degree+Requerments

1	2	3	4	**5**	6	7

Practice oriented   Equal emphasis   Research oriented

Percentage of faculty subscribing to each of the following orientations:

Psychodynamic/Psychoanalytic	5%
Applied behavioral analysis/Radical behavioral	10%
Family systems/Systems	40%
Existential/Phenomenological/Humanistic	35%
Cognitive/Cognitive-behavioral	25%
Multicultural/Diversity	75%

Courses required for incoming students to have completed prior to enrolling:
Bachelor's, but master's degree preferred

Recommended but not mandatory courses:
Not reported

GRE mean
Verbal 570   Quantitative 570
Analytical Writing not reported

GPA mean
Overall GPA 3.75

Number of applications/admission offers/incoming students in 2007
215 applied/9 admission offers/6 incoming

% of students receiving:
Full tuition waiver only: 100%
Assistantship/fellowship only: 25%
Both full tuition waiver & assistantship/fellowship: 75%

Approximate percentage of incoming students with a B.A./B.S. only: 10%   **Master's:** 90%

Approximate percentage of students who are Women: 100%   **Ethnic Minority:** 67%
International: not reported

Average years to complete the doctoral program (including internship): 6.5 years

Personal interview
Required in person

Attrition rate in past 7 years: 15%

Percentage of students applying for internship last year accepted into APPIC or APA internships: 75%

Formal tracks/concentrations: none

Research areas	# Faculty	# Grants
cognition and stereotypes		
cultural competence		
immigration		
multicultural counseling		
prevention		
racism and racial identity	2	0
sexual harassment	1	0
women and leadership	1	0

Clinical opportunities
Not reported

University of Denver (Ph.D.)

College of Education
Denver, CO 80208
phone#: (303) 871-2484
e-mail: mriva@du.edu
Web address:
www.du.edu/education/academicPrograms/cnp/

1	2	3	**4**	5	6	7
Practice oriented		Equal emphasis			Research oriented	

Percentage of faculty subscribing to each of the following orientations:
Psychodynamic/Psychoanalytic   25%
Applied behavioral analysis/Radical behavioral   0%
Family systems/Systems   15%
Existential/Phenomenological/Humanistic   25%
Cognitive/Cognitive-behavioral   35%

Courses required for incoming students to have completed prior to enrolling: None

Recommended but not mandatory courses:
Learning, personality, statistics

GRE mean
Verbal 600   Quantitative 600
Analytical Writing 4.7

GPA mean
Overall GPA 3.5

Number of applications/admission offers/incoming students in 2007
95 applied/12 admission offers/7 incoming

% of students receiving:
Full tuition waiver only: 30%
Assistantship/fellowship only: 60%
Both full tuition waiver & assistantship/fellowship: 10%

Approximate percentage of incoming students with a B.A./B.S. only: 0%   **Master's:** 100%

Approximate percentage of students who are Women: 80%   **Ethnic Minority:** 20%

Average years to complete the doctoral program (including internship): 5 years

Personal interview
Preferred in person but telephone acceptable

Attrition rate in past 7 years: not reported

Percentage of students applying for internship last year accepted into APPIC or APA internships: 100%

Formal tracks/concentrations: none

Research areas	# Faculty	# Grants
PTSD	1	1
social support	1	1
ethics	1	0
group counseling	1	0
multicultural counseling	1	1
job satisfaction in work settings	1	1

Clinical opportunities
placements working with racial/ethnic minorities
counseling centers
hospital settings
mental health centers
Veteran Administration Hospital
conducting counseling groups
psychological/neuropsychological assessment

University of Florida (Ph.D.)

Department of Psychology
Gainesville, FL 32611
phone#: (352) 392-0601
e-mail: kgr1@ufl.edu
Web address: www.psych.ufl.edu/

1	2	3	4	**5**	6	7
Practice oriented		Equal emphasis			Research oriented	

Percentage of faculty subscribing to each of the following orientations:
Psychodynamic/Psychoanalytic   0%
Applied behavioral analysis/Radical behavioral   0%
Family systems/Systems   25%
Existential/Phenomenological/Humanistic   25%
Cognitive/Cognitive-behavioral   50%

Courses required for incoming students to have completed prior to enrolling:
Undergraduate 4-year degree in psychology or related field

Recommended but not mandatory courses:
Statistics, research design/methods, personality, abnormal

GRE mean
Verbal 573   Quantitative 667
Analytical Writing not reported
Advanced Psychology not used

GPA mean
Overall GPA 3.8   Psychology GPA 3.9
Junior/Senior GPA 3.8

Number of applications/admission offers/incoming students in 2007
157 applied/7 admission offers/6 incoming

% of students receiving:
Full tuition waiver only: 0%
Assistantship/fellowship only: 0%
Both full tuition waiver & assistantship/fellowship: 100%

Approximate percentage of incoming students with a B.A./B.S. only: 50%   **Master's:** 50%

Approximate percentage of students who are Women: 57%   **Ethnic Minority:** 24%   **International:** 16%

Average years to complete the doctoral program (including internship): 6 years

Personal interview
Preferred in person but telephone acceptable

Attrition rate in past 7 years: 10%

Percentage of students applying for internship last year accepted into APPIC or APA internships: 100%

Formal tracks/concentrations: none

Research areas	# Faculty	# Grants
health psychology	2	1
constructivist psychology	1	0
discrimination/stigma	1	0
eating disorders	1	0
elderly	1	0
gender and emotion	1	1
mental health of minority clients	1	0
personality and mental health	1	0
sexual orientation	1	0
women	1	0

Clinical opportunities
anxiety disorder clinic
career counseling center
community mental health
crisis intervention center
domestic violence clinic
family medical practice
forensics hospital
hospice
nursing facility
pediatric/psychiatric
  assessment and treatment
prison
rural health care clinic
sexual offender
substance abuse clinic
university counseling center

Fordham University (Ph.D.)

Division of Psychological and Educational Services
Graduate School of Education
113 West 60th Street
New York, NY 10023
phone#: (212) 636-6460
e-mail: mjackson@fordham.edu
Web address: www.fordham.edu/gse

1	2	3	**4**	5	6	7
Practice oriented			Equal emphasis			Research oriented

Percentage of faculty subscribing to each of the following orientations:

Psychodynamic/Psychoanalytic	35%
Applied behavioral analysis/Radical behavioral	20%
Family systems/Systems	16%
Existential/Phenomenological/Humanistic	60%
Cognitive/Cognitive-behavioral	100%

Courses required for incoming students to have completed prior to enrolling:
15 credits in psychology, developmental, experimental, abnormal, personality

Recommended but not mandatory courses:
Qualitative research methods

GRE mean
Verbal 574   Quantitative 610
Analytical Writing 4.4

GPA mean
Overall GPA 3.7

Number of applications/admission offers/incoming students in 2007
103 applied/21 admission offers/12 incoming

% of students receiving:
Full tuition waiver only: 0%
Assistantship/fellowship only: 50%
Both full tuition waiver & assistantship/fellowship: 1%

Approximate percentage of incoming students with a B.A./B.S. only: 50%   **Master's:** 50%

Approximate percentage of students who are Women: 66%   **Ethnic Minority:** 33%   **International:** 11%

Average years to complete the doctoral program (including internship): 7 years

Personal interview
Preferred in person but telephone acceptable

Attrition rate in past 7 years: 8%

Percentage of students applying for internship last year accepted into APPIC or APA internships: 84%

Formal tracks/concentrations: none

Research areas	# Faculty	# Grants
career development	3	1
criminal behavior	1	1
health psychology	2	1
multicultural counseling	5	0
supervision	3	2

Clinical opportunities
college counseling centers
community mental health centers
on-campus clinical/research center
psychological services institute

University of Georgia (Ph.D.)

Department of Counseling and Human Development Services
Athens, GA 30602
phone#: (706) 542-1812
e-mail: edelgado@uga.edu
Web address:
www.coe.uga.edu/chds/counselingpsych/index.html

1	2	3	**4**	5	6	7

Practice oriented	Equal emphasis	Research oriented

Percentage of faculty subscribing to each of the following orientations:

Psychodynamic/Psychoanalytic	20%
Applied behavioral analysis/Radical behavioral	0%
Family systems/Systems	20%
Existential/Phenomenological/Humanistic	10%
Cognitive/Cognitive-behavioral	50%

Courses required for incoming students to have completed prior to enrolling:
Research methods, statistics, interpersonal relationships, individual assessment, vocational development, theories of counseling, individual counseling practicum, group counseling, multicultural counseling (master's degree required)

Recommended but not mandatory courses: None

GRE mean
Verbal + Quantitative 1100
Analytical Writing 3.5

GPA mean
Overall GPA undergraduate 3.0 Graduate 3.5

Number of applications/admission offers/incoming students in 2007
90 applied/20 admission offers/11 incoming

% of students receiving:
Full tuition waiver only: 0%
Assistantship/fellowship only: 0%
Both full tuition waiver & assistantship/fellowship: 100%

Approximate percentage of incoming students with a B.A./B.S. only: 0%   **Master's:** 100%

Approximate percentage of students who are Women: 75%   **Ethnic Minority:** 45%   **International:** 8%

Average years to complete the doctoral program (including internship): 4 years

Personal interview
Preferred in person

Attrition rate in past 7 years: 11%

Percentage of students applying for internship last year accepted into APPIC or APA internships: 80%

Formal tracks/concentrations: marriage and family therapy, supervision, psychological assessment (learning disabilities)

Research areas	# Faculty	# Grants
accident trauma	1	0
attributions and therapy	2	0
empowering schools	2	1
juvenile delinquency/aggression	2	2
men's development/gender	1	0
minority male adolescents	1	1
multicultural counseling	3	2
preventing violence and aggression in schools	2	3
school counselor education	2	0
substance abuse	1	0
young adult development	2	0

Clinical opportunities

adolescents	juvenile offenders
college students	school-age children
departmental captive clinic	supervision
homeless shelter	

Georgia State University (Ph.D.)

Department of Counseling and Psychological Services
Atlanta, GA 30303
phone#: (404) 651-2550
e-mail: bchung@gsu.edu
Web address: education.gsu.edu/cps/781.html

1	2	3	**4**	5	6	7

Practice oriented	Equal emphasis	Research oriented

Percentage of faculty subscribing to each of the following orientations:

Psychodynamic/Psychoanalytic	33%
Applied behavioral analysis/Radical behavioral	0%
Family systems/Systems	0%
Existential/Phenomenological/Humanistic	33%
Cognitive/Cognitive-behavioral	33%

Courses required for incoming students to have completed prior to enrolling:
M.A. in counseling or clinical psychology

Recommended but not mandatory courses: None

GRE mean
Verbal 550   Quantitative 600
Advanced Psychology not reported
Analytical Writing 4.9

GPA mean
Overall GPA 3.6

Number of applications/admission offers/incoming students in 2007
66 applied/8 admission offers/7 incoming

% of students receiving:
Full tuition waiver only: 0%
Assistantship/fellowship only: 0%
Both full tuition waiver & assistantship/fellowship: 100%

Approximate percentage of incoming students with a B.A./B.S. only: 0%   **Master's:** 100%

Approximate percentage of students who are Women: 80%   **Ethnic Minority:** 40%   **International:** 8%

Average years to complete the doctoral program (including internship): 5 years

Personal interview
Preferred in person but telephone acceptable

Attrition rate in past 7 years: 0.05%

Percentage of students applying for internship last year accepted into APPIC or APA internships: 100%

Formal tracks/concentrations: none

Research areas	# Faculty	# Grants
career development	1	0
forensics	1	0
gender/multicultural	2	0
stress/coping	2	1
traumatology	1	0
rehabilitation	1	0
consultation	1	1

Clinical opportunities

behavioral medicine	multicultural counseling
college counseling	stress management
forensic	

University of Houston (Ph.D.)

Counseling Psychology Program
Houston, TX 77004-5874
phone#: (713) 743-5019
e-mail: epsy@uh.edu
Web address: www.coe.uh.edu/degrees.cfm?ID=28

1	2	3	4	**5**	6	7
Practice oriented		Equal emphasis				Research oriented

Percentage of faculty subscribing to each of the following orientations:

Psychodynamic/Psychoanalytic	25%
Applied behavioral analysis/Radical behavioral	0%
Family systems/Systems	25%
Existential/Phenomenological/Humanistic	25%
Cognitive/Cognitive-behavioral	25%

Courses required for incoming students to have completed prior to enrolling: None

Recommended but not mandatory courses: None

GRE mean
Verbal 530   Quantitative 620
Analytical Writing 4.5

GPA mean
Overall master's GPA 3.5

Number of applications/admission offers/incoming students in 2007
60 applied/13 admission offers/6 incoming

% of students receiving:
Full tuition waiver only: 0%
Assistantship/fellowship only: 14%
Both full tuition waiver & assistantship/fellowship: 86%

Approximate percentage of incoming students with a B.A./B.S. only: 16%   **Master's:** 84%

Approximate percentage of students who are Women: 85%   **Ethnic Minority:** 34%   **International:** 0%

Average years to complete the doctoral program (including internship): 6 years

Personal interview
Preferred in person but telephone acceptable

Attrition rate in past 7 years: 10%

Percentage of students applying for internship last year accepted into APPIC or APA internships: 90%

Formal tracks/concentrations: none

Research areas	# Faculty	# Grants
adult attachment/adult survivors of childhood trauma	2	1
career counseling/ cross-cultural counseling	2	0
children/adolescents disorders	1	1
gender identity in men	1	0
mental health policy	1	0
telehealth	2	0
racial identity	2	1
group therapy	1	1

Clinical opportunities

child guidance center	chronic inpatient
family therapy	behavioral medicine
crisis intervention program	forensics
university counseling center	posttraumatic stress disorder
VA hospital	school districts
substance abuse	medical schools
gerontology	pediatric hospitals

Howard University (Ph.D.) (2006 data)

School of Education
2441 Fourth Street, NW
Washington DC 20059
phone#: (202) 806-7351 or (202) 806-7350
e-mail: adferguson@howard.edu
Web address: www.howard.edu/schooleducation/
Departments/HDPES/CPsychology/index.htm

1	2	3	**4**	5	6	7

Clinically oriented   Equal emphasis   Research oriented

Percentage of faculty subscribing to each of the following orientations:

Psychodynamic/Psychoanalytic	0%
Applied behavioral analysis/Radical behavioral	0%
Family systems/Systems	0%
Existential/Phenomenological/Humanistic	50%
Cognitive/Cognitive-behavioral	50%

Courses required for incoming students to have completed prior to enrolling:

Equivalent of Howard University Counseling Psychology master's (48–52 credit hours) or undergraduate degree in psychology.

Recommended but not mandatory courses:

Evaluated on a case-by-case basis based on above criteria.

GRE mean

Verbal 477.5   Quantitative 535
Analytical 506.5
Analytical Writing not reported

GPA mean

Overall master's GPA 3.8

Number of applications/admission offers/incoming students in 2005

12 applied/5 admission offers/4 incoming

% of students receiving:

Full tuition waiver only: 2%
Assistantship/fellowship only: 2%
Both full tuition waiver & assistantship/fellowship: 2%

Approximate percentage of incoming students with a B.A./B.S. only: 0%   Master's: 100%

Approximate percentage of students who are Women: 95%   Ethnic Minority: 100%

International: not reported

Average years to complete the doctoral program (including internship): 5 years

Personal interview

Required in person; but telephone acceptable for overseas candidates

Attrition rate in past 7 years: not reported

Percentage of students applying for internship last year accepted into APPIC or APA internships: 75%

Formal tracks/concentrations: none

Research areas	# Faculty	# Grants
addiction among African American and Bedouin Arabs	3	1
hope in counseling	1	0
multicultural competencies	1	1
racism stress	1	1
spirituality in counseling	2	0
videotapes in training	1	1
worldview, racial identity and self-efficacy	1	0

Clinical opportunities

Howard University (HU) Cancer Center
HU Center on Sickle Cell Anemia
HU Genome Center
HU Student Counseling Center

University of Illinois at Urbana–Champaign (Ph.D.)

Department of Educational Psychology
Champaign, IL 61820
phone#: (888) 843-3779
e-mail: hneville@uiuc.edu
Web address:
www.ed.uiuc.edu/edpsy/programs/phd.html

1	2	3	4	5	**6**	7

Practice oriented   Equal emphasis   Research oriented

Percentage of faculty subscribing to each of the following orientations:

Psychodynamic/Psychoanalytic	0%
Applied behavioral analysis/Radical behavioral	0%
Family systems/Systems	0%
Existential/Phenomenological/Humanistic	0%
Cognitive/Cognitive-behavioral	0%
Eclectic	100%

Courses required for incoming students to have completed prior to enrolling: None

Recommended but not mandatory courses:

Undergraduate psychology degree

GRE mean

Verbal 607   Quantitative 683
Analytical Writing not reported

GPA mean

Overall GPA 3.81

Number of applications/admission offers/incoming students in 2007

65 applied/4 admission offers/3 incoming

% of students receiving:

Full tuition waiver only: 0%
Assistantship/fellowship only: 0%
Both full tuition waiver & assistantship/fellowship: 100%

Approximate percentage of incoming students who entered with a B.A./B.S. only: 47%   Master's: 53%

Approximate percentage of students who are Women: 77%   Ethnic Minority: 32%   International:

Average years to complete the doctoral program (including internship): 6.5 years

Personal interview

Preferred in person but telephone acceptable

Attrition rate in past 7 years: not reported

Percentage of students applying for internship last year accepted into APPIC or APA internships: 100%

Formal tracks/concentrations: none

Research areas	# Faculty	# Grants
cancer control	1	1
cancer survivorship	1	1
eating disorders	1	0
ethnic/racial identity	2	0
Latina populations	1	1
personality assessment	1	1
racial and sexual violence	2	0
racism	2	3
vocational psychology	2	1

Clinical opportunities

child/adolescent
health psychology
mental health counseling
rehabilitation counseling
undergraduate counseling

VA medical center
medical/hospital
community mental health

Indiana State University (Ph.D.)

Department of Counseling
Terre Haute, IN 47809
phone#: (812) 237-2870
e-mail: jcampbell2@isugw.indstate.edu
Web address: counseling.indstate.edu/dcp/
default.htm

1	2	**3**	4	5	6	7

Practice oriented · Equal emphasis · Research oriented

Percentage of faculty subscribing to each of the following orientations:

Psychodynamic/Psychoanalytic	0%
Applied behavioral analysis/Radical behavioral	0%
Family systems/Systems	40%
Existential/Phenomenological/Humanistic	40%
Cognitive/Cognitive-behavioral	40%

Courses required for incoming students to have completed prior to enrolling:
Master's degree in counseling/psychology, including graduate courses in techniques of counseling, practicum, psychological assessment, and career development

Recommended but not mandatory courses:
Not reported

GRE mean
Not reported

GPA mean
Not reported

Number of applications/admission offers/incoming students in 2007
32 applied/11 admission offers/8 incoming

% of students receiving:
Full tuition waiver only: 0%
Assistantship/fellowship only: 0%
Both full tuition waiver & assistantship/fellowship: 100%

Approximate percentage of incoming students with a B.A./B.S. only: 0%   **Master's:** 100%

Approximate percentage of students who are
Women: 67%   **Ethnic Minority:** 29%   **International:** 10%

Average years to complete the doctoral program (including internship): 4.8 years

Personal interview
Preferred in person but telephone acceptable

Attrition rate in past 7 years: 5%

Percentage of students applying for internship last year accepted into APPIC or APA internships: 88%

Formal tracks/concentrations: none

Research areas	# Faculty	# Grants
AIDS/HIV	1	0
vocational assessment	2	0
counseling/supervision process	3	0
family therapy	3	1
health psychology	1	0
men's studies	2	0
personality assessment	1	0
program evaluation	1	0
psychology philosophy	1	0
school counseling	1	1
values/learning skills	1	0

Clinical opportunities

community mental health
 centers
local hospitals
marriage and family clinics

corrections
university counseling center
VA medical center

Indiana University (Ph.D.)

Department of Counseling and Educational Psychology
Wright Education Building, Room 4003
Bloomington, IN 47405
phone#: (812) 856-8300
e-mail: cep@indiana.edu
Web address:
www.indiana.edu/~counsel/cphdhome.html

1	2	3	**4**	5	6	7

Practice oriented · Equal emphasis · Research oriented

Percentage of faculty subscribing to each of the following orientations:

Psychodynamic/Psychoanalytic	0%
Applied behavioral analysis/Radical behavioral	0%
Family systems/Systems	30%
Existential/Phenomenological/Humanistic	30%
Cognitive/Cognitive-behavioral	40%

Courses required for incoming students to have completed prior to enrolling: None

Recommended but not mandatory courses:
Statistics and research methods

GRE mean
Verbal 600   Quantitative 614
Analytical Writing 4.81

GPA mean
Overall Undergraduate GPA 3.48
Overall Graduate GPA 3.87

Number of applications/admission offers/incoming students in 2007
Not reported

% of students receiving:
Full tuition waiver only: 0%
Assistantship/fellowship only: 0%
Both full tuition waiver & assistantship/fellowship: 100%

Approximate percentage of incoming students with a B.A./B.S. only: 10% **Master's:** 90%

Approximate percentage of incoming students who are Women: 75% **Ethnic Minority:** 11% **International:** 22%

Average years to complete the doctoral program (including internship): 4 years

Personal interview
Preferred in person but telephone acceptable

Attrition rate in past 7 years: 1.1%

Percentage of students applying for internship last year accepted into APPIC or APA internships: 100%

Formal tracks/concentrations: none

Research areas	# Faculty	# Grants
at-risk youth	1	2
counselor training	5	0
elementary school counseling	2	1
group counseling	2	0
human sexuality	0	0
marriage/family counseling	2	3
multicultural counseling	2	0
women's vocational behavior	1	0

Clinical opportunities
Not reported

University of Iowa (Ph.D.)

Division of Psychological and Quantitative
Foundations
Iowa City, IA 52242
phone#: (319) 335-5295
e-mail: william-liu@uiowa.edu
Web address: www.education.uiowa.edu/counspsy/

1	2	3	4	5	6	7
Practice oriented		Equal emphasis			Research oriented	

Percentage of faculty subscribing to each of the following orientations:

Psychodynamic/Psychoanalytic	25%
Applied behavioral analysis/Radical behavioral	0%
Family systems/Systems	25%
Existential/Phenomenological/Humanistic	0%
Cognitive/Cognitive-behavioral	50%

Courses required for incoming students to have completed prior to enrolling:
None

Recommended but not mandatory courses:
As much core psychology as possible

GRE mean
Verbal 519   Quantitative 625
Analytical Writing 5.0

GPA mean
Overall GPA 3.58

Number of applications/admission offers/incoming students in 2007
90 applied/10 admission offers/7 incoming

% of students receiving:
Full tuition waiver only: 0%
Assistantship/fellowship only: 40%
Both full tuition waiver & assistantship/fellowship: 60%

Approximate percentage of incoming students with a B.A./B.S. only: 25% **Master's:** 75%

Approximate percentage of students who are Women: 67% **Ethnic Minority:** 35% **International:** 2%

Average years to complete the doctoral program (including internship): 7 years

Personal interview
Interview required

Attrition rate in past 7 years: 5%

Percentage of students applying for internship last year accepted into APPIC or APA internships: 50%

Formal tracks/concentrations: none

Research areas	# Faculty	# Grants
child/adolescent health	1	1
college student suicide	1	0
ethics	2	1
multicultural	2	1
psychosocial oncology	2	1
public health	2	0
men	3	0
spirituality	2	0
mood and anxiety disorders	1	0
career	1	1

Clinical opportunities

community mental health	university counseling
hospitals	centers
specialty settings	VA medical center
prisons	women's center
public schools	homeless shelter

Iowa State University (Ph.D.)

Department of Psychology
Ames, IA 50011-3180
phone#: (515) 294-1743
e-mail: nascott@iastate.edu
Web address: www.psychology.iastate.edu

1	2	3	4	**5**	6	7
Practice oriented		Equal emphasis				Research oriented

Percentage of faculty subscribing to each of the following orientations:

Psychodynamic/Psychoanalytic   0%
Applied behavioral analysis/Radical behavioral   0%
Family systems/Systems   20%
Existential/Phenomenological/Humanistic   20%
Cognitive/Cognitive-behavioral   60%

Courses required for incoming students to have completed prior to enrolling:

A minimum of 15 credits in psychology, including statistics, psychological measurement, abnormal, developmental, social, and research methods

Recommended but not mandatory courses:

Brain and behavior, learning/cognition; most successful applicants have a diversified psychology major

GRE mean

Verbal 579   Quantitative 702
Advanced Psychology 706
Analytical Writing 4.79

GPA mean

Overall GPA 3.78   Psychology GPA 3.87
Junior/Senior GPA 3.87

Number of applications/admission offers/incoming students in 2007

68 applied/7 admission offers/5 incoming

% of students receiving:

Full tuition waiver only: 0%
Assistantship/fellowship only: 0%
Both full tuition waiver & assistantship/fellowship: 100%

Approximate percentage of incoming students with a B.A./B.S. only 40%   **Master's:** 60%

Approximate percentage of students who are Women: 77%   **Ethnic Minority:** 7%
International: 13%

Average years to complete the doctoral program (including internship): 6 years

Personal interview

Preferred in person but telephone acceptable

Attrition rate in past 7 years: 0%

Percentage of students applying for internship last year accepted into APPIC or APA internships: 100%

Formal tracks/concentrations: None

Research areas	# Faculty	# Grants
attachment and adjustment of international students	1	0
attachment and discrimination	1	0
ethics and legal issues	1	0
gender roles	1	1
multicultural	1	0
psychology and religion	1	1
assessment with sex offenders	1	1

social support	1	1
women in science	1	1
vocational interest assessment	2	0

Clinical opportunities

ADHD assessment clinic
community mental health center
mental health unit
private group practices
university counseling center
VA medical center
Youth and Shelter Services Agency

University of Kansas (Ph.D.)

Department of Psychology and Research in Education
Counseling Psychology Program
Lawrence, KS 66045
phone#: (785) 864-3931
e-mail: preadmit@ku.edu
Web address: soe.ku.edu/pre/cpsy/

1	2	3	**4**	5	6	7
Practice oriented		Equal emphasis				Research oriented

Percentage of faculty subscribing to each of the following orientations:

Psychodynamic/Psychoanalytic   30%
Applied behavioral analysis/Radical behavioral   0%
Family systems/Systems   20%
Existential/Phenomenological/Humanistic   30%
Cognitive/Cognitive-behavioral   60%

Courses required for incoming students to have completed prior to enrolling: None

Recommended but not mandatory courses:

Basic courses in psychology (e.g., social, personality, abnormal, experimental)

GRE mean

Verbal 544   Quantitative 614
Advanced Psychology not required
Analytical Writing 4.7

GPA mean

Overall GPA 3.65

Number of applications/admission offers/incoming students in 2007

70 applied/11 admission offers/8 incoming

% of students receiving:

Full tuition waiver only: 0%
Assistantship/fellowship only: 12%
Both full tuition waiver & assistantship/fellowship: 75%

Approximate percentage of incoming students with a B.A./B.S. only: 63%   **Master's:** 37%

Approximate percentage of students who are Women: 63%   **Ethnic Minority:** 12%   **International:** 0%

Average years to complete the doctoral program (including internship): 6.1 years

Personal interview

Required in person or by phone

Attrition rate in past 7 years: 10%

Percentage of students applying for internship last year accepted into APPIC or APA internships: 100%

Formal tracks/concentrations: none

Research areas	# Faculty	# Grants
creativity	1	1
positive psychology	3	1
therapy outcome and process	1	0
vocational decision making	1	2
women and science careers	3	1

Clinical opportunities
Not reported

University of Kentucky (Ph.D.)

Department of Educational and Counseling Psychology
Lexington, KY 40506
phone#: (606) 257-7881
e-mail: westil3@pop.uky.edu
Web address:
www.uky.edu/Education/EDP/counphd.html

1	2	3	4	5	**6**	7
Practice oriented		Equal emphasis			Research oriented	

Percentage of faculty subscribing to each of the following orientations:

Psychodynamic/Psychoanalytic	0%
Applied behavioral analysis/Radical behavioral	30%
Family systems/Systems	20%
Existential/Phenomenological/Humanistic	10%
Cognitive/Cognitive-behavioral	40%

Courses required for incoming students to have completed prior to enrolling: None

Recommended but not mandatory courses:
Prefer master's degree in behavioral science

GRE mean
Verbal + Quantitative 1100
Analytical Writing not reported

GPA mean
Overall GPA 3.4   Psychology GPA 3.6
Junior/Senior GPA 3.5

Number of applications/admission offers/incoming students in 2007
43 applied/10 admission offers/6 incoming

% of students receiving:
Full tuition waiver only: 0%
Assistantship/fellowship only: 45%
Both full tuition waiver & assistantship/fellowship: 25%

Approximate percentage of incoming students with a B.A./B.S. only: 0%   **Master's:** 100%

Approximate percentage of students who are Women: 60%   **Ethnic Minority:** 25%   **International:** 0%

Average years to complete the doctoral program (including internship): 5.1 years

Personal interview
Preferred in person but telephone acceptable

Attrition rate in past 7 years: not reported

Percentage of students applying for internship last year accepted into APPIC or APA internships: 90%

Formal tracks/concentrations: Each student required to create a specialization.

Research areas	# Faculty	# Grants
behavioral	2	1
family	2	0
gender	2	1
multicultural	2	0

Clinical opportunities
community mental health   residential treatment facility
counseling center   rural mental health centers
federal prison   VA hospital

Lehigh University (Ph.D.)

Counseling Psychology, School Psychology, and Special Education
Bethlehem, PA 18015-4792
phone#: (610) 758-3250
e-mail: ars1@lehigh.edu
Web address:
www.lehigh.edu/collegeofeducation/degree_programs/
counseling_psych/degrees/phd/phd_philosophy.htm

1	2	3	**4**	5	6	7
Practice oriented		Equal emphasis			Research oriented	

Percentage of faculty subscribing to each of the following orientations:

Psychodynamic/Psychoanalytic	25%
Applied behavioral analysis/Radical behavioral	0%
Family systems/Systems	25%
Existential/Phenomenological/Humanistic	25%
Cognitive/Cognitive-behavioral	25%

Courses required for incoming students to have completed prior to enrolling: None

Recommended but not mandatory courses:
Psychology related

GRE mean
Verbal 540   Quantitative 587
Analytical Writing not reported

GPA mean
Overall GPA 3.7

Number of applications/admission offers/incoming students in 2007
78 applied/8 admission offers/4 incoming

% of students receiving:
Full tuition waiver only: 20%
Assistantship/fellowship only: 0%
Both full tuition waiver & assistantship/fellowship: 80%

Approximate percentage of incoming students with a B.A./B.S. only: 50%   **Master's:** 50%

Approximate percentage of students who are Women: 70%   **Ethnic Minority:** 40%
International: not reported

Average years to complete the doctoral program (including internship): 6 years

Personal interview
Preferred in person but telephone acceptable

Attrition rate in past 7 years: not reported

Percentage of students applying for internship last year accepted into APPIC or APA internships: 100%

Formal tracks/concentrations: none

Research areas	# Faculty	# Grants
cross-cultural	1	1
family systems	1	1
supervision/training	1	1
vocational psychology	1	1

Clinical opportunities
not reported

Louisiana Tech University (Ph.D.)

Department of Psychology and Behavioral Sciences
P.O. Box 10048
Ruston, LA 71272
phone#: (318) 257-4315
e-mail: dthomas@latech.edu
Web address: www.latech.edu/tech/education/
psychology/cphd/index.php

1	2	3	**4**	5	6	7
Practice oriented		Equal emphasis			Research oriented	

Percentage of faculty subscribing to each of the following orientations:
Psychodynamic/Psychoanalytic   10%
Applied behavioral analysis/Radical behavioral   0%
Family systems/Systems   20%
Existential/Phenomenological/Humanistic   20%
Cognitive/Cognitive-behavioral   50%

Courses required for incoming students prior to enrolling: None

Courses recommended but not mandatory:
None

GRE mean
Verbal 520   Quantitative 610
Analytical Writing not used for admission purposes

GPA mean
Overall GPA 3.6

Number of applications/admission offers/incoming students in 2007
32 applied/8 admission offers/7 incoming

% of students receiving:
Full tuition waiver only: 0%
Assistantship/fellowship only: 95%
Both full tuition waiver & assistantship/fellowship: 5%

Approximate percentage of incoming students with a B.A./B.S. only: 60%   **Master's:** 40%

Approximate percentage of students who are Women: 85%   **Ethnic Minority:** 15%   **International:** 0%

Average years to complete the doctoral program (including internship): 5–6 years

Personal interview
In-person interview strongly preferred; telephone acceptable

Attrition rate in past 7 years: 16%

Percentage of students applying for internship last year accepted into APPIC or APA internships: 50%

Formal tracks/concentrations: none

Research areas	# Faculty	# Grants
career development	1	0
family therapy and child custody	1	0
lesbian/gay/bisexual	0	0
relationships & gender roles	1	0
body image	1	0
psychological reactance theory	1	0
sleep and academic performance	1	0

Clinical opportunities
children's home   medical center
community health centers   prison settings
developmental center   university counseling center
in-house clinic   VA medical centers

University of Louisville (Ph.D.)

Department of Educational and Counseling Psychology
Louisville, KY 40292
phone#: (502) 852-6884
e-mail: kathleen.kirby@gmail.com
Web address: www.louisville.edu/education/degrees/
phd-cps-counselingpsychology.html

1	2	3	**4**	5	6	7
Practice oriented		Equal emphasis			Research oriented	

Percentage of faculty subscribing to each of the following orientations:
Psychodynamic/Psychoanalytic   37%
Applied behavioral analysis/Radical behavioral   30%
Family systems/Systems   20%
Existential/Phenomenological/Humanistic   3%
Cognitive/Cognitive-behavioral   100%

Courses required for incoming students to have completed prior to enrolling:
abnormal, development, statistics or methodology, social

Recommended but not mandatory courses:
Psycholinguistics, sociology, anthropology, psychology, biology, physiology, ABA

GRE mean
Verbal 580   Quantitative 634
Analytical Writing not reported

GPA mean
Overall master's GPA 3.9

Number of applications/admission offers/incoming students in 2007
49 applied/10 admission offers/8 incoming

% of incoming students receiving:
Full tuition waiver only: 0%
Assistantship/fellowship only: 0%
Both full tuition waiver & assistantship/fellowship: 100%

Approximate percentage of incoming students with a B.A./B.S. only: 50%   **Master's:** 50%

Approximate percentage of students who are Women: 75%   **Ethnic Minority:** 12.5%
International: 12.5%

Average years to complete the doctoral program (including internship): 5.2 years entering with master's; 7 years entering with bachelors

Personal interview
No preference given

Attrition rate in past 7 years: 17%

Percentage of students applying for internship last year accepted into APPIC or APA internships: 89%

Formal tracks/concentrations: none

Research areas	# Faculty	# Grants
divorce adjustment	1	2
drug and alcohol abuse	2	1
evolutionary psychology	2	0
GBLT	1	1
school adjustment of special populations	1	0
school violence	1	2
stress and parenting	1	0
positive psychology	1	3
prevention-school based	3	5
AD/HD	2	15

Clinical opportunities

developmental disabilities
child treatment
college counseling center
school-based services
sex offender treatment
hospital based services
health psychology

healthy lifestyle/positive psychology
group interventions
prison settings
psychological assessment/ neuropsychology
vocational psychology

Loyola University of Chicago (Ph.D.)

School of Education
820 North Michigan Avenue
Chicago, IL 60611

phone#: (312) 915-6836
e-mail: sspeigh@luc.edu
Web address: www.luc.edu/education/academics _communitycounsel_phd.shtml

1	2	3	**4**	5	6	7
Practice oriented		Equal emphasis			Research oriented	

Percentage of faculty subscribing to each of the following orientations:

Psychodynamic/Psychoanalytic	0%
Applied behavioral analysis/Radical behavioral	0%
Family systems/Systems	25%
Existential/Phenomenological/Humanistic	25%
Cognitive/Cognitive-behavioral	50%

Courses required for incoming students to have completed prior to enrolling:
Master's degree in counseling, psychology, or related field

Recommended but not mandatory courses: None

GRE mean
Verbal 620   Quantitative 600
Advanced Psychology 550
Analytical Writing not reported

GPA mean
Overall GPA 3.5   Psychology GPA 3.8
Junior/Senior GPA 3.8

Number of applications/admission offers/incoming students in 2007
55 applied/5 admission offers/4 incoming

% of students receiving:
Full tuition waiver only: 0%
Assistantship/fellowship only: 0%
Both full tuition waiver & assistantship/fellowship: 100%

Approximate percentage of incoming students with a B.A./B.S. only: 0%   **Master's:** 100%

Approximate percentage of students who are Women: 60%   **Ethnic Minority:** 40%   **International:** 2%

Average years to complete the doctoral program (including internship): 6 years

Personal interview
Required in person

Attrition rate in past 7 years: 9%

Percentage of students applying for internship last year accepted into APPIC or APA internships: 100%

Formal tracks/concentrations: none

Research areas	# Faculty	# Grants
adolescent risk behavior	1	1
child/adolescent development	2	0
counseling process	1	0
counseling supervision	1	0
multicultural counseling	2	0
vocational psychology	1	1

Clinical opportunities

hospitals   universities
clinics

Marquette University (Ph.D.)

Department of Counseling and Educational
Psychology
146 Schroeder Complex
Milwaukee, WI 53201
phone#: (414) 288-5790
E-mail: todd.campbell@marquette.edu
Web address: www.marquette.edu/education/pages/
programs/coep/index.shtml

1	2	3	4	**5**	6	7
Practice oriented		Equal emphasis				Research oriented

Percentage of faculty subscribing to each of the following orientations:

Psychodynamic/Psychoanalytic   28%
Applied behavioral analysis/Radical behavioral   14%
Family systems/Systems   14%
Existential/Phenomenological/Humanistic   57%
Cognitive/Cognitive-behavioral   57%

Courses required for incoming students to have completed prior to enrolling: None

Recommended but not mandatory courses:
Psychology or counseling majors are recommended.

GRE mean
Verbal 520   Quantitative 660
Psychology advanced test not required
Analytical Writing 5.0

GPA mean
Overall GPA 3.8

Number of applications/admission offers/incoming students in 2007
72 applied/8 admission offers/5 incoming

% of students receiving:
Full tuition waiver only: 0%
Assistantship/fellowship only: 2%
Both full tuition waiver & assistantship/fellowship: 0%
(37.5% of students receive a partial tuition wavier)

Approximate percentage of incoming students with a B.A./B.S. only: 40%   **Master's:** 60%

Approximate percentage of students who are Women: 50%   **Ethnic Minority:** 12%   **International:** 2%

Average years to complete the doctoral program (including internship): 6 years

Personal interview
Preferred in person but telephone acceptable

Attrition rate in past 7 years: 9%

Percentage of students applying for internship last year accepted into APPIC or APA internships: 75%

Formal tracks/concentrations: addiction-mental health, child/adolescent, multicultural counseling

Research areas	# Faculty	# Grants
addictions	1	4
child maltreatment	2	0
multicultural	4	0
parenting	1	3
program evaluation in education	2	1
psychotherapy process	3	0
strengths, optimal functioning	3	0
clinical supervision	2	0

Clinical opportunities

addiction   clinical supervision
diverse populations   university counseling
homelessness   department of corrections
trauma   community mental health
parenting   medical centers
childhood disorders   schools
health/medical psychology   community clinics
neuropsychology

University of Maryland College Park (Ph.D.)

Department of Psychology and College of Education
College Park, MD 20742
e-mail: cgorham@psyc.umd.edu, boblent@umd.edu
Web address:
www.bsos.umd.edu/psyc/counseling/counsel2.htm

1	2	3	4	**5**	6	7
Practice oriented		Equal emphasis				Research oriented

Percentage of faculty subscribing to each of the following orientations:

Psychodynamic/Psychoanalytic   38%
Applied behavioral analysis/Radical behavioral   0%
Family systems/Systems   0%
Existential/Phenomenological/Humanistic   0%
Cognitive/Cognitive-behavioral   25%
Interpersonal   13%
Feminist   13%

Courses required for incoming students to have completed prior to enrolling:
No specific courses but we require a minimum of 15 credits of coursework in psychology

Recommended but not mandatory courses:
Statistics, core psychology

GRE mean
Verbal 621   Quantitative 693
Analytical Writing not reported

GPA mean
Overall Undergraduate GPA 3.59
Overall master's GPA 3.9

Number of applications/admission offers/incoming students in 2007
214 applied/11 admission offers/6 incoming

% of students receiving:
Full tuition waiver only: 0%
Assistantship/fellowship only: 0%
Both full tuition waiver & assistantship/fellowship: 100%

Approximate percentage of incoming students with a B.A./B.S. only: 17%   **Master's:** 83%

Approximate percentage of students who are Women: 79%   **Ethnic Minority:** 32%   **International:** 8%

Average years to complete the doctoral program (including internship): 6 years

Personal interview
Telephone required

Attrition rate in past 7 years: 9%

Percentage of students applying for internship last year accepted into APPIC or APA internships: 100%

Formal tracks/concentrations: none

Research areas	# Faculty	# Grants
AIDS/HIV	1	0
career counseling	3	0
career/vocational psychology	3	0
counseling process	3	0
counseling relationship	3	0
countertransference	2	0
domestic violence	1	0
dreams (their use in therapy)	1	0
health	2	0
interpersonal relationships	1	0
multicultural	3	0
supervision/training	3	0

Clinical opportunities
multicultural   consultation
group   career
individual   supervision practica

McGill University (Ph.D.)

Department of Educational and Counseling Psychology
Faculty of Education
3700 McTavish Street
Montreal, Quebec H3A 1Y2, Canada
phone#: (514) 398-4245
e-mail: ada.sinacore@mcgill.ca (program director)
diane.bernier@mcgill.ca (program coordinator)
Web address: www.mcgill.ca/edu-ecp/programs/counselling/

1	2	3	**4**	5	6	7
Practice oriented			Equal emphasis			Research oriented

Percentage of faculty subscribing to each of the following orientations:

Psychodynamic/Psychoanalytic	40%
Applied behavioral analysis/Radical behavioral	0%
Family systems/Systems	20%
Existential/Phenomenological/Humanistic	60%
Cognitive/Cognitive-behavioral	60%
Feminist/multicultural	40%

Courses required for incoming students to have completed prior to enrolling:
Undergraduate degree in psychology including courses in developmental, history, personality, abnormal, social, statistics. Master's degree in either counseling psychology or clinical psychology.

Recommended but not mandatory courses:
None

GRE mean
Not reported

GPA mean
Overall GPA 3.7

Number of applications/admission offers/incoming students in 2007:
17 applied/7 admission offers/6 incoming

% of students receiving:
Full tuition waiver only: 5%
Assistantship/fellowship only: 75%
Both full tuition waiver & assistantship/fellowship: 0%

Approximate percentage of incoming students with a B.A./B.S. only: 0%   **Master's:** 100%

Approximate percentage of students who are Women: 80%   **Ethnic Minority:** 15%
International: not reported

Average years to complete the doctoral program (including internship): 6.2 years

Personal interview
Preferred in person but telephone acceptable

Attrition rate in past 7 years: 22%

Percentage of students applying for internship last year accepted into APPIC or APA internships: 50%

Formal tracks/concentrations: psychotherapy, multiculturalism, supervision

Research areas	# Faculty	# Grants
development and training	1	0
feminism multicultural pedagogy	2	0
psychotherapy	2	2

Clinical opportunities
behavioral therapy clinic   psychiatry clinic
children's behavior clinic   psychotherapy clinic
eating disorders

University of Memphis (Ph.D.)

Department of Counseling, Educational Psychology and Research
Ball Education Building, Room 100
Memphis, TN 38152
phone#: (901) 678-2841
e-mail: slease@memphis.edu
Web address: coe.memphis.edu/cepr/PHD-counseling-psychology.htm

1	2	3	**4**	5	6	7
Practice oriented		Equal emphasis			Research oriented	

Percentage of faculty subscribing to each of the following orientations:

Psychodynamic/Psychoanalytic	0%
Applied behavioral analysis/Radical behavioral	0%
Family systems/Systems	57%
Existential/Phenomenological/Humanistic	50%
Cognitive/Cognitive-behavioral	71%
Feminist	33%
Constructivist	33%

Courses required for incoming students to have completed prior to enrolling:

Master's degree in counseling, psychology, or related field. Must have theories of counseling, group counseling, career counseling, statistics/research, practicum.

Recommended but not mandatory courses:

Psychological assessment, psychopathology

GRE mean

Verbal 560   Quantitative 520
Analytical Writing Not used

GPA mean

Overall GPA 3.82

Number of applications/admission offers/incoming students in 2007

applied not reported/admission offers not reported/8 incoming

% of students receiving:

Full tuition waiver only: 0%
Assistantship/fellowship only: 0%
Both full tuition waiver & assistantship/fellowship: 100%

Approximate percentage of incoming students with a B.A./B.S. only: 0%   Master's: 100%

Approximate percentage of students who are Women: 61%   Ethnic Minority: 22%   International: 17%

Average years to complete the doctoral program (including internship): 4.5 years

Personal interview

Preferred in person but telephone acceptable

Attrition rate in past 7 years: 2%

Percentage of students applying for internship last year accepted into APPIC or APA internships: 92%

Formal tracks/concentrations: diversity, international studies

Research areas	# Faculty	# Grants
AIDS/HIV counseling	1	0
at-risk families and children	2	1
consultation	2	1
gays, lesbians, and bisexuals	3	1
crisis/trauma	2	0
disabled persons	4	3
international psychology	2	2
multicultural counseling	5	0
professional development	2	0
psychological resources	1	0
vocational psychology	2	0
health psychology	1	1

Clinical opportunities

adolescents	inpatients
assessment	outpatients
children	rehabilitation
couples/families	substance abuse unit
domestic violence	university students
forensic psychology	

University of Miami (Ph.D.)

Department of Educational and Psychological Studies
P.O. Box 248065
Coral Gables, FL 33124-2040
phone#: (305) 284-3001
e-mail: blewis@miami.edu
Web address: www.education.miami.edu/program/Programs.asp?Program_ID=47

1	2	3	**4**	5	6	7
Practice oriented		Equal emphasis			Research oriented	

Percentage of faculty subscribing to each of the following orientations:

Psychodynamic/Psychoanalytic	14%
Applied behavioral analysis/Radical behavioral	0%
Family systems/Systems	50%
Existential/Phenomenological/Humanistic	20%
Cognitive/Cognitive-behavioral	60%

Courses required for incoming students to have completed prior to enrolling:

Standard curriculum for master's in counseling

Recommended but not mandatory courses:

None

GRE mean

Verbal 580   Quantitative 624
Analytical Writing not reported

GPA mean

Overall GPA 3.4   Psychology GPA 3.9

Number of applications/admission offers/incoming students in 2007

92 applied/9 admission offers/5 incoming

% of students receiving:

Full tuition waiver only: 0%
Assistantship/fellowship only: 0%
Both full tuition waiver & assistantship/fellowship: 100%

Approximate percentage of incoming students with a B.A./B.S. only: 17%   Master's: 83%

Approximate percentage of students who are Women: 78%   Ethnic Minority: 43%
International: not reported

Average years to complete the doctoral program (including internship): 6 years

Personal interview
Preferred in person but telephone acceptable

Attrition rate in past 7 years: 13.6%

Percentage of students applying for internship last year accepted into APPIC or APA internships: 100%

Formal tracks/concentrations: multicultural counseling, health psychology, family therapy

Research areas	# Faculty	# Grants
couple violence	1	0
ethnic minorities	3	1
families	3	1
health psychology	3	1

Clinical opportunities
Tailored to students' interests

University of Minnesota–Department of Educational Psychology (Ph.D.)

Counseling and Student Personnel Psychology
250 Education Sciences Building
56 East River Road
Minneapolis, MN 55455
phone#: (612) 624-6827
e-mail: cspp@umn.edu
Web address: education.umn.edu/EdPsych/CSPP/

1	2	3	**4**	5	6	7
Practice oriented		Equal emphasis			Research oriented	

Percentage of faculty subscribing to each of the following orientations:

Psychodynamic/Psychoanalytic	25%
Applied behavioral analysis/Radical behavioral	10%
Family systems/Systems	30%
Existential/Phenomenological/Humanistic	60%
Cognitive/Cognitive-behavioral	60%

Courses required for incoming students to have completed prior to enrolling:
None

Recommended but not mandatory courses:
Foundational courses in undergraduate psychology

GRE mean
Verbal 534   Quantitative 620
Analytical Writing 4.5

GPA mean
Overall GPA 3.33

Number of applications/admission offers/incoming students in 2007
46 applied/12 admission offers/7 incoming

% of students receiving:
Full tuition waiver only: 0%
Assistantship/fellowship only: 10%
Both full tuition waiver & assistantship/fellowship: 90%

Approximate percentage of incoming students with a B.A./B.S. only: 0%   **Master's:** 100%

Approximate percentage of students who are Women: 71%   **Ethnic Minority:** 43%
International: 14%

Average years to complete the doctoral program (including internship): 5 years

Personal interview
Interview not required

Attrition rate in past 7 years: 15%

Percentage of students applying for internship last year accepted into APPIC or APA internships: 100%

Formal tracks/concentrations: none

Research areas	# Faculty	# Grants
burnout prevention	2	0
career development	2	4
genetic counseling	1	1
high-risk adolescents	2	1
international counseling	4	1
master therapist	2	1
multicultural counseling	4	4
multicultural integrative therapy	1	0
prevention	1	1
school counseling	3	2
supervision	2	1
therapist development	2	2
therapy outcome	1	0

Clinical opportunities
Multiple practicum sites in the Twin Cities

University of Minnesota–Department of Psychology (Ph.D.)

75 East River Road
Minneapolis, MN 55455
phone#: (612) 625-3873
e-mail: counpsy@umn.edu
Web address:
www.psych.umn.edu/areas/counseling/index.htm

1	2	3	4	5	6	**7**
Practice oriented		Equal emphasis			Research oriented	

Percentage of faculty subscribing to each of the following orientations:

Psychodynamic/Psychoanalytic	33%
Applied behavioral analysis/Radical behavioral	0%
Family systems/Systems	0%
Existential/Phenomenological/Humanistic	0%
Cognitive/Cognitive-behavioral	66%

Courses required for incoming students to have completed prior to enrolling:
Broad base of scientific training in psychology with a background in statistics

Recommended but not mandatory courses:
See above

GRE mean
Verbal 659   Quantitative 706
Advanced Psychology not required
Analytical Writing 5.0

GPA mean
Overall GPA 3.48   Psychology GPA 3.83

Number of applications/admission offers/incoming students in 2007
86 applied/7 admission offers/5 incoming

% of students receiving:
Full tuition waiver only: 0%
Assistantship/fellowship only: 0%
Both full tuition waiver & assistantship/fellowship: 100%

Approximate percentage of incoming students with a B.A./B.S. only: 29%   **Master's:** 71%

Approximate percentage of students who are Women: 77%   **Ethnic Minority:** 19%
International: 27%

Average years to complete the doctoral program (including internship): 6 years

Personal interview
Interview not required

Attrition rate in past 7 years: 10%

Percentage of students applying for internship last year accepted into APPIC or APA internships: 100%

Formal tracks/concentrations: none

Research areas	# Faculty	# Grants
acculturation	1	0
Asian American identity	1	0
career development and choice	1	1
coping with stressful life events	1	1
cultural socialization	1	0
ethnic and racial identity	1	0
interest measurement	1	1
international adoption	1	1
interpersonal relations	1	0
multicultural counseling	1	0
occupational health psychology	1	0
stressful life events	1	0
personality and adjustment	1	0
posttraumatic growth	1	0
racism and discrimination	1	0
sexual assault recovery	1	0
values and work adjustment	1	0

Clinical opportunities
We use about 30 locations as practica and advanced practica locations. The sites are matched with students' interests.

University of Missouri–Columbia (Ph.D.)

Educational, School, and Counseling Psychology
Columbia, MO 65211-2130
phone#: (573) 882-7731
e-mail: HeppnerM@Missouri.edu

Web address: education.missouri.edu/ESCP/_ESCP/program_areas/counseling_psychology/index.php

1	2	3	**4**	5	6	7
Practice oriented		Equal emphasis			Research oriented	

Percentage of faculty subscribing to each of the following orientations:

Psychodynamic/Psychoanalytic	30%
Family systems/Systems	30%
Existential/Phenomenological/Humanistic	50%
Cognitive/Cognitive-behavioral	50%
Interpersonal	30%
Feminist	30%

Courses required for incoming students to have completed prior to enrolling:
If entering without a master's degree, 15 hours of prerequisite course work, including statistics, personality, social, and developmental

Recommended but not mandatory courses:
None

GRE mean
Verbal 540   Quantitative 610
Analytical Writing not reported
Advanced Psychology not reported

GPA mean
Overall GPA 3.5

Number of applications/admission offers/incoming students in 2007
97 applied/10 admission offers/9 incoming

% of students receiving:
Full tuition waiver only: 0%
Assistantship/fellowship only: 0%
Both full tuition waiver & assistantship/fellowship: 100%

Approximate percentage of incoming students with a B.A./B.S. only: 33%   **Master's:** 66%

Approximate percentage of students who are Women: 55%   **Ethnic Minority:** 33%
International: 11%

Average years to complete the doctoral program (including internship): 6 years

Personal interview
Preferred in person but telephone acceptable

Attrition rate in past 7 years: 11%

Percentage of students applying for internship last year accepted into APPIC or APA internships: 100%

Formal tracks/concentrations: multicultural minor; teaching minor; statistics minor, sports psychology, career development

Research areas	# Faculty	# Grants
addictions	2	0
African American adolescents	1	2
career development	5	2
counseling process	3	2

counseling supervision	2	1
counseling/therapy integration	1	0
disability	1	0
eating disorders	1	1
gender	2	0
group process	2	1
health psychology	2	1
identity development	1	0
multicultural counseling	5	2
perfectionism	1	0
problem solving	3	2
rape	1	1
scale construction	4	3

Clinical opportunities

cognitive-behavioral	state prison
family counseling center	university/college
learning disabilities clinic	counseling centers
rural community mental	university career center
health centers	university medical clinics
psychiatric clinic	VA hospital
psychology clinic	women's center
rehabilitation	women's shelters
state hospital	

University of Missouri–Kansas City (Ph.D.)

Division of Counseling, Educational Psychology, and Exercise Science
School of Education, Room 215
5100 Rockhill Road
Kansas City, MO 64110
phone#: (816) 235-2722
e-mail: umkccepsy@umkc.edu
Web address: education.umkc.edu/CEP/phd/index.asp

1	2	3	**4**	5	6	7
Practice oriented		Equal emphasis			Research oriented	

Percentage of faculty subscribing to each of the following orientations:

Psychodynamic/Psychoanalytic	10%
Applied behavioral analysis/Radical behavioral	5%
Family systems/Systems	20%
Existential/Phenomenological/Humanistic	25%
Cognitive/Cognitive-behavioral	40%

Courses required for incoming students to have completed prior to enrolling:
Undergraduate psychology major or master's degree in counseling or psychology

Recommended but not mandatory courses:
None

GRE mean
Not reported

GPA mean
Not reported

Number of applications/admission offers/incoming students in 2007
82 applied/6 admission offers/6 incoming

% of students receiving:
Full tuition waiver only: 0%
Assistantship/fellowship only: 0%
Both full tuition waiver & assistantship/fellowship: 100%

Approximate percentage of incoming students with a B.A./B.S. only: 83%   Master's: 17%

Approximate percentage of students who are
Women: 75%   Ethnic Minority: 37.5%
International: not reported

Average years to complete the doctoral program (including internship): 6 years

Personal interview
Preferred in person but telephone acceptable

Attrition rate in past 7 years: not reported

Percentage of students applying for internship last year accepted into APPIC or APA internships: 100%

Formal tracks/concentrations: none

Research areas	# Faculty	# Grants
AIDS	1	1
behavioral medicine	4	3
cross-cultural counseling	4	2
family systems theory	1	0
health psychology	3	0
interpersonal relations	3	0
professional issues	3	0
psychopathology prevention	3	0
psychotherapy process	3	0
sports psychology	1	0
stress and coping	1	0
substance abuse	1	0
supervision	2	0
vocational interests	1	0

Clinical opportunities
Not reported

University of Nebraska–Lincoln (Ph.D.)

Department of Educational Psychology
38 Teachers College Hall
Lincoln, NE 68588-0345
phone#: (402) 472-0573
e-mail: mscheel2@unl.edu
Web address:
cehs.unl.edu/edpsych/graduate/copsych.shtml

1	2	3	**4**	5	6	7
Practice oriented		Equal emphasis			Research oriented	

Percentage of faculty subscribing to each of the following orientations:

Psychodynamic/Psychoanalytic	20%
Applied behavioral analysis/Radical behavioral	0%
Family systems/Systems	20%
Existential/Phenomenological/Humanistic	20%
Cognitive/Cognitive-behavioral	40%

Courses required for incoming students to have completed prior to enrolling:
Bachelor's in a closely related area or master's in counseling or closely related field

Recommended but not mandatory courses:
None

GRE mean
Verbal 550   Quantitative 550

GPA mean
Overall GPA 3.5

Number of applications/admission offers/incoming students in 2007
42 applied/6 admission offers/5 incoming

% of students receiving:
Full tuition waiver only: 0%
Assistantship/fellowship only: 0%
Both full tuition waiver & assistantship/fellowship: 100%

Approximate percentage of incoming students with a B.A./B.S. only: 10%   **Master's:** 90%

Approximate percentage of students who are Women: 70%   **Ethnic Minority:** 30%   **International:** 10%

Average years to complete the doctoral program (including internship): 5 years

Personal interview
Preferred in person but telephone acceptable

Attrition rate in past 7 years: not reported

Percentage of students applying for internship last year accepted into APPIC or APA internships: 100%

Formal tracks/concentrations: multicultural counseling; gender; couple and family counseling

Research areas	# Faculty	# Grants
family counseling	1	0
multicultural	3	0
gender	2	0
vocational	3	1
immigrant and refugees	1	1
psychotherapy process	1	0

Clinical opportunities

couple and family counseling	psychological assessment
health psychology	vocational counseling
multicultural counseling	immigrants and refugees
	adolescence in schools

New Mexico State University (Ph.D.)

Department of Counseling and Educational Psychology
MSC 3CEP
P.O. Box 30001
Las Cruces, NM 88003-8001
phone#: (505) 646-2121
e-mail: eadams@nmsu.edu
Web address: education.nmsu.edu/cep/phd/index.html

1	2	3	**4**	5	6	7
Practice oriented		Equal emphasis			Research oriented	

Percentage of faculty subscribing to each of the following orientations:

Psychodynamic/Psychoanalytic	22%
Applied behavioral analysis/Radical behavioral	0%
Family systems/Systems	11%
Existential/Phenomenological/Humanistic	33%
Cognitive/Cognitive-behavioral	22%

Courses required for incoming students to have completed prior to enrolling: None

Recommended but not mandatory courses:
Counseling practicum, human development, multicultural, counseling theory and techniques, family therapy, group work, career/life planning, counseling research, diagnosis, addictions

GRE mean
Verbal + Quantitative 1000
Analytical Writing 4.5

GPA mean
Master's GPA 3.76

Number of applications/admission offers/incoming students in 2007
30 applied/19 admission offers/6 incoming

% of students receiving:
Full tuition waiver only: 0%
Assistantship/fellowship only: 80%
Both full tuition waiver & assistantship/fellowship: 20%

Approximate percentage of incoming students with a B.A./B.S. only: 0%   **Master's:** 100%

Approximate percentage of students who are Women: 54%   **Ethnic Minority:** 46%   **International:** 4%

Average years to complete the doctoral program (including internship): 5 years

Personal interview
Preferred in person but telephone acceptable

Attrition rate in past 7 years: 8%

Percentage of students applying for internship last year accepted into APPIC or APA internships: 100%

Formal tracks/concentrations: multicultural counseling, supervision/training, health psychology

Research areas	# Faculty	# Grants
acculturation	3	0
career	2	0
family systems	1	0
gender	3	0
social identity	3	0
multicultural curriculum development	1	0
interpersonal relationship enhancement	1	1
health psychology	1	1
LGBT	3	1

Clinical opportunities

community organizations	minorities
departmental training center	rural
families	substance abuse
groups	university counseling center
low income	vocational career development
medically underserved	

New York University (Ph.D.)

Department of Applied Psychology
East Building, 4th Floor
239 Greene Street
New York, NY 10003
phone#: (212) 998-5559
e-mail: mm13@nyu.edu
Web address: steinhardt.nyu.edu/education/appsych/
index.php/program/24/

1	2	3	4	**5**	6	7
Practice oriented			Equal emphasis			Research oriented

Percentage of faculty subscribing to each of the following orientations:

Psychodynamic/Psychoanalytic	44%
Applied behavioral analysis/Radical behavioral	14%
Family systems/Systems	14%
Existential/Phenomenological/Humanistic	14%
Cognitive/Cognitive-behavioral	14%

Courses required for incoming students to have completed prior to enrolling:
18 credits of prerequisites in psychology at undergraduate or graduate level. Not necessary to complete prerequisites before enrollment.

Recommended but not mandatory courses:
Basic areas in psychology course work

GRE mean
Verbal + Quantitative 1213

GPA mean
Overall GPA 3.6

Number of applications/admission offers/incoming students in 2007
169 applied/6 admission offers/4 incoming

% of students receiving:
Full tuition waiver only: 0%
Assistantship/fellowship only: 0%
Both full tuition waiver & assistantship/fellowship: 100%

Approximate percentage of incoming students with a B.A./B.S. only: 50%   **Master's:** 50%

Approximate percentage of students who are Women: 76%   **Ethnic Minority:** 44%
International: 7%

Average years to complete the doctoral program (including internship): 7 years

Personal interview
Required

Attrition rate in past 7 years: 5%

Percentage of students applying for internship last year accepted into APPIC or APA internships: 100%

Formal tracks/concentrations: none

Research areas	# Faculty	# Grants
group process	1	0
multicultural counseling	2	0
psychoanalytic constructs	1	0
psychopathology and differential diagnosis	2	0
religion and spirituality	1	1
women's development/health	2	2
work as a developmental context	1	0
LGBT	1	1
positive psychology	1	1

Clinical opportunities
Wide range of specialized practica and externship sites are available in the New York metropolitan area

University of North Dakota (Ph.D.)

Department of Counseling
Box 8255
Grand Forks, ND 58202-8255
phone#: (701) 777-2729
fax#: (701) 777-3184
e-mail: cl.juntunen@und.edu
Web address: www.counseling.und.edu/docbrochure
_brokendown/phdcoverpage.htm

1	2	3	**4**	5	6	7
Practice oriented			Equal emphasis			Research oriented

Percentage of faculty subscribing to each of the following orientations:

Psychodynamic/Psychoanalytic	40%
Applied behavioral analysis/Radical behavioral	0%
Family systems/Systems	20%
Existential/Phenomenological/Humanistic	40%
Cognitive/Cognitive-behavioral	50%
Feminist	50%

Courses required for incoming students to have completed prior to enrolling:
20 semester hours of undergraduate psychology including statistics, research methods, abnormal, developmental, personality

Recommended but not mandatory courses:
Research methods, master's level practicum, 60 hours supervised practice (for post-master's applicants)

GRE mean
Verbal 545   Quantitative 590
Advanced Psychology 607
Analytical Writing 4.8

GPA mean
Overall 3.5

Number of applications/admission offers/incoming students in 2007
38 applied/12 admission offers/8 incoming

% of students receiving:
Full tuition waiver only: 0%
Assistantship/fellowship only: 0%
Both full tuition waiver & assistantship/fellowship: 100%

Approximate percentage of incoming students with a B.A./B.S. only: 50% **Master's:** 50%

Approximate percentage of students who are Women: 75% **Ethnic Minority:** 15% **International:** 5%

Average years to complete the doctoral program (including internship): 5 years

Personal interview
Preferred in person but telephone acceptable

Attrition rate in past 7 years: 7%

Percentage of students applying for internship last year accepted into APPIC or APA internships: 90%

Formal tracks/concentrations: none

Research areas	# Faculty	# Grants
body image	1	0
career development	2	0
domestic violence	1	0
gay, lesbian, bisexual	2	1
gender and intimacy	1	1
geriatric psychology	1	1
group identity development	1	0
healthy relationships	1	0
HIV prevention	1	1
immigrant and refugee mental health	1	0
multicultural counseling	1	0
Native American career development	1	0
poverty	1	0
resiliency in adolescence	1	0
rural mental health	2	0
sizism	1	0
social support and chronic illness	1	0
student self-efficacy	1	0
supervisor strategies	2	0
vocational interests testing	1	1
white privilege	1	0
women/career development	1	0

Clinical opportunities
variety of community and academic settings

University of North Texas (Ph.D.)
Department of Psychology
P.O. Box 311280
Denton, TX 76203-3587
phone#: (940) 565-2671
e-mail: amym@unt.edu
Web address: www.psyc.unt.edu/gradcounseling.shtml

1	2	3	**4**	5	6	7
Practice oriented		Equal emphasis			Research oriented	

Percentage of faculty subscribing to each of the following orientations:
Psychodynamic/Psychoanalytic 30%
Applied behavioral analysis/Radical behavioral 0%
Family systems/Systems 40%
Existential/Phenomenological/Humanistic 40%
Cognitive/Cognitive-behavioral 20%

Courses required for incoming students to have completed prior to enrolling:
Statistics and three of the following: experimental, cognition, learning, perception, motivation, physiological, psychological measurement, or research thesis

Recommended but not mandatory courses:
Social, physiological, tests and measurements

GRE mean
Not reported

GPA mean
Overall GPA 3.5 on last 60 hours for bachelor's or overall GPA 3.5 for master's Psychology

Number of applications/admission offers/incoming students in 2007
97 applied/14 admission offers/8 incoming

% of students receiving:
Full tuition waiver only: 0%
Assistantship/fellowship only: 50%
Both full tuition waiver & assistantship/fellowship: 0%

Approximate percentage of incoming students with a B.A./B.S. only: 75% **Master's:** 25%

Approximate percentage of students who are Women: 71% **Ethnic Minority:** 6% **International:** 1%

Average years to complete the doctoral program (including internship): 5.9 years

Personal interview
Preferred in person but telephone acceptable

Attrition rate in past 7 years: 10%

Percentage of students applying for internship last year accepted into APPIC or APA internships: 100%

Formal tracks/concentrations: marriage & family, aging, sport psychology

Research areas	# Faculty	# Grants
counseling and therapy	1	0
eating disorders	3	0
gerontology	1	0
marriage and family	3	1
minority and cross-cultural	2	0
professional issues	3	0
sports psychology	2	1
vocational development	3	0

Clinical opportunities

external agencies after completing required on-campus practica

psychology clinic
university counseling and testing services

University of Northern Colorado (Psy.D.)

School of Applied Psychology and Counselor Education
248 McKee Hall, Campus Box 131
Greeley, CO 80639
phone#: (970) 351-2209
e-mail: brian.johnson@unco.edu
Web address: www.unco.edu/cebs/counspsych/

1	2	**3**	4	5	6	7
Practice oriented		Equal emphasis			Research oriented	

Percentage of faculty subscribing to each of the following orientations:

Psychodynamic/Psychoanalytic	0%
Applied behavioral analysis/Radical behavioral	10%
Family systems/Systems	30%
Existential/Phenomenological/Humanistic	30%
Cognitive/Cognitive-behavioral	30%

Courses required for incoming students to have completed prior to enrolling:
Either a bachelor's or master's degree in psychology or a closely related field.

Recommended but not mandatory courses: None

GRE mean
Verbal 550   Quantitative 550
Recommended GRE total 1000
Analytical Writing 5.0

GPA mean
Overall GPA 3.6–3.8

Number of applications/admission offers/incoming students in 2007
67 applied/11 admission offers/8 incoming

% of students receiving:
Full tuition waiver only: 0%
Assistantship/fellowship only: 50%
Both full tuition waiver & assistantship/fellowship: 25%

Approximate percentage of incoming students with a B.A./B.S. only: 25%   **Master's:** 75%

Approximate percentage of students who are Women: 65%   **Ethnic Minority:** 10%   **International:** 10%

Average years to complete the doctoral program (including internship): 4–5 years

Personal interview
Preferred in person but telephone is acceptable

Attrition rate in past 7 years: 13%

Percentage of students applying for internship last year accepted into APPIC or APA internships: 60%

Formal tracks/concentrations: none

Research areas	# Faculty	# Grants
child psychology	8	1
college student adjustment	2	1
counseling process	1	0
eating disorders	2	0
family dynamics	4	1
multicultural	6	0

Clinical opportunities

clinical hypnosis
cognitive/academic assessment
personality assessment
neuropsychological assessment

individual therapy
couples and family therapy
group therapy
play therapy
clinical supervision

University of Notre Dame (Ph.D.)

Department of Psychology
Notre Dame, IN 46556
phone#: (574) 631-6650
fax#: (574) 631-8883
e-mail: JudyA.Spiro.2@nd.edu
Web address: psychology.nd.edu/graduate-studies/counseling

1	2	3	4	5	**6**	7
Practice oriented		Equal emphasis			Research oriented	

Percentage of faculty subscribing to each of the following orientations:

Psychodynamic/Psychoanalytic	0%
Applied behavioral analysis/Radical behavioral	10%
Family systems/Systems	20%
Existential/Phenomenological/Humanistic	10%
Cognitive/Cognitive-behavioral	60%

Courses required for incoming students to have completed prior to enrolling:
Undergraduate psychology major, statistics, methodology, and research experience

Recommended but not mandatory courses: None

GRE mean
Verbal + Quantitative 1250

GPA mean
Overall GPA 3.8   Psychology GPA 3.8

Number of applications/admission offers/incoming students in 2007
150 applied/6 admission offers/3 incoming

% of students receiving:
Full tuition waiver only: 0%
Assistantship/fellowship only: 0%
Both full tuition waiver & assistantship/fellowship: 100%

Approximate percentage of incoming students with a B.A./B.S. only: 90%   **Master's:** 10%

Approximate percentage of students who are Women: 74%   **Ethnic Minority:** 48%
International: 4%

Average years to complete the doctoral program (including internship): 7 years

Personal interview
Preferred in person but telephone acceptable

Attrition rate in past 7 years: 19%

Percentage of students applying for internship last year accepted into APPIC or APA internships: 100%

Formal tracks/concentrations: none

Research areas	# Faculty	# Grants
behavioral medicine	1	1
health psychology	1	1
marital interaction	1	1
multicultural counseling	2	1
narrative psychology	1	1
social/clinical interface	2	0
depression	3	1

Clinical opportunities
juvenile justice center
local community mental
   health center
community outpatient
   hospital
university counseling center

University of Oklahoma (Ph.D.)
Department of Educational Psychology
Norman, OK 73019-0260
phone#: (405) 325-5974
e-mail: cstoltenberg@ou.edu or gpoedpsych@ou.edu
Web address:
www.ou.edu/education/cpp/CP/descCP.htm

1	2	3	**4**	5	6	7
Practice oriented			Equal emphasis			Research oriented

Percentage of faculty subscribing to each of the following orientations:
Psychodynamic/Psychoanalytic	57%
Applied behavioral analysis/Radical behavioral	14%
Family systems/Systems	71%
Existential/Phenomenological/Humanistic	57%
Cognitive/Cognitive-behavioral	86%
Narrative	28%
Feminist	28%

Courses required for incoming students to have completed prior to enrolling:
Algebra, 2 semesters of English grammar and composition, 18 semester hours in psychology or related area

Recommended but not mandatory courses:
None

GRE mean
Verbal 560   Quantitative 600
Analytical Writing not reported

GPA mean
Overall 3.5

Number of applications/admission offers/incoming students in 2007
65 applied/8 admission offers/8 incoming

% of students receiving:
Full tuition waiver only: 0%
Assistantship/fellowship only: 0%
Both full tuition waiver & assistantship/fellowship: 90%

Approximate percentage of incoming students with a B.A./B.S. only: 33%   **Master's:** 67%

Approximate percentage of students who are Women: 60%   **Ethnic Minority:** 20%
International: 5%

Average years to complete the doctoral program (including internship): 5 years

Personal interview
Preferred in person but telephone acceptable

Attrition rate in past 7 years: 5%

Percentage of students applying for internship last year accepted into APPIC or APA internships: 89%

Formal tracks/concentrations: marriage and family

Research areas	# Faculty	# Grants
American Indians	3	0
assessment	3	0
career	2	0
child treatment	4	0
clinical supervision	3	0
counseling process and outcomes	5	0
ecopsychology	2	0
gender	4	0
health psychology	3	0
marriage and family	4	0
multicultural counseling	4	0
narrative	1	0
relational health	2	0
trauma/violence	2	0

Clinical opportunities
child abuse and neglect
child study center
community mental health
correctional facilities
health sciences center/
   medical clinics
Indian health service clinic
psychiatric hospitals
rehabilitation clinics
university counseling center
VA hospital
schools

Oklahoma State University (Ph.D.)

School of Applied Health and Educational Psychology
Stillwater, OK 74078
phone#: (405) 744-6040
e-mail: carvin@okstate.edu
Web address:
www.okstate.edu/education/sahep/cpsy/index.html

1	2	3	**4**	5	6	7
Practice oriented		Equal emphasis			Research oriented	

Percentage of faculty subscribing to each of the following orientations:

Psychodynamic/Psychoanalytic	10%
Applied behavioral analysis/Radical behavioral	0%
Family systems/Systems	20%
Existential/Phenomenological/Humanistic	40%
Cognitive/Cognitive-behavioral	30%

Courses required for incoming students to have completed prior to enrolling:
Bachelor's or master's degree in psychology or related area

Recommended but not mandatory courses:
Statistics, research design

GRE mean
We recommend 500 for Verbal and 500 for Quantitative
Analytical Writing 4.5

GPA mean
Not reported

Number of applications/admission offers/incoming students in 2007
36 applied/13 admission offers/8 incoming

% of students receiving:
Full tuition waiver only: 10%
Assistantship/fellowship only: 80%
Both full tuition waiver & assistantship/fellowship: 10%

Approximate percentage of incoming students with a B.A./B.S. only: 27%   **Master's:** 73%

Approximate percentage of students who are Women: 60%   **Ethnic Minority:** 30%
International: 5%

Average years to complete the doctoral program (including internship): 4–5 years

Personal interview
Preferred in person but telephone acceptable

Attrition rate in past 7 years: 3%

Percentage of students applying for internship last year accepted into APPIC or APA internships: 100%

Formal tracks/concentrations: none

Research areas	# Faculty	# Grants
American Indian	3	0
at-risk youth	2	0
career	4	1
health psychology	2	0
LGBT	1	0
multicultural	4	0
professional	2	0
psychological assessment	1	0
rural mental health	1	0
sports psychology	1	0
supervision	3	0
women/gender issues	2	0

Clinical opportunities

correctional psychology unit
domestic violence center
Indian health services
inpatient hospital
marriage and family clinic
outpatient hospital
rural mental health clinic
university counseling
  centers
youth and family services

University of Oregon (Ph.D.)

Counseling Psychology Program
5251 University of Oregon
Eugene, OR 97403-5251
phone#: (541) 346-2456
e-mail: cpsy@uoregon.edu
Web address:
counpsych.uoregon.edu/programdescription.htm

1	2	3	4	**5**	6	7
Practice oriented		Equal emphasis			Research oriented	

Percentage of faculty subscribing to each of the following orientations:

Psychodynamic/Psychoanalytic	0%
Applied behavioral analysis/Radical behavioral	0%
Family systems/Systems	50%
Existential/Phenomenological/Humanistic	25%
Cognitive/Cognitive-behavioral	100%

Courses required for incoming students to have completed prior to enrolling:
No specific courses required

Recommended but not mandatory courses:
Some background in psychology

GRE mean
Verbal 550   Quantitative 560
Analytical Writing 4.75

GPA mean
Overall 3.54

Number of applications/admission offers/incoming students in 2007
130 applied/admission offers not reported/7 incoming

% of students receiving:
Full tuition waiver only: 0%
Assistantship/fellowship only: 0%
Both full tuition waiver & assistantship/fellowship: 100%

Approximate percentage of incoming students with a B.A./B.S. only: 80%   **Master's:** 20%

Approximate percentage of students who are Women: 75%   **Ethnic Minority:** 47%   **International:** 5%

Average years to complete the doctoral program (including internship): 5.5 years

Personal interview
Preferred in person but telephone acceptable

Attrition rate in past 7 years: 11%

Percentage of students applying for internship last year accepted into APPIC or APA internships: 100%

Formal tracks/concentrations: none

Research areas	# Faculty	# Grants
child and family psychology	3	2
college student development	2	0
domestic violence	1	0
multicultural	4	1
prevention research	4	2
social support and interactions	3	0
treatment outcomes	4	1
vocational psychology	2	0

Clinical opportunities

child–family	inpatient settings
community prevention	VA hospital
counseling centers	

Our Lady of the Lake University (Psy.D.)

School of Professional Studies
Graduate Admissions Office
411 SW 24th Street
San Antonio, TX 78207-4689
phone#: (210) 431-3914
e-mail: bobem@lake.ollusa.edu
Web address:
www.ollusa.edu/s/346/ollu.aspx?pgid=1745

1	**2**	3	4	5	6	7
Practice oriented		Equal emphasis			Research oriented	

Percentage of faculty subscribing to each of the following orientations:

Psychodynamic/Psychoanalytic	20%
Applied behavioral analysis/Radical behavioral	0%
Family systems/Systems	80%
Existential/Phenomenological/Humanistic	0%
Cognitive/Cognitive-behavioral	0%

Courses required for incoming students to have completed prior to enrolling:
Master's or bachelor's degree in psychology or closely related area

Recommended but not mandatory courses: None

GRE mean
Verbal 510   Quantitative 500
Analytical Writing not reported

GPA mean
Not reported

Number of applications/admission offers/incoming students in 2007
45 applied/7 admission offers/4 incoming

% of students receiving:
Full tuition waiver only: 10%
Assistantship/fellowship only: 20%
Both full tuition waiver & assistantship/fellowship: 10%

Approximate percentage of incoming students with a B.A./B.S. only: 0%   **Master's:** 100%

Approximate percentage of students who are Women: 86%   **Ethnic Minority:** 43%
International: 3%

Average years to complete the doctoral program (including internship): 5.5 years

Personal interview
Required in person

Attrition rate in past 7 years: 17.5%

Percentage of students applying for internship last year accepted into APPIC or APA internships: 100%

Formal tracks/concentrations: health psychology

Research areas	# Faculty	# Grants
brief therapy	3	2
ethics	1	0
reimbursement	1	0

Clinical opportunities

community counseling	Spanish-speaking
health psychology	population
school-age population	

Pennsylvania State University (Ph.D.)

Department of Counselor Education, Counseling Psychology, and Rehabilitation Services
University Park, PA 16802
phone#: (814) 865-8304
e-mail: CnPsydoc@psu.edu
Web address: http://www.ed.psu.edu/cnpsy/

1	2	3	**4**	5	6	7
Practice oriented		Equal emphasis			Research oriented	

Percentage of faculty subscribing to each of the following orientations:

Psychodynamic/Psychoanalytic	30%
Applied behavioral analysis/Radical behavioral	0%
Family systems/Systems	30%
Existential/Phenomenological/Humanistic	30%
Cognitive/Cognitive-behavioral	0%

Courses required for incoming students to have completed prior to enrolling:
theories of counseling/psychotherapy, assessment, statistics/research design, career counseling, multicultural counseling, group counseling, counselor skills training

Recommended but not mandatory courses:
Development, core courses in psychology

GRE mean
Verbal 560   Quantitative 568   Analytical 457
Analytical Writing not reported

GPA mean
Overall master's GPA 3.78

Number of applications/admission offers/incoming students in 2007
80 applied/8 admission offers/5 incoming

% of students receiving:
Full tuition waiver only: 0%
Assistantship/fellowship only: 0%
Both full tuition waiver & assistantship/fellowship: 100%

Approximate percentage of incoming students with a B.A./B.S. only: 0%   **Master's:** 100%

Approximate percentage of students who are Women: 76%   **Ethnic Minority:** 35%
International: 8%

Average years to complete the doctoral program (including internship): 6.1 years

Personal interview
Preferred in person but telephone acceptable

Attrition rate in past 7 years: 10%

Percentage of students applying for internship last year accepted into APPIC or APA internships: 100%

Formal tracks/concentrations: none

Research areas	# Faculty	# Grants
family systems	2	1
lesbian/gay/bisexual	1	0
perfectionism	1	0
psychotherapy	1	0

Clinical opportunities
Not reported

Purdue University (Ph.D.)

Department of Educational Studies
BRNG Hall, 100 N. University St.,
West Lafayette, IN 47907-2098
phone#: (765) 494-9748 (Secretary: Ros Bol)
e-mail: pistole@purdue.edu
Web address:
www.edst.purdue.edu/cd/psychology/index.html

1	2	3	4	5	6	7

Practice oriented   Equal emphasis   Research oriented

Percentage of faculty subscribing to each of the following orientations:
Psychodynamic/Psychoanalytic	25%
Applied behavioral analysis/Radical behavioral	0%
Family systems/Systems	25%
Existential/Phenomenological/Humanistic	0%
Cognitive/Cognitive-behavioral	75%

Courses required for incoming students to have completed prior to enrolling: None

Recommended but not mandatory courses:
Undergraduate psychology, statistics, research design

GRE mean
Verbal 547   Quantitative 624
Advanced Psychology not used
Analytical Writing 4.6

GPA mean
Overall GPA 3.5

Number of applications/admission offers/incoming students in 2007
35 applied/10 admission offers/4 incoming

% of students receiving:
Full tuition waiver only: 0%
Assistantship/fellowship only: 0%
Both full tuition waiver & assistantship/fellowship: 100%

Approximate percentage of incoming students with a B.A./B.S. only: 50%   **Master's:** 50%

Approximate percentage of students who are Women: 70%   **Ethnic Minority:** 9%   **International:** 21%

Average years to complete the doctoral program (including internship): 5 years

Personal interview
Preferred in person but telephone acceptable

Attrition rate in past 7 years: 0%

Percentage of students applying for internship last year accepted into APPIC or APA internships: 100%

Formal tracks/concentrations: none

Research areas	# Faculty	# Grants
adult attachment theory	1	1
career and talent development	1	0
grief and bereavement	1	1
adjustment of international students/immigration	1	1
therapeutic assessment	1	0
gambling	1	0

Clinical opportunities
university clinic	college counseling centers
hospitals	community mental health

University of St. Thomas (Psy.D.)

Graduate School of Professional Psychology
TMH451, 1000 La Salle Avenue
Minneapolis, MN 55403-2005
phone#: (651) 962-4650
e-mail: GradPsych@St.Thomas.Edu
Web address: www.stthomas.edu/gradpsych/
programs/psyd/default.html

1	2	3	4	5	6	7

Practice oriented   Equal emphasis   Research oriented

Percentage of faculty subscribing to each of the following orientations:

Psychodynamic/Psychoanalytic	10%
Applied behavioral analysis/Radical behavioral	0%
Family systems/Systems	20%
Existential/Phenomenological/Humanistic	10%
Cognitive/Cognitive-behavioral	40%

Courses required for incoming students to have completed prior to enrolling:
M.A. program in counseling psychology or equivalent

Recommended but not mandatory courses:
Abnormal, statistics, research design, personality, developmental

GRE mean
Verbal 500   Quantitative 500
Analytical Writing 3.5

GPA mean
Overall GPA 3.2

Number of applications/admission offers/incoming students in 2007
37 applied/16 admission offers/14 incoming

% of students receiving:
Full tuition waiver only: 0%
Assistantship/fellowship only: 12%
Both full tuition waiver & assistantship/fellowship: 0%

Approximate percentage of incoming students with a B.A./B.S. only: 0%   **Master's:** 100%

Approximate percentage of students who are Women: 70%   **Ethnic Minority:** 9%   **International:** 6%

Average years to complete the doctoral program (including internship): 4.5 years

Personal interview
Preferred in person

Attrition rate in past 7 years: 6%

Percentage of students applying for internship last year accepted into APPIC or APA internships: 40%

Formal tracks/concentrations: none

Research areas	# Faculty	# Grants
counseling process	2	0
cultural sensitive therapy	2	0
interprofessional ethics	1	0
licensure and regulatory boards	1	0
master therapists	1	0
religion and psychotherapy	1	0

Clinical opportunities
full range of diagnostic disorders in a variety of settings

Seton Hall University (Ph.D.)

Department of Professional Psychology and
Family Therapy
College of Education
400 South Orange Avenue
South Orange, NJ 07079

phone#: (973) 275-2740
e-mail: palmerla@shu.edu
Web address: education.shu.edu/academicprograms/profpsych/phd_counsel/index.html

1	2	3	**4**	5	6	7
Practice oriented		Equal emphasis			Research oriented	

Percentage of faculty subscribing to each of the following orientations:

Psychodynamic/Psychoanalytic	25%
Applied behavioral analysis/Radical behavioral	0%
Family systems/Systems	0%
Existential/Phenomenological/Humanistic	25%
Cognitive/Cognitive-behavioral	50%

Courses required for incoming students to have completed prior to enrolling:
Group counseling, abnormal, test and measurement, counseling skills

Recommended but not mandatory courses: None

GRE mean
Verbal 482   Quantitative 521
Analytical Writing 4.4

GPA mean
Overall GPA 3.78

Number of applications/admission offers/incoming students in 2007
106 applied/10 admission offers/8 incoming

% of students receiving:
Full tuition waiver only: 0%
Assistantship/fellowship only: 100%
Both full tuition waiver & assistantship/fellowship: 0%

Approximate percentage of incoming students with a B.A./B.S. only: 0%   **Master's:** 100%

Approximate percentage of students who are Women: 70%   **Ethnic Minority:** 37.5%   **International:** 8%

Average years to complete the doctoral program (including internship): 5 years

Personal interview
Preferred in person but telephone acceptable

Attrition rate in past 7 years: 11%

Percentage of students applying for internship last year accepted into APPIC or APA internships: 100%

Formal tracks/concentrations: neuropsychology, multicultural, assessment, infant mental health, couples and families

Research areas	# Faculty	# Grants
career development	1	0
multicultural counseling	3	0
neuropsychology	1	0
psychological trauma	1	0
resiliency	1	0
student well-being	1	0

health and coping	1	0
spirituality	1	0
the advising relationship	1	0

Clinical opportunities

The university does not run any specialty clinics. The program has developed an extensive offering of diverse clinical training opportunities in the greater New York area.

Southern Illinois University (Ph.D.)

Department of Psychology
Carbondale, IL 62901
phone#: (618) 453-3564
e-mail: gradpsyc@siu.edu (graduate secretary)
chwalisz@siu.edu (program director)
Web address:
www.psychology.siu.edu/counseling/index.html

1	2	3	**4**	5	6	7
Practice oriented		Equal emphasis			Research oriented	

Percentage of faculty subscribing to each of the following orientations:

Psychodynamic/Psychoanalytic	0%
Applied behavioral analysis/Radical behavioral	0%
Family systems/Systems	0%
Existential/Phenomenological/Humanistic	67%
Cognitive/Cognitive-behavioral	33%

Courses required for incoming students to have completed prior to enrolling: None

Recommended but not mandatory courses:

At least 1 statistics course; if student was not an undergraduate psychology major, we look for coursework in core areas of psychology

GRE mean

Verbal 528   Quantitative 593
Analytical Writing 5.38

GPA mean

Overall GPA 3.65

Number of applications/admission offers/incoming students in 2007

93 applied/8 admission offers/4 incoming

% of students receiving:

Full tuition waiver only: 0%
Assistantship/fellowship only: 0%
Both full tuition waiver & assistantship/fellowship: 100%

Approximate percentage of incoming students with a B.A./B.S. only: 90%   Master's: 10%

Approximate percentage of students who are Women: 80%   Ethnic Minority: 35%   International: 8%

Average years to complete the doctoral program (including internship): 5.5 years

Personal interview

Preferred in person but telephone acceptable

Attrition rate in past 7 years: 8%

Percentage of students applying for internship last year accepted into APPIC or APA internships: 100%

Formal tracks/concentrations: none

Research areas	# Faculty	# Grants
academic self-concept, and achievement	1	0
adjustment to brain injury/disability	1	0
career assessment and counseling	2	1
career choice and development	2	1
caregiver burden	1	1
counseling supervision	1	0
expectations about counseling	1	0
gender/cultural influences	3	2
health psychology	1	0
occupational stress and health	1	0
psychological measurement	1	0
student development	1	0
qualitative research methodology	1	0
racial/ethnic identity	3	0
self-efficacy	1	0
sexual harassment	1	0
spiritual/religious issues	1	0
stress and coping	2	0
women in management	1	0
workplace violence	1	0

Clinical opportunities

career development	university counseling center
marriage and family	community clinics
rural mental health	VA hospital
partial hospitalization	vocational rehabilitation
psychiatric (inpatient)	substance abuse
state correctional system (medium security facility)	stress management
	sexuality counseling
student health service	

University of Southern Mississippi (Ph.D.)

Department of Psychology
118 College Dr. #5025
Hattiesburg, MS 39406-0001
phone#: (601) 266-4602
e-mail: m.leach@usm.edu
Web address:
www.usm.edu/counselingpsy/doc/dochome.html

1	2	3	**4**	5	6	7
Practice oriented		Equal emphasis			Research oriented	

Percentage of faculty subscribing to each of the following orientations:

Psychodynamic/Psychoanalytic	10%
Applied behavioral analysis/Radical behavioral	0%
Family systems/Systems	20%
Existential/Phenomenological/Humanistic	20%
Cognitive/Cognitive-behavioral	50%

Courses required for incoming students to have completed prior to enrolling: None

Recommended but not mandatory courses:
Statistics, personality, testing and assessment

GRE mean
Verbal 550   Quantitative 550
Analytical Writing Data: 3.5–4.0

GPA mean
Overall GPA 3.40   Overall master's GPA 3.70

Number of applications/admission offers/incoming students in 2007
52 applied/14 admission offers/5 incoming

% of students receiving:
Full tuition waiver only: 0%
Assistantship/fellowship only: 0%
Both full tuition waiver & assistantship/fellowship: 100%

Approximate percentage of incoming students with a B.A./B.S. only: 75%   **Master's:** 25%

Approximate percentage of students who are Women: 75%   **Ethnic Minority:** 40%
International: 0% this year; previous: 15%

Average years to complete the doctoral program (including internship): 5 post BA/BS; 4 post master's

Personal interview
Preferred in person but telephone acceptable

Attrition rate in past 7 years: 10%

Percentage of students applying for internship last year accepted into APPIC or APA internships: 100%

Formal tracks/concentrations: none

Research areas	# Faculty	# Grants
anger	1	1
attachment	3	0
body image	1	0
constructivist therapy	1	0
diversity	3	0
eating disorders	1	0
empirically supported treatments	2	0
forgiveness	1	0
international counseling issues	1	0
motivational interviewing	1	0
parenting	1	0
spirituality	2	1
suicide	1	0
vocational	1	0

Clinical opportunities
alcohol and drug treatment
community mental health center
counseling assessment center
counseling training clinic
inpatient
outpatient
university counseling center
university medical center (Jackson, MS)
VA hospital (Biloxi, MS)
National Guard Youth Challenge Program

University of Tennessee–Knoxville (Ph.D.)

Department of Psychology
312 Austin Peay Building
Knoxville, TN 37996-0900
phone#: (865) 974-3328
e-mail: cjogle@utk.edu
Web address: psychology.utk.edu

1	2	3	**4**	5	6	7
Practice oriented		Equal emphasis			Research oriented	

Percentage of faculty subscribing to each of the following orientations:

Psychodynamic/Psychoanalytic	20%
Applied behavioral analysis/Radical behavioral	0%
Family systems/Systems	14%
Existential/Phenomenological/Humanistic	29%
Cognitive/Cognitive-behavioral	43%

Courses required for incoming students to have completed prior to enrolling:
An undergraduate degree is required, but no particular courses.

Recommended but not mandatory courses: None

GRE mean
Verbal 540   Quantitative 580
Analytical Writing not reported

GPA mean
Overall GPA 3.35 (Undergraduate); 3.78 (Graduate)

Number of applications/admission offers/incoming students in 2007
57 applied/10 admission offers/5 incoming

% of students receiving:
Full tuition waiver only: 0%
Assistantship/fellowship only: 0%
Both full tuition waiver & assistantship/fellowship: 100%

Approximate percentage of incoming students with a B.A./B.S. only: 40%   **Master's:** 60%

Approximate percentage of students who are:
Women: 80%   **Ethnic Minority:** 20%   **International:** 0%

Average years to complete the doctoral program (including internship): 6 years

Personal interview:
Interview not required

Attrition rate in past 7 years: 10%

Percentage of students applying for internship last year accepted into APPIC or APA internships: 60%

Formal tracks/concentrations: none

Research areas	# Faculty	# Grants
careers	3	0
counseling process	3	0

Clinical opportunities
assistantship available in department's psychological clinic

Tennessee State University (Ph.D.)

Department of Psychology
Nashville, TN 37209-1561
phone#: (615) 963-5141
e-mail: cblazina@tnstate.edu
Web address:
www.tnstate.edu/interior.asp?ptid=1&mid=878

1	2	3	**4**	5	6	7
Practice oriented		Equal emphasis			Research oriented	

Percentage of faculty subscribing to each of the following orientations:

Psychodynamic/Psychoanalytic	60%
Applied behavioral analysis/Radical behavioral	0%
Family systems/Systems	20%
Existential/Phenomenological/Humanistic	17%
Cognitive/Cognitive-behavioral	20%

Courses required for incoming students to have completed prior to enrolling:
Learning; statistics; research methodology; counseling; intellectual assessment; personality theory, developmental or psychometrics (2 out of 3); master's-level practicum; history & systems of psychology

Recommended but not mandatory courses: none

GRE mean
Verbal 500   Quantitative 500
Analytical Writing not reported

GPA mean
Overall GPA 3.25

Number of applications/admission offers/incoming students in 2007
45 applied/11 admission offers/4 incoming

% of students receiving:
Full tuition waiver only: 0%
Assistantship/fellowship only: 10%
Both full tuition waiver & assistantship/fellowship: 100%

Approximate percentage of incoming students with a B.A./B.S. only: 0%   **Master's:** 100%

Approximate percentage of students who are Women: 66.6%   **Ethnic Minority:** 33.3%
International: 1%

Average years to complete the doctoral program (including internship): 4 years

Personal interview
Preferred in person but telephone acceptable

Attrition rate in past 7 years: not reported

Percentage of students applying for internship last year accepted into APPIC or APA internships: 100%

Formal tracks/concentrations: none

Research areas	# Faculty	# Grants
decision making	1	0
eating disorders	2	1
men's issues	1	0
multicultural concerns	2	1
teaching of psychology	1	0

Clinical opportunities
adult, child, and adolescent psychiatry
behavioral health
forensics
university counseling center
community mental health
VA hospital

Texas A&M University (Ph.D.)

Department of Educational Psychology
College Station, TX 77843
phone#: (979) 845-1833
e-mail: cpsy@tamu.edu
Web address: cpsy.tamu.edu

1	2	3	**4**	5	6	7
Practice oriented		Equal emphasis			Research oriented	

Percentage of faculty subscribing to each of the following orientations:

Psychodynamic/Psychoanalytic	20%
Multicultural/Feminist	40%
Cognitive/Cognitive-behavioral	20%

Courses required for incoming students prior to enrolling: None

Courses recommended but not mandatory:
Courses in psychology, statistics, and research methods

GRE mean
Verbal 560   Quantitative 560
Analytical Writing not reported

GPA mean
Overall GPA 3.8   Psychology GPA 3.5
Junior/Senior GPA 3.5

Number of applications/admission offers/incoming students in 2007
65 applied/12 admission offers/10 incoming

% of students receiving:
Full tuition waiver only: 0%
Assistantship/fellowship only: 50%
Both full tuition waiver & assistantship/fellowship: 50%

Approximate percentage of incoming students with a B.A./B.S. only: 80%   **Master's:** 20%

Approximate percentage of students who are:
Women: 80%   **Ethnic Minority:** 59%   **International:** 5%

Average years to complete the doctoral program (including internship): 6 years

Personal interview
Required in person

Attrition rate in past 7 years: 6%

Percentage of students applying for internship last year accepted into APPIC or APA internships: 85%

Formal tracks/concentrations: clinical geropsychology, multicultural counseling, public health, Mexican American health/mental health research

Research areas	# Faculty	# Grants
geropsychology	1	0
rehabilitation/caregivers	1	3
methods in psychological research	1	0
multicultural training	2	0
acculturation process	1	0
racial/ethnic minority groups	3	1
public health	2	1

Clinical opportunities
university counseling centers
VA hospitals
community health clinics

University of Texas at Austin
Department of Educational Psychology
D 5800
Austin, TX 78712
phone#: (512) 471-4409
e-mail: bennie.crum@mail.utexas.edu
Web address:
edpsych.edb.utexas.edu/admissions/counseling.php

1	2	3	4	**5**	6	7

Practice oriented	Equal emphasis	Research oriented

Percentage of faculty subscribing to each of the following orientations:

Psychodynamic/Psychoanalytic	22%
Applied behavioral analysis/Radical behavioral	11%
Existential/Phenomenological/Humanistic	22%
Interpersonal/Constructivist	11%
Cognitive/Cognitive-behavioral	11%
Multicultural	22%

Courses required for incoming students to have completed prior to enrolling:
bachelor's degree

Recommended but not mandatory courses: None

GRE mean
Verbal + Quantitative 1231
Analytical Writing not reported

GPA mean
Overall GPA 3.4

Number of applications/admission offers/incoming students in 2007
165 applied/10 admission offers/9 incoming

% of students receiving:
Full tuition waiver only: 0%
Assistantship/fellowship only: 67%
Both full tuition waiver & assistantship/fellowship: 33%

Approximate percentage of incoming students with a B.A./B.S. only: 83%   **Master's:** 17%

Approximate percentage of students who are Women: 64%   **Ethnic Minority:** 31%   **International:** 5%

Average years to complete the doctoral program (including internship): 6 years

Personal interview
Preferred in person but telephone acceptable

Attrition rate in past 7 years: 10%

Percentage of students applying for internship last year accepted into APPIC or APA internships: 92%

Formal tracks/concentrations: assessments, health psychology, multicultural counseling

Research areas	# Faculty	# Grants
depression	1	0
attachment	1	0
psychology of men and masculinity	1	0
multicultural/cross-cultural	3	0
psychoanalysis	2	0

Clinical opportunities
adolescent and adult inpatient and outpatient
community practicum
correctional facilities
immigrant/refugee clinic
inpatient units at state and VA hospitals
long-term outpatient psychotherapy
university counseling centers

Texas Tech University (Ph.D.)
Department of Psychology
Lubbock, TX 79409
phone#: (806) 742-3711, ext. 231
e-mail: sheila.garos@ttu.edu
Web address: www.depts.ttu.edu/psy/psy.php?page
=graduate/counseling/counseling

1	2	3	**4**	5	6	7

Practice oriented	Equal emphasis	Research oriented

Percentage of faculty subscribing to each of the following orientations:

Psychodynamic/Psychoanalytic	20%
Applied behavioral analysis/Radical behavioral	0%
Family systems/Systems	10%
Existential/Phenomenological/Humanistic	35%
Cognitive/Cognitive-behavioral	35%

Courses required for incoming students to have completed prior to enrolling:
18 undergraduate hours in psychology and statistics

Recommended but not mandatory courses: None

GRE mean
Verbal 529   Quantitative 627
Analytical Writing 5.0

GPA mean
Overall GPA 3.68

Number of applications/admission offers/incoming students in 2007
84 applied/11 admission offers/6 incoming

% of students receiving:
Full tuition waiver only: 0%
Assistantship/fellowship only: 0%
Both full tuition waiver & assistantship/fellowship: 100%

Approximate percentage of incoming students with a B.A./B.S. only: 80%   Master's: 20%

Approximate percentage of students who are Women: 80%   Ethnic Minority: 30%   International: 0%

Average years to complete the doctoral program (including internship): 6 years

Personal interview
Required in person

Attrition rate in past 7 years: 20%

Percentage of students applying for internship last year accepted into APPIC or APA internships: 75%

Formal tracks/concentrations: none

Research areas	# Faculty	# Grants
Asian Americans	1	0
behavioral addictions	1	0
cardiac rehabilitation	1	0
coping and stress	2	0
cultural differences in the self	1	0
depression	1	0
family	2	0
forensic/correctional	1	1
gender and women	2	0
group therapy	1	0
health psychology	4	0
multicultural counseling	1	0
positive psychology	1	0
professional issues	1	0
relationships	1	0
religion	1	0
sexual behavior	1	0
vocational	2	0

Clinical opportunities

inpatient psychiatric unit
child advocacy center
community mental health
outpatient psychology clinic
health sciences center/
    cancer center
public school district
neuropsychological
    assessment
personality assessment
psychiatric prison unit
university counseling center

Texas Woman's University (Ph.D.)

Department of Psychology and Philosophy
P.O. Box 425470
Denton, TX 76204
phone#: (940) 898-2303
e-mail: rnutt@mail.twu.edu

Web address:
www.twu.edu/as/psyphil/Counseling_Doctoral.htm

1	2	3	4	5	6	7
Practice oriented		Equal emphasis			Research oriented	

Percentage of faculty subscribing to each of the following orientations:

Psychodynamic/Psychoanalytic	10%
Applied behavioral analysis/Radical behavioral	10%
Family systems/Systems	50%
Existential/Phenomenological/Humanistic	100%
Cognitive/Cognitive-behavioral	40%

Courses required for incoming students to have completed prior to enrolling:
Development, statistics, learning, experimental

Recommended but not mandatory courses: None

GRE mean
Verbal 560   Quantitative 560
Analytical Writing not reported

GPA mean
Psychology GPA 3.7   Junior/Senior GPA 3.5

Number of applications/admission offers/incoming students in 2007
Not reported

% of students receiving:
Full tuition waiver only: 0%
Assistantship/fellowship only: 20%
Both full tuition waiver & assistantship/fellowship: 0%

Approximate percentage of incoming students with a B.A./B.S. only: 50%   Master's: 50%

Approximate percentage of students who are Women: 80%   Ethnic Minority: 38%   International: 4%

Average years to complete the doctoral program (including internship): 6 years

Personal interview
Preferred in person but telephone acceptable

Attrition rate in past 7 years: 2%

Percentage of students applying for internship last year accepted into APPIC or APA internships: 100%

Formal tracks/concentrations: family psychology, special populations/diversity/gender

Research areas	# Faculty	# Grants
career development	3	1
ethics and regulation	2	0
gender	4	1
infidelity	1	1
marriage	3	0
sexual harassment	3	1

Clinical opportunities
university counseling center
community mental health
domestic violence agencies
hospitals

University of Utah (Ph.D.)

Department of Educational Psychology
1705E Campus Center Drive, Room 327
Salt Lake City, UT 84112-9255
phone#: (801) 581-7148
e-mail: paul.gore@ed.utah.edu
Web address: cp.ed.utah.edu

1	2	3	**4**	5	6	7
Practice oriented		Equal emphasis			Research oriented	

Percentage of faculty subscribing to each of the following orientations:

Psychodynamic/Psychoanalytic	13%
Applied behavioral analysis/Radical behavioral	0%
Family systems/Systems	0%
Existential/Phenomenological/Humanistic	2%
Cognitive/Cognitive-behavioral	25%
Feminist/Multicultural	9%
Interpersonal	15%

Courses required for incoming students to have completed prior to enrolling:

Undergraduate and/or graduate preparation in psychology is required but no specific courses are required.

Recommended but not mandatory courses:

Experimental, personality, developmental, physiological, abnormal, statistics, research methods, social, and learning

GRE mean

Verbal 550   Quantitative 600   Analytical not reported
Advanced Psychology not required
Analytical Writing 4.7

GPA mean

Overall GPA 3.7

Number of applications/admission offers/incoming students in 2007

60 applied/13 admission offers/7 incoming

% of students receiving:

Full tuition waiver only: 0%
Assistantship/fellowship only: 0%
Both full tuition waiver & assistantship/fellowship: 100%

Approximate percentage of incoming students with a B.A./B.S. only: 52%   Master's: 48%

Approximate percentage of students who are Women: 66%   Ethnic Minority: 22%   International: 5%

Average years to complete the doctoral program (including internship): 6.5 years

Personal interview

Interview not required

Attrition rate in past 7 years: 10%

Percentage of students applying for internship last year accepted into APPIC or APA internships: 90%

Formal tracks/concentrations: none

Research areas	# Faculty	# Grants
abuse	2	1
adolescent mood disorders	1	0
applied gerontology	1	0
children and adolescents	3	2
gender and women's	2	0
human emotion	1	0
ethics	1	0
lesbian, gay, bisexual, transgender	2	0
multicultural counseling	3	0
professional education/training	1	0
psychotherapy process/outcome	1	0
substance abuse	1	1
career development	2	0

Clinical opportunities

community mental health
drug and alcohol treatment
ethnic student center
family medicine health center
gerontology services

sexual abuse treatment
university counseling center
VA hospital
pain clinic
women's resource center

Virginia Commonwealth University (Ph.D.)

Department of Psychology
Richmond, VA 23284-2018
phone#: 804-828-8222
e-mail: sdanish@vcu.edu (Director)
Web address:
www.has.vcu.edu/psy/counseling/index.html

1	2	3	4	**5**	6	7
Practice oriented		Equal emphasis			Research oriented	

Percentage of faculty subscribing to each of the following orientations:

Psychodynamic/Interpersonal	30%
Applied behavioral analysis/Radical behavioral	0%
Family systems/Systems	10%
Existential/Phenomenological/Humanistic	8%
Cognitive-behavioral/Feminist	28%
Developmental	8%

Courses required for incoming students to have completed prior to enrolling:

18 undergraduate credit hours in psychology, including statistics and research methods

Recommended but not mandatory courses: None

GRE mean

Verbal 570   Quantitative 610
Analytical Writing 5.0

GPA mean

Overall GPA 3.54

Number of applications/admission offers/incoming students in 2007

153 applied/10 admission offers/7 incoming

% of students receiving:
Full tuition waiver only: 0%
Assistantship/fellowship only: 0%
Both full tuition waiver & assistantship/fellowship: 100%

Approximate percentage of incoming students with a B.A./B.S. only: 63%

Approximate percentage of students who are Women: 100% **Ethnic Minority:** 29% **International:** 0%

Average years to complete the doctoral program (including internship): 5 years

Personal interview
Preferred in person but telephone acceptable

Attrition rate in past 7 years: 12.7%

Percentage of students applying for internship last year accepted into APPIC or APA internships: 100%

Formal tracks/concentrations: health psychology

Research areas	# Faculty	# Grants
career intervention	1	2
minority mental health	3	0
forgiveness/religious values	2	0
health psychology	5	5
interventions	1	1
prevention	2	2
leadership and group dynamics	1	0
marital and family enrichment	2	0
teaching of life skills/community	1	1

Clinical opportunities

college mental health center	juvenile correctional system
university counseling center	state psychiatric hospital
child treatment center	substance abuse
federal correctional center	VA hospital
rehabilitation medicine unit	

Washington State University (Ph.D.)

Department of Educational Leadership and Counseling Psychology
Pullman, WA 99164
phone#: (509) 335-7016 or 335-9195
e-mail: gradstudies@wsu.edu and
church@mail.wsu.edu
Web address:
www.educ.wsu.edu/elcp/documents/CCounPsy.html

1	2	3	4	5	6	7

Practice oriented	Equal emphasis	Research oriented

Percentage of faculty subscribing to each of the following orientations:

Psychodynamic/Psychoanalytic	0%
Applied behavioral analysis/Radical behavioral	0%
Family systems/Systems	10%
Existential/Phenomenological/Humanistic	40%
Cognitive/Cognitive-behavioral	50%

Courses required for incoming students to have completed prior to enrolling: None

Recommended but not mandatory courses: None

GRE mean
Verbal 490   Quantitative 560   Analytical 554
Analytical Writing not reported
Advanced Psychology not reported

GPA mean
Overall GPA 3.66
Overall master's GPA 3.88

Number of applications/admission offers/incoming students in 2007
56 applied/13 admission offers/8 incoming

% of students receiving:
Full tuition waiver only: 0%
Assistantship/fellowship only: 0%
Both full tuition waiver & assistantship/fellowship: 80%

Approximate percentage of incoming students with a B.A./B.S. only: 50% **Master's:** 50%

Approximate percentage of students who are Women: 77% **Ethnic Minority:** 40%
International: 8.5%

Average years to complete the doctoral program (including internship): 6 years

Personal interview
Interview not required

Attrition rate in past 7 years: 5%

Percentage of students applying for internship last year accepted into APPIC or APA internships: 90%

Formal tracks/concentrations: none

Research areas	# Faculty	# Grants
acculturation/ethnic identity	3	0
cross-cultural/multicultural	3	1
disabilities	1	1
eating disorders	1	0
hypnosis and attentional processes	2	1
measurement/assessment	3	1
personality	1	0
resiliency	1	0
social influence	1	0
supervision	1	0
vocational	2	0

Clinical opportunities
not reported

West Virginia University (Ph.D.)

Department of Counseling, Rehabilitation Counseling, and Counseling Psychology
P.O. Box 6122
Morgantown, WV 26506-6122
phone#: (304) 293-3807 x1209
e-mail: sherry.cormier@mail.wvu.edu
Web address: www.hre.wvu.edu/crc/counseling
_psychology/index.htm

1	2	**3**	4	5	6	7
Practice oriented			Equal emphasis			Research oriented

Percentage of faculty subscribing to each of the following orientations:

Psychodynamic/Psychoanalytic	20%
Applied behavioral analysis/Radical behavioral	0%
Family systems/Systems	20%
Existential/Phenomenological/Humanistic	40%
Cognitive/Cognitive-behavioral	20%

Courses required for incoming students to have completed prior to enrolling:

Master's degree in counseling psychology, clinical psychology, or related field

Recommended but not mandatory courses:

Supervised field experience, multivariate methods, psychopharmacology

GRE mean

Verbal 520   Quantitative 617
Analytical Writing 4.5

GPA mean

Overall GPA 3.25
Overall graduate GPA 3.7

Number of applications/admission offers/incoming students in 2007

25 applied/14 admission offers/7 incoming

% of students receiving:

Full tuition waiver only: 25%
Assistantship/fellowship only: 0%
Both full tuition waiver & assistantship/fellowship: 75%

Approximate percentage of incoming students with a B.A./B.S. only: 0%   Master's: 100%

Approximate percentage of students who are Women: 30%   Ethnic Minority: 14%
International: not reported

Average years to complete the doctoral program (including internship): 5.5 years

Personal interview

Required in person

Attrition rate in past 7 years: 5%

Percentage of students applying for internship last year accepted into APPIC or APA internships: 90%

Formal tracks/concentrations: none

Research areas	# Faculty	# Grants
clinical supervision	1	0
consulting models	1	0
group counseling	1	0
injured athletes	1	0
personality assessment	2	0
psychiatric rehabilitation	1	0
psychology and mental health	3	0
psychology of disability	1	0
psychotherapeutic techniques	3	0
rehab counseling and psychology	2	0
self-efficacy and health	2	0
vocational counseling	2	0

Clinical opportunities

community agencies
correctional facilities

counseling centers
VA hospital

Western Michigan University (Ph.D.)

Department of Counselor Education and
Counseling Psychology
3102 Sangren Hall
Kalamazoo, MI 49008-5195
phone#: (269) 387-5100
e-mail: carolyn.cardwell@wmich.edu
Web address: www.wmich.edu/coe/cecp/

1	2	3	4	**5**	6	7
Practice oriented			Equal emphasis			Research oriented

Percentage of faculty subscribing to each of the following orientations:

Psychodynamic/Psychoanalytic	13%
Applied behavioral analysis/Radical behavioral	0%
Family systems/Systems	20%
Existential/Phenomenological/Humanistic	88%
Cognitive/Cognitive-behavioral	88%

Courses required for incoming students to have completed prior to enrolling:

Undergraduate degree required; master's degree preferred

Recommended but not mandatory courses:

Psychology or social science major

GRE mean

Verbal + Quantitative 1000
Analytical Writing not reported
Advanced Psychology not reported

GPA mean

Overall graduate GPA 3.5
Overall undergraduate GPA 3.5

Number of applications/admission offers/incoming students in 2007

70 applied/12 admission offers/9 incoming

% of students receiving:

Full tuition waiver only: 0%
Assistantship/fellowship only: 33%
Both full tuition waiver & assistantship/fellowship: 67%

Approximate percentage of incoming students with a B.A./B.S. only:10%   Master's: 90%

Approximate percentage of students who are Women: 70%   Ethnic Minority: 34%   International: 9%

Average years to complete the doctoral program (including internship): 5 years

Personal interview

Required in person

Attrition rate in past 7 years: 6%

Percentage of students applying for internship last year accepted into APPIC or APA internships: 100%

Formal tracks/concentrations: none

Research areas	# Faculty	# Grants
families	1	1
group work	1	1
multicultural concerns	4	0
psychological assessment	2	0
treatment	3	0

Clinical opportunities
In-house clinic and local hospitals, agencies, and schools

University of Wisconsin–Madison (Ph.D.)

Department of Counseling Psychology
321 Education Building, 1000 Bascom Mall
Madison, WI 53706
phone#: (608) 263-2746
e-mail: counpsych@education.wisc.edu
Web address:
www.education.wisc.edu/CP/doctoralprogram.htm

1	2	3	4	**5**	6	7

Practice oriented — Equal emphasis — Research oriented

Percentage of faculty subscribing to each of the following orientations:

Psychodynamic/Psychoanalytic	30%
Applied behavioral analysis/Radical behavioral	0%
Family systems/Systems	10%
Existential/Phenomenological/Humanistic	40%
Cognitive/Cognitive-behavioral	30%
Multicultural	100%

Courses required for incoming students to have completed prior to enrolling:
Master's degree in counseling, including multicultural counseling and career psychology

Recommended but not mandatory courses: None

GRE mean
Verbal not reported   Quantitative not reported
Analytical Writing not reported

GPA mean
Junior/Senior GPA 3.6

Number of applications/admission offers/incoming students in 2007
75 applied/12 admission offers/8 incoming

% of students receiving:
Full tuition waiver only: 0%
Assistantship/fellowship only: 0%
Both full tuition waiver & assistantship/fellowship: 100%

Approximate percentage of incoming students with a B.A./B.S. only: 0%   **Master's:** 95%

Approximate percentage of students who are Women: 60%   **Ethnic Minority:** 25%
International: Not reported

Average years to complete the doctoral program (including internship): 6 years

Personal interview
Telephone required

Attrition rate in past 7 years: 4%

Percentage of students applying for internship last year accepted into APPIC or APA internships: 75%

Formal tracks/concentrations: none

Research areas	# Faculty	# Grants
academic retention	2	0
career development	2	0
clinical supervision	1	1
corporate systems	1	0
ethnic identity	4	2
gender	4	0
group	1	0
multidisciplinary environments	2	1
multiethnic/cultural environments	5	3
process-outcome	3	0
school counseling	2	2

Clinical opportunities
not reported

University of Wisconsin–Milwaukee (Ph.D.)

Department of Educational Psychology
P.O. Box 413
Milwaukee, WI 53201
phone#: (414) 229-6830
e-mail: nadya@uwm.edu
Web address: www.soe.uwm.edu/pages/welcome/
Departments/Educational_Psychology/Degrees
_Programs_of_Study/Counseling

1	2	3	4	5	**6**	7

Practice oriented — Equal emphasis — Research oriented

Percentage of faculty subscribing to each of the following orientations:

Psychodynamic/Psychoanalytic	0%
Applied behavioral analysis/Radical behavioral	0%
Developmental Systems	20%
Interpersonal	20%
Existential/Phenomenological/Humanistic	0%
Cognitive/Cognitive-behavioral	60%

Courses required for incoming students to have completed prior to enrolling:
Group counseling, listening skills, statistics, multicultural counseling, theories of counseling, cognition, career development, personality

Recommended but not mandatory courses:
Cognition, personality

315

GRE mean
Verbal 466   Quantitative 523   Analytical 599
Analytical Writing 4.2
Advanced Psychology not reported

GPA mean
Overall GPA 3.8

Number of applications/admission offers/incoming students in 2007
41 applied/12 admission offers/6 incoming

% of students receiving:
Full tuition waiver only: 0%
Assistantship/fellowship only: 0%
Both full tuition waiver & assistantship/fellowship: 80%

Approximate percentage of incoming students with a B.A./B.S. only: 16%   **Master's:** 84%

Approximate percentage of students who are Women: 66%   **Ethnic Minority:** 39%   **International:** 8%

Average years to complete the doctoral program (including internship): 5.2 years

Personal interview
Preferred in person but telephone acceptable

Attrition rate in past 7 years: 5%

Percentage of students applying for internship last year accepted into APPIC or APA internships: 66%

Formal tracks/concentrations: none

Research areas	# Faculty	# Grants
youth addictions	1	2
barriers for women in math/science	1	1
hypnosis and hypnotizability	1	0
international research	1	2
intervention programming	1	1
masculinity and male gender role	1	0
counseling training	1	0
multicultural counseling	2	2
pediatric behavioral health	1	0
vocational development	2	2

Clinical opportunities
children's hospital
community mental health
counseling center
family services
inpatient psychiatric
medical college
VA hospital
day treatment for adolescents
eating disorders clinic

Counseling Psychology Programs That Have Been Discontinued

Michigan State University (accredited, inactive)

Ohio State University (accredited, inactive)

University of Southern California (accredited, inactive)

Stanford University (accredited, inactive)

Temple University (accredited, inactive)

Counseling Psychology Programs Not Reporting Information

Howard University

A P P E N D I X   A
TIME LINE

Freshman and Sophomore Years

1. Take the core psychology courses—introduction, statistics, research methods, abnormal, physiological.
2. Find out about faculty interests and research.
3. Make preliminary contact with faculty members whose research interests you.
4. Explore volunteer opportunities in clinical settings.
5. Investigate various career choices.
6. Join psychology student organizations and become an active member.
7. Attend departmental colloquia and social gatherings.
8. Enroll in courses helpful for graduate school, including biological sciences, mathematics, writing, and public speaking.
9. Learn to use library and electronic resources, such as scholarly journals and *PsycLit*.
10. Consider participating in your university's honors program, if you qualify.
11. Begin a career folder and place activities, honors, and other valuable reminders in it.
12. Discuss your career interests with faculty members and other mentors.

Junior Year

1. Take advanced psychology courses, for example, cognitive, developmental, psychological testing.
2. Begin clinical work, both volunteer and practicum.
3. Volunteer for research with faculty and begin researching a potential thesis/independent project.
4. Continue contact with faculty and upperclassmen.
5. Enroll in professional organizations, for example, student affiliate of American Psychological Association or American Psychological Society.
6. Apply for membership in your local Psi Chi chapter.
7. Visit your career services office on campus and determine how the staff can assist you in applying to graduate school.
8. Draft a curriculum vitae to determine your strengths and weaknesses.
9. Attend a state or regional psychology convention.
10. Peruse graduate school bulletins online to acquaint yourself with typical requirements, offerings, and policies.
11. Surf the Web. Become comfortable with leading Web sites on graduate school admissions.
12. Access the GRE bulletin and information online. Begin preparation for the GRE by purchasing a study guide, attending a preparation course, and taking practice tests.
13. Update your folder by putting your curriculum vita/resume and reminders of your activities and accomplishments in it.
14. Try to focus your interests in particular research areas, theoretical orientations, and clinical populations.
15. Consider serving as an officer in one of the student organizations on campus.
16. Meet with your advisor or mentor before summer to review your plan for graduate applications.

Application Year

June–August

1. Continue to acquire research competencies and clinical experiences.
2. Surf the Web and begin to gather information from program Web sites.
3. Begin to narrow down potential schools to 20–40.
4. Prepare intensively for the GREs.
5. Consider taking the GRE General Test if you are prepared; this will afford ample time to retake them in the fall if necessary.
6. Investigate financial aid opportunities for graduate students.
7. Set aside money for the cost of the GREs and applications.

August–September

1. Download program information and applications from program Web sites and/or write to schools for applications.
2. Review program information.
3. Consult with advisors regarding graduate programs, application procedures, faculty of interest.
4. Continue to study diligently for the GREs.
5. Update your curriculum vitae.
6. Investigate possible financial aid opportunities.
7. Begin a file in your institution's Office of Career Services/Planning.
8. Gather applications for salient fellowships and scholarships.

September–October

1. Take the GRE General Test (for first or second time).
2. Register for the GRE Psychology Subject Test administered in November and December.
3. Create a short list of schools using the worksheets.
4. Record the deadlines for submitting each application.
5. Choose the faculty at each program that most interest you.
6. Research your area of interest, focusing on the work of faculty with whom you would like to work.
7. Write to graduate faculty expressing interest in their work (if appropriate).
8. Request a copy of your own transcript and inspect it for any errors or omissions.
9. Begin first drafts of your personal statement and get feedback on it.
10. Update your CV or resume.

11. Calculate costs of applications and admission interviews and acquire the money for them.
12. Finalize the decision on whom you will ask for letters of recommendation.

October–November

1. Take the GRE Psychology Subject Test.
2. Take the MAT (only if necessary).
3. Prepare packets to distribute to your recommenders, including a complete vitae or resume.
4. Request letters of recommendation.
5. Arrange for the registrar to send your transcripts to schools.
6. Gather information on financial aid and loans available to graduate students.
7. Finalize your personal statements.

November–December

1. Complete applications.
2. Maintain a photocopy of each application for your records.
3. If the opportunity arises, visit professors with whom you have been in contact.
4. Submit applications.
5. Verify that the applications and all necessary materials have been received.
6. Request ETS forward your GRE scores to the appropriate institutions.

January–March

1. Wait patiently.
2. Insure that all of your letters of recommendation have been sent.
3. Be prepared for surprise telephone interviews.
4. Practice and prepare for admission interviews.
5. Travel to interviews as invited.
6. Develop contingency plans if not accepted into any programs.

April–May

1. If other programs make early offers, contact your top choices to determine the current status of your application.
2. Accept an offer of admission and promptly turn down less-preferred offers.
3. Finalize financial aid arrangements for next year.
4. Send official transcripts with Spring term grades to the program you plan to attend.
5. If not accepted to any schools, refer to Chapter 7.
6. Celebrate (if accepted) or regroup (if not accepted).
7. Inform people who wrote you letters of recommendation of the outcome.

A P P E N D I X   B

WORKSHEET FOR CHOOSING PROGRAMS

| Area of Interest | School | Research | | | Clinical | | | Self-Rating |
		# Faculty	Funded	Rank	Orien-tation	Res/Clin	Rank	

Area of Interest	School	Research			Clinical			
		# Faculty	Funded	Rank	Orien-tation	Res/Clin	Rank	Self-Rating

APPENDIX C

WORKSHEET
FOR ASSESSING
PROGRAM CRITERIA

School	Self-Rating	Courses	GRE-V	GRE-Q	GRE-S	GPA	Research	Clinical	Compete	Total

APPENDIX D

WORKSHEET FOR MAKING FINAL CHOICES

School	School Criteria	Research	Clinical	Theoretical Orientation	Financial Aid	Quality of Life

APPENDIX E
RESEARCH AREAS

	# Faculty	# Grants

Acceptance & Commitment Therapy

Georgia State University (Cl)	1	0
Illinois Institute of Technology (Cl)	1	0
Wichita State University (Cl)	1	0

Acculturation

New Mexico State University (Co)	3	0
University of Minnesota Dept of Psychology (Co)	1	0
Yeshiva University (PhD) (Cl)	2	3

Acquired Immune Deficiency Syndrome/HIV

Arizona State University (Co)	1	0
Argosy University–San Francisco	1	0
Carlos Albizu University–San Juan (Cl)	1	0
DePaul University (Cl)	1	3
George Washington University (Ph.D.) (Cl)	1	2
Georgia State University (Cl)	2	4
Indiana State University (Co)	1	0
Jackson State University (Cl)	3	3
Kent State University (Cl)	1	1
Loyola University–Chicago (Cl)	2	1
Ponce School of Medicine (Cl)	3	2
San Diego State University/University of California–San Diego (Cl)	7	1
Southern Illinois University (Cl)	1	0
Syracuse University (Cl)	2	2
University of Illinois at Chicago (Cl)	1	1
University of Maryland (Co)	1	0
University of Maryland–Baltimore (Cl)	2	1
University of Memphis (Co)	1	1
University of Miami (Cl)	6	2+
University of Missouri–Kansas City (Cl)	1	3
University of Missouri–Kansas City (Co)	1	1
University of North Dakota (Co)	1	1
University of North Texas (Cl)	1	0
University of Wyoming (Cl)	1	3
Virginia Consortium Program (Cl)	1	0
Virginia Polytechnic Institute and State University (Cl)	2	0
Western Michigan University (Cl)	1	1

Adjustment

Purdue University (Co)		
St. Louis University (Cl)	2	0
University of Northern Colorado (Co)	2	1

Adolescent/At-Risk Adolescent

Argosy University, Chicago (Psy.D.) (Cl)	1	0
Boston College (Co)	2	2
Carlos Albizu University–Miami Campus (Cl)	3	0
Carlos Albizu University–San Juan (Ph.D.) (Cl)	4	1
Catholic University of America (Cl)	3	1
Colorado State University (Co)	3	5
Emory University (Cl)	2	1
George Fox University (Cl)	1	0
George Washington University (Ph.D.) (Cl)	3	2
Howard University (Co)	3	1
Immaculata College (Cl)	2	0
Indiana University (Co)	1	2
Loyola University–Chicago (Cl)	6	4
Loyola University–Chicago (Co)	1	1
Northern Illinois University (Cl)	3	0
Northwestern University, Feinberg School of Medicine (Cl)	3	2

Note. Cl, Clinical; Co, Counseling; Cm, combined psychology programs.

	# Faculty	# Grants
Nova Southeastern University (Ph.D. & Psy.D.) (Cl)	5	0
Oklahoma State University (Co)	2	1
Ontario Institute for Studies in Education (Cm)	2	1
Purdue University (Cl)	1	0
Rosalind Franklin University of Medicine (Cl)	1	0
Rutgers University (Psy.D.) (Cl)	3	1
Seattle Pacific University (Cl)	3	1
Southern Illinois University (Cl)	2	0
Texas Tech University (Cl)	1	0
University of Cincinnati	5	3
University of Denver (Ph.D.) (Cl)	5	2
University of Georgia (Cl)	3	0
University of Georgia (Co)	2	0
University of Kentucky (Cl)	2	1
University of Massachusetts–Amherst (Cl)	4	3
University of Minnesota—Department of Educational Psychology (Co)	2	1
University of New Brunswick (Cl)	1	0
University of North Carolina at Chapel Hill (Cl)	3	3
University of North Carolina at Greensboro (Cl)	0	0
University of North Dakota (Co)	1	0
University of Pittsburgh (Cl)	8	28
University of South Florida (Cl)	4	2
University of Utah (Cl)	1	0
University of Vermont (Cl)	2	1
University of Virginia—Department of Human Services (Cl)	2	0
University of Virginia—Department of Psychology (Cl)	3	3
University of Wisconsin–Milwaukee (Co)	1	1
Virginia Commonwealth University (Cl)	5	4
Wichita State University (Cl)	1	2
Yeshiva University (Cm)	2	0
York University—Clinical-Developmental Area (Cl)	3	3

Affective Disorders/Depression/Mood Disorders

	# Faculty	# Grants
Alliant International University–Los Angeles (Psy.D.) (Cl)	1	0
American University (Cl)	1	0
Baylor University (Psy.D.) (Cl)	3	0
Binghamton University/State University of New York (Cl)	1	1
Boston University (Cl)	2	2
Brigham Young University (Cl)	1	1
Carlos Albizu University–Miami Campus (Cl)	3	0
Catholic University of America (Cl)	2	0
DePaul University (Cl)	2	2
Duke University (Cl)	4	4
Fairleigh Dickinson University (Cl)	0	0

Forest Institute of Professional Psychology (Cl)	2	1
George Washington University (Ph.D.) (Cl)	2	2
Hofstra University (Cm)	2	0
Idaho State University (Cl)	1	0
Illinois Institute of Technology (Cl)	1	1
Indiana State University (Cl)	2	0
Indiana University–Bloomington (Cl)	2	1
Jackson State University (Cl)	1	0
James Madison University (Cm)	1	0
Kent State University (Cl)	2	0
LaSalle University (Psy.D.) (Cl)	1	1
Louisiana State University (Cl)	1	1
Loyola University–Chicago (Cl)	0	0
Marquette University (Cl)	1	0
Northern Illinois University (Cl)	3	0
Northwestern University (Cl)	2	0
Ohio State University (Cl)	3	1
Oklahoma State University (Cl)	1	0
Pacific Graduate School of Psychology (Psy.D.) (Cl)	2	2
Pennsylvania State University (Cl)	2	0
Rutgers University (Ph.D.) (Cl)	0	0
St. Louis University (Cl)	2	0
San Diego State University/University of California–San Diego (Cl)	3	2
Simon Fraser University (Cl)	2	1
Southern Illinois University (Cl)	2	0
Stony Brook University/State University of New York (Cl)	1	4
Temple University (Cl)	1	1
Texas Tech University (Cl)	1	0
Texas Tech University (Co)	1	0
Uniformed Services University of Health Sciences (Cl)	1	2
University of Alabama (Cl)	1	0
University of Arizona (Cl)	2	1
University of Arkansas (Cl)	2	0
University at Buffalo/State University of New York (Cl)	2	1
University of California–Los Angeles (Cl)	2	3
University of Connecticut (Cl)	3	1
University of Colorado (Cl)	3	3
University of Georgia (Cl)	2	1
University of Hawaii at Manoa (Cl)	2	0
University of Houston (Cl)	3	2
University of Illinois at Chicago (Cl)	2	0
University of Iowa (Cl)	2	4
University of Kansas (Cl)	3	1
University of Maine (Cl)	1	0
University of Miami (Cl)	3	1
University of Minnesota (Cl)		
University of Montana (Cl)	1	0
University of Nevada–Reno (Cl)	1	0
University of North Carolina at Greensboro (Cl)	1	0
University of Notre Dame (Co)	3	1
University of Oregon (Cl)	3	2
University of Pennsylvania (Cl)	3	4
University of Pittsburgh (Cl)	6	22
University of Rochester (Cl)	1	1
University of South Dakota (Cl)	2	0

	# Faculty	# Grants
University of South Florida (Cl)	1	0
University of Texas at Austin (Co)	1	1
University of Texas at Austin (Cl)	1	0
University of Texas Southwestern Medical Center at Dallas (Cl)	5	4
University of Washington (Cl)	3	1
University of Waterloo (Cl)	1	1
University of Wisconsin–Madison (Cl)	4	1
University of Wisconsin–Milwaukee (Cl)	1	2
University of Wyoming (Cl)	3	2
Utah State University (Cm)	2	0
Vanderbilt University (Cl)	8	5
Virginia Polytechnic Institute and State University (Cl)	2	0
Western Michigan University (Cl)	2	1
Yale University (Cl)	3	0
Yeshiva University (Psy.D.) (Cl)	2	0
York University—Adult Clinical Program (Cl)	1	1

Aging/Gerontology/Adult Development

Adler School of Professional Psychology (Cl)	1	0
Argosy University–Atlanta (Psy.D.) (Cl)	0	0
Argosy University, Phoenix (Psy.D.) (Cl)	1	0
Arizona State University (Cl)	2	2
Boston University (Cl)	2	2
Carlos Albizu University–Miami Campus (Cl)	1	0
Carlos Albizu University–San Juan (Psy.D.) (Cl)	2	0
Carlos Albizu University–San Juan (Ph.D.) (Cl)	2	1
Case Western Reserve University (Cl)	2	1
Colorado State University (Co)	3	0
Columbia University, Teachers College (Cl)	1	1
Florida Institute of Technology (Cl)	1	2
Immaculata University (Psy.D.) (Cl)	1	0
Kent State University (Cl)	1	0
Loyola College in Maryland (Psy.D.) (Cl)	2	0
Loyola College–Chicago (Cl)	1	0
Marquette University (Cl)	1	0
Michigan State University (Cl)	1	0
Nova Southeastern University (Ph.D. & Psy.D.) (Cl)	1	0
Pacific Graduate School of Psychology (Cl)	1	1
Philadelphia College of Osteopathic Medicine (Psy.D.)(Cl)	1	0
Rosalind Franklin University of Medicine (Cl)	1	1
San Diego State University/University of California–San Diego (Cl)	8	1
Texas A&M University (Cl)	2	1
Texas A&M University (Co)	1	0
University of Alabama (Cl)	5	3
University of Alabama at Birmingham (Cl)	3	6
University of Connecticut (Cl)	1	0

University of Cincinnati (Cl)	2	0
University of Florida (Co)	1	0
University of Georgia (Cl)	1	3
University of Houston (Co)	2	1
University of Indianapolis (Psy.D.) (Cl)	2	1
University of Kansas (Cl)	1	0
University of Louisville (Cl)	2	1
University of Massachusetts at Amherst (Cl)	2	0
University of Missouri–St. Louis (Cl)	1	2
University of Montana (Cl)	1	1
University of Nevada–Reno (Cl)	2	4
University of New Brunswick (Cl)	1	0
University of North Dakota (Co)	1	1
University of North Texas (Cl)	1	1
University of North Texas (Co)	1	1
University of Ottawa (Cl)	1	1
University of Southern California (Cl)	4	13
University of Tulsa (Cl)	0	0
University of Utah (Co)	1	0
University of Victoria (Cl)	1	1
Washington University (Cl)	3	3
West Virginia University (Cl)	2	0
Western Michigan University (Cl)	1	1
Wheaton College (Cl)	1	1
Wright Institute (Psy.D.) (Cl)	1	0
Wright State University (Cl)	1	0
Xavier University (Cl)	2	0
Yeshiva University (Psy.D.) (Cl)	1	1
York University—Adult Clinical Program (Cl)	1	2

Aggression/Anger Control

Colorado State University (Co)	1	0
Hofstra University (Cm)	2	0
Kent State University (Cl)	1	1
Marywood University (Psy.D.) (Cl)	1	0
Philadelphia College of Osteopathic Medicine (Psy.D.) (Cl)	1	0
Purdue University (Cl)	3	1
University of Southern Mississippi (Co)	1	1
University of Arkansas (Cl)	3	1
University of Georgia (Cl)	2	1
University of Georgia (Co)	2	2
York University—Clinical-Developmental Area (Cl)	3	3

Anxiety Disorders/Panic Disorders

American University (Cl)	1	0
Auburn University (Cl)	2	0
Binghamton University/State University of New York (Cl)	2	1
Boston University (Cl)	7	5
Catholic University of America (Cl)	3	1
Central Michigan University (Cl)	1	1
Colorado State University (Co)	1	0
Concordia University (Cl)	2	3
Florida State University (Cl)	1	4
George Mason University (Cl)	1	0

	# Faculty	# Grants
George Washington University (Ph.D.) (Cl)	1	0
Georgia State University (Cl)	1	1
Indiana State University (Psy.D.) (Cl)	0	0
Kent State University (Cl)	2	0
LaSalle University (Psy.D.) (Cl)	1	0
Louisiana State University (Cl)	1	1
Loyola College in Maryland (Psy.D.) (Cl)	1	0
Miami University (Cl)	3	1
Northern Illinois University (Cl)	3	0
Northwestern University (Cl)	2	1
Nova Southeastern University (Ph.D. & Psy.D.) (Cl)	1	0
Ohio State University (Cl)	2	1
Oklahoma State University (Cl)	1	0
Ontario Institute for Studies in Education (Cm)	2	2
Pacific Graduate School of Psychology (Psy.D.) (Cl)	6	4
Pennsylvania State University (Cl)	7	3
Philadelphia College of Osteopathic Medicine (Psy.D.) (Cl)	7	0
Purdue University (Cl)	1	0
Rosalind Franklin University of Medicine (Cl)	1	1
Rutgers University (Psy.D.) (Cl)	3	1
St. John's University (Cl)	2	0
St. Louis University (Cl)	2	0
San Diego State University/University of California–San Diego (Cl)	4	1
Southern Illinois University (Cl)	3	0
Temple University (Cl)	2	5
Texas A&M University (Cl)	3	1
Texas Tech University (Cl)	1	1
University of Arkansas (Cl)	2	0
University at Albany/State University of New York (Cl)	1	0
University at Buffalo/State University of New York (Cl)	3	1
University of British Columbia (Cl)	3	5
University of California–Los Angeles (Cl)	1	4
University of Connecticut (Cl)	2	0
University of Delaware (Cl)	2	1
University of Florida (Cl)	2	3
University of Georgia (Cl)	2	1
University of Hawaii at Manoa (Cl)	1	1
University of Houston (Cl)	3	3
University of Illinois at Chicago (Cl)	3	1
University of Iowa (Co)	1	0
University of Kansas (Cl)	1	0
University of Louisville (Cl)	3	0
University of Maine (Cl)	2	1
University of Manitoba (Cl)	4	0
University of Maryland (Cl)	0	0
University of Minnesota (Cl)		
University of Missouri–Columbia (Cl)	2	1
University of Nebraska–Lincoln (Cl)	2	2
University of Nevada–Reno (Cl)	2	0
University of New Brunswick (Cl)	3	1
University of North Carolina at Chapel Hill (Cl)	1	0
University of North Dakota (Cl)	1	0
University of Oregon (Cl)	2	2
University of Pennsylvania (Cl)	2	5
University of Texas at Austin (Cl)	1	0
University of Toledo (Cl)	2	0
University of Vermont (Cl)	1	3
University of Virginia—Department of Psychology (Cl)	1	0
University of Washington (Cl)	3	1
University of Waterloo (Cl)	5	3
University of Wisconsin–Milwaukee (Cl)	3	3
University of Wyoming (Cl)	2	1
Vanderbilt University (Cl)	7	2
Virginia Commonwealth University (Cl)	2	1
Virginia Polytechnic Institute and State University (Cl)	3	1
West Virginia University (Cl)	2	0
Western Michigan University (Cl)	1	0
Yale University (Cl)	2	0
Yeshiva University (Psy.D.) (Cl)	1	0
York University—Adult Clinical Program (Cl)	1	1

Assessment/Diagnosis

	# Faculty	# Grants
Alliant International University–San Diego (Psy.D. & Ph.D.) (Cl)	4	0
Argosy University–Atlanta (Psy.D.) (Cl)	4	0
Argosy University–Twin Cities (Psy.D.) (Cl)	1	0
Azusa Pacific University (Psy.D.) (Cl)	2	0
Binghamton University/State University of New York (Cl)	4	0
Brigham Young University (Cl)	2	0
Catholic University of America (Cl)	2	0
Central Michigan University (Cl)	1	0
Colorado State University (Co)	3	0
Fairleigh Dickinson University (Cl)	6	2
Fordham University (Cl)	3	0
Gallaudet University (Cl)	2	1
George Washington University (Psy.D.) (Cl)	3	0
Indiana State University (Psy.D.) (Cl)	2	0
Jackson State University (Cl)	6	0
LaSalle University (Psy.D.) (Cl)	1	1
New School University (Cl)	2	1
Oklahoma State University (Co)	1	0
Pacific Graduate School of Psychology (Cl)	5	1
Philadelphia College of Osteopathic Medicine (Psy.D.)(Cl)	3	0
Roosevelt University (Psy.D.) (Cl)	3	0
St. Louis University (Cl)	2	0
San Diego State University/University of California–San Diego (Cl)	4	0
Southern Illinois University (Cl)	8	0
Texas A&M University (Cl)	3	0
Texas Tech University (Cl)	2	0
University of Alabama (Cl)	1	0
University of Buffalo/SUNY (Cm)	4	0
University of California–Santa Barbara (Cm)		

	# Faculty	# Grants
University of Colorado (Cl)	2	1
University of Detroit–Mercy (Cl)	1	0
University of Hartford (Psy.D.) (Cl)	1	0
University of Hawaii at Manoa (Cl)	7	2
University of Iowa (Cl)	2	2
University of Kentucky (Cl)	3	0
University of Massachusetts at Amherst (Cl)	1	1
University of Mississippi (Cl)	2	0
University of Montana (Cl)	2	1
University of Nevada–Reno (Cl)	3	0
University of North Carolina at Chapel Hill (Cl)	1	0
University of North Carolina at Greensboro (Cl)	1	0
University of Southern Mississippi (Co)	1	0
University of Toledo (Cl)	2	0
Virginia Consortium Program in Clinical Psychology (Cl)	5	0
Washington State University (Co)	3	1
Western Michigan University (Co)		
Widener University (Cl)	5	0
Yeshiva University (Cm)	3	0

Attachment

Catholic University of America (Cl)	2	0
City University of New York at City College (Cl)	3	1
Fordham University (Cl)	1	0
Iowa State University (Co)	2	0
Purdue University (Co)	1	1
University of Delaware (Cl)	2	2
University of Southern Mississippi (Co)	3	0
University of Texas–Austin (Co)	1	0
University of Wisconsin–Milwaukee (Cl)	2	0

Attention-Deficit/Hyperactivity Disorder

Argosy University–Schaumburg (Psy.D.) (Cl)	1	0
Argosy University–Phoenix (Cl)	1	0
Carlos Albizu University–San Juan (Ph.D.) (Cl)	1	0
Colorado State University (Co)	1	0
Emory University (Cl)	1	1
Illinois Institute of Technology (Cl)	1	0
Marquette University (Cl)	1	0
Michigan State University (Cl)	1	3
Nova Southeastern University (Ph.D. & Psy.D.) (Cl)	3	1
Ontario Institute for Studies in Education (Cm)	4	9
Pepperdine University (Cl)	1	2
Regent University (Cl)	1	1
University at Buffalo/State University of New York (Cl)	2	10
University of British Columbia (Cl)	1	3
University of California–Berkeley (Cl)	1	2
University of Central Florida (Cl)	1	0

University of Louisville (Co)	2	15
University of Maine (Cl)	1	0
University of Montana (Cl)	0	0
University of North Carolina at Greensboro (Cl)	1	2
University of Pittsburgh (Cl)	1	2
University of Rochester (Cl)	1	1
University of Texas at Austin (Cl)	1	1
University of Victoria (Cl)	1	1
University of Wyoming (Cl)	1	0
Utah State University (Cm)	1	0
Virginia Consortium Program in Clinical Psychology (Psy.D.) (Cl)	1	0
Virginia Polytechnic Institute and State University (Cl)	1	0
Yeshiva University (Cm)	2	0

Attitudes, Beliefs, and Values

Arizona State University (Co)	1	0
George Fox University (Psy.D.) (Cl)	1	0
Immaculata College (Cl)	1	0
Indiana State University (Co)	1	0
James Madison University (Cm)	3	2
University of Missouri Kansas City (Cl)	1	0

Autism/Pervasive Developmental Disorder

Binghamton University (Cl)	1	1
Brigham Young University (Cl)	1	1
Louisiana State University (Cl)	1	1
Rutgers University (Ph.D.) (Cl)	1	1
Rutgers University (Psy.D.) (Cl)	1	1
San Diego State University/University of California–San Diego (Cl)	2	0
St. John's University (Cl)	1	1
University at Albany/State University of New York (Cl)	1	3
University of California–Santa Barbara (Cm)		
University of Connecticut (Cl)	3	3
University of Illinois at Chicago (Cl)	1	4
University of Missouri–Columbia (Cl)	1	0
University of Pittsburgh (Cl)	3	16
University of Washington (Cl)	1	1
Vanderbilt University (Cl)	2	1
Virginia Polytechnic Institute and State University (Cl)	1	0
University of Rochester (Cl)	2	2
York University—Clinical-Developmental Area (Cl)	2	2

Behavior Therapy/Applied Behavioral Analysis

Eastern Michigan University (Cl)	2	0
Hofstra University (Cm)	3	0
Nova Southeastern University (Ph.D. & Psy.D.) (Cl)	8	0
Pacific University (Cl)	7	0
Rutgers University (Ph.D.) (Cl)	2	0

	# Faculty	# Grants
Rutgers University (Psy.D.) (Cl)	1	1
San Diego State University/University of California–San Diego (Cl)	4	0
University of Denver (Psy.D.) (Cl)	1	0
University of Hartford (Psy.D.) (Cl)	1	0
University of Kentucky (Co)	2	1
University of Manitoba (Cl)	3	2
University of Nevada–Reno (Cl)	3	0
University of North Carolina at Greensboro (Cl)	1	0
University of North Dakota (Cl)	2	0
Virginia Consortium Program in Clinical Psychology (Cl)	1	0
Western Michigan University (Cl)	2	0
Yeshiva University (Cl)	1	0
Yeshiva University (Cm)	3	0

Behavioral Genetics

Boston University (Cl)	1	1
Emory University (Cl)	2	1
Northwestern University (Cl)	1	0
Southern Illinois University (Cl)	1	0
University of Denver (Ph.D.) (Cl)	1	1
University of Illinois at Urbana–Champaign (Cl)	2	2
University of Minnesota (Cl)		
University of Pittsburgh (Cl)	4	11
University of Virginia (Cl)	2	1
Yale University (Cl)	1	0

Behavioral Medicine/Health Psychology

Adelphi University (Cl)	1	1
Alliant International University–Fresno (Ph.D.) (Cl)	4	0
Alliant International University–Fresno (Psy.D.) (Cl)	6	0
Alliant International University–Los Angeles (Ph.D. & Psy.D.) (Cl)	9	2
Alliant International University–San Diego (Ph.D. & Psy.D.) (Cl)	8	
Alliant International University–San Francisco (Ph.D.)(Cl)	3	0
Alliant International University–San Francisco (Psy.D.)(Cl)	4	0
Antioch/New England Graduate School (Cl)	1	1
Argosy University–Chicago (Psy.D.) (Cl)	4	3
Argosy University–Honolulu Campus (Psy.D.) (Cl)	1	0
Argosy University–Phoenix (Psy.D.) (Cl)	2	0
Arizona State University (Cl)	7	6
Arizona State University (Co)	1	0
Ball State University (Co)	2	0
Baylor University (Cl)	1	0
Binghamton University/State University of New York (Cl)	1	1
Bowling Green State University (Cl)	2	1
Brigham Young University (Cl)	2	1

	# Faculty	# Grants
California Institute of Integral Studies (Psy.D.) (Cl)	1	1
Case Western Reserve University (Cl)	1	1
Central Michigan University (Cl)	1	1
Chicago School of Professional Psychology (Cl)	1	0
Colorado State University (Co)	8	4
Concordia University (Cl)	2	1
Drexel University (Cl)	2	0
Duke University (Cl)	4	6
Eastern Michigan University (Cl)	1	0
Fairleigh Dickinson University (Cl)	3	0
Fielding Graduate Institute (Cl)	—	—
Florida Institute of Technology (Cl)	3	0
Fordham University (Cl)	2	2
Fordham University (Co)	2	1
Forest Institute	2	1
Fuller Theological Seminary (Ph.D. & Psy.D.) (Cl)	3	0
George Washington University (Ph.D.) (Cl)	1	0
Howard University (Cl)	3	3
Illinois Institute of Technology (Cl)	1	1
Indiana State University (Psy.D.) (Cl)	3	1
Indiana State University (Co)	1	0
Indiana University–Bloomington (Cl)	2	2
Indiana University of Pennsylvania (Cl)	2	0
Indiana University–Purdue University Indianapolis (Cl)	3	1
LaSalle University (Cl)	1	1
Loma Linda University (Ph.D. & Psy.D.) (Cl)	6	3
Loyola College in Maryland (Psy.D.) (Cl)	3	0
New Mexico State University (Co)	1	1
Nova Southeastern University (Ph.D. & Psy.D.) (Cl)	7	2
Ohio State University (Cl)	5	7
Ohio University (Cl)	4	6
Oklahoma State University (Cl)	2	0
Oklahoma State University (Co)	2	1
Pacific Graduate School of Psychology (Cl)	4	1
Pacific University (Cl)	1	0
Pennsylvania State University (Cl)	2	0
Roosevelt University (Psy.D.) (Cl)	4	1
Rosalind Franklin University of Medicine and Science (Cl)	1	0
Rutgers University (Ph.D.) (Cl)	5	1
Sam Houston State University (Cl)	1	1
San Diego State University/University of California–San Diego (Cl)	22	3
Seattle Pacific University (Cl)	2	0
Simon Fraser University (Cl)	1	1
Southern Illinois University (Cl)	2	0
Southern Illinois University (Co)	2	0
Spalding University (Psy.D.) (Cl)	2	1
St. John's University (Cl)	2	1
Texas A&M University (Cl)	2	1
Texas A&M University (Co)	2	1
Texas Tech University (Cl)	3	1
Texas Tech University (Co)	6	0
Uniformed Services University of Health Sciences (Cl)	1	3

	# Faculty	# Grants
University of Alabama (Cl)	3	2
University of Alabama at Birmingham (Cl)	2	2
University at Albany/State University of New York (Cl)	2	0
University at Buffalo/State University of New York (Cl)	2	2
University at Buffalo/State University of New York (Cm)	4	3
University of Arizona (Cl)	6	6
University of British Columbia (Cl)	1	3
University of California–Los Angeles (Cl)	5	12
University of Cincinnati (Cl)	5	3
University of Connecticut (Cl)	3	2
University of Florida (Cl)	3	3
University of Florida (Co)	2	1
University of Georgia (Cl)	2	0
University of Hawaii at Manoa (Cl)	1	0
University of Illinois at Chicago (Cl)	4	1
University of Illinois at Urbana (Cl)	3	8
University of Iowa (Cl)	3	4
University of Iowa (Co)	6	4
University of Kansas (Cl)	2	1
University of Kentucky (Cl)	2	1
University of Louisville (Cl)	3	1
University of Maine (Cl)	1	1
University of Manitoba (Cl)	2	1
University of Maryland–Baltimore County (Cl)	4	3
University of Maryland (Co)	2	0
University of Memphis (Cl)	4	1
University of Memphis (Co)	1	1
University of Miami (Cl)	14	2
University of Miami (Co)	2	1
University of Michigan (Cl)	2	0
University of Minnesota—Department of Psychology (Co)	1	0
University of Missouri–Columbia (Cl)	2	1
University of Missouri–Columbia (Co)	2	1
University of Missouri–Kansas City (Co)	3	0
University of Missouri–St. Louis (Cl)	1	1
University of Montana (Cl)	3	0
University of Nevada–Reno (Cl)	2	0
University of New Mexico (Cl)	3	0
University of North Carolina at Chapel Hill (Cl)	1	2
University of North Dakota (Cl)	2	0
University of Notre Dame (Co)	1	1
University of Ottawa (Cl)	2	1
University of Pittsburgh (Cl)	14	38
University of Rhode Island (Cl)	3	10
University of Saskatchewan (Cl)	3	2
University of South Dakota (Cl)	2	0
University of South Florida (Cl)	5	5
University of Southern California (Cl)	3	5
University of Tennessee (Cl)	3	1
University of Texas at Austin (Cl)	1	1
University of Texas Southwestern Medical Center at Dallas (Cl)	3	3
University of Utah (Cl)	2	1
University of Vermont (Cl)	3	2
University of Windsor (Cl)	3	5
University of Wisconsin–Madison (Cl)	3	
University of Wisconsin–Milwaukee (Cl)	2	0
University of Wisconsin–Milwaukee (Co)	1	0
Utah State University (Cm)	3	2
Vanderbilt University (Cl)	5	3
Virginia Commonwealth University (Cl)	5	3
Virginia Commonwealth University (Co)	5	5
Virginia Polytechnic Institute and State University (Cl)	3	2
Washington State University (Cl)	5	8
West Virginia University (Cl)	3	0
West Virginia University (Co)	2	0
Western Michigan University (Cl)	1	1
Yale University (Cl)	2	2
Yeshiva University (PhD) (Cl)	1	1
York University—Adult Clinical Program (Cl)	1	2

Biofeedback/Relaxation

Fuller Theological Seminary (Ph.D. & Psy.D.) (Cl)	1	0
George Washington University (Ph.D.) (Cl)	1	0
Hofstra University (Cm)	1	0
James Madison University (Cm)	1	1
Nova Southeastern University (Ph.D. & Psy.D.) (Cl)	2	0
Pennsylvania State University (Cl)	2	1
San Diego State University/University of California–San Diego (Cl)	1	0
Seattle Pacific University (Cl)	1	1
University of North Dakota (Cl)	1	0
Virginia Consortium Program in Clinical Psychology (Cl)	1	0

Brain Injury/Head Injury

Georgia State University (Cl)	3	1
James Madison University (Cm)	1	0
Southern Illinois University (Co)	1	0
University of Montana (Cl)	1	0
University of Victoria (Cl)	2	2

Child Abuse/Neglect/Sexual Abuse

Columbia University, Teachers College (Cl)	1	1
DePaul University (Cl)	1	1
Drexel University (Cl)	1	0
Marquette University (Co)	2	0
Ontario Institute for Studies in Education (Cm)	2	1
Pacific Graduate School of Psychology (Psy.D.) (Cl)	2	0
Philadelphia College of Osteopathic Medicine (Psy.D.)(Cl)	1	0
St. John's University (Cl)	1	2
Southern Illinois University (Cl)	1	0
Texas Tech University (Cl)	1	0

	# Faculty	# Grants
University of Iowa (Cl)	2	1
University of Michigan (Cl)	1	0
University of Nebraska–Lincoln (Cl)	2	2
University of Rochester (Cl)	1	2
University of Saskatchewan (Cl)	1	1
University of Utah (Co)	2	1
University of Victoria (Cl)	1	1
Virginia Consortium Program in Clinical Psychology (Cl)	1	0
York University—Clinical-Developmental Area (Cl)	3	2

Child/Child Clinical/Pediatric

Adler School of Professional Psychology (Cl)	2	0
Alliant International University–Los Angeles (Ph.D. & Psy.D.) (Cl)	3	
Alliant International University–Fresno (Cl)	2	
Alliant International University–San Diego (Ph.D. & Psy.D.) (Cl)	10	
American University (Cl)	1	0
Antioch/New England Graduate School (Cl)	2	0
Argosy University, Atlanta (Psy.D.) (Cl)	2	0
Argosy University, Honolulu (Psy.D.) (Cl)	3	0
Arizona State University (Cl)	5	15
Auburn University (Cl)	3	1
Azusa Pacific University (Psy.D.) (Cl)	2	1
Ball State University (Co)	2	0
Binghamton University/State University of New York (Cl)	3	3
Bowling Green State University (Cl)	2	1
Brigham Young University (Cl)	3	1
Carlos Albizu University–Miami Campus (Cl)	3	0
Catholic University of America (Cl)	4	1
Central Michigan University (Cl)	1	2
Chicago School of Professional Psychology (Cl)	1	0
Drexel University (Cl)	3	4
Eastern Michigan University (Cl)	3	0
Fairleigh Dickinson University (Cl)	2	0
Fordham University (Cl)	2	0
Fuller Theological Seminary (Ph.D. & Psy.D.) (Cl)	3	1
George Washington University (Ph.D. & Psy.D.) (Cl)	2	1
Georgia State University (Cl)	1	1
Hofstra University (Cm)	2	0
Illinois Institute of Technology (Cl)	4	2
Immaculata College (Cl)	2	0
Indiana State University (Psy.D.) (Cl)	1	0
Indiana University–Bloomington (Cl)	1	2
Jackson State University (Cl)	1	0
LaSalle University (Psy.D.) (Cl)	1	0
Loma Linda University (Ph.D. & Psy.D.) (Cl)	1	2
Loyola University–Chicago (Cl)	1	3
Loyola University–Chicago (Co)	2	0
Marquette University (Cl)	3	1
Miami University (Cl)	1	1
New School University (Cl)	1	1
Northwestern University Medical School (Cl)	3	1
Nova Southeastern University (Ph.D. & Psy.D.) (Cl)	5	0
Ohio State University (Cl)	3	4
Ohio University (Cl)	2	2
Oklahoma State University (Cl)	0	0
Ontario Institute for Studies in Education (Cm)	2	1
Pacific Graduate School of Psychology (Ph.D.) (Cl)	3	0
Pacific University (Psy.D.) (Cl)	4	6
Pennsylvania State University (Cl)	3	2
Roosevelt University (Psy.D.) (Cl)	4	1
St. Louis University (Cl)	2	1
San Diego State University/University of California–San Diego (Cl)	5	0
Seattle Pacific University (Cl)	3	3
Simon Fraser University (Cl)	3	6
Southern Illinois University (Cl)	3	0
Temple University (Cl)	1	3
Texas A&M University (Cl)	4	3
Texas Tech University (Cl)	2	2
University of Alabama (Cl)	4	1
University at Albany/State University of New York (Cl)	4	1
University of Arkansas (Cl)	2	0
University of Central Florida (Cl)	1	0
University of Cincinnati (Cl)	3	2
University of Colorado (Cl)	3	2
University of Delaware (Cl)	4	5
University of Florida (Cl)	5	7
University of Georgia (Cl)	6	4
University of Hartford (Psy.D.) (Cl)	2	0
University of Hawaii at Manoa (Cl)	3	4
University of Houston (Cl)	3	2
University of Houston (Co)	1	1
University of Kansas (Cl)	4	2
University of Kentucky (Cl)	2	1
University of Massachusetts at Amherst (Cl)	4	3
University of Memphis (Co & Cl)	2	1
University of Miami (Cl)	9	4
University of Michigan (Cl)	8	5
University of Mississippi (Cl)	3	0
University of Missouri–St. Louis (Cl)	2	1
University of Nebraska–Lincoln (Cl)	2	1
University of Nevada–Las Vegas (Cl)	2	1
University of New Mexico (Cl)	1	0
University of North Carolina at Chapel Hill (Cl)	1	2
University of North Carolina at Greensboro (Cl)	1	0
University of North Texas (Cl)	1	1
University of Northern Colorado (Co)	8	1
University of Oregon (Co)	3	2
University of Ottawa (Cl)	4	1
University of Pittsburgh (Cl)	14	45

	# Faculty	# Grants
University of Rhode Island (Cl)	1	0
University of South Dakota (Cl)	3	0
University of South Florida (Cl)	4	2
University of Southern Mississippi (Co & Cl)	3	0
University of Texas Southwestern Medical Center at Dallas (Cl)	1	0
University of Toledo (Cl)	3	0
University of Utah (Cl)	1	0
University of Utah (Co)	3	2
University of Virginia (Human Services) (Cl)	1	0
University of Virginia—Department of Psychology (Cl)	5	5
University of Washington (Cl)	3	3
University of Windsor (Cl)	4	3
University of Wisconsin–Milwaukee	4	3
Utah State University (Cm)	4	2
Virginia Commonwealth University (Cl)	5	4
Virginia Consortium Program in Clinical Psychology (Cl)	1	0
Virginia Polytechnic Institute and State University (Cl)	4	3
Washington State University (Cl)	4	4
West Virginia University (Cl)	1	0
Wheaton College (Psy.D.) (Cl)	3	0
Wichita State University (Cl)	1	2
Widener University (Cl)	4	1
Yeshiva University (Cm)	2	0

Chronic Illness

Drexel University (Cl)	1	0
Philadelphia College Osteopathic Medicine (Psy.D.) (Cl)	2	1
San Diego State University (Cl)	4	1
University of Kansas (Cl)	2	1
University of Michigan (Cl)	1	0
University of Manitoba (Cl)	1	0
University of North Dakota (Co)	1	0
University of Pittsburgh (Cl)	2	6
Wright State University (Psy.D.) (Cl)	1	0

Chronic/Severe Mental Illness

Case Western Reserve University (Cl)	1	0
Illinois Institute of Technology (Cl)	2	1
Indiana University–Purdue University Indianapolis (Cl)	2	3–4
Nova Southeastern University (Ph.D. & Psy.D.) (Cl)	2	0
Rutgers University (Psy.D.) (Cl)	2	1
University of Cincinnati (Cl)	4	3
Seattle Pacific University (Cl)	1	1
University of Houston (Cl)	3	1
University of Louisville (Cl)	1	0
University of Maryland (Cl)	1	2
University of Massachusetts at Boston (Cl)	1	1

University of Missouri–Kansas City (Cl)	1	1
University of Nebraska–Lincoln (Cl)	1	1
University of South Dakota (Cl)	2	0
Virginia Consortium Program (Psy.D.) (Cl)	1	0

Clinical Judgment/Decision Making

Ball State University (Co)	1	0
Indiana State University (Psy.D.) (Cl)	1	0
Indiana University of Pennsylvania (Cl)	1	0
San Diego State University/University of California–San Diego (Cl)	1	0
Southern Illinois University (Cl)	1	0
University of Alabama (Cl)	0	0
University of Detroit–Mercy (Cl)	1	0
University of Rhode Island (Cl)	1	0

Cognition/Social Cognition

Argosy University–Washington, DC Campus (Cl)	1	0
Arizona State University (Co)	1	0
Case Western Reserve University (Cl)	2	0
Catholic University of America (Cl)	3	0
Colorado State University (Co)	5	1
Concordia University (Cl)	4	5
Fuller Theological Seminary (Ph.D. & Psy.D.) (Cl)	1	0
Gallaudet University (Cl)	1	1
George Mason University (Cl)	4	0
Northwestern University (Cl)	2	1
Ontario Institute for Studies in Education (Cm)	3	2
Pennsylvania State University (Cl)	2	0
San Diego State University/University of California–San Diego (Cl)	13	0
Simon Fraser University (Cl)	5	6
University of Denver (Psy.D.) (Cl)	1	0
University of Pittsburgh (Cl)	4	10
University of Waterloo (Cl)	1	1
Yale University (Cl)	3	0

Cognitive Therapy/Cognitive-Behavioral Therapy

Arizona State University (Co)	1	0
Baylor University (Cl)	3	0
Brigham Young University (Cl)	1	1
Ontario Institute for Studies in Education (Cm)	2	2
Philadelphia College Osteopathic Medicine (Psy.D.) (Cl)	10	0
Texas Tech University (Cl)	3	0
University of Southern California (Cl)	3	1
University of Toledo (Cl)	2	0
University of Washington (Cl)	4	2
Xavier University (Cl)	5	0
York University—Clinical-Developmental Area (Cl)	2	1

	# Faculty	# Grants

Community Psychology

	# Faculty	# Grants
Adler School of Professional Psychology (Psy.D.) (Cl)	1	1
Antioch/New England Graduate School (Cl)	2	2
Arizona State University (Cl)	6	11
Boston University (Cl)	2	0
Bowling Green State University (Cl)	1	1
Catholic University of America (Cl)	1	2
Fairleigh Dickinson University (Cl)	3	0
George Washington University (Ph.D.) (Cl)	6	1
George Washington University (Psy.D.) (Cl)	3	1
JFK University (Psy.D.) (Cl)	2	0
Loyola University–Chicago (Cl)	3	0
Miami University (Cl)	4	3
Nova Southeastern University (Ph.D. & Psy.D.) (Cl)	3	0
Pace University (Psy.D.) (Cm)	1	0
Rutgers University (Psy.D.) (Cl)	2	1
St. Louis University (Cl)	1	0
San Diego State University/University of California–San Diego (Cl)	1	0
Southern Illinois University (Cl)	1	0
Texas Tech University (Cl)	1	0
University of Denver (Ph.D.) (Cl)	1	4
University of Hartford (Cl)	1	0
University of Hawaii (Cl)	2	3
University of Illinois at Chicago (Cl)	1	1
University of Illinois at Urbana–Champaign (Cl)	5	4
University of La Verne (Psy.D.) (Cl)	12	0
University of Manitoba (Cl)	1	0
University of Maryland–Baltimore County (Cl)	4	2
University of Mississippi (Cl)	2	0
University of North Dakota (Cl)	2	0
University of Pennsylvania (Cl)	1	0
University of Rhode Island (Cl)	1	4
University of South Carolina (Cl)	1	1
University of Texas Southwestern Medical Center at Dallas (Cl)	1	0
University of Virginia—Department of Psychology (Cl)	3	3
University of Windsor (Cl)	2	2
Virginia Commonwealth University (Cl)	5	3
Virginia Commonwealth University (Co)	1	1
Virginia Consortium Program in Clinical Psychology (Cl)	1	1
Wichita State University (Cl)	2	1

Conduct Disorder

	# Faculty	# Grants
Duke University (Cl)	2	3
Florida State University (Cl)	1	1
Miami University (Cl)	3	2
Michigan State University (Cl)	1	1
University of South Carolina (Cl)	1	1

Consultation

	# Faculty	# Grants
Arizona State University (Co)	2	0
Georgia State University (Co)	1	1
University of Memphis (Co)	1	1

Crisis Intervention

	# Faculty	# Grants
Brigham Young University (Co)	1	1
University of Memphis (Co)	2	0

Deafness/Hearing Impairment

	# Faculty	# Grants
Gallaudet University (Cl)	9	2

Death and Dying/Bereavement

	# Faculty	# Grants
Biola University (Ph.D.) (Cl)	1	0
Biola University (Psy.D.) (Cl)	1	0
Drexel University (Cl)	2	2
Indiana University of Pennsylvania (Cl)	1	0
Loyola University–Chicago (Cl)	1	0
Pacific Graduate School of Psychology (Ph.D.) (Cl)	3	0
Purdue University (Co)		
San Diego State University/University of California–San Diego (Cl)	2	0
University of Michigan (Cl)	2	2
University of Saskatchewan (Cl)	1	0
Adelphi University (Cl)	1	1
Catholic University of America (Cl)		
Concordia University (Cl)	3	5
Fordham University (Cl)	4	3
Fuller Theological Seminary (Ph.D. & Psy.D.) (Cl)	3	1
George Washington University (Ph.D. Psy.D.) (Cl)	2	2
Idaho State University (Cl)	1	1
Immaculata College (Cl)	3	0
Long Island University (Cl)	4	3
New School University (Cl)	1	0
Northern Illinois University (Cl)	3	1
Pacific Graduate School of Psychology (Ph.D.) (Cl)	4	0
Pennsylvania State University (Cl)	2	1
Purdue University (Cl)	2	2
Simon Fraser University (Cl)	6	6
Spalding University (Cl)	2	0
Stony Brook University/State University of New York (Cl)	1	1
University of Colorado (Cl)	3	1
University of Delaware (Cl)		
University of New Brunswick (Cl)	1	1
University of Texas Southwestern Medical Center at Dallas (Cl)	1	1
University of Utah (Cl)	4	2
University of Wisconsin–Milwaukee (Cl)	2	0
Auburn University (Cl)	1	1
Binghamton University/State University of New York (Cl)	1	2

	# Faculty	# Grants
Case Western Reserve University (Cl)	1	1
Georgia State University (Cl)	1	2
Long Island University–C.W. Post Campus (Cl)	1	0
Louisiana State University (Cl)	1	1
Pennsylvania State University (Cl)	3	1
Rutgers University (Psy.D.) (Cl)	3	2
San Diego State University (Cl)	2	0
University of Alabama at Birmingham (Cl)	6	16
University at Albany/State University of New York (Cl)	1	1
University of Denver (Ph.D.) (Cl)	1	4
University of Illinois at Chicago (Cl)	1	0
University of Manitoba (Cl)	3	0
University of Wyoming (Cl)	2	1
University of Texas at Austin (Cl)	1	1
Virginia Consortium Program in Clinical Psychology (Cl)	1	0
York University—Clinical-Developmental Area (Cl)	2	3

Disabilities/Disabled Persons

DePaul University (Cl)	2	2
Loyola University–Chicago (Cl)	1	2
Seattle Pacific University (Cl)	1	0
University of Memphis (Co)	4	3
University of Missouri–Columbia (Co)	1	0
Washington State University (Co)	1	1
West Virginia University (Co)	1	0

Disaster/Trauma

Alliant International University– Los Angeles (Ph.D.) (Cl)	1	0
Argosy University Chicago (Cl)	1	0
Chicago School of Professional Psychology (Cl)	1	0
Georgia State University (Co)	1	0
Idaho State University (Cl)	2	1
Long Island University (Cl)	1	1
Miami University (Cl)	2	0
Nova Southeastern University (Ph.D. & Psy.D.) (Cl)	7	0
Pacific University (Psy.D.) (Cl)	1	0
Philadelphia College of Osteopathic Medicine (Psy.D.) (Cl)	1	0
Sam Houston State University (Cl)	1	2
Seton Hall University (Co)	1	0
Temple University (Cl)	2	0
Texas Tech University (Cl)	2	0
University of British Columbia (Co)	2	1
University of Connecticut (Cl)	3	3
University of Denver (Ph.D.) (Cl)	3	1
University of Denver (Psy.D.) (Cl)	1	0
University of Georgia (Co)	1	0
University of Houston (Co)	2	1
University of Kansas (Cl)	2	1
University of Manitoba (Cl)	3	0

University of Massachusetts at Boston (Cl)	4	1
University of Memphis (Co)	2	0
University of Miami (Cl)	4	2+
University of Minnesota–Department of Psychology (Co)	1	0
University of Mississippi (Cl)	2	0
University of Missouri–Columbia (Co)	1	1
University of Missouri–Kansas City (Cl)	1	1
University of Missouri–St. Louis (Cl)	2	2
University of Nebraska–Lincoln (Cl)	1	1
University of North Dakota (Co)	2	0
University of North Texas (Cl)	2	0
University of Pittsburgh (Cl)	1	1
University of South Dakota (Cl)	5	2
University of Wyoming (Cl)	1	0
Yeshiva University (Psy.D.) (Cl)	2	0
York University—Adult Clinical Program (Cl)	1	0

Divorce/Child Custody

Colorado State University (Co)	3	0
Drexel University (Cl)	1	0
University of Louisville (Co)	1	2
University of Michigan (Cl)	1	1
University of Victoria (Cl)	1	1
Virginia Commonwealth University (Cl)	1	0

Dreams

Miami University (Cl)	1	0
University of Maryland (Co)	1	0

Eating Disorders/Body Image

American University (Cl)	1	0
Argosy University, Chicago (Psy.D.) (Cl)	1	0
Brigham Young University (Cl)	1	1
Colorado State (Cl)	1	0
Duke University (Cl)	1	0
Emory University (Cl)	1	0
Fairleigh Dickinson University (Cl)	0	0
Florida Institute of Technology (Cl)	1	0
Florida State University (Cl)	3	3
Hofstra University (Cm)	1	0
Indiana State University (Cl)	2	1
Indiana University–Bloomington (Cl)	1	0
Kent State University (Cl)	1	0
Louisiana State University (Cl)	1	1
Louisiana Tech University (Co)	1	0
Miami University (Cl)	1	0
Michigan State University (Cl)	1	2
Northeastern University (Cm)	1	1
Pacific Graduate School of Psychology (Psy.D.) (Cl)	2	1
Philadelphia College of Osteopathic Medicine (Psy.D.) (Cl)	1	0
Rutgers University (Ph.D.) (Cl)	1	1
Rutgers University (Psy.D.) (Cl)	1	1
St. Louis University (Cl)	1	1

	# Faculty	# Grants
Sam Houston State University (Cl)	1	0
Tennessee State University (Co)	2	1
Texas Tech University (Cl)	1	0
Uniformed Services University of Health Sciences (Cl)	1	1
University of Alabama at Birmingham (Cl)	1	1
University at Albany/State University of New York (Cl)	1	1
University of Central Florida (Cl)	2	0
University of Colorado (Cl)	0	0
University of Florida (Co)	1	1
University of Hawaii at Manoa (Cl)	2	0
University of Iowa (Cl)	1	0
University of Illinois at Chicago (Cl)	1	0
University of Illinois at Urbana–Champaign (Co)	1	0
University of Indianapolis (Cl)	1	0
University of Iowa (Cl)	1	pending
University of Kentucky (Cl)	1	1
University of Manitoba (Cl)	2	0
University of Minnesota (Cl)	2	1
University of Missouri–Columbia (Cl)	1	1
University of Missouri–Columbia (Co)	1	1
University of Missouri–Kansas City (Cl)	1	0
University of Nevada–Las Vegas (Cl)	1	0
University of New Mexico (Cl)	1	1
University of North Dakota (Co)	1	0
University of North Texas (Co)	3	0
University of Northern Colorado (Co)	2	0
University of Pittsburgh (Cl)	1	4
University of South Florida (Cl)	2	1
University of Southern Mississippi (Co)	2	0
University of Windsor (Cl)	2	1
Vanderbilt University (Cl)	3	2
Virginia Consortium Program in Clinical Psychology (Cl)	1	0
Virginia Polytechnic Institute and State University (Cl)	1	0
Washington State University (Co)	1	0
Yale University (Cl)	2	2
York University—Adult Clinical Program (Cl)	1	2

Emotion

Boston University (Cl)	3	1
Catholic University of America (Cl)	2	0
Georgia State University (Cl)	3	0
LaSalle University (Cl)	1	0
Michigan State University (Cl)	1	0
New School University (Cl)	1	0
Ontario Institute for Studies in Education (Cm)	3	3
Pennsylvania State University (Cl)	5	1
University of Arkansas (Cl)	3	0
University of California–Berkeley (Cl)	5	5
University of Delaware (Cl)	4	1
University of Georgia (Cl)	1	0

University of Illinois at Urbana–Champaign (Cl)	5	10
University of Mississippi (Cl)	2	1
University of Montana (Cl)	0	0
University of North Texas (Cl)	1	0
University of Pittsburgh (Cl)	5	19
University of South Florida (Cl)	2	0
University of Utah (Co)	1	0
University of Wisconsin–Milwaukee (Cl)	2	0
Vanderbilt University (Cl)	9	2
York University—Clinical-Developmental Area (Cl)	1	0

Epidemiology

University of Texas at Austin (Cl)	1	0
University of Virginia (Cl)	2	1

Ethical Issues

Auburn University (Co)	3	3
Colorado State University (Co)	1	0
Fairleigh Dickinson University (Cl)	2	0
Gallaudet University (Cl)	1	0
Immaculata University (Cl)	2	1
Indiana University of Pennsylvania (Cl)	1	0
Iowa State University (Co)	1	0
Loyola College in Maryland (Cl)	2	0
Loyola University–Chicago (Cl)	1	0
Our Lady of the Lake University (Co)	1	0
Rutgers University (Ph.D.) (Cl)	1	0
Rutgers University (Psy.D.) (Cl)	1	0
St. Louis University (Cl)	3	0
Texas Tech University (Cl)	1	0
Texas Woman's University (Co)	2	0
University of British Columbia (Co)	1	0
University of Denver (Co)	1	0
University of St. Thomas (Co)	1	0
Vanderbilt University (Cl)	1	0

Family/Family Therapy/Family Systems

Alliant International University–Fresno (Psy.D.) (Cl)	3	—
Alliant International University–Los Angeles (Psy.D.) (Cl)	8	—
Alliant International University–San Diego (Ph.D. & Psy.D.) (Cl)	10	—
Alliant International University–San Francisco (Ph.D.) (Cl)	6	0
Argosy University, Chicago (Psy.D.) (Cl)	1	3
Argosy University, Schaumberg (Psy.D.) (Cl)	1	0
Arizona State University (Cl)	4	4
Arizona State University (Co)	1	0
Azusa Pacific University (Cl)	2	0
Boston University (Cl)	2	1
Bowling Green State University (Cl)	2	0
Carlos Albizu University–San Juan (Psy.D.) (Cl)	3	0

	# Faculty	# Grants
Catholic University of America (Cl)	2	1
Chestnut Hill University (Cl)	1	1
Clark University (Cl)	3	2
Colorado State University (Co)	1	0
Drexel University (Cl)	2	1
Florida Institute of Technology (Cl)	2	0
Fordham University (Cl)	1	0
Fuller Theological Seminary (Ph.D. & Psy.D.) (Cl)	2	1
George Washington University (Cl)	2	1
Georgia State University (Cl)	2	4
Hofstra University (Cm)	1	0
Howard University (Cl)	2	0
Illinois Institute of Technology (Cl)	1	0
Immaculata University (Cl)	2	0
Indiana State University (Co)	2	3
Indiana University (Cl)	1	1
Indiana University (Co)	3	3
Indiana University of Pennsylvania (Cl)	1	0
James Madison University (Cm)	2	0
Kent State University (Cl)	2	2
Lehigh University (Co)	1	1
Louisiana Tech University (Co)	1	0
Marquette University (Cl)	2	1
McGill University (Cl)	2	1
Miami University (Cl)	3	1
Michigan State University (Cl)	3	1
New Mexico State University (Co)	1	0
Ohio University (Cl)	2	2
Pennsylvania State University (Cl)	2	1
Pennsylvania State University (Co)	2	0
Pepperdine University (Cl)	0	0
Purdue University (Cl)	2	1
Rutgers University (Psy.D.) (Cl)	4	2
St. Louis University (Cl)	3	0
Sam Houston State University (Cl)	1	1
San Diego State University/University of California–San Diego (Cl)	5	0
Seattle Pacific University (Cl)	2	0
Simon Fraser University (Cl)	3	3
Southern Illinois University (Cl)	1	0
Suffolk University (Cl)	3	0
Syracuse University (Cl)	1	2
Texas A&M University (Cl)	5	3
Texas Tech University (Co)	2	0
University at Albany/State University of New York (Co)	1	1
University of Arizona (Cl)	2	4
University of Arkansas (Cl)	2	0
University at Buffalo/State University of New York (Cm)	1	0
University of California–Los Angeles (Cl)	3	3
University of California–Santa Barbara (Cm)	—	—
University of Colorado (Cl)	1	1
University of Denver (Ph.D.) (Cl)	3	1
University of Denver (Psy.D.) (Cl)	2	0
University of Detroit–Mercy (Cl)	2	0
University of Georgia (Cl)	1	1
University of Houston (Cl)	3	2
University of Indianapolis (Cl)	1	1
University of Kentucky (Co)	2	0
University of Maryland–Baltimore County (Cl)	1	1
University of Massachusetts at Amherst (Cl)	2	2
University of Massachusetts at Boston (Cl)	3	2
University of Memphis (Co)	2	1
University of Miami (Cl)	1	1
University of Miami (Co)	2	1
University of Michigan (Cl)	6	3
University of Missouri–Kansas City (Co)	2	0
University of Nebraska–Lincoln (Co)	1	0
University of New Mexico (Cl)	2	3
University of North Carolina at Chapel Hill (Cl)	1	2
University of Northern Colorado (Co)	4	1
University of Ottawa (Cl)	1	1
University of Pennsylvania (Cl)	1	0
University of Pittsburgh (Cl)	14	45
University of Rhode Island (Cl)	1	0
University of South Florida (Cl)	1	0
University of Tennessee (Cl)	6	2
University of Utah (Cl)	4	2
University of Victoria (Cl)	1	1
University of Virginia–Department of Human Services (Cl)	1	0
University of Virginia–Department of Psychology (Cl)	2	2
Virginia Consortium Program in Clinical Psychology (Cl)	0	4
Wayne State University (Cl)	1	2
Western Michigan University (Co)		
Wheaton College (Cl)	4	0
Wright Institute (Cl)	1	0
Wright State University (Cl)	1	0
Yeshiva University (Cm)	2	0
Yeshiva University (Cl)	1	0

Forensic/Psychology and Law

	# Faculty	# Grants
Alliant International University–San Diego (Ph.D. & Psy.D.) (Cl)	3	0
Alliant International University–Fresno (Ph.D. & Psy.D.) (Cl)	1	—
Argosy University–Phoenix (Cl)	2	0
Azusa Pacific University (Cl)	3	1
Carlos Albizu University–Miami Campus (Cl)	1	0
Chicago School of Professional Psychology (Cl)	2	0
Fairleigh Dickinson University (Cl)	2	1
Feinberg School of Medicine (Cl)	2	1
Georgia State University (Co)	1	0
Northeastern University (Cm)	1	1
Nova Southeastern University (Ph.D. & Psy.D.) (Cl)	3	2
Pacific Graduate School of Psychology (Ph.D.)(Cl)	2	0
Pacific University (Cl)	2	0

	# Faculty	# Grants
Pepperdine University (Cl)	1	0
Sam Houston State University (Cl)	1	1
Simon Fraser University (Cl)	3	8
Texas Tech University (Co)	1	0
University of Alabama (Cl)	4	0
University of Denver (Psy.D.) (Cl)	2	0
University of Houston (Cl)	2	1
University of Indianapolis (Cl)	1	0
University of La Verne (Psy.D.) (Cl)	2	0
University of Louisville (Cl)	2	0
University of Maine (Cl)	3	0
University of Nebraska–Lincoln (Cl)	2	2
University of New Brunswick (Cl)	1	1
University of North Texas (Cl)	3	1
University of Ottawa (Cl)	1	0
University of Saskatchewan (Cl)	4	2
University of St. Thomas (Co)	1	0
University of Utah (Cl)	1	1
University of Virginia—Department of Human Services (Cl)	2	3
University of Wyoming (Cl)	1	0
Virginia Commonwealth University (Cl)	1	0
Virginia Commonwealth University (Co)	1	2
Virginia Consortium Program in Clinical Psychology (Cl)	1	0
West Virginia University (Cl)	1	0
Yeshiva University (Psy.D.) (Cl)	1	0

Forgiveness

University of Southern Mississippi (Co)	2	0
Virginia Commonwealth University (Co)	2	0

Gay/Lesbian/Bisexuality

Argosy University, Chicago (Psy.D.) (Cl)	2	0
Argosy University–Honolulu Campus (Cl)	2	0
Auburn University (Co)	2	0
George Mason University (Cl)	1	0
Louisiana Tech University (Co)	0	0
Loyola College in Maryland (Psy.D.) (Cl)	1	0
John F. Kennedy University (Cl)	1	0
Marshall University (Psy.D.) (Cl)	1	0
New Mexico State University (Co)	3	1
New York University (Co)	1	1
Oklahoma State University (Co)	1	0
Pennsylvania State University (Co)	1	0
University of California–Santa Barbara (Cm)	—	—
University of Louisville (Co)	1	1
University of Memphis (Co)	3	1
University of North Dakota (Co)	2	1
University of Utah (Co)	2	0
University of Vermont (Cl)	1	1

Gender Roles/Sex Differences

Alliant International University–San Francisco (Ph.D.) (Cl)	6	0

Alliant International University–San Francisco (Psy.D.) (Cl)	3	0
Arizona State University (Cl)	1	1
Arizona State University (Co)	2	0
Biola University (Psy.D.) (Cl)	2	1
Boston College (Co)	2	0
Boston University (Cl)	1	0
Brigham Young University (Cl)	2	1
Concordia University (Cl)	2	1
Georgia State University (Cl)	1	1
Indiana State University (Cl)	3	0
Indiana University of Pennsylvania (Cl)	1	0
Iowa State University (Co)	1	1
Louisiana Tech University (Co)	1	0
New Mexico State University (Co)	3	0
Nova Southeastern University (Ph.D. & Psy.D.) (Cl)	1	0
Oklahoma State University (Co)	2	0
Ontario Institute for Studies in Education (Cm)	1	1
Pace University (Psy.D.) (Cm)	2	0
Rutgers University (Psy.D.) (Cl)	1	0
St. John's University (Cl)	2	0
San Diego State University/University of California–San Diego (Cl)	2	0
Seattle Pacific University (Cl)	3	1
Southern Illinois University (Cl)	1	0
Southern Illinois University (Co)	3	0
Suffolk University (Cl)	1	0
Texas A&M University (Co)	4	1
Texas Tech University (Co)	2	0
Texas Woman's University (Co)	4	1
University of Florida (Co)	1	0
University of Georgia (Co)	1	0
University of Houston (Co)	1	0
University of Kentucky (Co)	2	1
University of La Verne (Psy.D.) (Cl)	2	0
University of Missouri–Columbia (Co)	2	0
University of Missouri–Kansas City (Cl)	1	0
University of Montana (Cl)	1	1
University of Nebraska–Lincoln (Cl)	2	0
University of North Dakota (Cl)	2	0
University of North Dakota (Co)	4	0
University of Oklahoma (Co)	4	0
University of Wisconsin–Madison (Co)	4	0
University of Wisconsin–Milwaukee (Co)	1	0
Vanderbilt University (Cl)	2	10
Virginia Consortium Program in Clinical Psychology (Cl)	3	0
Virginia Polytechnic Institute and State University (Cl)	1	0
Wheaton College (Cl)	2	1
Wright Institute (Cl)	3	0
Wright State University (Cl)	3	0

Group Process and Therapy

Adelphi University (Cl)	2	0
Antioch/New England Graduate School (Cl)	1	0
Arizona State University (Co)	1	0
Baylor University (Cl)	1	0

	# Faculty	# Grants
Brigham Young University (Cl)	3	1
Fuller Theological Seminary (Ph.D. & Psy.D.) (Cl)	1	0
George Washington University (Psy.D.) (Cl)	3	0
Indiana University (Co)	2	0
Marquette University (Cl)	1	0
New York University (Co)	1	0
Sam Houston State University (Cl)	1	0
Texas Tech University (Co)	1	0
University of Denver (Co)	1	0
University of Hartford (Cl)	1	0
University of Houston (Co)	1	1
University of Missouri–Columbia (Co)	2	1
University of North Dakota (Co)	1	0
University of Tennessee (Co)	1	0
University of Wisconsin–Madison (Co)	1	0
Virginia Commonwealth University (Co)	1	0
Washington State University (Co)	1	0
West Virginia University (Co)	1	0
Western Michigan University (Co)		

Homelessness

	# Faculty	# Grants
Azusa Pacific University (Cl)	1	0
Drexel University (Cl)	1	0
University of Michigan (Cl)	1	0

Hypnosis

	# Faculty	# Grants
Binghamton University/State University of New York (Cl)	1	1
Pennsylvania State University (Cl)	1	0
Seattle Pacific University (Cl)	2	0
University of Manitoba (Cl)	1	0
University of Wisconsin–Milwaukee (Co)	1	0
Virginia Polytechnic Institute and State University (Cl)	1	1
Washington State University (Co)	2	1

Infancy

	# Faculty	# Grants
Concordia University (Cl)	8	10
Emory University (Cl)	1	2
George Washington University (Psy.D.) (Cl)	1	1
Hofstra University (Cm)	1	0
Pace University (Psy.D.) (Cm)	3	0
University of Western Ontario (Cl)	2	1

Interpersonal Relations/Processes

	# Faculty	# Grants
Adelphi University (Cl)	1	1
Arizona State University (Co)	4	0
Catholic University of America (Cl)	2	0
Colorado State University (Co)	1	0
Idaho State University (Cl)	1	0
New Mexico State University (Co)	1	1

	# Faculty	# Grants
Sam Houston State University (Cl)	1	0
San Diego State University/University of California–San Diego (Cl)	1	0
University of Denver (Cl)	3	5
University of Maryland (Co)	1	0
University of Maryland–Baltimore County (Cl)	1	0
University of Minnesota–Department of Psychology (Co)	1	0
University of Missouri–Kansas City (Co)	3	0
University of North Carolina at Greensboro (Cl)		
University of North Dakota (Co)	1	0
University of Waterloo (Cl)	2	1
Virginia Consortium Program in Clinical Psychology (Cl)	2	0

Intervention

	# Faculty	# Grants
Argosy University–Chicago (Cl)	2	0
Florida State University (Cl)	2	1
University of Illinois at Urbana–Champaign (Cl)	2	2
University of Wisconsin–Milwaukee (Co)	1	1
Virginia Commonwealth University (Co)	1	1

Learning

	# Faculty	# Grants
Pace University (Psy.D.) (Cm)	1	0
Roosevelt University (Psy.D.) (Cl)	1	0
University New Mexico (Cl)	1	0
University of Wisconsin–Madison (Co)	2	0
Virginia Consortium Program in Clinical Psychology (Cl)	2	0

Learning Disabilities/Disorders

	# Faculty	# Grants
Argosy University–Phoenix (Cl)	1	0
Binghamton University/State University of New York (Cl)	1	1
Case Western Reserve University (Cl)	1	1
Colorado State University (Co)	1	0
Georgia State University (Cl) (dyslexia)	1	4
Marshall University (Psy.D.) (Cl)	1	0
Ontario Institute for Studies in Education (Cm)	4	4
Pace University (Psy.D.) (Cm)	1	0
Southern Illinois University (Cl)	2	1
University of Texas Southwestern Medical Center at Dallas (Cl)	1	0
University of Virginia—Department of Human Services (Cl)	1	0
University of Wisconsin–Milwaukee (Cl)	1	0
Virginia Consortium Program in Clinical Psychology (Cl)	2	0
Widener University (Psy.D.) (Cl)	3	0
Yeshiva University (Cm)	3	0

Managed Care/Health Care

	# Faculty	# Grants
Jackson State University (Cl)	3	0
University of Montana (Cl)	1	0

	# Faculty	# Grants

Marriage/Couples

Adelphi University (Cl)	1	1
Argosy University–Chicago (Cl)	1	0
Auburn University (Cl)	1	0
Binghamton University/State University of New York (Cl)	1	1
Catholic University of America (Cl)	1	1
Fordham University (Cl)	1	0
Fuller Theological Seminary (Ph.D. & Psy.D.) (Cl)	4	0
George Fox University (Psy.D.) (Cl)	1	1
Georgia State University (Cl)	1	0
Illinois Institute of Technology (Cl)	1	1
Indiana University (Co)	2	3
Indiana University–Bloomington (Cl)	1	1
Long Island University–C.W. Post Campus (Cl)	2	0
Regent University (Cl)	2	1
Rutgers University (Ph.D.) (Cl)	2	1
Rutgers University (Psy.D.) (Cl)	3	1
San Diego State University/University of California–San Diego (Cl)	5	0
San Houston State University (Cl)	1	1
Southern Illinois University (Cl)	1	0
Stony Brook University/State University of New York (Cl)	3	5
Temple University (Cl)	1	0
Texas A&M University (Cl)	5	3
Texas Woman's University (Co)	4	1
University of California–Los Angeles (Cl)	2	3
University of Denver (Ph.D.) (Cl)	2	5
University of Denver (Psy.D.) (Cl)	1	0
University of Delaware (Cl)	1	1
University of Detroit–Mercy (Cl)	2	0
University of Georgia (Cl)	1	1
University of Houston (Cl)	2	1
University of Iowa (Cl)	1	0
University of Kansas (Cl)	1	0
University of Nevada–Reno (Cl)	2	1
University of North Carolina at Chapel Hill (Cl)	1	2
University of North Texas (Co)	3	2
University of Notre Dame (Co)	1	1
University of Ottawa (Cl)	2	1
University of Rochester (Cl)	1	0
University of South Carolina (Cl)	4	0
University of Southern California (Cl)	4	3
University of Victoria (Cl)	1	1
Virginia Commonwealth University (Co)	2	0
Virginia Consortium Program in Clinical Psychology (Cl)	2	0
Virginia Polytechnic Institute and State University (Cl)	1	0
York University—Adult Clinical Program (Cl)	1	1

Memory

Binghamton University/State University of New York (Cl)	2	0
George Fox University (Psy.D.) (Cl)	2	1
Idaho State University (Cl)	1	2
Marquette University (Cl)	1	2
University of Montana (Cl)	1	0

Men's Issues

Argosy University–Shaumburg (Psy.D.) (Cl)	1	0
Colorado State University (Co)	1	0
Indiana State University (Co)	2	0
University of Iowa (Co)	3	0
University of Texas at Austin (Co)	1	0
University of Wisconsin–Milwaukee (Co)	1	0

Minority/Cross-Cultural/Diversity

Alliant International University–Fresno (Ph.D.) (Cl)	4	—
Alliant International University–Fresno (Psy.D.) (Cl)	3	—
Alliant International University–Los Angeles (Psy.D.) (Cl)	6	—
Alliant International University–Los Angeles (Ph.D.) (Cl)	3	—
Alliant International University–San Diego (Psy.D.) (Cl)	5	—
Alliant International University–San Diego (Ph.D.) (Cl)	4	—
Alliant International University–San Francisco (Ph.D.) (Cl)	4	—
Alliant International University–San Francisco (Psy.D.) (Cl)	11	—
Antioch/New England Graduate School (Cl)	1	0
Argosy University, Atlanta (Psy.D.) (Cl)	3	0
Argosy University, Chicago (Psy.D.)	3	1
Argosy University–Honolulu (Psy.D.) (Cl)	9	0
Argosy University, Schaumburg (Psy.D.)	2	1
Argosy University–Phoenix (Cl)	5	0
Argosy University–Twin Cities (Psy.D.) (Cl)	2	0
Argosy University–Washington, DC Campus (Cl)	1	0
Arizona State University (Cl)	6	11
Arizona State University (Co)	4	0
Azusa Pacific University (Psy.D.) (Cl)	2	0
Ball State University (Co)	4	1
Biola University (Ph.D.) (Cl)	4	0
Biola University (Psy.D.) (Cl)	4	0
Boston College (Co)	3	3
Boston University (Cl)	2	0
Brigham Young University (Co)	2	2
Carlos Albizu University–Miami Campus (Cl)	6	0
Central Michigan University (Cl)	1	0

	# Faculty	# Grants
Chicago School of Professional Psychology (Cl)	9	1
City University of New York at City College (Cl)	1	0
Colorado State University (Co)	6	3
Columbia University, Teachers College (Ph.D.) (Co)	2	0
DePaul University (Cl)	3	1
Eastern Michigan University (Cl)	2	0
Fairleigh Dickinson University (Cl)	2	0
Fordham University (Co)	5	0
Fuller Theological Seminary (Ph.D. & Psy.D.) (Cl)	2	0
Gallaudet University (Cl)	1	1
George Washington University (Ph.D.) (Cl)	4	3
Georgia State University (Cl)	3	0
Georgia State University (Co)	2	0
Howard University (Cl)	4	4
Immaculata University (Psy.D.) (Cl)	3	0
Indiana University (Co)	2	0
Indiana University of Pennsylvania (Cl)	3	0
Iowa State University (Co)	1	0
James Madison University (Cm)	4	1
Lehigh University (Co)	1	1
Long Island University (Cl)	4	0
Loyola College in Maryland (Psy.D.) (Cl)	3	0
Loyola University–Chicago (Cl)	4	3
Loyola University–Chicago (Co)	2	0
Marshall University (Cl)	1	0
Marquette University (Cl & Co)	4	0
Marywood University (Cl)	2	0
Miami University (Cl)	2	0
New York University (Co)	2	0
Northeastern University (Cm)	1	1
Northern Illinois University (Cl)	1	1
Nova Southeastern University (Ph.D. & Psy.D.) (Cl)	2	0
Oklahoma State University (Co)	7	8
Ontario Institute for Studies in Education (Cm)	3	3
Pace University (Psy.D.) (Cm)	2	0
Pacific Graduate School of Psychology (Psy.D.) (Cl)	5	1
Pennsylvania State University (Cl)	1	1
Pepperdine University (Psy.D.) (Cl)	1	1
Philadelphia College of Osteopathic Medicine (Psy.D.) (Cl)	4	0
Purdue University (Cl)	2	0
Purdue University (Co)	1	1
Rutgers University (Psy.D.) (Cl)	2	0
St. John's University (Cl)	7	1
St. Louis University (Cl)	1	0
San Diego State University/University of California–San Diego (Cl)	10	0
Seattle Pacific University (Cl)	5	0
Seton Hall University (Co)	3	0
Southern Illinois University (Co)	6	2
Temple University (Cl)	1	1
Tennessee State University (Co)	2	1
Texas A&M University (Co)	2	0
Texas Tech University (Cl)	2	3
Texas Tech University (Co)	3	0
University of Akron (Co)	2	0
University of Alabama (Cl)	2	2
University at Albany/State University of New York (Co)	24	2
University of British Columbia (Co)	1	2
University at Buffalo/State University of New York (Cm)	1	0
University of California–Berkeley (Cl)	1	1
University of California–Santa Barbara (Cm)	4	1
University of Central Florida (Cl)	1	0
University of Connecticut (Cl)	2	1
University of Denver (Ph.D.) (Cl)	2	2
University of Denver (Psy.D.) (Cl)	1	0
University of Denver (Co)	1	1
University of Florida (Co)	1	0
University of Georgia (Co)	4	3
University of Hawaii at Manoa (Cl)	4	3
University of Houston (Cl)	3	2
University of Houston (Co)	2	0
University of Illinois at Urbana–Champaign (Cl)	5	0
University of Illinois at Urbana–Champaign (Co)	2	2
University of Indianapolis (Cl)	2	1
University of Iowa (Co)	2	1
University of Kansas (Cl)	5	0
University of Kentucky (Co)	2	0
University of La Verne (Psy.D.) (Cl)	7	2
University of Maryland (Co)	3	0
University of Massachusetts at Boston (Cl)	3	0
University of Memphis (Co)	7	2
University of Miami (Co)	1	0
University of Minnesota (Cl)	—	—
University of Minnesota—Department of Educational Psychology (Co)	4	4
University of Minnesota—Department of Psychology (Co)	1	0
University of Mississippi (Cl)	1	0
University of Missouri–Columbia (Co)	6	4
University of Missouri–Kansas City (Co)	4	2
University of Missouri–St. Louis (Cl)	1	0
University of Montana (Cl)	1	0
University of Nebraska–Lincoln (Co)	1	0
University of Nevada–Reno (Cl)	4	2
University of New Mexico (Cl)	3	1
University of North Carolina at Chapel Hill (Cl)	2	0
University of North Dakota (Cl)	4	1
University of North Dakota (Co)	1	0
University of North Texas (Co)	2	1
University of Northern Colorado (Co)	6	0
University of Notre Dame (Co)	1	1
University of Oklahoma (Co)	4	0
University of Oregon (Cl)	1	1
University of Oregon (Co)	4	1
University of Ottawa (Cl)	1	0
University of Rhode Island (Cl)	1	0

	# Faculty	# Grants
University of St. Thomas (Co)	2	0
University of South Dakota (Cl)	7	2
University of Southern Mississippi (Co)	3	0
University of Texas at Austin (Cl)	1	0
University of Texas at Austin (Co)	3	1
University of Texas Southwestern Medical Center at Dallas (Cl)	2	0
University of Toledo (Cl)	2	0
University of Utah (Cl)	2	0
University of Utah (Co)	3	0
University of Victoria (Cl)	1	1
University of Virginia—Department of Human Services (Cl)	1	1
University of Virginia—Department of Psychology (Cl)	3	1
University of Washington (Cl)	5	4
University of Waterloo (Cl)	1	1
University of Wisconsin–Madison (Co)	9	5
University of Wisconsin–Milwaukee (Co)	2	2
University of Wisconsin–Milwaukee (Cl)	1	0
University of Wyoming (Cl)	1	1
Utah State University (Cm)	1	0
Virginia Commonwealth University (Cl)	2	1
Virginia Commonwealth University (Co)	3	0
Virginia Polytechnic Institute and State University (Cl)	2	1
Washington State University (Co)	3	1
West Virginia University (Cl)	1	0
Western Michigan University (Co)		
Wheaton College (Cl)	1	1
Wright Institute (Cl)	3	0
Wright State University (Cl)	5	2
Yeshiva University (Cl)	2	0
Yeshiva University (Cm)	3	0

MMPI

California Institute of Integral Studies (Psy.D.) (Cl)	1	1
Fordham University (Cl)	3	0
Kent State University (Cl)	2	2
Wichita State University (Cl)	1	0

Moral Development

Azusa Pacific University (Cl)	2	1
New School University (Cl)	1	0
St. John's University (Cl)	3	0
University of La Verne (Psy.D.) (Cl)	2	0

Motivation

Adelphi University (Cl)	1	0
Clark University (Cl)	1	1
James Madison University (Cm)	1	0
University of Rochester (Cl)	4	2

Narrative Psychology

University of Norte Dame (Co)	1	1
York University—Adult Clinical Program (Cl)	1	0

Neuroimaging/Functional Neuroimaging

Georgia State University (Cl)	3	1
University of Pittsburgh (Cl)	7	27
Vanderbilt University (Cl)	3	3

Neuropsychology

Adler School of Professional Psychology (Cl)	4	1
Argosy University, Atlanta (Ph.D.) (Cl)	3	0
Argosy University, Chicago (Psy.D.) (Cl)	3	0
Argosy University–Honolulu Campus (Cl)	2	0
Argosy University–Phoenix (Cl)	1	0
Azusa Pacific University (Psy.D.) (Cl)	1	0
Binghamton University/State University of New York (Cl)	1	2
Biola University (Ph.D.) (Cl)	1	0
Biola University (Psy.D.) (Cl)	1	1
Boston University (Cl)	3	2
Brigham Young University (Cl)	2	4
Carlos Albizu University–Miami Campus (Cl)	2	0
Central Michigan University (Cl)	1	1
Concordia University (Cl)	9	12
Drexel University (Cl)	6	4
Duke University (Cl)	1	1
Eastern Michigan University (Cl)	2	1
Emory University (Cl)	1	0
Florida Institute of Technology (Cl)	2	1
Fordham University (Cl)	2	1
Fielding Graduate University (Cl)	—	—
Fuller Theological Seminary (Ph.D. & Psy.D.) (Cl)	2	0
Gallaudet University (Cl)	1	1
George Fox University (Psy.D.) (Cl)	1	1
Georgia State University (Cl)	3	2
Howard University (Cl)	2	2
Immaculata University (Cl)	2	0
Indiana University–Purdue University Indianapolis (Cl)	2	3
Loma Linda University (Ph.D. & Psy.D.) (Cl)	2	0
Long Island University (Cl)	1	0
Louisiana State University (Cl)	1	0
Loyola College in Maryland (Psy.D.) (Cl)	2	0
Marquette University (Cl)	2	0
McGill University (Cl)	1	1
Michigan State University (Cl)	2	3
Northeastern University (Cm)	1	0
Northwestern University, Feinberg School of Medicine (Cl)	3	1
Nova Southeastern University (Ph.D. & Psy.D.) (Cl)	5	2

	# Faculty	# Grants
Ohio State University (Cl)	2	3
Ohio University (Cl)	1	1
Pacific Graduate School of Psychology (Cl)	2	1
Pacific University (Cl)	1	1
Pennsylvania State University (Cl)	2	1
Roosevelt University (Cl)		
Rosalind Franklin University of Medicine (Cl)	1	2
St. Louis University (Cl)	1	0
Sam Houston State University (Cl)	1	1
San Diego State University/University of California–San Diego (Cl)	7	0
Seton Hall University (Co)	1	0
Simon Fraser University (Cl)	3	5
Temple University (Cl)	1	2
Texas Tech University (Cl)	1	0
Uniformed Services University of Health Sciences (Cl)	1	1
University of Alabama at Birmingham (Cl)	3	2
University at Albany/State University of New York (Cl)	1	0
University of Arizona (Cl)	2	2
University of Cincinnati (Cl)	6	5
University of Connecticut (Cl)	4	3
University of Denver (Ph.D.) (Cl)	1	1
University of Florida (Cl)	8	7
University of Georgia (Cl)	1	2
University of Houston (Cl)	4	4
University of Illinois at Urbana–Champaign (Cl)	2	1
University of Indianapolis (Psy.D.) (Cl)	3	1
University of Kansas (Cl)	2	1
University of Kentucky (Cl)	2	1
University of Manitoba (Cl)	2	1
University of Michigan (Cl)	6	0
University of Missouri–Kansas City (Cl)	1	1
University of Montana (Cl)	1	0
University of Nevada–Las Vegas (Cl)	1	1
University of New Brunswick (Cl)	3	3
University of New Mexico (Cl)	2	4
University of North Texas (Cl)	1	0
University of Oregon (Cl)	2	2
University of Pittsburgh (Cl)	7	27
University of Saskatchewan (Cl)	1	1
University of South Carolina (Cl)	2	1
University of South Florida (Cl)	1	0
University of Southern California (Cl)	1	0
University of Texas at Austin (Cl)	2	1
University of Texas Southwestern Medical Center at Dallas (Cl)	4	4
University of Tulsa (Cl)	1	1
University of Utah (Cl)	1	2
University of Virginia (Cl)	1	0
University of Windsor (Cl)	4	4
University of Wisconsin–Milwaukee (Cl)	2	1
Vanderbilt University (Cl)	3	3
Virginia Consortium Program in Clinical Psychology (Cl)	1	2
Virginia Polytechnic Institute and State University (Cl)	2	0
Washington State University (Cl)	1	1
Washington University (Cl)	4	5
Wayne State University (Cl)	2	2
Western Michigan University (Cl)	1	0
Yeshiva University (Ph.D.) (Cl)	2	2
York University—Adult Clinical Program (Cl)	3	2

Object Relations

Biola University (Ph.D.) (Cl)	4	0
Biola University (Psy.D.) (Cl)	4	0
City University of New York at City College (Cl)	4	1

Organizational

Ball State University (Co)	1	0
Indiana State University (Cl)	1	1
Rutgers University (Psy.D.) (Cl)	1	0
Virginia Consortium Program in Clinical Psychology (Cl)	1	1

Pain Management

Binghamton University/State University of New York (Cl)	1	1
Forest Institute of Professional Psychology (Cl)	2	1
George Fox University (Psy.D.) (Cl)	1	1
Jackson State University (Cl)	3	1
Philadelphia College of Osteopathic Medicine (Psy.D.) (Cl)	1	0
Rosalind Franklin University of Medicine (Cl)	1	1
San Diego State University (Cl)	2	0
University of Alabama (Cl)	1	1
University of Florida (Cl)	2	3
University of Georgia (Cl)	1	1
University of Kansas (Cl)	1	0
University of Kentucky (Cl)	1	1
University of North Dakota (Cl)	1	0
University of Texas Southwestern Medical Center at Dallas (Cl)	1	1
Virginia Polytechnic Institute and State University (Cl)	2	0
West Virginia University (Cl)	1	0
York University—Adult Clinical Program (Cl)	1	1

Parent–Child Interactions/Parenting

Biola University (Ph.D.) (Cl)	3	0
Biola University (Psy.D.) (Cl)	3	0
Case Western Reserve University (Cl)	2	0
Catholic University of America (Cl)	2	1
Colorado State University (Co)	1	0
DePaul University (Cl)	1	1

	# Faculty	# Grants
Fielding Graduate University (Cl)	—	—
Fordham University (Cl)	2	0
Gallaudet University (Cl)	1	1
Georgia State University (Cl)	1	1
Idaho State University (Cl)	1	0
Indiana University of Pennsylvania (Cl)	4	1
James Madison University (Cm)	2	0
Long Island University–C.W. Post Campus (Cl)	1	0
Louisiana State University (Cl)	1	0
Marquette University (Co)	1	3
Miami University (Cl)	1	1
Northern Illinois University (Cl)	3	1
Ontario Institute for Studies in Education (Cm)	3	3
Pennsylvania State University (Cl)	3	2
Stony Brook University/State University of New York (Cl)	1	2
Texas Tech University (Cl)	1	0
University of Houston (Cl)	2	1
University of Indianapolis (Cl)	1	1
University of Louisville (Co)	1	0
University of Southern Mississippi (Co)	1	0
University of Virginia—Department of Human Services (Cl)	3	1
Virginia Consortium Program in Clinical Psychology (Cl)	3	1
Virginia Polytechnic Institute and State University (Cl)	2	1
Wheaton College (Cl)	3	0
Wright Institute (Psy.D.) (Cl)	6	0
Wright State University (Cl)	6	0
Yeshiva University (Psy.D.) (Cl)	1	0

Personality Assessment

	# Faculty	# Grants
Arizona State University (Cl)	1	0
Auburn University (Cl)	1	0
Baylor University (Psy.D.) (Cl)	3	0
Florida Institute of Technology (Cl)	3	0
George Washington University (Psy.D.) (Cl)	3	0
Immaculata University (Cl)	2	0
Indiana State University (Co)	1	0
New School University (Cl)	1	0
Northwestern University (Cl)	4	2
Pennsylvania State University (Cl)	3	1
Philadelphia College of Osteopathic Medicine (Psy.D.) (Cl)	3	0
Purdue University (Cl)	1	0
Southern Illinois University (Cl)	4	0
University of Akron (Co)	2	0
University of Illinois at Urbana–Champaign	1	1
University of Kentucky (Cl)	3	1
University of Minnesota (Cl)	—	—
University of North Dakota (Cl)	2	0
University of South Florida (Cl)	1	0
University of Utah (Cl)	3	0
West Virginia University (Co)	2	0

	# Faculty	# Grants
York University—Adult Clinical Program (Cl)	1	0

Personality Disorders

	# Faculty	# Grants
Argosy University, Chicago (Psy.D.) (Cl)	1	0
Binghamton University/State University of New York (Cl)	1	1
Boston University (Cl)	1	0
Case Western Reserve University (Cl)	1	6
Drexel University (Cl)	2	0
Eastern Michigan University (Cl)	1	0
Emory University (Cl)	3	2
Fordham University (Cl)	2	1
Indiana State University (Cl)	1	0
Miami University (Cl)	3	0
Northern Illinois University (Cl)	1	0
Pennsylvania State University (Cl)	2	0
Philadelphia College of Osteopathic Medicine (Psy.D.) (Cl)	1	0
St. Louis University (Cl)	2	0
University of Colorado (Cl)	0	0
University of Iowa (Cl)	1	1
University of Kentucky (Cl)	2	0
University of Michigan (Cl)	2	0
University of Minnesota (Cl)	—	—
University of Missouri–Columbia (Cl)	1	2
University of North Carolina at Greensboro (Cl)	1	0
University of North Dakota (Cl)	3	0
University of Tulsa (Cl)	2	0
University of Utah (Cl)	1	0
University of Virginia—Department of Psychology (Cl)	2	1
University of Wisconsin–Madison (Cl)	1	2

Personality/Temperament

	# Faculty	# Grants
Case Western Reserve University (Cl)	1	1
George Mason University (Cl)	1	1
Hofstra University (Cm)	2	0
Loyola University–Chicago (Cl)	2	0
Ohio State University (Cl)	1	0
Pennsylvania State University (Cl)	2	0
Purdue University (Cl)	3	0
Regent University (Cl)	1	1
University of Florida (Co)	1	0
University of Maryland (Cl)	1	0
University of Minnesota—Department of Psychology (Co)	1	0
Vanderbilt University (Cl)	1	1
Washington State University (Co)	1	0

Positive Psychology/Resilience

	# Faculty	# Grants
Carlos Albizu University–Miami Campus (Cl)	1	0
George Mason University (Cl)	3	0
Immaculata College (Cl)	2	0
Marywood University (Cl)	1	0
New York University (Co)	1	1

	# Faculty	# Grants
Pepperdine University (Psy.D.) (Cl)	2	1
Seton Hall University (Co)	1	0
Texas Tech University (Co)	1	0
University of Indianapolis (Psy.D) (Cl)	1	0
University of Kansas (Co)	3	1
University of Louisville (Co)	1	3
University of Montana (Cl)	2	0
Washington State University (Co)	1	0

Posttraumatic Stress Disorder

	# Faculty	# Grants
Alliant International University–Los Angeles (Ph.D. & Psy.D.) (Cl)	3	—
Alliant International University–San Diego (Ph.D. & Psy.D.) (Cl)	4	—
Argosy University–Honolulu Campus (Cl)	2	1
Binghamton University/State University of New York (Cl)	2	0
Duke University (Cl)	0	0
Eastern Michigan University (Cl)	2	1
Florida Institute of Technology (Psy.D.) (Cl)	1	0
Fuller Theological Seminary (Ph.D. & Psy.D.) (Cl)	2	0
Jackson State University (Cl)	1	0
LaSalle University (Cl)	1	0
Loyola College in Maryland (Cl)	4	0
Miami University (Cl)	1	1
Nova Southeastern University (Ph.D. & Psy.D.) (Cl)	4	0
Pace University (Psy.D.) (Cm)	1	0
Pepperdine University (Cl)	1	2
San Diego State University/University of California–San Diego (Cl)	1	0
University of Denver (Co)	1	1
University of Detroit–Mercy (Cl)	2	0
University of Indianapolis (Cl)	1	0
University of Minnesota–Department of Psychology (Co)	1	0
University of Mississippi (Cl)	1	0
University of Montana (Cl)	3	1
University of North Texas (Cl)	2	0
University of Tulsa (Cl)	2	0
West Virginia University (Cl)	1	0
Western Michigan University (Cl)	1	0
University of Wyoming (Cl)	1	1

Prevention

	# Faculty	# Grants
Arizona State University (Cl)	6	9
Binghamton University/State University of New York (Cl)	3	1
Boston College (Co)	3	2
DePaul University (Cl)		
Fordham University (Cl)	1	0
Hofstra University (Cm)	2	0
Indiana University of Pennsylvania (Cl)	1	0
Loyola University–Chicago (Cl)	3	2
New School University (Cl)	2	1
Northern Illinois University (Cl)	1	0
Rutgers University (Ph.D.) (Cl)	2	1
University at Albany/State University of New York (Co)	1	0
University of Central Florida (Cl)	1	0
University of Colorado (Cl)	3	0
University of Denver (Ph.D.) (Cl)	2	5
University of Georgia (Cl)	2	1
University of Minnesota—Department of Educational Psychology (Co)	1	0
University of Nevada–Reno (Cl)	4	2
University of Oregon (Co)	4	2
University of Pittsburgh (Cl)	3	9
University of South Carolina (Cl)	5	3
University of Vermont (Cl)	2	1
University of Virginia (Cl)	3	2
Vanderbilt University (Cl)	3	2
Virginia Commonwealth University (Co)	2	2
Virginia Consortium Program in Clinical Psychology (Cl)	1	3
Virginia Polytechnic Institute and State University (Cl)	4	3

Problem Solving

	# Faculty	# Grants
San Diego State University/University of California–San Diego (Cl)	4	0
Stony Brook University/State University of New York (Cl)	2	2
University of Missouri–Columbia (Co)	3	2

Professional Issues/Training

	# Faculty	# Grants
Indiana State University (Psy.D.) (Cl)	1	0
Indiana University of Pennsylvania (Cl)	5	1
Miami University (Cl)	2	1
Oklahoma State University (Co)	2	1
St. Louis University (Cl)	3	0
Texas Tech University (Co)	2	0
University of Alabama (Cl)	2	0
University of Georgia (Co)	4	0
University of Memphis (Co)	2	0
University of Missouri–Kansas City (Co)	3	0
University of North Texas (Co)	4	0
University of Utah (Co)	1	0
Yeshiva University (Cm)	3	0

Program Evaluation

	# Faculty	# Grants
Alliant International University–San Francisco (Ph.D.) (Cl)	1	—
Antioch/New England Graduate School (Psy.D.) (Cl)	2	0
Brigham Young (Co)	3	3
DePaul University (Cl)	3	1
George Mason University (Cl)	1	1
Indiana State University (Co)	1	0
Marquette University (Cl)	2	1
Miami University (Cl)	2	2
Pepperdine University (Cl)	1	1
Rutgers University (Ph.D.) (Cl)	1	1

	# Faculty	# Grants
Rutgers University (Psy.D.) (Cl)	1	1
Seattle Pacific University (Cl)	2	1
Spalding University (Cl)	1	0
University of Illinois at Urbana–Champaign (Cl)	4	3
University of Pittsburgh (Cl)	2	3
University of Toledo (Cl)	2	1
Western Michigan University (Cl)	1	0

Psychoanalysis/Psychodynamics

Adelphi University	8	3
California Institute of Integral Studies (Psy.D.) (Cl)	2	0
New School University (Cl)	2	0
New York University (Co)	1	0
Nova Southeastern University (Ph.D. & Psy.D.) (Cl)	3	0
Pacific University (Psy.D.) (Cl)	2	0
Rutgers University (Psy.D.) (Cl)	4	1
Seattle Pacific University (Cl)	1	0
University of Pennsylvania (Cl)	2	2
University of Texas at Austin (Co)	2	0
Virginia Consortium Program in Clinical Psychology (Cl)	1	0
Xavier University (Cl)	4	0
Yeshiva University (Cl)	5	0

Psychometrics/Measurement

Auburn University (Co)	2	0
Brigham Young University (Cl)	3	1
Northern Illinois University (Cl)	3	0
Pace University (Psy.D.) (Cm)	3	0
Ponce School of Medicine (Cl)	4	1
Southern Illinois University (Co)	1	0
University at Buffalo/State University of New York (Cl)	1	0

Psychoneuroimmunology

Arizona State University (Cl)	3	3
Ohio State University (Cl)	2	5
University of Kentucky (Cl)	1	1
University of Manitoba (Cl)	1	0
University of Maryland–Baltimore County (Cl)	1	0
University of Miami (Cl)	6	2
University of Pittsburgh (Cl)	3	9

Psychopathology—Adult Psychopathology

Binghamton University/State University of New York (Cl)	8	2
Brigham Young University (Cl)	2	0
Catholic University of America (Cl)	3	1
Central Michigan University (Cl)	1	1
Clark University (Cl)	2	1
Colorado State University (Co)	3	0

Concordia University (Cl)	2	1
Florida State University (Cl)	3	3
George Washington University (Psy.D.) (Cl)	4	0
Indiana State University (Cl)	2	0
Indiana University of Pennsylvania (Cl)	3	0
Loyola University–Chicago (Cl)	2	0
New School University (Cl)	2	0
New York University (Co)	2	0
Northern Illinois University (Cl)	3	0
Ohio University (Cl)	2	0
Pacific Graduate School of Psychology (Cl)	7	2
Pennsylvania State University (Cl)	5	1
Rosalind Franklin University of Medicine (Cl)	1	0
Rutgers University (Ph.D.) (Cl)	1	1
San Diego State University/University of California–San Diego (Cl)	3	0
Seattle Pacific University (Cl)	3	3
Simon Fraser University (Cl)	8	8
Stony Brook University/State University of New York (Cl)	1	3
University of Alabama (Cl)	3	2
University at Albany/State University of New York (Cl)	1	0
University of Colorado (Cl)	4	3
University of Connecticut (Cl)	5	2
University of Houston (Cl)	6	3
University of Iowa (Cl)	1	0
University of Kansas (Cl)	1	0
University of Kentucky (Cl)	4	0
University of Manitoba (Cl)	1	0
University of Miami (Cl)	6	2
University of Missouri–Kansas City (Co)	3	0
University of Nebraska–Lincoln (Cl)	3	2
University of North Dakota (Cl)	6	0
University of Southern Mississippi (Cl)	5	1
University of Tennessee (Cl)	4	1
University of Utah (Cl)	4	10
University of Virginia (Cl)	3	3
Vanderbilt University (Cl)	12	5
Virginia Commonwealth University (Cl)	1	1
Washington State University (Cl)	5	6
Washington University (Cl)	4	3
Yale University (Cl)	5	0

Psychopathology—Child/Developmental

Baylor University (Cl)	2	0
Brigham Young University (Cl)	2	0
Catholic University of America (Cl)	4	1
Duke University (Cl)	5	5
Indiana University of Pennsylvania (Cl)	1	0
Long Island University (Cl)	2	0
Loyola College in Maryland (Cl)	5	0
Loyola University–Chicago (Cl)	5	4
Miami University (Cl)	6	4
Ontario Institute for Studies in Education (Cm)	4	5
Philadelphia College of Osteopathic Medicine (Psy.D.) (Cl)	1	0

	# Faculty	# Grants
Rutgers University (Ph.D.) (Cl)	1	1
Simon Fraser University (Cl)	3	5
University at Buffalo/State University of New York (Cl)	31	1
University of Central Florida (Cl)	1	0
University of Connecticut (Cl)	7	3
University of Denver (Ph.D.) (Cl)	3	0
University of Georgia (Cl)	2	1
University of Kentucky (Cl)	1	1
University of Manitoba (Cl)	1	0
University of Massachusetts at Amherst (Cl)	1	1
University of Miami (Cl)	5	2
University of Minnesota (Cl)	—	—
University of Montana (Cl)	2	1
University of Oregon (Cl)	2	1
University of Pittsburgh (Cl)	14	45
University of Southern California (Cl)	3	3
University of Southern Mississippi (Cl)	3	0
University of Tennessee (Cl)	3	1
University of Tulsa (Cl)	2	1
University of Vermont (Cl)	4	2
University of Wisconsin–Madison (Cl)	4	—
Virginia Consortium Program in Clinical Psychology (Cl)	3	0
West Virginia University (Cl)	1	0
Yale University (Cl)	2	0

Psychopharmacology

	# Faculty	# Grants
Argosy University–Phoenix (Cl)	1	0
Idaho State University (Cl)	1	2
San Diego State University/University of California–San Diego (Cl)	6	2
University of Georgia (Cl)	1	0
University of Minnesota (Cl)		
University of Nevada–Las Vegas (Cl)	1	0
University of Pennsylvania (Cl)	1	1
University of Pittsburgh (Cl)	4	14
Vanderbilt University (Cl)	2	2

Psychophysiology

	# Faculty	# Grants
Binghamton University/State University of New York (Cl)	2	0
Howard University (Cl)	1	0
Louisiana State University (Cl)	1	0
Pennsylvania State University (Cl)	2	0
Rutgers University (Psy.D.) (Cl)	1	0
San Diego State University/University of California–San Diego (Cl)	5	0
Syracuse University (Cl)	3	2
University of Alabama at Birmingham (Cl)	1	1
University of Delaware (Cl)	3	1
University of Illinois at Urbana–Champaign (Cl)	3	8
University of Kentucky (Cl)	2	1
University of Maryland (Cl)	2	0
University of Minnesota (Cl)	—	—

	# Faculty	# Grants
University of North Dakota (Cl)	1	0
University of Pennsylvania (Cl)	3	3
University of Pittsburgh (Cl)	5	16
Vanderbilt University—Department of Psychology (Cl)	6	2
Virginia Commonwealth University (Cl)	2	0

Psychotherapists

	# Faculty	# Grants
Argosy University Chicago (Cl)	2	1
California Institute of Integral Studies (Psy.D.) (Cl)	1	0
University of Minnesota Dept of Education (Co)	2	2
University of Massachusetts at Amherst (Cl)	1	1

Psychotherapy/Process and Outcome

	# Faculty	# Grants
Adelphi University (Cl)	3	2
Argosy University–Chicago (Cl)	1	0
Argosy Twin Cities (PsyD) (Cl)	2	0
Argosy University, Schaumberg (Psy.D.)	2	1
Carlos Albizu University–Miami Campus (Cl)	6	0
Catholic University of America (Cl)	3	0
City University of New York at City College (Cl)	3	0
Colorado State University (Co)	1	0
Columbia University, Teachers College (Cl)	3	1
Drexel University (Cl)	5	1
Fairleigh Dickinson University (Cl)	4	0
George Mason University (Cl)	1	0
Hofstra University (Cm)	1	2
Immaculata College (Cl)	2	0
James Madison University (Cm)	1	0
Loma Linda University (Ph.D. & Psy.D.) (Cl)	1	0
Loyola College in Maryland (Cl)	1	0
Loyola University–Chicago (Cl)	4	1
Loyola University–Chicago (Co)	1	0
Marshall University (Psy.D.) (Cl)	1	0
Marquette University (Cl)	6	0
Marquette University (Co)	3	0
McGill University (Cl)	1	1
McGill University (Co)	2	1
Miami University (Cl)	3	0
New School University (Cl)	3	1
Northwestern University (Cl)	1	0
Nova Southeastern University (Ph.D. & Psy.D.) (Cl)	8	1
Pacific Graduate School of Psychology (Ph.D.) (Cl)	2	0
Pennsylvania State University (Cl)	4	3
Pennsylvania State University (Co)	1	0
Pepperdine University (Cl)	6	1
Philadelphia College of Osteopathic Medicine (Psy.D.) (Cl)	1	0
Rutgers University (Ph.D.) (Cl)	5	3
Rutgers University (Psy.D.) (Cl)	3	1

	# Faculty	# Grants
San Diego State University/University of California–San Diego (Cl)	4	0
Stony Brook University/State University of New York (Cl)	2	2
Southern Illinois University (Co)	1	0
Texas A&M University (Cl)	7	2
University of Alabama (Cl)	2	0
University at Albany/State University of New York (Co)	1	1
University of British Columbia (Co)	1	0
University of California–Santa Barbara (Cm)	—	—
University of Colorado (Cl)	4	2
University of Delaware (Cl)	2	2
University of Denver (Ph.D.) (Cl)	2	4
University of Detroit–Mercy (Cl)	4	0
University of Georgia (Co)	2	0
University of Hartford (Cl)	4	1
University of Hawaii at Manoa (Cl)	4	4
University of Illinois at Urbana–Champaign (Cl)	1	1
University of Kansas (Cl)	3	0
University of Kansas (Co)	1	1
University of La Verne (Psy.D.) (Cl)	3	0
University of Maine (Cl)	3	0
University of Manitoba (Cl)	3	0
University of Maryland (Cl)	2	2
University of Massachusetts at Amherst (Cl)	1	1
University of Memphis (Cl)	3	0
University of Michigan (Cl)	5	0
University of Minnesota—Department of Educational Psychology (Co)	2	0
University of Missouri–Columbia (Co)	1	0
University of Missouri–Kansas City (Co)	3	0
University of Montana (Cl)	3	0
University Nebraska–Lincoln (Cl)	1	0
University of Northern Colorado (Co)	1	0
University of North Texas (Co)	6	0
University of Oregon (Co)	4	1
University of Ottawa (Cl)	1	0
University of Saskatchewan (Cl)	2	1
University of Tennessee (Co)	4	1
University of Toledo (Cl)	3	1
University of Utah (Co)	1	0
University of Washington (Cl)	1	1
University of Windsor (Cl)	3	2
University of Wisconsin–Madison (Co)	3	0
University of Wisconsin–Milwaukee (Cl)	2	4
Vanderbilt University (Cl)	2	2
Virginia Commonwealth University (Cl)	3	3
Virginia Consortium Program in Clinical Psychology (Cl)	2	0
Virginia Polytechnic Institute and State University (Cl)	2	1
Washington University (Cl)	4	2
West Virginia University (Co)	3	0
Western Michigan University (Cl)	4	0
Wright Institute (Cl)	3	0

	# Faculty	# Grants
Yeshiva University (Psy.D.) (Cl)	3	0
York University—Adult Clinical Program (Cl)	4	2

Rehabilitation

	# Faculty	# Grants
Ball State University (Co)	2	1
Georgia State University (Co)	2	0
Illinois Institute of Technology (Cl)	2	1
Texas A&M University	1	3
University of British Columbia (Co)	1	1
University at Buffalo/State University of New York (Cm)	2	0
University of New Brunswick (Cl)	1	1
University of Texas Southwestern Medical Center at Dallas (Cl)	1	1
West Virginia University (Co)	4	0

Religion/Spirituality

	# Faculty	# Grants
Azusa Pacific University (Cl)	4	1
Biola University (Ph.D.) (Cl)	4	2
Biola University (Psy.D.) (Cl)	4	2
Bowling Green State University (Cl)	2	1
Brigham Young University (Co)	6	3
California Institute of Integral Studies (Psy.D.) (Cl)	4	1
Columbia University, Teachers College (Cl)	1	1
Fuller Theological Seminary (Ph.D. & Psy.D.) (Cl)	7	0
George Fox University (Cl)	1	1
Iowa State University (Co)	1	1
Loma Linda University (Ph.D. & Psy.D.) (Cl)	2	0
Loyola College in Maryland (Cl)	2	0
New York University (Co)	1	1
Regent University (Cl)	4	3
Seattle Pacific University (Cl)	3	1
Seton Hall University (Co)	1	0
Southern Illinois University (Cl)	1	0
Southern Illinois University (Co)	1	0
Texas Tech University (Co)	1	0
University at Albany/State University of New York (Co)	1	0
University of Detroit–Mercy (Cl)	3	0
University of Iowa	2	0
University of Maryland–Baltimore County (Cl)	1	0
University of Southern Mississippi (Co)	2	1
University of St. Thomas (Co)	1	0
Virginia Commonwealth University (Co)	2	0
Virginia Consortium Program in Clinical Psychology (Cl)	1	0
West Virginia University (Co)	1	0
Wheaton College (Cl)	4	0

Research Methodology

	# Faculty	# Grants
Marshall University (Psy.D.) (Cl)	1	0
Sam Houston State University (Cl)	1	0

	# Faculty	# Grants
Southern Illinois University (Co)	1	0
Texas A&M University (Co)	1	0

Rural Mental Health/Psychology

	# Faculty	# Grants
Marshall University (Psy.D.) (Cl)	2	1
Oklahoma State University (Co)	1	0
Pennsylvania State University (Cl)	1	1
University of Florida (Cl)	1	2
University of Mississippi (Cl)	2	0
University of North Dakota (Cl)	2	2
University of North Dakota (Co)	2	0
University of South Dakota (Cl)	6	0
Utah State University (Cm)	2	1
Wheaton College (Cl)	2	0

Schizophrenia/Psychoses/Severe Mental Illness

	# Faculty	# Grants
Boston University (Cl)	1	1
Drexel University (Cl)	0	0
Emory University (Cl)	2	1
Hofstra University (Cm)	2	1
Indiana University–Bloomington (Cl)	2	4
Kent State University (Cl)	1	1
Long Island University–C.W. Post Campus (Cl)	1	0
Rosalind Franklin University of Medicine (Cl)	1	0
St. John's University (Cl)	1	0
San Diego State University/University of California–San Diego (Cl)	7	2
University of California–Los Angeles (Cl)	3	5
University of Central Florida (Cl)	1	0
University of Georgia (Cl)	1	0
University of Hawaii at Manoa (Cl)	5	1
University of Houston (Cl)	2	1
University of Illinois at Chicago (Cl)	1	4
University of Illinois at Urbana–Champaign (Cl)	2	5
University of Indianapolis (Psy.D.) (Cl)		
University of Manitoba (Cl)	1	0
University of Michigan (Cl)	1	0
University of Minnesota (Cl)	—	—
University of Missouri–Columbia (Cl)	1	0
University of Montana (Cl)	1	0
University of North Carolina at Chapel Hill (Cl)	1	2
University of North Carolina at Greensboro (Cl)	1	1
University of North Texas (Cl)	2	0
University of Pittsburgh (Cl)	1	1
University of Virginia—Department of Psychology (Cl)	2	0
University of Wisconsin–Madison (Cl)	2	3
University of Wyoming (Cl)	1	0
Vanderbilt University (Cl)	1	1
Virginia Consortium Program in Clinical Psychology (Cl)	2	2

	# Faculty	# Grants
York University—Adult Clinical Program (Cl)	2	1

School/Education

	# Faculty	# Grants
Azusa Pacific University (Cl)	2	1
Brigham Young University (Co)	3	2
Boston College (Co)	4	6
Colorado State University (Co)	1	0
Duke University (Cl)	2	2
Florida State University (Cm)	3	1
George Fox University (Cl)	1	1
Immaculata College (Cl)	2	0
Indiana State University (Co)	1	1
Indiana University (Co)	2	1
Marywood University (Psy.D.) (Cl)	3	0
Miami University (Cl)	4	3
Ontario Institute for Studies in Education (Cm)	5	7
Roosevelt University (Psy.D.) (Cl)	1	0
Southern Illinois University (Co)	2	0
University of California–Los Angeles (Cl)	1	1
University of California–Santa Barbara (Cm)	—	—
University of Georgia (Co)	2	1
University of Kansas (Cl)	2	1
University of Louisville (Co)	1	0
University of Minnesota—Department of Educational Psychology (Co)	3	2
University of Waterloo (Cl)	3	1
University of Virginia–Department of Human Services (Cl)	4	1
University of Wisconsin–Madison (Co)	0	2
Utah State University (Cm)	1	0

Self-Esteem/Self-Efficacy

	# Faculty	# Grants
Catholic University of America (Cl)	1	0
George Mason University (Cl)	1	0
Marquette University (Cl)	1	0
University of Detroit–Mercy (Cl)	2	0
University of North Dakota (Co)	1	1

Sexuality/Dysfunction and Deviation

	# Faculty	# Grants
Argosy University, Atlanta (Psy.D.) (Cl)	2	0
Auburn University (Cl)	1	0
California Institute of Integral Studies (Psy.D.) (Cl)	1	0
Carlos Albizu University–San Juan (Psy.D.) (Cl)	2	0
East Michigan University (Cl)	1	0
Hofstra University (Cm)	1	0
Indiana University (Co)	3	0
Indiana University–Bloomington (Cl)	1	3
Loyola College in Maryland (Cl)	2	0
Loyola University–Chicago (Cl)	1	0
San Diego State University/University of California–San Diego (Cl)	1	0
Southern Illinois University (Co)	1	0
Texas Tech University (Co)	1	0

	# Faculty	# Grants
Uniformed Services University of Health Sciences (Cl)	1	0
University of British Columbia (Cl)	1	1
University of Florida (Co)	1	0
University of Montana (Cl)	0	0
University of New Brunswick (Cl)	3	2
University of Ottawa (Cl)	1	1
University of Texas at Austin (Cl)	1	1
University of Utah (Cl)	1	0
Western Michigan University (Cl)	1	1
University of Waterloo (Cl)	1	1

Sleep Disorders

	# Faculty	# Grants
San Diego State University/University of California–San Diego (Cl)	4	0
Southern Illinois University (Cl)	1	0
University of Arizona (Cl)	1	2
University of California–Berkeley (Cl)	1	1
University of Texas Southwestern Medical Center at Dallas (Cl)	1	1
Yeshiva University (Cl)	1	0

Social–Psychological Approaches

	# Faculty	# Grants
Arizona State University (Co)	2	0
Ball State University (Co)	3	0
George Mason University (Cl)	4	0
Loyola College in Maryland (Psy.D.) (Cl)	1	0
Xavier University (Cl)	1	0
Yale University (Cl)	1	0

Social Skills/Competence

	# Faculty	# Grants
Binghamton University/State University of New York (Cl)	1	0
Carlos Albizu University–San Juan (Ph.D.) (Cl)	1	0
Concordia University (Cl)	1	1
Drexel University (Cl)	2	2
Duke University (Cl)	0	0
Florida State University (Cl)	1	1
Indiana University–Bloomington (Cl)	3	2
James Madison University (Cm)	4	0
Louisiana State University (Cl)	2	1
Purdue University (Cl)	2	0
San Diego State University/University of California–San Diego (Cl)	1	0
University of Alabama (Cl)	2	1
University of Houston (Cl)	4	3
University of Maine (Cl)	4	2
University of Michigan (Cl)	2	1
University of Mississippi (Cl)	3	0
University of Nevada–Reno (Cl)	1	0
University of Nevada–Reno (Cl)	3	0
University of Ottawa (Cl)	2	2
Virginia Commonwealth University (Co)	1	1
Virginia Polytechnic Institute and State University (Cl)	3	0

	# Faculty	# Grants
York University—Clinical-Developmental Area (Cl)	3	3

Social Support

	# Faculty	# Grants
DePaul University (Cl)	1	1
Fordham University (Cl)	2	0
Illinois Institute of Technology (Cl)	1	0
Iowa State University (Co)	1	1
University of Denver (Co)	1	1
University of Oregon (Co)	3	0
University of Pittsburgh (Cl)	1	4

Sports Psychology

	# Faculty	# Grants
Carlos Albizu University–San Juan (Cl)	1	0
Carlos Albizu University–San Juan (Psy.D.) (Cl)	2	0
Catholic University of America (Cl)	1	0
LaSalle University (Psy.D.) (Cl)	1	0
Oklahoma State University (Co)	1	0
Rosalind Franklin University of Medicine (Cl)	1	0
St. Louis University (Cl)	1	0
Spalding University (Psy.D.) (Cl)	2	0
University of Manitoba (Cl)	1	1
University of Missouri–Kansas City (Co)	1	0
University of North Texas (Co)	2	1
West Virginia University (Co)	1	0

Statistics

	# Faculty	# Grants
Fairleigh Dickinson University (Cl)	2	0
Loma Linda University (Ph.D. & Psy.D.) (Cl)	3	0
University of Nevada–Las Vegas (Cl)	1	0
University of Pittsburgh (Cl)	2	2
Vanderbilt University (Cl)	2	1
Xavier University (Cl)	2	0

Stigma

	# Faculty	# Grants
Argosy University, Chicago Northwest (Psy.D.)	1	1
Jackson State University (Cl)	2	0
University of California–Berkeley (Cl)	1	1
University of Florida (Co)	1	0
University of Hartford (Psy.D.) (Cl)	1	1

Stress and Coping

	# Faculty	# Grants
American University (Cl)	1	0
Catholic University of America (Cl)	3	1
Colorado State University (Co)	2	0
Columbia University, Teachers College (Cl)	2	1
Duke University (Cl)	4	4
Fairleigh Dickinson University (Cl)	2	0
Fordham University (Cl)	2	1

	# Faculty	# Grants
Forest Institute of Professional Psychology (Cl)	2	1
Fuller Theological Seminary (Ph.D. & Psy.D.) (Cl)	1	0
George Fox University (Psy.D.) (Cl)	1	1
George Mason University (Cl)	2	0
George Washington University (Ph.D.) (Cl)	3	1
Georgia State University (Co)	2	1
Indiana State University (Cl)	2	0
Indiana University–Bloomington (Cl)	1	1
Kent State University (Cl)	4	2
Louisiana State University (Cl)	1	0
Marywood University (Psy.D.) (Cl)	3	0
St. John's University (Cl)	1	1
St. Louis University (Cl)	2	0
San Diego State University/University of California–San Diego (Cl)	13	0
Seattle Pacific University (Cl)	1	0
Seton Hall University (Co)	1	0
Simon Fraser University (Cl)	1	1
Southern Illinois University (Cl)	1	0
Southern Illinois University (Co)	3	0
Texas Tech University (Co)	2	0
Uniformed Services University of Health Sciences (Cl)	3	7
University of British Columbia (Co)	1	2
University of Georgia (Cl)	1	1
University of Kansas (Cl)	2	1
University of Louisville (Cl)	2	0
University of Massachusetts at Amherst (Cl)	1	1
University of Miami (Cl)	9	2
University of Minnesota (Cl)	—	—
University of Minnesota Department of Psychology (Co)	1	1
University of Missouri–Kansas City (Co)	1	0
University of North Dakota (Cl)	6	0
University of North Texas (Cl)	2	1
University of Oregon (Cl)	1	0
University of Pittsburgh (Cl)	4	15
University of Texas at Austin (Cl)	1	1
University of Tulsa (Cl)	3	0
University of Utah (Cl)	2	0
Virginia Commonwealth University (Cl)	2	0
Virginia Polytechnic Institute and State University (Cl)	1	0
Widener University (Psy.D.) (Cl)	2	2
Wright Institute (Psy.D.) (Cl)	1	0
Wright State University (Cl)	1	0
Yeshiva University (Cl)	4	1
York University—Clinical-Developmental Area (Cl)	1	0

Substance Abuse/Addictive Behaviors

	# Faculty	# Grants
Alliant International University–Los Angeles (Cl)	1	—
Alliant International University–San Diego (Psy.D.) (Cl)	3	0
Alliant International University–San Francisco Bay (Psy.D.) (Cl)	5	—
Alliant International University–San Francisco Bay (Cl)	2	—
American University (Cl)	2	2
Argosy University, Chicago Northwest (Cl)	1	0
Argosy University, Chicago Northwest (Psy.D.) (Cl)	1	1
Argosy University, San Francisco (Cl)	1	0
Arizona State University (Cl)	2	4
Auburn University (Co)	3	1
Binghamton University/State University of New York (Cl)	1	1
Boston University (Cl)	1	1
Bowling Green State University (Cl)	1	0
Colorado State University (Co)	4	3
East Michigan University (Cl)	1	0
Drexel University (Cl)	2	2
Florida State University (Cl)	2	1
Fordham University (Cl)	2	1
Georgia State University (Cl)	1	1
Fuller Theological Seminary (Ph.D. & Psy.D.) (Cl)	1	0
Hofstra University (Cm)	3	1
Idaho State University (Cl)	3	1
Indiana State University (Psy.D.) (Cl)	1	1
Indiana University–Bloomington (Cl)	1	1
Jackson State University (Cl)	2	0
Marquette University (Cl)	1	0
Marquette University (Co)	1	4
Michigan State University (Cl)	1	1
Oklahoma State University (Cl)	1	0
Pacific Graduate School of Psychology (Psy.D.) (Cl)	2	0
Philadelphia College of Osteopathic Medicine (Psy.D.) (Cl)	1	0
Rutgers University (Ph.D.) (Cl)	3	2
Rutgers University (Psy.D.) (Cl)	4	2
St. John's University (Cl)	1	0
Sam Houston State University (Cl)	1	1
San Diego State University/University of California–San Diego (Cl)	12	5
Seattle Pacific University (Cl)	1	1
Southern Illinois University (Cl)	1	1
Syracuse University (Cl)	2	4
Texas A&M University (Cl)	1	1
Texas Tech University (Cl)	1	1
Texas Tech University (Co)	1	0
Uniformed Services University of Health Sciences (Cl)	1	3
University of Alabama at Birmingham (Cl)	3	2
University at Albany/State University of New York (Cl)	2	1
University of Arkansas (Cl)	2	2
University at Buffalo/State University of New York (Cl)	5	8
University of California–Santa Barbara (Cm)	—	—
University of Central Florida (Cl)	1	0
University of Cincinnati (Cl)	4	4
University of Colorado (Cl)	2	2

	# Faculty	# Grants
University of Detroit–Mercy (Cl)	1	1
University of Georgia (Cl)	3	0
University of Georgia (Co)	1	0
University of Hartford (Psy.D.) (Cl)	1	0
University of Hawaii at Manoa (Cl)	1	3
University of Illinois at Chicago (Cl)	4	6
University of Iowa (Cl)	1	0
University of Kentucky (Cl)	4	2
University of Louisville (Cl)	1	0
University of Louisville (Co)	2	1
University of Maryland (Cl)	3	4
University of Maryland–Baltimore County (Cl)	2	2
University of Massachusetts at Amherst (Cl)	1	0
University of Memphis (Cl)	2	3
University of Michigan (Cl)	2	2
University of Minnesota—Department of Educational Psychology (Co)	—	—
University of Mississippi (Cl)	1	1
University of Missouri–Columbia (Cl)	5	10
University of Missouri–Columbia (Co)	2	0
University of Missouri–Kansas City (Co)	1	0
University of Montana (Cl)	2	1
University of Nevada–Reno (Cl)	2	1
University of New Brunswick (Cl)	1	1
University of New Mexico (Cl)	6	8
University of North Carolina at Chapel Hill (Cl)	1	1
University of North Dakota (Cl)	1	0
University of Pennsylvania (Cl)	1	1
University of Pittsburgh (Cl)	8	21
University of South Dakota (Cl)	2	1
University of South Florida (Cl)	2	5
University of Southern California (Cl)	4	2
University of Southern Mississippi (Co)	2	2
University of Texas at Austin (Cl)	1	1
University of Utah (Co)	1	1
University of Victoria (Cl)	1	1
University of Washington (Cl)	3	3
University of Western Ontario (Cl)	1	1
University of Windsor (Cl)	2	1
University of Wisconsin–Madison (Cl)	3	0
University of Wisconsin–Milwaukee (Cl)	1	2
University of Wisconsin–Milwaukee (Co)	2	—
Wright Institute (Psy.D.) (Cl)	2	0
University of South Mississippi (Co)	1	0
University of Wyoming (Cl)	1	1
Utah State University (Cm)	1	1
Vanderbilt University (Cl)	3	0
Virginia Commonwealth University (Cl)	1	1
Virginia Consortium Program in Clinical Psychology (Cl)	1	3
Virginia Polytechnic Institute and State University (Cl)	2	3
Wright Institute (Cl)	2	0
Yale University (Cl)	1	2
York University—Adult Clinical Program (Cl)	1	0

Suicide

Catholic University of America (Cl)	2	1
Florida State University (Cl)	1	0
Howard University (Cl)	1	0
James Madison University (Cm)	1	0
Marshall University (Psy.D.) (Cl)	1	0
Texas Tech University (Cl)	2	3
University of Akron (Co)	2	0
University of Illinois (Cl)	1	1
University of Iowa (Co)	1	0
University of Maryland–Baltimore County (Cl)	1	0
University of Nevada–Reno (Cl)	1	0
University of North Dakota (Cl)	1	1
University of South Florida (Cl)	1	2
University of Washington (Cl)	1	1
West Virginia University (Cl)	1	1
Yeshiva University (Cl)	1	0

Supervision/Mentoring/Training

Antioch/New England Graduate School (Psy.D.) (Cl)	2	0
Arizona State University (Co)	4	0
Catholic University of America (Cl)	1	0
Colorado State University (Co)	2	0
Florida Institute of Technology (Cl)	1	0
Fordham University (Co)	3	2
George Fox University (Cl)	1	0
Howard University (Cl)	4	2
Indiana State University (Co)	5	0
James Madison University (Cm)	1	0
Lehigh University (Co)	1	1
Loyola University–Chicago (Co)	1	0
Marquette University (Co)	2	0
Marywood University (Psy.D.) (Cl)	4	0
McGill University (Cl)	1	0
Oklahoma State University (Co)	3	0
Pepperdine University (Psy.D.) (Cl)	1	0
Philadelphia College of Osteopathic Medicine (Psy.D.) (Cl)	1	0
Seattle Pacific University (Cl)	1	0
Southern Illinois University (Co)	1	0
Spalding University (Psy.D.) (Cl)	1	0
University at Albany/State University of New York (Co)	2	0
University of Hartford (Psy.D.) (Cl)	1	0
University of Manitoba (Cl)	1	0
University of Maryland (Co)	3	0
University of Missouri–Columbia (Co)	2	1
University of Missouri–Kansas City (Co)	2	0
University of Virginia–Department of Human Services (Cl)	4	6
University of Wisconsin–Madison (Co)	1	1
Washington State University (Co)	1	0
West Virginia University (Co)	1	0

Violence/Abuse/Sexual Abuse

Argosy University, Schaumburg (Psy.D.) (Cl)	2	0

	# Faculty	# Grants
Boston College (Co)	3	2
Boston University (Cl)	1	0
Catholic University of America (Cl)	1	1
Central Michigan University (Cl)	1	0
Colorado State University (Co)	2	0
Columbia University, Teachers College (Co)	1	0
DePaul University (Cl)		
Drexel University (Cl)	2	1
Duke University (Cl)	0	0
Fairleigh Dickinson University (Cl)	3	0
Fielding Graduate Institute (Cl)	—	—
Florida Institute of Technology (Cl)	1	1
George Mason University (Cl)	1	0
Idaho State University (Cl)	1	2
Indiana University of Pennsylvania (Cl)	1	0
LaSalle University (Psy.D.) (Cl)	1	1
Long Island University–C.W. Post Campus (Cl)	2	0
Loyola College in Maryland (Psy.D.) (Cl)	1	0
Miami University (Cl)	4	2
Michigan State University (Cl)	4	2
Northern Illinois University (Cl)	3	1
Nova Southeastern University (Ph.D. & Psy.D.) (Cl)	7	0
Ohio University (Cl)	1	1
Oklahoma State University (Cl)	0	0
Pennsylvania State University (Cl)	2	0
St. John's University (Cl)	1	0
St. Louis University (Cl)	2	1
Sam Houston State University (Cl)	2	1
Simon Fraser University (Cl)	5	5
Southern Illinois University (Cl)	1	0
Southern Illinois University (Co)	2	0
Texas Women's University (Co)	3	1
University of Alabama (Cl)	2	2
University of California–Santa Barbara (Cm)	—	—
University of Colorado (Cl)	2	0
University of Denver (Ph.D.) (Cl)	1	1
University of Georgia (Cl)	8	2
University of Houston (Co)	1	1
University of Illinois at Urbana–Champaign (Co)	2	0
University of Kansas (Cl)	3	1
University of Kentucky (Cl)	1	2
University of Manitoba (Cl)	5	0
University of Maryland (Co)	1	0
University of Maryland–Baltimore County (Cl)	1	1
University of Miami (Co)	1	0
University of Michigan (Cl)	1	1
University of Minnesota Dept of Psychology (Co)	1	0
University of Mississippi (Cl)	2	0
University of Missouri–Columbia (Co)	1	1
University of Montana (Cl)	1	1
University of Nevada–Reno (Cl)	2	0
University of North Dakota (Co)	1	0
University of North Texas (Cl)	2	0
University of Oregon (Co)	1	0
University of South Carolina (Cl)	2	1
University of South Dakota (Cl)	2	0
University of Southern California (Cl)	3	2
University of Toledo (Cl)	1	0
University of Vermont (Cl)	2	0
University of Virginia—Department of Human Services (Cl)	2	1
University of Virginia—Department of Psychology (Cl)	4	2
University of Washington (Cl)	2	1
York University—Clinical-Developmental Area (Cl)	4	3

Vocational Interests/Career Development

Argosy University, Chicago (Cl)	1	0
Arizona State University (Co)	3	1
Ball State University (Co)	4	0
Boston College (Co)	1	3
Colorado State University (Co)	2	0
Florida State University (Cm)	2	2
Fordham University (Co)	3	1
Georgia State University (Co)	1	0
Indiana State University (Co)	2	0
Indiana University (Co)	1	0
Iowa State University (Co)	3	1
Lehigh University (Co)	1	1
Louisiana Tech University (Co)	1	0
Loyola University–Chicago (Co)	1	1
New Mexico State University (Co)	2	0
New York University (Co)	1	0
Oklahoma State University (Co)	4	1
Purdue University (Co)	1	0
Seattle Pacific University (Cl)	3	0
Seton Hall University (Co)	1	0
Southern Illinois University (Co)	4	2
Texas Tech University (Co)	2	0
Texas Woman's University (Co)	3	1
University of Akron (Co)	2	0
University at Albany/State University of New York (Co)	1	0
University of British Columbia (Co)	3	4
University at Buffalo/State University of New York (Cm)	2	0
University of California–Santa Barbara (Cm)		
University of Denver (Co)	1	1
University of Illinois at Urbana–Champaign (Co)	2	1
University of Iowa (Co)	1	1
University of Kansas (Co)	1	2
University of Louisville (Co)	1	2
University of Maryland (Co)	4	2
University of Memphis (Co)	2	0
University of Minnesota—Department of Educational Psychology (Co)	2	4
University of Minnesota—Department of Psychology (Co)	1	1
University of So. Mississippi (Co)	1	0
University of Missouri–Columbia (Co)	5	2
University of Missouri–Kansas City (Co)	1	0
University of Nebraska–Lincoln (Co)	1	0

	# Faculty	# Grants
University of North Dakota (Co)	2	0
University of North Texas (Co)	3	1
University of Oregon (Co)	2	0
University of Tennessee (Co)	2	0
University of Utah (Co)	2	0
University of Wisconsin–Madison (Co)	2	0
University of Wisconsin–Milwaukee (Co)	2	0
Virginia Commonwealth University (Co)	1	2
Washington State University (Co)	2	0
West Virginia University (Co)	2	0
Yeshiva University (Cm)	2	0

Weight Management

University of Florida (Cl)	1	1
University of Pittsburgh (Cl)	1	4
Yeshiva University (Ph.D.)(Cl)	1	0

Women's Studies/Issues

Alliant International University–Fresno (Psy.D.) (Cl)	3	
Alliant International University–Los Angeles (Ph.D. & Psy.D.) (Cl)	3	
Alliant International University–San Diego (Ph.D. & Psy.D.) (Cl)	2	1
Alliant International University–San Francisco (Ph.D.) (Cl)	4	0
Antioch/New England Graduate School (Cl)	2	0
Arizona State University (Co)	7	1
Ball State University (Co)	2	0
Boston University (Cl)	1	0
Brigham Young University (Co)	2	1
Colorado State University (Co)	3	1
Columbia University, Teachers College (Ph.D.) (Co)	1	0
Fairleigh Dickinson University (Cl)	3	0
Indiana State University (Psy.D.) (Cl)	2	0
Indiana University (Co)	1	0
Indiana University of Pennsylvania (Cl)	2	0
Iowa State University (Co)	1	1
Loyola College in Maryland (Psy.D.) (Cl)	2	0
Marshall University (Psy.D.) (Cl)	1	0
Ohio State University (Co)	2	0
Oklahoma State University (Co)	2	0
San Diego State University (Cl)	3	0
Seattle Pacific University (Cl)	2	1
Southern Illinois University (Co)	1	0
Texas Tech University (Co)	2	0
University at Albany/State University of New York (Co)	2	0
University of Akron (Co)	3	0
University of British Columbia (Co)	1	0
University of Florida (Co)	1	0
University of Georgia (Cl)	2	0
University of Illinois at Urbana–Champaign (Cl)	3	2
University of Indianapolis (Psy.D.) (Cl)	1	0
University of Kansas (Cl)	1	0

	# Faculty	# Grants
University of Kansas (Co)	3	1
University of Maine (Cl)	1	0
University of Missouri–St. Louis (Cl)	1	0
University of Nevada–Las Vegas (Cl)	1	0
University of New Brunswick (Cl)		
University of North Dakota (Cl)	2	0
University of North Dakota (Co)	1	0
University of Utah (Cl)	2	0
University of Wisconsin–Milwaukee (Co)	1	1
Virginia Consortium Program in Clinical Psychology (Cl)	4	0
West Virginia (Cl)	1	0

Miscellaneous

abortion—Southern Illinois University (Cl)	1	0
action research—Miami University (Cl)	2	1
adoption—Rutgers University (Psy.D.) (Cl)	1	1
Auburn University (Co)	1	0
altruism—Columbia University, Teachers College (Cl)	1	0
behavior control—Emory University (Cl)	1	0
University of Maryland (Cl)	2	1
behavioral dentistry—West Virginia; University (Cl)	1	0
biopsychology—Loma Linda University (Cl)	2	2
Indiana University–Purdue		
biopsychosocial—Fuller Theological Seminary (Cl)	4	2
bipolar disorder—University of California–Berkeley	1	1
brief therapy—Our Lady of the Lake University (Co)	3	2
burnout prevention—University of Minnesota—Department of Educational Psychology (Co)	2	0
caregiver burden—Southern Illinois University (Co)	1	1
change processes—Adelphi University (Cl)	2	0
chronic fatigue syndrome—DePaul University (Cl)	1	3
University of Mississippi (Cl)	1	0
college student development—University of Oregon (Co)	2	0
computer based research—University of Mississippi (Cl)	1	1
conscious/unconscious processes—Drexel University (Cl)	1	0
University of Michigan (Cl)	1	0
constructivist psychology—University of Florida (Co)	1	0
University of Southern Mississippi (Co)	1	0
corporate systems—University of Wisconsin–Madison (Co)	1	0
countertransference—University of Maryland	2	0
creativity—Adelphi University (Cl)	1	1
University of Kansas (Co)	1	1

	# Faculty	# Grants
critical incidence response—University of Detroit–Mercy (Cl)	2	0
data-based case management—University of Hawaii at Manoa (Cl)	0	2
dementia—University of Texas Southwestern Medical Center at Dallas (Cl)	1	1
disability psychology—JFK University (Cl) 1	1	0
dissociative disorders—Rutgers University (Psy.D.) (Cl)	1	0
diversity issues in the military—Regent University (Cl)	1	0
educational outcomes—Colorado State	1	1
emotional social development—University of Missouri Kansas City (Cl)	2	1
empirically supported treatments—University of Southern Mississippi (Co)	2	0
epidemiology—Florida State University (Cl);	1	1
Yale University (Cl)	1	0
evolutionary psychology—University of Louisville (Co)	2	0
existential-humanistic—Immaculata College (Cl)	2	0
experiential therapy—Argosy University, Schaumburg (Psy.D.)	3	1
extracurricular activities—Loyola University–Chicago (Cl)	1	0
fear conditioning—Marquette University (Cl)	1	0
fear conditioning and extinction—Ponce School of Medicine	1	1
feminism—Rutgers (Psy.D.) (Cl)	1	0
feminism pedagogy and multicultural pedagogy—McGill University	2	0
fetal alcohol disorder—University of Victoria (Cl);	1	1
Miami University (Cl)	1	0
friendship—Indiana State University (Psy.D.) (Cl);	2	1
University of North Dakota (Cl)	2	0
gambling—Loyola College–Maryland (Psy.D.)(Cl);	1	1
University of Windsor (Cl)	0	3
genetic counseling—University of Minnesota—Department of Educational Psychology (Cl)	1	1
genetics—University of Colorado at Boulder (Cl)	1	1
gifted/talented children—Florida State University	2	2
habit behaviors—Western Michigan University (Cl)	1	0
health care administration—University of Nevada–Reno (Cl)	1	1
health care compliance—University of Hawaii at Manoa (Cl)	2	0
helping behavior—University of Detroit–Mercy (Cl)	1	0
help-seeking—Marquette University (Cl)	1	1
human error—Hofstra University (Cm)	1	0
hypothyroidism—Ontario Institute for Studies in Education (Cm)	1	1
identity development—University of Detroit–Mercy (Cl)	2	0
incest survivors—University of Nevada–Reno (Cl)	2	0
infertility—University of British Columbia (Co)	1	0
inner city children—University of Michigan (Cl)	4	2
inner-city children—Drexel University (Cl)	4	2
instrument validation—Carlos Albizu University (PhD) (Cl)	2	0
international adoption—University of Minnesota Dept of Psychology (Co)	1	1
Jungian and feminist topics—California Institute of Integral Studies (Psy.D.) (Cl)	1	0
leadership—Northeastern University (Cm);	3	1
Virginia Commonwealth University (Co)	1	0
media and psychology—University of Massachusetts at Boston (Cl)	1	0
medical illness/comorbidity—Pacific Graduate School of Professional Psychology (Cl)	2	1
mental health policy—University of Houston (Co)	1	0
mental health systems—University of Hawaii at Manoa (Cl)	5	6
migraines—Yeshiva University (PhD) (Cl)	1	3
mindfulness interventions—La Salle University (Psy.D.) (Cl)	2	1
multidisciplinary environments—University of Wisconsin–Madison (Co)	1	1
multisystemic therapy—University of Missouri–Columbia (Cl)	1	1
music apperception test development—California Institute of Integral Studies (Psy.D.)		
Native American vocational development—Brigham Young (Co)	1	1
nonverbal communication—Loyola College in Maryland (Cl)	1	0
nutrition—San Diego State University/University of California–San Diego (Cl)	1	0
obsessive-compulsive disorder—University of Virginia (Cl);	1	2
University of Waterloo (Cl)	0	2
patient non-adherence—Philadelphia College of Osteopathic Medicine (Psy.D.) (Cl)	1	0
perception/eye movement—University of Detroit–Mercy (Cl)	1	1
perfectionism—University of Missouri–Columbia (Co)	1	0
philosophical issues—Indiana State University (Co);	1	5

	# Faculty	# Grants
Rutgers University (Psy.D.) (Cl)	2	0
Rutgers University (Ph.D.) (Cl)	1	0
play therapy—Alliant International University–Fresno (Psy.D. & Ph.D.) (Cl)	1	
poverty—Marshall University (Psy.D.) (Cl)	1	0
University of Colorado (Cl); University of North Dakota (Co)	1	1
pregnancy—DePaul University (Cl);	2	1
Virginia Commonwealth University (Cl)	1	1
psychological games—JFK University (Cl)	1	0
psychological reactance—Louisiana Tech University (Co)	1	0
psychological resources—University of Memphis (Co)	1	0
psychologies of peace and war— Seattle Pacific University (Cl)	1	0
psychology and the arts—Rutgers (Psy.D.) (Cl)	1	0
psychology of humor—San Diego State University (Cl)	1	0
psychology of immigration—JFK University (Cl)	1	0
rational-emotive therapy—Hofstra University (Cm)	1	0
reimbursement issues—Our Lady of the Lake University (Psy.D.) (Co)	1	0
retention—Arizona State University (Co)	4	1
risk and resilience—Columbia University (Cl); Boston College	2	2
Rorschach—Argosy Twin Cities (PsyD) (Cl);	2	1
Sam Houston State University (Cl)	0	0
scale construction—University of Missouri–Columbia (Co)	4	3
self help—Wichita State University (Cl)	1	5
self psychology—Seattle Pacific University (Cl)	1	0
self-determination theory—University of Waterloo (Co)	1	1
self-efficacy—Southern Illinois University (Co)	1	0
sex offenders—Simon Fraser University (Cl)	2	2
shame—George Fox University (Cl)	1	0
shyness—Virginia Polytechnic Institute and State University (Cl)	1	0
sizism—University of North Dakota (Co)	1	0
social identity—New Mexico University (Co)	3	0
social influence—Washington State University (Co);	1	1
Sam Houston State University (Cl)	0	0
social policies—City University of New York at City College (Cl)	1	0
social/clinical psychology interface— University of Notre Dame (Co)	2	0
somatization disorders—Rutgers University (Cl)	1	1
stereotypes—University of Massachusetts–Boston (Cl)	0	0
student self-efficacy—University of North Dakota (Co)	1	0
student well being—Seton Hall University (Co)	1	0
symbolic play—Yeshiva University (Cm)	1	0
teaching—Wichita State University (Cl)	1	1
Tennessee State University (Co)	1	0
telehealth/technology—University of Houston (Co)	2	0
terrorism—Pacific Graduate School of Professional Psychology (PsyD) (Cl)	2	2
treatment cost effectiveness—American University (Cl); Western Michigan University (Co)	1	0
treatment development—University of Nevada–Reno (Cl)	3	1
treatment dissemination—University of Missouri–Columbia (Cl)	1	1
unconscious processes and motivation—Adelphi University (Cl);	1	3
University Indianapolis (Cl)	0	5–6
utilization of health services—Loyola College–Chicago (Cl)	1	0
verbal behavior—University of Nevada–Reno (Cl)	4	0
white privilege—University of North Dakota (Cl)	1	0

APPENDIX F

SPECIALTY CLINICS AND PRACTICA SITES

Acquired Immune Deficiency Syndrome (AIDS)/HIV

Argosy University–Phoenix (Cl)
Argosy University–Twin Cities (Cl)
Azusa Pacific University (Cl)
California Institute of Integral Studies (Psy.D.) (Cl)
George Washington University (Ph.D.) (Cl)
Georgia State University (Cl)
University of La Verne (Cl)
Loyola University–Chicago (Cl)
Pacific Graduate School of Psychology (Cl)
Pepperdine University (Cl)
Rutgers University (Psy.D.) (Cl)
University of Illinois at Chicago (Cl)
University of Miami (Cl)
University of Nevada–Reno (Cl)
University of Vermont (Cl)
Virginia Polytechnic Institute and State University (Cl)
Wright State University (Cl)

Adolescent Psychotherapy/At-Risk Adolescents/Delinquency

Alliant International University–Fresno (Ph.D. & Psy.D.) (Cl)
Argosy University–Honolulu Campus (Cl)
Auburn University (Cl)
Binghamton University/State University of New York (Cl)
Boston University (Cl)
Brigham Young University (Cl)
Colorado State University (Co)
Concordia University (Cl)
Duke University (Cl)
Florida State University (Cl)

George Fox University (Cl)
George Washington University (Ph.D. & Psy.D.) (Cl)
Marshall University (Cl)
Miami University (Cl)
Northwestern University, Feinberg School of Medicine (Cl)
Pepperdine University (Psy.D.) (Cl)
Rutgers University (Ph.D.) (Cl)
Rutgers University (Psy.D.) (Cl)
Southern Illinois University (Cl)
Tennessee State University (Co)
University at Albany/State University of New York (Cl & Co)
University of Denver (Ph.D.) (Cl)
University of Georgia (Co)
University of Maine (Cl)
University of Massachusetts at Amherst (Cl)
University of Memphis (Co)
University of Montana (Cl)
University of Pittsburgh (Cl)
University of Saskatchewan (Cl)
University of South Florida (Cl)
University of Texas at Austin (Co)
University of Utah (Cl)
University of Vermont (Cl)
University of Waterloo (Cl)
Virginia Commonwealth University (Co)
Virginia Consortium Program in Clinical Psychology (Cl)
Yale University (Cl)
Yeshiva University (Cl & Cm)

Aging/Gerontology

Alliant International University–Los Angeles (Ph.D. & Psy.D) (Cl)
Argosy University–Chicago (Cl)

Note. Cl, Clinical; Co, Counseling; Cm, combined psychology programs.

355

Argosy University–Washington, DC Campus (Cl)
Arizona State University (Cl)
Azusa Pacific University (Cl)
Baylor University (Psy.D.) (Cl)
Binghamton University (Cl)
Boston University (Cl)
California Institute of Integral Studies (Cl)
Case Western Reserve University (Cl)
Catholic University of American (Cl)
Central Michigan University (Cl)
City University of New York at City College (Cl)
Concordia University (Cl)
Duke University (Cl)
Fairleigh Dickinson University (Cl)
Fuller Theological Seminary (Ph.D. & Psy.D.) (Cl)
George Fox University (Cl)
Loyola College in Maryland (Psy.D.) (Cl)
Marywood University (Cl)
Marquette University (Cl)
Miami University (Cl)
Michigan State University (Cl)
Ohio State University (Cl)
Pacific Graduate School of Psychology (Ph.D. & Psy.D) (Cl)
Pepperdine University (Cl)
Philadelphia College of Osteopathic Medicine (Cl)
Rutgers University (Psy.D.) (Cl)
Suffolk University (Cl)
University of Alabama (Cl)
University of Arizona (Cl)
University of Houston (Cl)
University of Iowa (Cl)
University of Louisville (Cl)
University of Massachusetts at Amherst (Cl)
University of Minnesota (Cl)
University of Missouri–St. Louis (Cl)
University of Nevada–Reno (Cl)
University of Ottawa (Cl)
University of Southern California (Cl)
University of Utah (Co)
Virginia Polytechnic Institute and State University (Cl)
Wayne State University (Cl)
West Virginia University (Cl)
Wright Institute (Cl)
Yeshiva University (Ph.D. & Psy.D) (Cl)
York University–Adult Clinical Program (Cl)

Illinois Institute of Technology (Cl)
LaSalle University (Cl)
Miami University (Cl)
Michigan State University (Cl)
Northwestern University (Cl)
Nova Southeastern University (Ph.D. & Psy.D.) (Cl)
Ohio State University (Cl)
Purdue University (Cl)
Rutgers University (Ph.D.) (Cl)
Rutgers University (Psy.D.) (Cl)
Temple University (Cl)
University of Arizona (Cl)
University at Buffalo/State University of New York (Cl)
University of California–Los Angeles (Cl)
University of Delaware (Cl)
University of Georgia (Cl)
University of Hartford (Cl)
University of Houston (Cl)
University of Illinois at Chicago (Cl)
University of Illinois at Urbana–Champaign (Cl)
University of Iowa (Cl)
University of Louisville (Cl)
University of Manitoba (Cl)
University of Memphis (Cl)
University of Minnesota (Cl)
University of Montana (Cl)
University of Nevada–Reno (Cl)
University of North Dakota (Cl)
University of North Texas (Cl)
University of Oregon (Cl)
University of Ottawa (Cl)
University of Pittsburgh (Cl)
University of South Florida (Cl)
University of Texas at Austin (Cl)
University of Texas Southwestern Medical Center at Dallas (Cl)
University of Vermont (Cl)
University of Virginia—Department of Psychology (Cl)
University of Western Ontario (Cl)
University of Wyoming (Cl)
Vanderbilt University—Department of Psychology (Cl)
Virginia Commonwealth University (Cl)
Virginia Polytechnic Institute and State University (Cl)
Wichita State University (Cl)
Wright Institute (Cl)
Yeshiva University (Psy.D.)(Cl)
York University—Adult Clinical Program (Cl)

Affective Disorders/Depression/Mood Disorders

Baylor University (Cl)
Binghamton University/State University of New York (Cl)
Boston University (Cl)
Case Western Reserve University (Cl)
Duke University (Cl)
George Washington University (Ph.D.) (Cl)
Georgia State University (Cl)

Anxiety Disorders/Panic Disorders

Argosy University–Washington, DC Campus (Cl)
Auburn University (Cl)
Baylor University (Psy.D.) (Cl)
Binghamton University/State University of New York (Cl)
Case Western Reserve University (Cl)
Eastern Michigan University (Cl)
Fairleigh Dickinson University (Cl)

Florida State University (Cl)
George Washington University (Ph.D.) (Cl)
Georgia State University (Cl)
Howard University (Cl)
Idaho State University (Cl)
Indiana University–Bloomington (Cl)
LaSalle University (Cl)
Louisiana State University (Cl)
Miami University (Cl)
Michigan State University (Cl)
Northern Illinois University (Cl)
Northwestern University (Cl)
Nova Southeastern University (Ph.D. & Psy.D.) (Cl)
Ohio State University (Cl)
Oklahoma State University (Cl)
Ontario Institute for Studies in Education (Cm)
Pacific Graduate School of Psychology (Ph.D. & Psy.D) (Cl)
Purdue University (Cl)
Roosevelt University (Cl)
Rosalind Franklin University of Medicine and Science (Cl)
Rutgers University (Ph.D.) (Cl)
Rutgers University (Psy.D.) (Cl)
St. Louis University (Cl)
San Diego State University/University of California–
    San Diego (Cl)
Syracuse University (Cl)
Temple University (Cl)
University at Albany/State University of New York (Cl)
University at Buffalo/State University of New York (Cl)
University of Alabama (Cl)
University of California–Los Angeles (Cl)
University of Connecticut (Cl)
University of Delaware (Cl)
University of Florida (Cl & Co)
University of Georgia (Cl)
University of Hartford (Cl)
University of Houston (Cl)
University of Illinois at Chicago (Cl)
University of Illinois at Urbana–Champaign (Cl)
University of Kansas (Cl)
University of Louisville (Cl)
University of Maine (Cl)
University of Manitoba (Cl)
University of Memphis (Cl)
University of Minnesota (Cl)
University of Missouri–St. Louis (Cl)
University of Nebraska–Lincoln (Cl)
University of Nevada–Las Vegas (Cl)
University of Nevada–Reno (Cl)
University of North Carolina at Chapel Hill (Cl)
University of North Dakota (Cl)
University of Oregon (Cl)
University of Ottawa (Cl)
University of Pittsburgh (Cl)
University of South Florida (Cl)
University of Texas at Austin (Cl)
University of Toledo (Cl)

University of Utah (Cl)
University of Vermont (Cl)
University of Virginia—Department of Psychology (Cl)
University of Washington (Cl)
University of Wyoming (Cl)
Vanderbilt University—Department of Psychology (Cl)
Virginia Commonwealth University (Cl)
Virginia Polytechnic Institute and State University (Cl)
West Virginia University (Cl)
Wichita State University (Cl)
Yale University (Cl)
Yeshiva University (Ph.D. & Psy.D.) (Cl)
York University—Adult Clinical Program (Cl)

Assessment/Testing

Adelphi University (Cl)
American University (Cl)
Antioch/New England Graduate School (Psy.D.) (Cl)
Argosy University–Atlanta (Cl)
Arizona State University (Cl)
Catholic University of America (Cl)
Central Michigan University (Cl)
DePaul University (Cl)
Emory University (Cl)
Fairleigh Dickinson University (Cl)
Fuller Theological Seminary (Ph.D. & Psy.D.) (Cl)
Gallaudet University (Cl)
George Fox University (Cl)
George Mason University (Cl)
George Washington University (Ph.D. & Psy.D.) (Cl)
Georgia State University (Cl)
Indiana University–Bloomington (Cl)
Indiana University of Pennsylvania (Cl)
James Madison University (Cm)
LaSalle University (Cl)
Loyola University–Chicago (Cl)
Miami University (Cl)
Michigan State University (Cl)
Northern Illinois University (Cl)
Nova Southeastern University (Ph.D. & Psy.D.) (Cl)
Pacific Graduate School of Psychology (Cl)
Pepperdine University (Cl)
Purdue University (Cl)
Rutgers University (Ph.D.) (Cl)
Rutgers University (Psy.D.) (Cl)
St. Louis University (Cl)
University of British Columbia (Cl)
University of Colorado (Cl)
University of Delaware (Cl)
University of Denver (Psy.D.) (Cl)
University of Denver (Co)
University of Florida (Co)
University of Georgia (Cl)
University of Hawaii at Manoa (Cl)
University of Houston (Cl)
University of Illinois at Urbana–Champaign (Cl)

University of Kentucky (Cl)
University of Louisville (Cl)
University of Mississippi (Cl)
University of Missouri–Columbia (Cl)
University of Montana (Cl)
University of Nebraska–Lincoln (Co)
University of North Carolina at Chapel Hill (Cl)
University of North Dakota (Cl)
University of Pennsylvania (Cl)
University of Pittsburgh (Cl)
University of South Florida (Cl)
University of Toledo (Cl)
University of Virginia—Department of Human Services (Cl)
University of Wisconsin–Madison (Cl)
Virginia Commonwealth University (Cl)
Virginia Consortium Program in Clinical Psychology (Cl)
Widener University (Cl)
Wright Institute (Cl)

Attention-Deficit/Hyperactivity Disorder

Auburn University (Cl)
Case Western Reserve University (Cl)
George Washington University (Ph.D.) (Cl)
Indiana State University (Psy.D.)(Cl)
Iowa State University (Co)
Marquette University (Cl)
Miami University (Cl)
Northern Illinois University (Cl)
Ontario Institute for Studies in Education (Cm)
Pepperdine University (Cl)
Purdue University (Cl)
Rutgers University (Psy.D.) (Cl)
University of Arkansas (Cl)
University at Buffalo/State University of New York (Cl)
University of Georgia (Cl)
University of Maine (Cl)
University of Minnesota (Cl)
University of North Texas (Cl)
University of Pittsburgh (Cl)
University of Rochester (Cl)
University of South Florida (Cl)
Virginia Polytechnic Institute and State University (Cl)
York University—Clinical Developmental Area (Cl)

Behavioral Medicine/Health Psychology

Alliant International University–Fresno (Ph.D. & Psy.D) (Cl)
Antioch/New England Graduate School (Cl)
Argosy University–Atlanta (Cl)
Argosy University–Chicago (Cl)
Argosy University–Schaumburg (Cl)
Arizona State University (Cl)
Azusa Pacific University (Cl)
Baylor University (Cl)
Binghamton University/State University of New York (Cl)

Boston University (Cl)
Bowling Green State University (Cl)
California Institute of Integral Studies (Cl)
Chicago School of Professional Psychology (Cl)
Drexel University (Cl)
Duke University (Cl)
Eastern Michigan University (Cl)
Emory University (Cl)
Fairleigh Dickinson University (Cl)
Florida Institute of Technology (Cl)
Florida State University (Cl)
Forest Institute of Professional Psychology (Cl)
George Fox University (Cl)
George Washington University (Ph.D.) (Cl)
Georgia State University (Cl)
Georgia State University (Co)
Howard University (Cl)
Illinois Institute of Technology (Cl)
Indiana State University (Cl)
Indiana University (Cl)
Indiana University–Bloomington (Cl)
Indiana University of Pennsylvania (Cl)
Indiana University–Purdue University Indianapolis (Cl)
Jackson State University (Cl)
Kent State University (Cl)
LaSalle University (Cl)
Loma Linda University (Ph.D. & Psy.D.) (Cl)
Louisiana State University (Cl)
Louisiana Tech University (Co)
Loyola College in Maryland (Psy.D.) (Cl)
Loyola University–Chicago (Cl)
Marywood University (Cl)
Marquette University (Co)
Northwestern University (Cl)
Ohio State University (Cl)
Oklahoma State University (Cl)
Our Lady of the Lake University (Co)
Pacific Graduate School of Psychology (Cl)
Pepperdine University (Cl)
Regent University (Cl)
Roosevelt University (Cl)
Rosalind Franklin University of Medicine and Science (Cl)
Rutgers University (Ph.D.) (Cl)
Rutgers University (Psy.D.) (Cl)
San Diego State University/University of California–San Diego (Cl)
Seattle Pacific University (Cl)
Spalding University (Cl)
Syracuse University (Cl)
St. Louis University (Cl)
Tennessee State University (Co)
Texas Tech University (Co)
University of Alabama (Cl)
University of Alabama at Birmingham (Cl)
University at Albany/State University of New York (Cl)
University of Arizona (Cl)
University of British Columbia (Cl)

University of Cincinnati (Cl)
University of Connecticut (Cl)
University of Delaware (Cl)
University of Denver (Psy.D.) (Cl)
University of Florida (Co)
University of Georgia (Cl)
University of Hawaii at Manoa (Cl)
University of Houston (Cl)
University of Illinois at Chicago (Cl)
University of Illinois at Urbana–Champaign (Co)
University of Iowa (Cl)
University of Kansas (Cl)
University of Kentucky (Cl)
University of Louisville (Cl)
University of Maine (Cl)
University of Manitoba (Cl)
University of Memphis (Cl)
University of Miami (Cl)
University of Mississippi (Cl)
University of Missouri–Columbia (Cl)
University of Missouri–St. Louis (Cl)
University of Nebraska–Lincoln (Co)
University of Nevada–Reno (Cl)
University of New Brunswick (Cl)
University of New Mexico (Cl)
University of North Carolina at Chapel Hill (Cl)
University of North Dakota (Cl)
University of Pittsburgh (Cl)
University of Rhode Island (Cl)
University of Saskatchewan (Cl)
University of South Florida (Cl)
University of Tennessee (Cl)
University of Texas at Austin (Cl)
University of Texas Southwestern Medical Center at Dallas (Cl)
University of Utah (Cl)
University of Vermont (Cl)
University of Virginia—Department of Human Services (Cl)
University of Virginia—Department of Psychology (Cl)
University of Wisconsin–Milwaukee (Cl)
Utah State University (Cm)
Vanderbilt University—Department of Psychology (Cl)
Virginia Commonwealth University (Cl)
Virginia Polytechnic Institute and State University (Cl)
Washington State University (Cl)
Wayne State University (Cl)
West Virginia University (Cl)
Widener University (Cl)
Yale University (Cl)
Yeshiva University (Ph.D.) (Cl)
York University—Adult Clinical Program (Cl)

Biofeedback

Forest Institute of Professional Psychology (Cl)
Nova Southeastern University (Ph.D. & Psy.D.) (Cl)
Widener University (Cl)

Child/Pediatric

Adelphi University (Cl)
Alliant International University–Fresno (Ph.D. & Psy.D) (Cl)
Alliant International University–San Francisco (Ph.D. & Psy.D.) (Cl)
Antioch/New England Graduate School (Cl)
Argosy University–Atlanta (Cl)
Argosy University–Chicago (Cl)
Argosy University–Honolulu Campus (Cl)
Argosy University–Phoenix (Cl)
Argosy University–Schaumberg (Cl)
Argosy University–Washington, DC Campus (Cl)
Arizona State University (Cl)
Azusa Pacific University (Cl)
Baylor University (Cl)
Binghamton University–State University of New York (Cl)
Boston College (Co)
Biola University (Ph.D.) (Cl)
Biola University (Psy.D.) (Cl)
Bowling Green State University (Cl)
California Institute of Integral Studies (Cl)
Case Western Reserve University (Cl)
Central Michigan University (Cl)
Chicago School of Professional Psychology (Cl)
City University of New York at City College (Cl)
Columbia University, Teachers College (Cl)
Concordia University (Cl)
DePaul University (Cl)
Drexel University (Cl)
Duke University (Cl)
Florida State University (Cl)
Forest Institute of Professional Psychology (Cl)
Fuller Theological Seminary (Ph.D. & Psy.D.) (Cl)
George Fox University (Cl)
George Washington University (Ph.D.) (Cl)
Georgia School of Professional Psychology (Cl)
Georgia State University (Cl)
Illinois Institute of Technology (Cl)
Illinois School of Professional Psychology–Chicago
Jackson State University (Cl)
Kent State University (Cl)
LaSalle University (Cl)
Loma Linda University (Cl)
Louisiana Tech University (Co)
Loyola College in Maryland (Cl)
Marywood University (Cl)
Marquette University (Cl)
Miami University (Cl)
McGill University (Cl & Co)
Northern Illinois University (Cl)
Northwestern University, Feinberg School of Medicine (Cl)
Nova Southeastern University (Ph.D. & Psy.D.) (Cl)
Ohio State University (Cl)
Ohio University (Cl)
Ontario Institute for Studies in Education (Cm)
Pace University (Psy.D.) (Cm)

Pacific Graduate School of Psychology (Cl)
Pepperdine University (Cl)
Purdue University (Cl)
Queen's University (Cl)
Regent University (Cl)
Roosevelt University (Cl)
St. John's University (Cl)
San Diego State University/University of California–San Diego (Cl)
Seattle Pacific University (Cl)
Suffolk University (Cl)
Texas Tech University (Co)
Uniformed Services University of Health Sciences (Cl)
University at Albany–State University of New York (Cl)
University of Arkansas (Cl)
University of British Columbia (Cl)
University at Buffalo/State University of New York (Cl)
University of California–Los Angeles (Cl)
University of Central Florida (Cl)
University of Cincinnati (Cl)
University of Connecticut (Cl)
University of Delaware (Cl)
University of Denver (Ph.D.) (Cl)
University of Florida (Cl)
University of Florida (Co)
University of Georgia (Cl)
University of Hartford (Cl)
University of Hawaii at Manoa (Cl)
University of Houston (Cl)
University of Houston (Co)
University of Illinois at Urbana–Champaign (Cl)
University of Illinois at Urbana–Champaign (Co)
University of Iowa (Cl)
University of Kansas (Cl)
University of Kentucky (Cl)
University of La Verne (Cl)
University of Louisville (Cl)
University of Louisville (Co)
University of Maine (Cl)
University of Manitoba (Cl)
University of Maryland–Baltimore County (Cl)
University of Massachusetts at Amherst (Cl)
University of Memphis (Co)
University of Miami (Cl)
University of Michigan (Cl)
University of Minnesota (Cl)
University of Mississippi (Cl)
University of Missouri–Columbia (Cl)
University of Missouri–St. Louis (Cl)
University of Montana (Cl)
University of Nevada–LasVegas (Cl)
University of New Mexico (Cl)
University of North Carolina at Chapel Hill (Cl)
University of North Texas (Cl)
University of Oklahoma (Co)
University of Oregon (Cl)
University of Oregon (Co)

University of Pittsburgh (Cl)
University of Rhode Island (Cl)
University of Rochester (Cl)
University of Saskatchewan (Cl)
University of South Florida (Cl)
University of Southern Mississippi (Cl)
University of Texas at Austin (Cl)
University of Texas Southwestern Medical Center at Dallas (Cl)
University of Toledo (Cl)
University of Utah (Cl)
University of Vermont (Cl)
University of Victoria (Cl)
University of Virginia (Human Services) (Cl)
University of Virginia—Department of Psychology (Cl)
University of Washington (Cl)
University of Waterloo (Cl)
University of Wisconsin–Milwaukee (Cl)
University of Wisconsin–Milwaukee (Co)
Utah State University (Cm)
Vanderbilt University—Department of Psychology (Cl)
Virginia Commonwealth University (Cl)
Virginia Commonwealth University (Co)
Virginia Polytechnic Institute and State University (Cl)
Wright Institute (Cl)
Wright State University (Cl)
Yale University (Cl)
Yeshiva University (Cl & Cm)
York University—Clinical-Developmental Area (Cl)

Chronic/Severe Mental Illness

Alliant International University–Los Angeles (Ph.D. & Psy.D) (Cl)
Argosy University–Chicago (Cl)
Argosy University–Schaumberg (Cl)
California Institute of Integral Studies (Cl)
Azusa Pacific University (Cl)
Fuller Theological Seminary (Ph.D. & Psy.D.) (Cl)
Indiana University–Purdue University Indianapolis (Cl)
Northeastern University (Cm)
Northwestern University, Feinberg School of Medicine (Cl)
Pepperdine University (Cl)
Roosevelt University (Cl)
Seattle Pacific University (Cl)
University of Alabama (Cl)
University of California–Los Angeles (Cl)
University of Cincinnati (Cl)
University of Connecticut (Cl)
University of Hartford (Cl)
University of Hawaii at Manoa (Cl)
University of Kentucky (Cl)
University of Maryland–Baltimore County (Cl)
University of Mississippi (Cl)
University of Nebraska–Lincoln (Cl)
University of Pittsburg (Cl)
University of South Dakota (Cl)

University of Texas at Austin (Cl)
University of Vermont (Cl)
Utah State University (Cm)
Virginia Commonwealth University (Cl)

Cognitive/Cognitive-Behavioral Therapy

American University (Cl)
Antioch/New England Graduate School (Cl)
Argosy University–Chicago (Cl)
Central Michigan University (Cl)
Concordia University (Cl)
Drexel University (Cl)
Duke University (Cl)
Emory University (Cl)
Fielding Graduate Institute (Cl)
George Mason University (Cl)
Georgia State University (Co)
Idaho State University (Cl)
Long Island University (Cl)
McGill University (Co)
Nova Southeastern University (Ph.D. & Psy.D.) (Cl)
Pepperdine University (Cl)
Philadelphia College of Osteopathic Medicine (Cl)
St. John's University (Cl)
San Diego State University/University of California–
    San Diego (Cl)
University of Colorado (Cl)
University of Denver (Psy.D.) (Cl)
University of Georgia (Cl)
University of Houston (Cl)
University of Iowa (Cl)
University of Kentucky (Cl)
University of Manitoba (Cl)
University of Massachusetts at Amherst (Cl)
University of Minnesota (Cl)
University of Missouri–Columbia (Co)
University of North Carolina at Chapel Hill (Cl)
University of Northern Colorado (Co)
University of Oregon (Cl)
University of Pennsylvania (Cl)
University of Pittsburgh (Cl)
University of Texas Southwestern Medical Center at Dallas
    (Cl)
University of ToledoUniversity of Utah (Cl)
University of Wisconsin–Madison (Cl)
Widener University (Cl)
Yeshiva University (Cl)

Community Psychology

Adler School of Professional Psychology (Cl)
Antioch/New England Graduate School (Cl)
Argosy University–Chicago (Cl)
Argosy University–Schaumberg (Cl)
Azusa Pacific University (Cl)

Baylor University (Cl)
Brigham Young University (Cl)
Boston College (Co)
Boston University (Cl)
Bowling Green State University (Cl)
California Institute of Integral Studies (Cl)
Chicago School of Professional Psychology (Cl)
DePaul University (Cl)
Fairleigh Dickinson University (Cl)
George Fox University (Cl)
George Mason University (Cl)
Georgia State University (Cl)
Howard University (Cl)
Northwest (Cl)
Indiana State University (Co)
Indiana University (Cl)
Iowa State University (Co)
Loma Linda University (Ph.D. & Psy.D.) (Cl)
Louisiana Tech University (Co)
Marshall University (Cl)
Marywood University (Cl)
Marquette University (Co)
Miami University (Cl)
New Mexico State University (Co)
Nova Southeastern University (Cl)
Our Lady of the Lake University (Co)
Pepperdine University (Cl)
Rutgers University (Ph.D.) (Cl)
Rutgers University (Psy.D.) (Cl)
Seattle Pacific University (Cl)
Southern Illinois University (Co)
Stony Brook University (Cl)
Syracuse University (Cl)
Tennessee State University (Co)
Texas A&M University (Cl)
Texas Tech University (Co)
University at Buffalo/State University of New York (Cl)
University of Arizona (Cl)
University of Arkansas (Cl)
University of California–Los Angeles (Cl)
University of California–Santa Barbara (Cm)
University of Cincinnati (Cl)
University of Florida (Co)
University of Illinois at Urbana–Champaign (Cl)
University of Iowa (Co)
University of Kansas (Cl)
University of Kentucky (Cl)
University of Kentucky (Co)
University of Maine (Cl)
University of Manitoba (Cl)
University of Minnesota (Cl)
University of Mississippi (Cl)
University of Montana (Cl)
University of New Brunswick (Cl)
University of North Dakota (Cl)
University of Oregon (Co)
University of Ottawa (Cl)

University of Pennsylvania (Cm)
University of Rhode Island (Cl)
University of South Carolina (Cl)
University of South Dakota (Cl)
University of Southern California (Cl)
University of Southern Mississippi (Co)
University of Texas at Austin (Cl)
University of Texas at Austin (Co)
University of Texas Southwestern Medical Center at Dallas (Cl)
University of Utah (Co)
University of Virginia—Department of Psychology (Cl)
University of Washington (Cl)
University of Wisconsin–Milwaukee (Co)
Utah State University (Cm)
Virginia Commonwealth University (Cl)
Virginia Commonwealth University (Co)
Wayne State University (Cl)
West Virginia University (Co)

Conduct Disorder

Antioch/New England Graduate School (Cl)
Binghamton University (Cl)
George Washington University (Ph.D.) (Cl)
Miami University (Cl)
Purdue University (Cl)
Rutgers University (Ph.D.) (Cl)
Rutgers University (Psy.D.) (Cl)
Temple University (Cl)
University of Alabama (Cl)
University of Delaware (Cl)
University of Houston (Cl)
University of Miami (Cl)
University of Minnesota (Cl)
University of Pittsburgh (Cl)
University of Tennessee (Cl)
Virginia Polytechnic Institute and State University (Cl)
Yale University (Cl)

Consultation

University of Maryland (Co)
Miami University (Cl)
Nova Southeastern University (Ph.D. & Psy.D) (Cl)
University of Mississippi (Cl)
Virginia Polytechnic Institute and State University (Cl)

Correctional Psychology/Prisons

Adler School of Professional Psychology (Cl)
Argosy University–Honolulu Campus (Cl)
Argosy University–Schaumburg (Cl)
Binghamton University/SUNY (Cl)
George Fox University (Cl)

Indiana State University (Co)
Loyola College–Maryland (Psy.D.) (Cl)
Oklahoma State University (Co)
Seattle Pacific University (Cl)
Southern Illinois University (Cl)
Southern Illinois University (Co)
Texas Tech University (Co)
University of Florida (Co)
University of Iowa (Co)
University of Kentucky (Co)
University of Louisville (Co)
University of Missouri–Columbia (Co)
University of Texas–Austin
University of Virginia—Department of Human Services (Cl)
Virginia Commonwealth University (Cl & Co)
West Virginia University (Co)

Crisis Intervention

Argosy University–Atlanta (Cl)
Argosy University–Chicago (Cl)
Baylor University (Cl)
California Institute of Integral Studies (Psy.D.) (Cl)
Georgia School of Professional Psychology (Cl)
Howard University (Cl)
Indiana University–Purdue University Indianapolis (Cl)
Northwestern University (Cl)
Nova Southeastern University (Ph.D. & Psy.D.) (Cl)
Ohio State University (Cl)
Syracuse University (Cl)
University of Houston (Co)
University of Maine (Cl)
University of Minnesota (Cl)
University of South Dakota (Cl)
University of Texas at Austin (Cl)
University of Virginia—Department of Human Services (Cl)
Wright Institute (Cl)
Wright State University (Cl)

Deafness

Gallaudet University (Cl)
Louisiana State University (Cl)
University of Texas Southwestern Medical Center at Dallas (Cl)

Developmental Disabilities/Autism

Adler School of Professional Psychology (Cl)
Argosy University–Honolulu Campus (Cl)
Auburn University (Cl)
Binghamton University (Cl)
George Washington University (Ph.D. & Psy.D.) (Cl)
Georgia State University (Cl)
Long Island University–C.W. Post Campus (Cl)

Louisiana State University (Cl)
Miami University (Cl)
Northeastern University (Cm)
Northern Illinois University (Cl)
Ontario Institute for Studies in Education (Cm)
Pacific Graduate School of Psychology (Psy.D.) (Cl)
Rutgers University (Ph.D.) (Cl)
Rutgers University (Psy.D.) (Cl)
University of Alabama (Cl)
University at Albany/State University of New York (Cl)
University of California–Los Angeles (Cl)
University of California–Santa Barbara (Cm)
University of Cincinnati (Cl) (developmental disorders)
University of Connecticut (Cl)
University of Delaware (Cl)
University of Denver (Ph.D.) (Cl)
University of Georgia (Cl)
University of Hawaii at Manoa (Cl)
University of Louisville (Co)
University of Maine (Cl)
University of Manitoba (Cl)
University of Memphis (Cl)
University of Miami (Cl)
University of Milwaukee (Cl)
University of Mississippi (Cl)
University of North Carolina at Chapel Hill (Cl)
University of Pittsburgh (Cl)
University of Rochester (Cl)
University of Saskatchewan (Cl)
University of Texas Southwestern Medical Center at Dallas (Cl)
Vanderbilt University (Cl)
University of Washington (Cl)
University of Wyoming (Cl)
York University (Cl)

Disabilities/Disabled Persons

Alliant International University–Fresno (Ph.D. & Psy.D.) (Cl)
Alliant International University–San Francisco (Ph.D. & Psy.D.) (Cl)
Argosy School of Professional Psychology (Cl)
Ontario Institute for Studies in Education (Cm)
Utah State University (Cm)

Disaster/Trauma/Torture

University of Connecticut (Cl)
University of Denver (Psy.D.) (Cl)
Marquette University (Co)
University of Missouri–St. Louis (Cl)
University of Montana (Cl)
University of South Dakota (Cl)
Virginia Consortium Program in Clinical Psychology (Cl)

Dissociative Disorder/Multiple Personality Disorder

Boston University (Cl)
George Washington University (Ph.D.) (Cl)
Rutgers University (Psy.D.) (Cl)
University of Georgia (Cl)

Divorce/Child Custody

Alliant International University—San Diego (Cl)
University of Houston (Cl)
Virginia Commonwealth University (Cl)

Eating Disorders/Body Image

Alliant International University–Fresno (Ph.D. & Psy.D.) (Cl)
Argosy University–Chicago (Cl)
Baylor University (Cl)
Boston University (Cl)
Brigham Young University (Cl & Co)
Duke University (Cl)
Florida Institute of Technology (Cl)
George Washington University (Ph.D.) (Cl)
Kent State University (Cl)
Long Island University–C.W. Post Campus (Cl)
Louisiana State University (Cl)
Loyola College in Maryland (Psy.D.) (Cl)
Loyola University–Chicago (Cl)
McGill University (Co)
Michigan State University (Cl)
Ohio State University (Cl)
Pepperdine University (Psy.D.) (Cl)
Roosevelt University (Psy.D.) (Cl)
Rutgers University (Ph.D. & Psy.D.) (Cl)
St. Louis University (Cl)
University at Albany/State University of New York (Cl)
University of California–Santa Barbara (Cm)
University of Central Florida (Cl)
University of Georgia (Cl)
University of Hawaii at Manoa (Cl)
University of Iowa (Cl)
University of Maine (Cl)
University of Manitoba (Cl)
University of Memphis (Cl)
University of Miami (Cl)
University of Minnesota (Cl)
University of Mississippi (Cl)
University of Pittsburgh (Cl)
University of South Florida (Cl)
University of Vermont (Cl)
Utah State University (Cm)
Yale University (Cl)
York University—Adult Clinical Program (Cl)

Family Therapy/Systems

Adelphi University (Cl)
Alliant International University–Fresno (Ph.D. & Psy.D) (Cl)
Antioch/New England Graduate School (Cl)
Argosy University–Chicago (Cl)
Argosy University–San Francisco (Cl)
Argosy University–Schaumburg (Cl)
Arizona State University (Cl)
Azusa Pacific University (Cl)
Baylor University (Cl)
Binghamton University/State University of New York (Cl)
Biola University (Ph.D.) (Cl)
Biola University (Psy.D.) (Cl)
Boston University (Cl)
Bowling Green State University (Cl)
Brigham Young University (Cl & Co)
California Institute of Integral Studies (Psy.D.) (Cl)
Carlos Albizu–San Juan (Psy.D.) (Cl)
Catholic University of America (Cl)
City University of New York at City College (Cl)
Clark University (Cl)
Colorado State University (Co)
Concordia University (Cl)
DePaul University (Cl)
Drexel University (Cl)
Fairleigh Dickinson University (Cl)
Florida Institute of Technology (Psy.D.) (Cl)
Fuller Theological Seminary (Ph.D. & Psy.D.) (Cl)
George Mason University (Cl)
George Washington University (Ph.D. & Psy.D.) (Cl)
Georgia State University (Cl)
Howard University (Cl)
Idaho State University (Cl)
Indiana State University (Co)
Indiana University of Pennsylvania (Cl)
Iowa University (Co)
James Madison University (Cm)
Long Island University (Cl)
Long Island University–C.W. Post Campus (Cl)
Louisiana State University (Cl)
Loyola College in Maryland (Psy.D.) (Cl)
Loyola University–Chicago (Cl)
Marquette University (Cl)
Miami University (Cl)
Michigan State University (Cl)
New Mexico State University (Co)
Northeastern University (Cm)
Northern Illinois University (Cl)
Northwestern University (Cl)
Nova Southeastern University (Ph.D. & Psy.D.) (Cl)
Ohio State University (Cl)
Ohio University (Cl)
Oklahoma State University (Cl)
Oklahoma State University (Co)
Ontario Institute for Studies in Education (Cm)
Pacific Graduate School of Psychology (Cl)

Philadelphia College of Osteopathic Medicine (Psy.D.) (Cl)
Purdue University (Cl)
Rutgers University (Ph.D.) (Cl)
Rutgers University (Psy.D.) (Cl)
St. John's University (Cl)
St. Louis University (Cl)
San Diego State University/University of California–San Diego (Cl)
Southern Illinois University (Cl)
Southern Illinois University (Co)
Spalding University (Psy.D.) (Cl)
Syracuse University (Cl)
Texas A&M University (Cl)
University of Akron (Co)
University of Arizona (Cl)
University of California–Los Angeles (Cl)
University of California–Santa Barbara (Cm)
University of Central Florida (Cl)
University of Colorado (Cl)
University of Delaware (Cl)
University of Denver (Ph.D.) (Cl)
University of Florida (Co)
University of Georgia (Cl)
University of Hartford (Psy.D.) (Cl)
University of Houston (Co)
University of Illinois at Urbana–Champaign (Cl)
University of La Verne (Cl)
University of Manitoba (Cl)
University of Maryland–Baltimore County (Cl)
University of Memphis (Cl & Co)
University of Miami (Cl)
University of Michigan (Cl)
University of Minnesota (Cl)
University of Mississippi (Cl)
University of Missouri–Columbia (Co)
University of Missouri–St. Louis (Cl)
University of Montana (Cl)
University of Nebraska–Lincoln (Co)
University of Northern Colorado (Co)
University of Oregon (Cl)
University of Oregon (Co)
University of Ottawa (Cl)
University of Pittsburgh (Cl)
University of Rhode Island (Cl)
University of South Carolina (Cl)
University of South Florida (Cl)
University of Texas Southwestern Medical Center at Dallas (Cl)
University of Toledo (Cl)
University of Utah (Cl)
University of Utah (Co)
University of Victoria (Cl)
University of Virginia—Department of Human Services (Cl)
University of Virginia—Department of Psychology (Cl)
University of Washington (Cl)
University of Wisconsin–Madison (Cl)
University of Wisconsin–Milwaukee (Cl) (Co)

Vanderbilt University—Department of Psychology (Cl)
Widener University (Psy.D.) (Cl)
Wright Institute (Cl)
Wright State University (Cl)
Yeshiva University (Cl) (Psy.D.)
Yeshiva University (Cm)

Forensic

Alliant International University–Fresno (Ph.D. & Psy.D.) (Cl)
Alliant International University–San Francisco (Ph.D. &
   Psy.D.) (Cl)
Antioch/New England Graduate School (Cl)
Argosy University–Atlanta (Cl)
Argosy University–Chicago (Cl)
Argosy University–San Francisco (Cl)
Argosy University–Schaumburg (Cl)
Argosy University–Washington, DC Campus (Cl)
Azusa Pacific University (Cl)
California Institute of Integral Studies (Psy.D.) (Cl)
Carlos Albizu University–San Juan (Psy.D.) (Cl)
Central Michigan University (Cl)
Chicago School of Professional Psychology (Cl)
Drexel University (Cl)
Florida Institute of Technology (Cl)
Forest Institute of Professional Psychology (Cl)
Fuller Theological Seminary (Ph.D. & Psy.D.) (Cl)
George Washington University (Ph.D.) (Cl)
Georgia State University (Co)
Indiana State University (Psy.D.) (Cl)
Jackson State University (Cl)
James Madison University (Cm)
Kent State University (Cl)
Long Island University (Cl)
Loyola College in Maryland (Psy.D.) (Cl)
Northern Illinois University (Cl)
Nova Southeastern University (Ph.D. & Psy.D.) (Cl)
Pacific Graduate School of Psychology (Cl)
Pepperdine University (Cl)
Regent University (Cl)
Rutgers University (Psy.D.) (Cl)
Southern Illinois University (Cl)
Suffolk University (Cl)
Tennessee State University (Co)
Texas A&M University (Cl)
University of Alabama (Cl)
University of British Columbia (Cl)
University of Florida (Cl & Co)
University of Hartford (Psy.D.) (Cl)
University of Houston (Cl & Co)
University of Illinois at Urbana–Champaign (Cl)
University of Kansas (Cl)
University of La Verne (Cl)
University of Louisville (Cl)
University of Maryland–Baltimore County (Cl)
University of Memphis (Co)
University of Minnesota (Cl)

University of Nebraska–Lincoln (Cl)
University of New Mexico (Cl)
University of North Texas (Cl)
University of Saskatchewan (Cl)
University of South Dakota (Cl)
University of Texas Southwestern Medical Center at Dallas
   (Cl)
University of Utah (Cl)
University of Victoria (Cl)
University of Virginia (Human Services) (Cl)
University of Virginia—Department of Psychology (Cl)
West Michigan University (Cl)
West Virginia University (Cl)
Widener University (Psy.D.) (Cl)
Wright Institute (Cl)
Wright State University (Cl)
York University—Adult Clinical Program (Cl)

Gay/Lesbian/Bisexual/Transgender

Alliant International University–San Francisco (Ph.D. &
   Psy.D.) (Cl)
Alliant International University–Fresno (Ph.D. & Psy.D.) (Cl)
Antioch/New England Graduate School (Cl)
Argosy University–Chicago (Cl)
Argosy University–Washington, DC Campus (Cl)
California Institute of Integral Studies (Psy.D.) (Cl)
Chicago School of Professional Psychology (Cl)
Pacific Graduate School of Psychology (Cl)
University of Pittsburgh (Cl)
Wright Institute (Psy.D.) (Cl)
Wright State University (Cl)
York University—Clinical-Developmental Area (Cl)

Group Therapy

Adelphi University (Cl)
Antioch/New England Graduate School (Cl)
Argosy–Chicago (Cl)
Baylor University (Cl)
Catholic University of America (Cl)
DePaul University (Cl)
Fuller Theological Seminary (Ph.D. & Psy.D.) (Cl)
George Mason University (Cl)
George Washington University (Ph.D.) (Cl)
Georgia State University (Cl)
Long Island University–C.W. Post Campus (Cl)
Miami University (Cl)
Michigan State University (Cl)
New Mexico State University (Co)
Nova Southeastern University (Ph.D. & Psy.D.) (Cl)
Pepperdine University (Cl)
Rutgers University (Psy.D.) (Cl)
St. John's University (Cl)
University of Colorado (Cl)
University of Denver (Psy.D.) (Cl)

University of Illinois at Urbana–Champaign (Cl)
University of Louisville (Co)
University of Maryland (Co)
University of Miami (Cl)
University of Ottawa (Cl)
University of Pittsburgh (Cl)
Widener University (Cl)
Wright Institute (Psy.D.) (Cl)
Wright State University (Cl)

Hypnosis

Rutgers University (Psy.D.) (Cl)
University of Denver (Psy.D.) (Cl)
University of Tennessee (Cl)
University of Waterloo (Cl)

Impulse Control/Aggression/Anger Control

Baylor University (Cl)
George Washington University (Ph.D.) (Cl)
Long Island University–C.W. Post Campus (Cl)
Rutgers University (Psy.D.) (Cl)
University of Georgia (Cl)

Infancy/Postpartum

Chicago School of Professional Psychology (Cl)
Rutgers University (Psy.D.) (Cl)
University of Iowa (Cl)

Inpatient Psychology/Psychiatry

Alliant International University–Alameda (Ph.D. & Psy.D.)
   (Cl)
Argosy University–Atlanta (Cl)
Argosy University–Schaumburg (Cl)
Azusa Pacific University (Cl)
Biola University (Ph.D.) (Cl)
Biola University (Psy.D.) (Cl)
Boston College (Co)
Chicago School of Professional Psychology (Cl)
Colorado State University (Co)
Duke University (Cl)
East Michigan University (Cl)
Florida State University (Cl)
Fuller Theological Seminary (Ph.D. & Psy.D.) (Cl)
George Fox University (Cl)
Indiana State University (Co)
Jackson State University (Cl)
James Madison University (Cm)
Long Island University (Cl)
Loyola College in Maryland (Psy.D.) (Cl)
Marshall University (Psy.D.) (Cl)
Marywood University (Psy.D.) (Cl)
Miami University (Cl)

McGill University (Cl & Co)
Ohio University (Cl)
Oklahoma State University (Co)
Pacific Graduate School of Psychology (Ph.D. & Psy.D.)
   (Cl)
Pepperdine University (Psy.D.) (Cl)
Ponce School of Medicine (Cl)
Regent University (Cl)
Roosevelt University (Psy.D.) (Cl)
Southern Illinois University (Co)
Suffolk University (Cl)
Texas Tech University (Co)
University of California–Santa Barbara (Cm)
University of Denver (Ph.D.) (Cl & Co)
University of Florida (Cl & Co)
University of Iowa (Co)
University of Kentucky (Co)
University of Louisville (Co)
University of Massachusetts at Amherst (Cl)
University of Memphis (Co)
University of Missouri–Columbia (Cl & Co)
University of New Brunswick (Cl)
University of New Mexico (Cl)
University of Oregon (Co)
University of Pittsburgh (Cl)
University of Southern Mississippi (Co)
University of Texas at Austin (Co)
University of Texas Southwestern Medical Center at Dallas
   (Cl)
University of Utah (Cl & Co)
University of Victoria (Cl)
University of Virginia—Department of Human Services (Cl)
University of Wisconsin–Milwaukee (Cl & Co)
University of Wyoming (Cl)
Virginia Commonwealth University (Cl & Co)
Washington State University (Cl)

Interpersonal Therapy

Emory University (Cl)
Fuller Theological Seminary (Ph.D. & Psy.D) (Cl)
University of Colorado
University of Louisville (Cl)
Yale University (Cl)

Learning Disabilities

Binghamton University/SUNY (Cl)
George Washington University (Psy.D.) (Cm)
James Madison University (Cm)
Ontario Institute for Studies in Education (Cm)
St. Louis University (Cl)
University of Houston (Cl)
University of Missouri–Columbia (Co)
University of Wisconsin–Milwaukee (Cl)
York University—Clinical-Developmental Area (Cl)

Marital/Couples

Argosy International University–Chicago (Cl)
Arizona State University (Cl)
Binghamton University/State University of New York (Cl)
Boston University (Cl)
Carlos Albizu University–San Juan (Psy.D.) (Cl)
Catholic University of America (Cl)
Clark University (Cl)
Concordia University (Cl)
Forest Institute of Professional Psychology (Cl)
Fuller Theological Seminary (Ph.D. & Psy.D.) (Cl)
George Mason University (Cl)
George Washington University (Ph.D.) (Cl)
Illinois Institute of Technology (Cl)
Indiana State University (Co)
Indiana University–Bloomington (Cl)
Kent State University (Cl)
Long Island University–C.W. Post Campus (Cl)
Michigan State University (Cl)
Northwestern University (Cl)
Oklahoma State University (Cl)
Oklahoma State University (Co)
Pepperdine University (Cl)
Rutgers University (Psy.D.) (Cl)
St. Louis University (Cl)
Southern Illinois University (Co)
Stony Brook University/State University of New York (Cl)
Syracuse University (Cl)
University of Arizona (Cl)
University of California–Los Angeles (Cl)
University of Colorado (Cl)
University of Delaware (Cl)
University of Denver (Ph.D.) (Cl)
University of Georgia (Cl)
University of Manitoba (Cl)
University of Memphis (Co)
University of Miami (Cl)
University of Montana (Cl)
University of Nevada–Reno (Cl)
University of North Carolina at Chapel Hill (Cl)
University of North Dakota (Cl)
University of Northern Colorado (Co)
University of Oregon (Cl)
University of Ottawa (Cl)
University of Rhode Island (Cl)
University of Southern California (Cl)
University of Tennessee (Cl)
University of Texas at Austin (Cl)
University of Virginia (Human Services) (Cl)
University of Virginia—Department of Psychology (Cl)
University of Wisconsin–Milwaukee (Cl)
University of Washington (Cl)
Virginia Polytechnic Institute and State University (Cl)
Widener University (Cl)
Wright Institute (Cl)

Wright State University (Cl)
Yeshiva University (Cl)

Mental Retardation

Ontario Institute for Studies in Education (Cm)
University of Mississippi (Cl)
University of Vermont (Cl)

Minority/Cross-Cultural/Multicultural

Alliant International University–San Francisco (Ph.D. & Psy.D.) (Cl)
Alliant International University–Fresno (Ph.D. & Psy.D.) (Cl)
Argosy University–San Francisco (Cl)
Biola University (Ph.D.) (Cl)
Biola University (Psy.D.) (Cl)
California Institute of Integral Studies (Psy.D.) (Cl)
Catholic University of America (Cl)
Chicago School of Professional Psychology (Cl)
DePaul University (Cl)
Fairleigh Dickinson University (Cl)
Forest Institute of Professional Psychology (Cl)
George Fox University (Cl)
George Washington University (Ph.D.) (Cl)
Georgia State University (Co)
Howard University (Cl)
Illinois Institute of Technology (Cl)
Marquette University (Co)
Michigan State University (Cl)
Miami University (Cl)
New Mexico State University (Co)
Northeastern University (Cm)
Nova Southeastern University (Ph.D. & Psy.D.) (Cl)
Oklahoma State University (Co)
Our Lady of the Lake University (Co)
Pacific Graduate School of Psychology (Psy.D.) (Cl)
Pepperdine University (Psy.D.) (Cl)
Philadelphia College of Osteopathic Medicine (Psy.D.) (Cl)
Rutgers University (Ph.D.) (Cl)
Rutgers University (Psy.D.) (Cl)
Seattle University (Cl)
St. Louis University (Cl)
University at Albany/State University of New York (Cl)
University of California–Los Angeles (Cl)
University of Connecticut (Cl)
University of Denver (Co)
University of Denver (Ph.D.) (Cl)
University of Hawaii at Manoa (Cl)
University of Houston (Cl)
University of Illinois–Urbana (Cl)
University of Maryland (Co)
University of Massachusetts at Amherst (Cl)
University of Miami (Cl)
University of Nebraska–Lincoln (Cl)
University of Nebraska–Lincoln (Co)

University of New Mexico (Cl)
University of North Dakota (Cl)
University of Pittsburgh (Cl)
University of South Dakota (Cl)
University of Southern California (Cl)
University of Utah (Cl & Co)
University of Washington (Cl)
Utah State University (Cm)
Wayne State University (Cl)
Widener University (Cl)
Wright Institute (Cl)
Wright State University (Cl)
Yeshiva University (Cl & Cm)

Neuropsychology/Clinical Neuropsychology/Brain Injury

Adelphi University (Cl)
Alliant International University–Fresno (Ph.D. & Psy.D.) (Cl)
Alliant International University–San Francisco (Ph.D. & Psy.D.) (Cl)
Antioch/New England Graduate School (Cl)
Argosy University–Atlanta (Cl)
Argosy University–Chicago (Cl)
Argosy University–Phoenix (Cl)
Argosy University–San Francisco (Cl)
Argosy University–Schaumburg (Cl)
Argosy University, Washington, DC Campus (Cl)
Baylor University (Cl)
Binghamton University/State University of New York (Cl)
Boston University (Cl)
Brigham Young University (Cl)
California Institute of Integral Studies (Cl)
Catholic University of America (Cl)
Central Michigan University (Cl)
Colorado State (Co)
Drexel University (Cl)
Duke University (Cl)
East Michigan University (Cl)
Emory University (Cl)
Fairleigh Dickinson University (Cl)
Florida Institute of Technology (Cl)
Forest Institute of Professional Psychology (Cl)
Fuller Theological Seminary (Ph.D. & Psy.D.) (Cl)
George Fox University (Psy.D.) (Cl)
George Washington University (Cl)
Georgia State University (Cl)
Howard University (Cl)
Idaho University (Cl)
Illinois Institute of Technology (Cl)
Indiana University–Bloomington (Cl)
Indiana University–Purdue University Indianapolis (Cl)
James Madison University (Cm)
Kent State University (Cl)
Loma Linda University (Cl)
Long Island University (Cl)
Long Island University–C.W. Post Campus (Cl)

Louisiana State University (Cl)
Loyola University–Chicago (Cl)
Marquette University (Cl & Co)
Northwestern University (Cl)
Northwestern University, Feinberg School of Medicine (Cl)
Nova Southeastern (Ph.D. & Psy.D.) (Cl)
Ohio State University (Cl)
Ohio University (Cl)
Ontario Institute for Studies in Education (Cm)
Pace University (Psy.D.) (Cm)
Pacific Graduate School of Psychology (Ph.D. & Psy.D) (Cl)
Pepperdine University (Cl)
Regent University (Cl)
Roosevelt University (Psy.D.) (Cl)
Rosalind Franklin University of Medicine and Science (Cl)
Rutgers University (Psy.D.) (Cl)
St. John's University (Cl)
St. Louis University (Cl)
San Diego State University/University of California–San Diego (Cl)
Seattle Pacific University (Cl)
Southern Illinois University (Cl)
Suffolk University (Cl)
Syracuse University (Cl)
Temple University (Cl)
Texas A&M University (Cl)
Texas Tech University (Co)
University of Alabama at Birmingham (Cl)
University of Alabama at Tuscaloosa (Cl)
University at Albany/State University of New York (Cl)
University at Albany/State University of New York (Co)
University of Arizona (Cl)
University of Arkansas (Cl)
University of Central Florida (Cl)
University of Cincinnati (Cl)
University of Connecticut (Cl)
University of Denver (Ph.D.) (Cl & Co)
University of Florida (Cl)
University of Georgia (Cl)
University of Hawaii at Manoa (Cl)
University of Houston (Cl)
University of Illinois at Urbana–Champaign (Cl)
University of Iowa (Cl)
University of Kentucky (Cl)
University of Louisville (Co)
University of Manitoba (Cl)
University of Maryland–Baltimore County (Cl)
University of Memphis (Cl)
University of Miami (Cl)
University of Minnesota (Cl)
University of Montana (Cl)
University of Nebraska–Lincoln (Cl)
University of New Brunswick (Cl)
University of New Mexico (Cl)
University of Oregon (Cl)
University of Pittsburgh (Cl)
University of Rochester (Cl)

University of Saskatchewan (Cl)
University of South Carolina (Cl)
University of South Florida (Cl)
University of Texas at Austin (Cl)
University of Texas Southwestern Medical Center at Dallas (Cl)
University of Vermont (Cl)
University of Victoria (Cl)
University of Virginia—Department of Human Services (Cl)
University of Virginia—Department of Psychology (Cl)
University of Washington (Cl)
University of Waterloo (Cl)
University of Wisconsin–Madison (Cl)
University of Wisconsin–Milwaukee (Cl)
Utah State University (Cm)
Vanderbilt University—Department of Psychology (Cl)
Virginia Commonwealth University (Cl)
Virginia Polytechnic Institute and State University (Cl)
Washington State University (Cl)
Wayne State University (Cl)
Widener University (Cl)
Wright Institute (Cl)
Wright State University (Cl)
Yeshiva University (Cl)
York University—Adult Clinical Program (Cl)

Obsessive–Compulsive Disorder

Case Western Reserve University (Cl)
George Washington University (Cl)
Indiana University–Bloomington (Cl)
Louisiana State University (Cl)
Rutgers University (Ph.D.) (Cl)
Rutgers University (Psy.D.) (Cl)
University of Manitoba (Cl)
University of Minnesota (Cl)
University of North Dakota (Cl)
University of Pittsburgh (Cl)
University of Virginia—Department of Psychology (Cl)

Organizational

Chicago School of Professional Psychology (Cl)
Rutgers University (Psy.D.) (Cl)
Widener University (Cl)

Pain Management

Argosy University–Phoenix (Cl)
Binghamton University/State University of New York (Cl)
Forest Institute of Professional Psychology (Cl)
George Fox University (Cl)
Illinois Institute of Technology (Cl)
Marquette University (Cl)
Nova Southeastern University (Ph.D. & Psy.D.) (Cl)
Ohio University (Cl)

Pacific Graduate School of Psychology (Psy.D.) (Cl)
University of Alabama (Cl)
University of Florida (Cl)
University of Missouri–Kansas City (Cl)
University of Montana (Cl)
University of Ottawa (Cl)
University of Pittsburgh (Cl)
University of Utah (Co)
Virginia Commonwealth University (Cl)

Parent–Child Interaction/Parent Training

Arizona State University (Cl)
Central Michigan University (Cl)
Idaho State University (Cl)
Long Island University–C.W. Post Campus (Cl)
Miami University (Cl)
Northern Illinois University (Cl)
Nova Southeastern University (Ph.D. & Psy.D.) (Cl)
St. Louis University (Cl)
University of Alabama (Cl)
University at Buffalo/State University of New York (Cl)
University of Florida (Cl)
University of Ottawa (Cl)
University of Pittsburgh (Cl)
University of Virginia—Department of Human Services (Cl)
West Virginia University (Cl)
Yeshiva University (Cl & Cm)

Personality Disorders

Antioch/New England Graduate School (Cl)
Argosy University–Chicago (Cl)
Baylor University (Cl)
Case Western Reserve University (Cl)
George Washington University (Ph.D.) (Cl)
Georgia State University (Cl)
Loyola University–Chicago (Cl)
Northern Illinois University (Cl)
Purdue University (Cl)
Rutgers University (Ph.D.) (Cl)
Rutgers University (Psy.D.) (Cl)
St. Louis University (Cl)
Texas Tech University (Co)
University of Georgia (Cl)
University of Minnesota (Cl)
University of Montana (Cl)
University of Nevada–Reno (Cl)
University of North Dakota (Cl)
University of Northern Colorado (Co)
University of Pittsburgh (Cl)
University of Tennessee (Cl)
University of Texas Southwestern Medical Center at Dallas (Cl)
University of Utah (Cl)
University of Washington (Cl)

Vanderbilt University—Department of Psychology (Cl)
Wright State University (Ph.D. & Psy.D) (Cl)

Posttraumatic Stress Disorder/Trauma

Argosy University–Washington, DC Campus (Cl)
Auburn University (Cl)
Florida Institute of Technology (Cl)
Miami University (Cl)
Pacific Graduate School of Psychology (Psy.D.) (Cl)
Pepperdine University (Cl)
University of Houston (Cl)
University of Mississippi (Cl)
University of Missouri–St. Louis (Cl)
University of Nevada–Reno (Cl)
University of North Texas (Cl)
University of Ottawa (Cl)
Western Michigan University (Cl)

Prevention

Argosy University–Chicago (Cl)
Arizona State University (Cl)
Clark University (Cl)
Miami University (Cl)
University of Illinois at Chicago (Cl)
University of Maryland–Baltimore County (Cl)
University of Missouri–Columbia (Cl)
University of Vermont (Cl)
Virginia Polytechnic Institute and State University (Cl)

Primary Care

Colorado State University (Co)
Loma Linda University (Cl)
West Virginia University (Cl)

Private Practice

Brigham Young University (Cl)
Chicago School of Professional Psychology (Cl)
Loyola College in Maryland (Psy.D.) (Cl)

Psychiatric Emergency Care

University of Maryland–Baltimore County (Cl)
University of Texas Southwestern Medical Center at Dallas (Cl)

Psychoanalytic/Psychodynamic Therapy

Adelphi University (Cl)
American University (Cl)
Antioch/New England Graduate School (Cl)
Argosy University–Chicago (Cl)

Central Michigan University (Cl)
Columbia University, Teachers College (Cl)
Concordia University (Cl)
Emory University (Cl)
Fielding Graduate Institute (Cl)
George Washington University (Ph.D.) (Cl)
Long Island University–C.W. Post Campus (Cl)
Nova Southeastern University (Ph.D. & Psy.D.) (Cl)
Rutgers University (Psy.D.) (Cl)
St. John's University (Cl)
St. Louis University (Cl)
University of Colorado (Cl)
University of Denver (Psy.D.) (Cl)
University of Massachusetts at Amherst (Cl)
University of Minnesota (Cl)
University of Pennsylvania (Cl)
University of Rochester (Cl)
University of Toledo (Cl)
Widener University (Psy.D.) (Cl)
Wright Institute (Cl)
Wright State University (Cl)
Yeshiva University (Cl)

Psychotherapy Integration

Adelphi University (Cl)
George Mason University (Cl)
Loyola College–Chicago (Cl)
McGill University (Co)

Rehabilitation

Antioch/New England Graduate School (Cl)
Argosy University–Atlanta (Cl)
Argosy University–Chicago (Cl)
Argosy University–Schaumburg (Cl)
Auburn University (Co)
Georgia State University (Cl)
Illinois School of Professional Psychology–Chicago Campus (Psy.D. & Ph.D.) (Cl)
Jackson State University (Cl)
Pepperdine University (Cl)
Southern Illinois University (Cl)
Southern Illinois University (Co)
University of Hawaii at Manoa (Cl)
University of Houston (Cl)
University of Illinois at Urbana–Champaign (Co)
University of Maryland–Baltimore County (Cl)
University of Memphis (Co)
University of Missouri–Columbia (Cl)
University of Missouri–Columbia (Co)
University of Texas Southwestern Medical Center at Dallas (Cl)
University of Victoria (Cl)
University of Washington (Cl)
Virginia Commonwealth University (Co)

Wayne State University (Cl)
Wright Institute (Cl)
Wright State University (Cl)
York University—Clinical-Developmental Area (Cl)

Religion/Spirituality

Argosy University–Chicago (Cl)
Biola University (Ph.D.) (Cl)
Biola University (Psy.D.) (Cl)
Pepperdine University (Cl)
Regent University (Cl)
Seattle Pacific University (Cl)

Rural Mental Health/Psychology

Antioch/New England Graduate School (Cl)
Baylor University (Cl)
Chicago School of Professional Psychology (Cl)
George Fox University (Cl)
Indiana State University (Psy.D.) (Cl)
Marshall University (Psy.D.) (Cl)
Miami University (Cl)
New Mexico State University (Co)
Oklahoma State University (Co)
Southern Illinois University (Co)
Texas A&M University (Cl)
University of Florida (Co)
University of Kentucky (Co)
University of Missouri–Columbia (Co)
University of Montana (Cl)
University of North Dakota (Cl)
University of South Dakota (Cl)
University of Wyoming (Cl)

Schizophrenia/Psychosis/Serious Mental Illness

Argosy University–San Francisco (Cl)
Baylor University (Cl)
Binghamton University/State University of New York (Cl)
Boston University (Cl)
Case Western Reserve University (Cl)
George Washington University (Ph.D. & Psy.D.) (Cl)
Howard University (Cl)
Indiana University–Bloomington (Cl)
Kent State University (Cl)
Louisiana State University (Cl)
Northwestern University (Cl)
Pepperdine University (Cl)
Rutgers University (Psy.D.) (Cl)
University of Houston (Cl)
University of Louisville (Cl)
University of Minnesota (Cl)
University of Montana (Cl)
University of Pittsburgh (Cl)

University of Texas at Austin (Cl)
University of Virginia—Department of Psychology (Cl)
Vanderbilt University—Department of Psychology (Cl)
Wright Institute (Cl)
Wright State University (Cl)

School/Educational

Adler School of Professional Psychology (Cl)
Alliant International University–Fresno (Ph.D. & Psy.D.) (Cl)
Alliant International University–Los Angeles (Ph.D. & Psy.D) (Cl)
Argosy University–Atlanta (Cl)
Argosy University–Chicago (Cl)
Argosy University–Honolulu Campus (Cl)
Argosy University–Phoenix (Cl)
Argosy University–San Francisco (Cl)
Argosy University–Washington, DC Campus (Cl)
Azusa Pacific University (Cl)
Baylor University (Cl)
Binghamton University/State University of New York (Cl)
Boston College (Co)
Bowling Green State University (Cl)
Brigham Young University (Cl)
Central Michigan University (Cl)
Chicago School of Professional Psychology (Cl)
Clark University (Cl)
Duke University (Cl)
George Fox University (Cl)
Georgia State University (Co)
Indiana University (Cl)
Indiana University–Bloomington (Cl)
Indiana University–Purdue University Indianapolis (Cl)
Long Island University–C.W. Post Campus (Cl)
Louisiana State University (Cl)
James Madison University (Cm)
Marquette University (Co)
Marshall University (Psy.D.) (Cl)
Miami University (Cl)
Ohio State University (Cl)
Ohio University (Cl)
Our Lady of the Lake University (Co)
Pepperdine University (Psy.D.) (Cl)
Roosevelt University (Psy.D.) (Cl)
Rutgers University (Psy.D.) (Cl)
San Diego University (Cl)
Suffolk University (Cl)
Syracuse University (Cl)
Texas Tech University (Co)
University of Arkansas (Cl)
University at Buffalo/State University of New York (Cm)
University of California–Los Angeles (Cl)
University of California–Santa Barbara (Cm)
University of Cincinnati (Cl)
University of Georgia (Co)
University of Illinois at Urbana–Champaign (Co)

University of Iowa (Co)
University of Louisville (Co)
University of Maryland–Baltimore County (Cl)
University of Memphis (Cl & Co)
University of Nebraska–Lincoln
University of New Mexico (Cl)
University of North Carolina at Greensboro (Cl)
University of Virginia (Human Services) (Cl)
University of Washington (Cl)
University of Waterloo (Cl)
Utah State University (Cm)
Virginia Commonwealth University (Cl)
West Virginia University (Cl)
Western Michigan University (Cl & Co)
Widener University (Cl)
Yeshiva University (Cl & Cm)
York University—Clinical-Developmental Area (Cl)

Sex Therapy/Deviation and Dysfunction

Adler School of Professional Psychology (Cl)
Argosy University–Chicago (Cl)
Baylor University (Psy.D.) (Cl)
Carlos Albizu University (Psy.D.) (Cl)
Idaho State University (Cl)
Ohio State University (Cl)
Rutgers University (Ph.D.) (Cl)
Rutgers University (Psy.D.) (Cl)
Southern Illinois University (Co)
University of Florida (Co)
University of Louisville (Co)
University of Ottawa (Cl)
University of Rhode Island (Cl)
University of Utah (Cl)
Widener University (Cl)

Sleep Disorders

University of Alabama (Cl)
University of Arizona (Cl)
University of Texas Southwestern Medical Center at Dallas (Cl)

Smoking Cessation

Indiana University–Bloomington (Cl)
University of Illinois at Chicago (Cl)
University of Kansas (Cl)
University of Mississippi (Cl)
University of Pittsburgh (Cl)
University of Rochester (Cl)

Sports Psychology

Argosy University–Chicago (Cl)
Carlos Albizu University–San Juan (Cl)
University of Manitoba (Cl)

Stress

Georgia State University (Co)
Indiana University of Pennsylvania (Cl)
Long Island University–C.W. Post Campus (Cl)
Loyola College in Maryland (Psy.D.) (Cl)
Nova Southeastern University (Ph.D. & Psy.D.) (Cl)
Southern Illinois University (Co)
University of Connecticut (Cl)
University of Georgia (Cl)
University of Wisconsin–Milwaukee (Cl)

Substance Abuse/Addiction

Adelphi University (Cl)
Antioch/New England Graduate School (Cl)
Argosy University–Atlanta (Cl)
Argosy University–Honolulu Campus (Cl)
Argosy University–Phoenix (Cl)
Argosy University–San Francisco (Cl)
Argosy University–Schaumburg (Cl)
Argosy University–Washington, DC Campus (Cl)
Auburn University (Co)
Azusa Pacific University (Cl)
Baylor University (Cl)
Binghamton University (Cl)
Duke University (Cl)
Fairleigh Dickinson University (Cl)
George Fox University (Cl)
George Washington University (Ph.D. (Cl)
Howard University (Cl)
Idaho State University (Cl)
Long Island University (Cl)
Loyola University–Chicago (Cl)
Marquette University (Co)
New Mexico State University (Co)
Nova Southeastern University (Ph.D. & Psy.D.) (Cl)
Ohio University (Cl)
Oklahoma State University (Cl)
Pacific Graduate School of Psychology (Psy.D.) (Cl)
Pepperdine University (Cl)
Rutgers University (Ph.D.) (Cl)
Southern Illinois University (Cl)
Southern Illinois University (Co)
Syracuse University (Cl)
University at Albany/State University of New York (Cl)
University at Albany/State University of New York (Co)
Texas A&M University (Cl)
Uniformed Services University of Health Sciences (Cl)
University of Arkansas (Cl)
University of Central Florida (Cl)
University of Colorado (Cl)
University of Connecticut (Cl)
University of Florida (Co)
University of Georgia (Cl)
University of Hawaii at Manoa (Cl)
University of La Verne (Cl)

University of Maryland–Baltimore County (Cl)
University of Memphis (Cl)
University of Memphis (Co)
University of Miami (Cl)
University of Minnesota (Cl)
University of Mississippi (Cl)
University of Montana (Cl)
University of Nebraska–Lincoln (Cl)
University of Nevada–Reno (Cl)
University of New Mexico (Cl)
University of North Dakota (Cl)
University of Pittsburgh (Cl)
University of South Dakota (Cl)
University of South Florida (Cl)
University of Southern Mississippi (Co)
University of Tennessee (Cl)
University of Utah (Cl & Co)
University of Vermont (Cl)
University of Washington (Cl)
University of Wisconsin–Madison (Cl)
Vanderbilt University (Cl)
Virginia Commonwealth University (Cl & Co)
Virginia Polytechnic Institute and State University (Cl)
Wayne State University (Cl)
Wright Institute (Cl)
Wright State University (Cl)
Yale University (Cl)
York University—Adult Clinical Program (Cl)

Suicide/Prevention

Baylor University (Cl)
University of Houston (Cl)
University of Pittsburgh (Cl)

Supervision

Antioch/New England Graduate School (Cl)
Binghamton University/State University of New York (Cl)
Fuller Theological Seminary (Ph.D. & Psy.D.) (Cl)
Georgia State University (Cl)
James Madison University (Cm)
Marquette University (Co)
University of California–Los Angeles (Cl)
University of Denver (Psy.D.) (Cl)
University of Georgia (Cl)
University of Georgia (Co)
University of Manitoba (Cl)
University of Maryland (Co)
University of Massachusetts at Amherst (Cl)
University of Northern Colorado (Co)

Veterans Hospital/Medical Center

Argosy University–Honolulu Campus (Cl)
Brigham Young University (Cl)
Chicago School of Professional Psychology (Cl)

Indiana State University (Co)
Iowa State University (Co)
Louisiana Tech University (Co)
Pacific Graduate School of Psychology (Ph.D. & Psy.D) (Cl)
Pepperdine University (Psy.D.) (Cl)
Regent University (Cl)
Roosevelt University (Psy.D.) (Cl)
Southern Illinois University (Co)
Tennessee State University (Co)
Texas A&M University (Co)
Uniformed Services University of Health Sciences (Cl)
University at Albany/State University of New York (Co)
University of Denver (Co)
University of Houston (Co)
University of Illinois at Urbana–Champaign (Co)
University of Iowa (Co)
University of Kentucky (Co)
University of Missouri–Columbia (Cl)
University of Missouri–Columbia (Co)
University of Oregon (Co)
University of Pittsburgh (Cl)
University of Southern Mississippi (Co)
University of Texas at Austin (Co)
University of Utah (Co)
Virginia Commonwealth University (Co)
West Virginia University (Co)

Victim/Violence/Sexual Abuse

Antioch/New England Graduate School (Psy.D.) (Cl)
Argosy University–Chicago (Cl)
Baylor University (Cl)
Boston College (Co)
Boston University (Cl)
Carlos Albizu University–San Juan (Psy.D.) (Cl)
Carlos Albizu University–San Juan (Ph.D.) (Cl)
Clark University (Cl)
Florida Institute of Technology (Cl)
Fuller Theological Seminary (Ph.D. & Psy.D.) (Cl)
George Washington University (Ph.D.) (Cl)
Georgia State University (Cl)
Howard University (Cl)
Long Island University–C.W. Post Campus (Cl)
Loyola University–Chicago (Cl)
Michigan State University (Cl)
Northern Illinois University (Cl)
Nova Southeastern University (Ph.D. & Psy.D) (Cl)
Oklahoma State University (Co)
Pacific Graduate School of Psychology (Psy.D.) (Cl)
Rutgers University (Psy.D.) (Cl)
Southern Illinois University (Cl)
Texas Woman's University (Co)
University of Delaware (Cl)
University of Florida (Co)
University of Georgia (Cl)
University of Houston (Cl)
University of Manitoba (Cl)

University of Maryland–Baltimore County (Cl)
University of Memphis (Co)
University of Miami (Cl)
University of Mississippi (Cl)
University of Montana (Cl)
University of Nebraska–Lincoln (Cl)
University of Nevada–Reno (Cl)
University of North Dakota (Cl)
University of Pittsburgh (Cl)
University of Utah (Co)
University of Virginia—Department of Psychology (Cl)

Vocational/Career Development

Florida State University (Cm)
New Mexico State University (Co)
Southern Illinois University (Co)
Temple University (Co)
Uniformed Services University of Health Sciences (Cl)
University of California–Santa Barbara (Cm)
University of Florida (Co)
University of Georgia (Co)
University of Louisville (Co)
University of Maryland (Co)
University of Missouri–Columbia (Co)
University of Nebraska–Lincoln (Co)
University of Texas Southwestern Medical Center at Dallas (Cl)

Weight Management

University of Florida (Cl)
University of Illinois at Chicago (Cl)
University of Kansas (Cl)
University of Pittsburgh (Cl)
University of South Florida (Cl)
Yeshiva University (Cl)

Women's Studies/Issues

Alliant International University–Fresno (Ph.D. & Psy.D.) (Cl)
Alliant International University–San Francisco (Ph.D. & Psy.D.) (Cl)
University of Iowa (Co)
University of Missouri–Columbia (Co)
University of Utah (Co)
Wright State University (Cl)

Miscellaneous

adoption—Pepperdine University (Cl)
attachment disorder—Miami University (Cl)
behavioral analysis—Arizona State University (Cl)
behavior genetics—University of Oregon (Cl)
behavioral dentistry—West Virginia University (Cl)
creative & expressive arts—Chicago School of Professional Psychology (Cl)
data management systems—Virginia Polytechnic Institute and State University (Cl)
dual diagnosis clinic—University of Hawaii at Manoa (Cl)
factitious disorders—University of Alabama (Cl)
gambling—University of Memphis (Cl)
homeless shelter—University of Georgia (Co), University of Iowa (Co)
hypnosis—University of Northern Colorado (Co)
humanistic/experiential therapy—Pepperdine University (Cl), American University (Cl)
interpersonal therapy—Emory University (Cl), Fuller Theological Seminary (Ph.D. & Psy.D) (Cl)
low income populations—New Mexico State University (Co)
immigrants—Florida State University (Cl), University of Texas–Austin (Co)
military settings—Uniformed Services University of Health Sciences (Cl)
mindfulness—University of Colorado (Cl)
National Guard Youth Challenge Program—University of Southern Mississippi (Co)
nursing facility—University of Florida (Co)
play therapy—Baylor University (Psy.D.) (Cl), Michigan State University (Cl)
positive psychology—University of Louisville (Co)
program evaluation—George Mason University (Cl)
psychopharmacology/medication management—Forest Institute of Professional Psychology (Psy.D.) (Cl)
selective mutism—University of South Florida (Cl)
shyness—Pacific Graduate School of Psychology (Cl)
social skills—University of Mississippi (Cl)
somatization disorders—Rutgers University (Ph.D.) (Cl)
systems management—Virginia Polytechnic Institute and State University (Cl)
TA Gestalt training—Fielding Graduate University (Cl)
underserved populations—Forest Institute of Professional Psychology (Cl), New Mexico State University (Co)

A P P E N D I X   G
PROGRAM CONCENTRATIONS AND TRACKS

Adult/Aging/Geropsychology

Antioch University New England (Psy.D.)
Argosy University–Atlanta Campus (Psy.D.)
Boston University (Cl)
Case Western Reserve University (Cl)
Catholic University of America (Cl)
Duke University (Cl)
Howard University (Cl)
George Washington University (Psy.D.)
Marquette University (Cl)
Miami University (Cl)
Northwestern University (Cl)
Ohio State University (Cl)
Purdue University (Cl)
Seton Hall University (Co)
Southern Illinois University (Cl)
Spalding University (Psy.D.) (Cl)
Texas A&M University (Co)
University of Alabama at Birmingham (Cl)
University of Alabama at Tuscaloosa (Cl)
University of Central Florida (Cl)
University of Houston (Cl)
University of Indianapolis (Psy.D.) (Cl)
University of Iowa (Cl)
University of Kansas (Cl)
University of La Verne (Psy.D.) (Cl)
University of Massachusetts at Amherst (Cl)
University of Miami (Cl)
University of Missouri–Columbia (Cl)
University of Nebraska–Lincoln (Cl)
University of North Carolina at Chapel Hill (Cl)
University of North Texas (Co)
University of Pittsburgh (Cl)
University of Southern California (Cl)
University of Southern Mississippi (Cl)
University of Utah (Cl)

University of Washington (Cl)
University of Windsor (Cl)
University of Wisconsin–Madison (Cl)
Vanderbilt University (Psychology and Human
    Development) (Cl)
Xavier University (Psy.D.) (Cl)
Yeshiva University (Psy.D.) (Cl)
York University (Cl)

Assessment

Antioch University New England (Psy.D.)
George Washington University (Psy.D.) (Cl)
Kent State University (Cl)
University of Florida (Co)
University of Texas–Austin (Co)
University of Massachusetts at Amherst (Cl)

Child/Pediatric

Adler School of Professional Psychology (Cl)
Alliant International University–Fresno (Psy.D. & Ph.D.) (Cl)
Alliant International University–San Francisco Bay (Psy.D. &
    Ph.D.) (Cl)
Antioch University New England (Psy.D.)
Argosy University Chicago (Cl)
Argosy University, Hawaii Campus (Psy.D.)
Arizona State University (Cl)
Auburn University (Cl)
Boston University (Cl)
Bowling Green State University (Cl)
Brigham Young University (Cl)
Carlos Albizu University–Miami Campus (Psy.D.) (Cl)
Case Western Reserve University (Cl)
Catholic University of America (Cl)
Chicago School of Professional Psychology (Psy.D.) (Cl)

DePaul University (Cl)
Duke University (Cl)
George Washington University (Psy.D.) (Cl)
Howard University (Cl)
Indiana State University (Psy.D.) (Cl)
Indiana University of Pennsylvania (Psy.D.) (Cl)
Loyola University of Chicago (Cl)
Marquette University (Cl & Co)
Massachusetts School of Professional Psychology (Psy.D.) (Cl)
Northwestern University, Feinberg School of Medicine (Cl)
Ohio University (Cl)
Oklahoma State University (Cl)
Pacific University (Cl)
Purdue University (Cl)
Simon Fraser University (Cl)
Spalding University (Psy.D.) (Cl)
St. John's University (Cl)
Suffolk University (Cl)
Columbia University–Teachers College (Cl)
Southern Illinois University (Cl)
Ohio State University (Cl)
University of Alabama at Birmingham (Cl)
University of Alabama at Tuscaloosa (Cl)
University of Central Florida (Cl)
University of Connecticut (Cl)
University of Denver (Cl) (Ph.D. & Psy.D.)
University of Florida (Cl)
University of Georgia (Cl)
University of Hartford (Psy.D.) (Cl)
University of Indianapolis (Psy.D.) (Cl)
University of Iowa (Cl)
University of Kansas (Cl)
The University of Memphis (Cl)
University of Miami (Cl)
University of Missouri–Columbia (Cl)
University of Missouri–St. Louis (Cl)
University of Montana (Cl)
University of North Carolina at Chapel Hill (Cl)
University of North Carolina at Greensboro (Cl)
University of South Florida (Cl)
University of Southern Mississippi (Cl)
University of Texas Southwestern Medical Center at Dallas (Cl)
University of Virginia–Department of Human Services (Cl)
University of Washington (Cl)
University of Windsor (Cl)
Virginia Commonwealth University (Cl)
Wayne State University (Cl)
West Virginia University (Cl)
Xavier University (Psy.D.) (Cl)
Yeshiva University (Psy.D.) (Cm)

Child & Family

Adler School of Professional Psychology (Cl)
Alliant International University–San Diego (Psy.D. & Ph.D.) (Cl)

Argosy University–Atlanta Campus (Psy.D.) (Cl)
Alliant International University–San Francisco Bay (Psy.D. & Ph.D.) (Cl)
Argosy University–Washington DC Campus (Psy.D) (Cl)
Argosy University–Twin Cities Campus (Psy.D.) (Cl)
Florida Institute of Technology (Psy.D.) (Cl)
Fordham University (Cl)
Forest Institute of Professional Psychology (Cl)
Kent State University (Cl)
La Salle University (Psy.D.) (Cl)
Miami University (Cl)
Regent University (Cl)
University of Houston (Cl)
University of Massachusetts at Amherst (Cl)
The University of Montana (Cl)
University of North Texas (Co)
University of Nebraska–Lincoln (Cl)
University of Rhode Island (Cl)
University of South Carolina (Cl)
University of Southern California (Cl)
University of Toledo (Cl)
University of Utah (Cl)
Vanderbilt University (Psychology and Human Development) (Cl)

Cognitive/Cognitive-Behavioral

American University (Cl)
Concordia University (Cl)
Pepperdine University (Psy.D.) (Cl)
University of Toledo (Cl)

Community

Arizona State University (Cl)
Bowling Green State University (Cl)
DePaul University (Cl)
Georgia State University (Cl)
Pepperdine University (Psy.D.) (Cl)
Rutgers, The State University of New Jersey (Psy.D.)(Cl)
University of Maryland, Baltimore County (Cl)
Wayne State University (Cl)

Family/Marriage & Family

Alliant International University–Los Angeles (Psy.D. & Ph.D.) (Cl)
Alliant International University–San Diego (Psy.D. & Ph.D.) (Cl)
Alliant International University–San Francisco Bay (Psy.D. & Ph.D.) (Cl)
Argosy University Chicago (Cl)
Argosy University, Hawaii Campus (Psy.D.) (Cl)
Azusa Pacific University (PsyD) (Cl)
Ball State University (Co)
Catholic University of America (Cl)
Chestnut Hill University (Psy.D.) (Cl)

Forest Institute of Professional Psychology (Cl)
Fuller Theological Seminary (Ph.D. & Psy.D.) (Cl)
Indiana University of Pennsylvania (Psy.D.) (Cl)
Loma Linda University (Cl)
Massachusetts School of Professional Psychology (Psy.D.) (Cl)
Pepperdine University (Psy.D.) (Cl)
Regent University (Cl)
Seton Hall University (Co)
Spalding University (Psy.D.) (Cl)
Texas Woman's University (Co)
University of Florida (Co)
University of Toledo (Cl)
University of Miami (Co)
University of Nebraska–Lincoln (Co)
University of Virginia–Department of Human Services (Cl)
Widener University (Psy.D.) (Cl)

Forensic/Psychology & Law

Alliant International University–Fresno (Psy.D. & Ph.D.) (Cl)
Alliant International University–San Diego (Psy.D. & Ph.D.) (Cl)
Alliant International University–San Francisco Bay (Psy.D. & Ph.D.) (Cl)
Argosy University, Chicago (Cl)
Argosy University, Washington DC Campus (Psy.D) (Cl)
Argosy University, Twin Cities Campus (Psy.D.) (Cl)
Azusa Pacific University (Psy.D.) (Cl)
Carlos Albizu University–Miami Campus (Psy.D.) (Cl)
Chicago School of Professional Psychology (Psy.D.) (Cl)
City University of New York at City College (Cl)
Drexel University (Cl)
Fielding Graduate University (Cl)
Florida Institute of Technology (Psy.D.) (Cl)
Fordham University (Cl)
Forest Institute of Professional Psychology (Cl)
Indiana State University (Psy.D.) (Cl)
Loma Linda University (Cl)
Massachusetts School of Professional Psychology (Psy.D.) (Cl)
Pacific University (Cl)
Pepperdine University (Psy.D.) (Cl)
Simon Fraser University (Cl)
Spalding University (Psy.D.) (Cl)
University of Alabama at Tuscaloosa (Cl)
University of Denver (Psy.D.) (Cl)
University of La Verne (Psy.D.) (Cl)
University of Nebraska–Lincoln (Cl)
University of Virginia–Department of Human Services (Cl)
Widener University (Psy.D.) (Cl)

Gender Studies

City University of New York at City College (Cl)
University of Missouri–St. Louis (Cl)
University of Nebraska–Lincoln (Co)

Generalist

Argosy University–Phoenix (Psy.D.) (Cl)
Baylor University (Psy.D.) (Cl)
Carlos Albizu University–Miami Campus (Psy.D.) (Cl)
Chicago School of Professional Psychology (Psy.D.) (Cl)
Georgia State University (Cl)
Illinois Institute of Technology (Cl)
Kent State University (Cl)
La Salle University (Psy.D.) (Cl)
Simon Fraser University (Cl)
University of Cincinnati (Cl)
University of Georgia (Cl)
University of Hartford (Psy.D.) (Cl)
University of Indianapolis (Psy.D.) (Cl)
University of Kentucky (Cl)
University of Maine (Cl)
University of Maryland, Baltimore County (Cl)
University of Tulsa (Cl)
West Virginia University (Cl)

Health/Behavioral Medicine

Alliant International University–Fresno (Psy.D. & Ph.D.) (Cl)
Alliant International University–Los Angeles (Psy.D. & Ph.D.) (Cl)
Alliant International University–San Diego (Psy.D. & Ph.D.) (Cl)
Alliant International University–San Francisco Bay (Psy.D. & Ph.D.) (Cl)
Antioch University New England (Psy.D.)
Argosy University, Atlanta Campus (Psy.D.) (Cl)
Argosy University, Chicago (Cl)
Argosy University, Hawaii Campus (Psy.D.)
Antioch University New England (Psy.D.)
Argosy University, Twin Cities Campus (Psy.D.) (Cl)
Argosy University, Washington DC Campus (Psy.D) (Cl)
Arizona State University (Cl)
Bowling Green State University (Cl)
Chicago School of Professional Psychology (Psy.D.) (Cl)
City University of New York at City College (Cl)
Drexel University (Cl)
Duke University (Cl)
Fielding Graduate University (Cl)
Florida Institute of Technology (Psy.D.) (Cl)
Fordham University (Cl)
Indiana State University (Psy.D.) (Cl)
Indiana University of Pennsylvania (Psy.D.) (Cl)
Kent State University (Cl)
La Salle University (Psy.D.) (Cl)
Loma Linda University (Cl)
Massachusetts School of Professional Psychology (Psy.D.) (Cl)
New Mexico University (Co)
Ohio University (Cl)
Ohio State University (Cl)
Oklahoma State University (Cl)

Our Lady of the Lake University (Psy.D.) (Co)
Ponce School of Medicine (Cl)
Regent University (Cl)
Rosalind Franklin University of Medicine and Science (Cl)
Spalding University (Psy.D.) (Cl)
Syracuse University (Cl)
Texas A&M University (Co)
University of Alabama at Tuscaloosa (Cl)
University of Cincinnati (Cl)
University of Connecticut (Cl)
University of Florida (Cl)
University of Indianapolis (Psy.D.) (Cl)
University of Iowa (Cl)
University of Kansas (Cl)
University of Kentucky (Cl)
University of Maryland, Baltimore County (Cl)
The University of Memphis (Cl)
University of Miami (Cl & Co)
University of Missouri Kansas City (Cl)
University of Missouri–St. Louis (Cl)
University of Pittsburgh (Cl)
University of South Florida (Cl)
University of Texas–Austin (Co)
University of Texas Southwestern Medical Center at Dallas (Cl)
University of Utah (Cl)
University of Wyoming (Cl)
Utah State University (Cm)
Virginia Commonwealth University (Cl)
Wayne State University (Cl)
West Virginia University (Cl)
Widener University (Psy.D.) (Cl)
York University (Cl)

Human Development/ Developmental/Lifespan

Concordia University (Cl)
West Virginia University (Cl)
University of Delaware (Cl)
University of Maine (Cl)
University of Minnesota (Cl)
University of Pittsburgh (Cl)
University of Rochester (Cl)
University of Victoria (Cl)
York University (Clinical-Developmental Psychology) (Cl)

Multicultural/Cross-Cultural/Diversity

Alliant International University–Los Angeles (Psy.D. & Ph.D.) (Cl)
Alliant International University–San Diego (Psy.D. & Ph.D.) (Cl)
Alliant International University–San Francisco Bay (Psy.D. & Ph.D.) (Cl)
Argosy University, Chicago (Cl)
Argosy University, Hawaii Campus (Psy.D.) (Cl)

Argosy University, Washington DC Campus (Psy.D) (Cl)
Ball State University (Co)
Catholic University of America (Cl)
Chicago School of Professional Psychology (Psy.D.) (Cl)
JFK University (Cl)
Marquette University (Co)
McGill University (Co)
New Mexico State University (Co)
Pacific University (Cl)
Pepperdine University (Cl)
Seton Hall University (Co)
Texas A&M University (Co)
Texas Woman's University (Co)
University of La Verne (Psy.D.) (Cl)
University of Memphis (Co)
University of Miami (Co)
University of Missouri–Columbia (Co)
University of Nebraska–Lincoln (Co)
University of Texas–Austin (Co)
Widener University (Psy.D.) (Cl)

Neuropsychology

Adler School of Professional Psychology (Cl)
Argosy University, Atlanta Campus (Psy.D.) (Cl)
Argosy University, Washington DC Campus (Psy.D) (Cl)
Boston University (Cl)
Brigham Young University (Cl)
Concordia University (Cl)
Carlos Albizu University–Miami Campus (Psy.D.) (Cl)
Drexel University (Cl)
Fielding Graduate University (Cl)
Florida Institute of Technology (Psy.D.) (Cl)
Fordham University (Cl)
Forest Institute of Professional Psychology (Cl)
Georgia State University (Cl)
Loma Linda University (Cl)
Loyola University of Chicago (Cl)
Northwestern University, Feinberg School of Medicine (Cl)
Pacific University (Cl)
Ponce School of Medicine (Cl)
Rosalind Franklin University of Medicine and Science (Cl)
Seton Hall University (Co)
Simon Fraser University (Cl)
Suffolk University (Cl)
University of Alabama at Birmingham (Cl)
University of Cincinnati (Cl)
University of Colorado at Boulder (Cl)
University of Connecticut (Cl)
University of Florida (Cl)
University of Georgia (Cl)
University of Houston (Cl)
University of Iowa (Cl)
University of Kentucky (Cl)
University of Montana (Cl)
University of Ottawa (Cl)
University of Rhode Island (Cl)

University of South Florida (Cl)
University of Texas Southwestern Medical Center at Dallas
(Cl)
University of Utah (Cl)
University of Victoria (Cl)
University of Windsor (Cl)
Virginia Consortium Program in Clinical Psychology
(Psy.D.) (Cl)
Wayne State University (Cl)
Widener University (Psy.D.) (Cl)

Organizational/Consulting

Pacific University (Cl)
Regent University (Cl)
Widener University (Psy.D.) (Cl)

Psychoanalytic/Psychodynamic Therapy

Alliant International University–San Diego (Psy.D. & Ph.D.)
(Cl)
Alliant International University–San Francisco Bay (Psy.D. &
Ph.D.) (Cl)
Pepperdine University (Psy.D.) (Cl)
University of Toledo (Cl)
Widener University (Psy.D.) (Cl)

Sport Psychology/Clinical Sport

La Salle University (Psy.D.) (Cl)
Rutgers, The State University of New Jersey (Psy.D.) (Cl)
University of Denver (Psy.D.) (Cl)
University of Missouri–Columbia (Co)
University of North Texas (Co)

Substance Abuse/Addiction

Adler School of Professional Psychology (Cl)
Immaculata University (Psy.D.) (Cl)
Marquette University (Co)
Syracuse University (Cl)
University of South Florida (Cl)

Supervision/Clinical Supervision

Yeshiva University (Psy.D.)
McGill University (Co)
New Mexico State University (Co)
University of Florida (Co)

Trauma/Disaster

Argosy University–Twin Cities Campus (Psy.D.)
Miami University (Cl)

University of Denver (Psy.D.) (Cl)
University of Missouri–St. Louis (Cl)
University of South Dakota (Cl)

Miscellaneous

AD/HD—University of North Carolina at Greensboro (Cl)
Adlerian psychotherapy—Adler School of Professional
Psychology (Cl)
applied methodology—University of Rhode Island (Cl)
applied behavior analysis—West Virginia University (Cl);
Eastern Michigan University (Cl)
behavioral genetics—University of Colorado at Boulder (Cl)
career development—University of Missouri–Columbia (Co)
clinical and health research—Concordia University (Cl)
close relationship—Stony Brook University/State University
of New York (Cl)
group—Widener University (Psy.D.) (Cl), Adler School of
Professional Psychology (Cl)
health service administration & business—Xavier University
(Psy.D.) (Cl)
human factors—University of Cincinnati (Cl)
humanistic existential—Pepperdine University (Psy.D.) (Cl)
infant mental health—Seton Hall University (Co)
integrated health care—Forest Institute of Professional
Psychology (Cl)
international studies—University of Memphis (Co)
leadership—Fuller Theological Seminary (Psy.D.) (Cl)
medical clinical—Uniformed Services University of Health
Sciences (Cl); University of Alabama at Birmingham
(Cl)
military clinical—Uniformed Services University of Health
Sciences (Cl)
pediatric health—Loma Linda University (Cl); University of
Miami (Cl)
personality—University of Iowa (Cl); University of South
Florida (Cl)
primary care psychology—Adler School of Professional
Psychology (Cl)
psychological testing—Immaculata University (Psy.D.) (Cl);
Chestnut Hill University (Psy.D.) (Cl)
psychopathology—Rosalind Franklin University of Medicine
and Science (Cl)
psychotherapy research—University of Memphis (Cl);
McGill University (Co)
public health—Loma Linda University (Cl)
rehabilitation—Illinois Institute of Technology (Cl)
rural/minority—Utah State University (Cm)
severe mental illness—Xavier University (Psy.D.) (Cl)
statistics—University of Missouri–Columbia (Co)
teaching—University of Missouri–Columbia (Co)

REFERENCES

Accredited doctoral programs in professional psychology: 2006. (2006). *American Psychologist, 61,* 991–1005.

Actkinson, T. R. (2000, Winter). Master's and myth. *Eye on Psi Chi, 4,* 19–25.

American Psychological Association. (1986). *Careers in psychology.* Washington, DC: Author.

American Psychological Association. (2007). *Graduate study in psychology.* Washington, DC: Author.

American Psychological Association. (2002). Ethical principles of psychologists and code of conduct. *American Psychologist, 57,* 1060–1073.

American Psychological Association Research Office. (1999). *Demographic characteristics of Division 12 and Division 17 members: 1997.* Washington, DC: Author.

American Psychological Association Research Office. (2000). *1998–1999 Survey of Graduate Departments of Psychology.* Washington, DC: Author.

American Psychological Association Research Office. (2003). *2001 doctorate employment survey.* Washington, DC: Author.

American Psychological Association. (2006). *The APAGS resource guide for LGBT students in psychology.* Washington, DC: Author.

Anderson, N., & Shackleton, V. (1990). Decision making in the graduate selection interview: A field study. *Journal of Occupational Psychology, 63,* 63–76.

APA Practice Directorate. (1991). *Summary of psychology licensing or certification laws.* Washington, DC: Author.

APPIC. (2006). *APPIC Match: 2000–2006 match rates by doctoral program.* Washington, DC: Association of Psychology Postdoctoral and Internship Centers. Also at www.appic.org/downloads/APPIC_match_2000-06 _by_state.pdf

Appleby, D. C., & Appleby, K. M. (2003, August). *The "kisses of death" in the graduate school applications process.* Poster presented at the annual convention of the American Psychological Association, Toronto.

Appleby, D., Keenan, J., & Mauer, B. (1999, Spring). Applicant characteristics valued by graduate programs in psychology. *Eye on Psi Chi, 3,* 39.

Asher, D. (2000) *Graduate admissions essays: How to write your way into the graduate program of your choice.* Berkeley, CA: Ten Speed Press.

Association of State and Provincial Psychology Boards and National Register of Health Service Providers in Psychology. (2005). *Doctoral psychology programs meeting designation criteria.* Washington, DC: National Register.

Astin, A. W., Green, K. C., & Korn, W. S. (1987). *The American freshman: Twenty-year trends 1966–85.* University of California, Cooperative Institutional Research Program, American Council on Education.

Ault, R. L. (1993). To waive or not to waive? Students' misconceptions about the confidentiality choice for letters of recommendation. *Teaching of Psychology, 20,* 44–45.

Barron, J. (1986). Search for survival and identity—and power. *The Clinical Psychologist, 39,* 61–63.

Bartsch, R. A., Warren, T. D., Sharp, A. D., & Green, M. A. (2003). Assessment of psychology graduate program information on the Web. *Teaching of Psychology, 30,* 167–170.

Bechtoldt, H., Norcross, J. C., Wyckoff, L. A., Pokrywa, M. L., & Campbell, L. F. (2001). Theoretical orientations and employment settings of clinical and counseling psychologists: A comparative study. *The Clinical Psychologist, 54*(1), 3–6.

Bernal, M. E., Sirolli, A. A., Weisser, S. K., Ruiz, J. A., Chamberlain, V. J., & Knight, G. P. (1999). Relevance of multicultural training to students' applications to clinical psychology programs. *Cultural Diversity and Ethnic Minority Psychology, 5,* 43–55.

Bernstein, B. L., & Kerr, B. (1993). Counseling psychology and the scientist–practitioner model: Implementation and implications. *The Counseling Psychologist, 21,* 136–151.

Bersoff, D. N., Goodman-Delahunty, J., Grisso, J. T., Hans, V. P., Poythress, N. G., & Roesch, R. G. (1997). Training in law and psychology: Models from the Villanova Conference. *American Psychologist, 52,* 1301–1310.

Beutler, L. E., & Fisher, D. (1994). Combined specialty training in counseling, clinical, and school psychology: An idea whose time has returned. *Professional Psychology: Research and Practice, 25,* 62–69.

Biaggio, M., Orchard, S., Larson, J., Petrino, K., & Mihara, R. (2003). Guidelines for gay/lesbian/bisexual-affirmative educational practices in graduate psychology programs. *Professional Psychology: Research & Practice, 34,* 548–554.

Boitano, J. J. (1999, August). *Graduate training in neuroscience.* Paper presented at the 107th annual convention of the American Psychological Association, Boston, MA.

Bolles, R. N. (2006). *What color is your parachute? A practical manual for job-hunters and career-changes* (2006 ed.). Berkeley, CA: Ten Speed Press.

Bonifzi, D. Z., Crespy, S. D., & Reiker, P. (1997). Value of a master's degree for gaining admission to doctoral programs in psychology. *Teaching of Psychology, 24,* 176–182.

Bottoms, B. L., & Nysse, K. L. (1999, Fall). Applying to graduate school: Writing a compelling personal statement. *Eye on Psi Chi, 4,* 20–22.

Boudreau, R. A., Killip, S. M., MacInnis, S. H., Milloy, D. G., & Rogers, T. B. (1983). An evaluation of Graduate Record Examinations as predictors of graduate success in a Canadian context. *Canadian Psychology, 24,* 191–199.

Brems, C., & Johnson, M. E. (1997). Comparison of recent graduates of clinical versus counseling psychology programs. *Journal of Psychology, 131,* 91–99.

Briihl, D. S., & Wasieleski, D. T. (2004). A survey of master's-level psychology programs: Admissions criteria and program policies. *Teaching of Psychology, 31,* 252–256.

Bullock, M. (1997, July/August). Federal funding is available for psychology graduate students. *Psychological Science Agenda,* p. 4.

Burgess, D., Keeley, J., & Blashfield, R. (2006, August). *Full disclosure data on clinical psychology doctorate programs: The need to be fuller and more disclosing.* Poster presented at the 114th annual convention of the American Psychological Association, New Orleans.

Buskist, W., & Mixon, A. (1998). *Master's programs in psychology and counseling psychology.* Needham Heights, MA: Allyn & Bacon.

Cashin, J. R., & Landrum, R. E. (1991). Undergraduate students' perceptions of graduate admissions in psychology. *Psychological Reports, 69,* 1107–1110.

Castle, P. H., & Norcross, J. C. (2002, August). *Empirical data and integrative perspectives on combined doctoral programs.* Paper presented at the 110th annual convention of the American Psychological Association, Chicago, IL.

Ceci, S. J., & Peters, D. (1984). Letters of reference: A naturalistic study of the effects of confidentiality. *American Psychologist, 39,* 29–31.

Chanatry, J. A. (2007). *Medical school admission requirements (MSAR) 2008–2009: The most authoritative guide to U.S. and Canadian medical schools* (58th ed.). Association of American Medical Colleges.

Chapman, C. P., & Lane, H. C. (1997). Perceptions about the use of letters of recommendation. *The Advisor, 17,* 31–36.

Chernyshenko, O. S., & Ones, D. S. (1999). How selective are psychology graduate programs? The effect of the selection ratio on GRE score validity. *Educational and Psychological Measurement, 59,* 951–961.

Cobb, H. C., Reeve, R. E., Shealy, C. N., Norcross, J. C., et al. (2004). Overlap among clinical, counseling, and school psychology: Implications for the profession and combined-integrated training. *Journal of Clinical Psychology, 60,* 939–956.

Collins, L. H. (2001, Winter). Does research experience make a significant difference in graduate admissions? *Eye on Psi Chi, 5,* 26–28.

Conway, J. B. (1988). Differences among clinical psychologists: Scientists, practitioners, and scientist–practitioners. *Professional Psychology: Research and Practice, 19,* 642–655.

Corcoran, K. J., Michels, J. L., & Ahina, L. K. (1999, August). *Clinical surfing: Clinical psychology doctoral programs on the web.* Paper presented at the 107th annual convention of the American Psychological Association, Boston, MA.

Coyle, S. L., & Bae, Y. (1987). *Summary report 1986: Doctorate recipients from United States universities.* Washington, DC: National Academy Press.

Crowe, M. B., Grogan, J. M., Jacobs, R. R., Lindsay, C. A., & Mack, M. M. (1985). Delineation of the roles of clinical psychology: A survey of practice in psychology. *Professional Psychology: Research and Practice, 16,* 124–137.

Dattilio, F. (1992). Doctoral studies for master's level licensed psychologists. *The Pennsylvania Psychologist Quarterly, 52*(2), 7, 11.

Dollinger, S. J. (1989). Predictive validity of the Graduate Record Examination in a clinical psychology program. *Professional Psychology: Research and Practice, 20,* 56–58.

Drummond, F., Rodolfa, E., & Smith, D. (1981). A survey of APA- and non-APA-approved internship programs. *American Psychologist, 36,* 411–414.

Eddy, B., Lloyd, P. J., & Lubin, B. (1987). Enhancing the application to doctoral professional programs: Suggestions from a national survey. *Teaching of Psychology, 14,* 160–163.

Educational Testing Service (ETS). (1984). *Analysis of score change patterns of examinees repeating the GRE General test.* Princeton, NJ: Educational testing Service.

Educational Testing Service. (1995). *Practicing to take the GRE Psychology Test* (3rd ed.). Princeton, NJ: Author.

Elam, C. L., et al. (1998). Letters of recommendation: Medical school admission committee members' recommendations. *The Advisor, 18,* 4–6.

Farry, J., Norcross, J. C., Mayne, T. J., & Sayette, M. A. (1995, August). *Acceptance rates and financial aid in clinical psychology: An update.* Poster presented at the 103rd annual convention of the American Psychological Association, New York, NY.

Fauber, R. L. (2006). Graduate admissions in clinical psychology: Observations on the present and thoughts on the future. *Clinical Psychology: Science and Practice, 13*, 227–234.

Fennell, K., & Kohout, J. (2002). *Characteristics of graduate departments of psychology: 1999–2000.* Washington, DC: American Psychological Association.

Ferrari, J. R., & Hemovich, V. B. (2004). Student-based psychology journals: Perceptions by graduate program directors. *Teaching of Psychology, 31*, 272–275.

Fitzgerald, L. F., & Osipow, S. H. (1986). An occupational analysis of counseling psychology. How special is the specialty? *American Psychologist, 41*, 535–544.

Fretz, B. R. (1976, Spring). Finding careers with a bachelor's degree in psychology. *Psi Chi Newsletter, 2*, 5–13.

Fretz, B. R., & Stang, D. J. (1980). *Preparing for graduate study in psychology: Not for seniors only!* Washington, DC: American Psychological Association.

Gaddy, C. D., Charlot-Swilley, D., Nelson, P. D., & Reich, J. N. (1995). Selected outcomes of accredited programs. *Professional Psychology: Research and Practice, 26*, 507–513.

Gartner, J. D. (1986). Antireligious prejudice in admissions to doctoral programs in clinical psychology. *Professional Psychology: Research and Practice, 17*, 473–475.

Gehlman, S., Wicherski, M., & Kohout, J. (1995). *Characteristics of graduate departments of psychology: 1993–1994.* Washington, DC: American Psychological Association Research Office.

Goldberg, E. L., & Alliger, G. M. (1992). Assessing the validity of the GRE for students in psychology: A validity generalization approach. *Educational and Psychological Measurement, 52*, 1019–1027.

Golding, J. M., Lang, K., Eymard, L. A., & Shadish, W. R. (1988). The buck stops here: A survey of the financial status of Ph.D. graduate students in psychology, 1966–1987. *American Psychologist, 43*, 1089–1091.

Goliszek, A. (2000). *The complete medical school preparation and admissions guide.* New York: Healthnet Press.

Gordon, R. A. (1990). Research productivity in master's-level psychology programs. *Professional Psychology: Research and Practice, 21*, 33–36.

Graduate Record Examinations. (2007). *2007–2008 GRE information and registration bulletin.* Princeton, NJ: Educational Testing Service.

Grote, C. L., Robiner, W. N., & Haut, A. (2001). Disclosure of negative information in letters of recommendation: Writers' intentions and readers' experiences. *Professional Psychology: Research and Practice, 32*, 655–661.

Halgin, R. P. (1986). Advising undergraduates who wish to become clinicians. *Teaching of Psychology, 13*, 7–12.

Hall, J. E., Wexelbaum, S. F., & Boucher, A. P. (2007). Looking ahead: Planning for a successful career as a psychologist. *Eye on Psi Chi, 12(2)*, 10–12.

Hayes, S. C., & Hayes, L. J. (1989). Writing your vitae. *APS Observer, 2(3)*, 15–17.

Heppner, P. P., & Downing, N. E. (1982). Job interviewing for new psychologists: Riding the emotional rollercoaster. *Professional Psychology, 13*, 334–341.

Hersh, J. B., & Poey, K. (1984). A proposed interviewing guide for intern applicants. *Professional Psychology, 15*, 3–5.

Hershey, J. M., Kopplin, D. A., & Cornell, J. F. (1991). Doctors of psychology. Their career experiences and attitudes toward degree and training. *Professional Psychology: Research and Practice, 22*, 351–356.

Hines, D. (1985). Admissions criteria for ranking master's-level applicants to clinical doctoral programs. *Teaching of Psychology, 13*, 64–66.

Holmes, C. B., & Beishline, M. J. (1996, August). *Doctoral admission rates for students with GRE scores below 1000.* Poster presented at the 104th annual meeting of the American Psychological Association, Toronto.

Huss, M. T., Randall, B. A., Patry, M., Davis, S. F., & Hansen, D. J. (2002). Factors influencing self-rated preparedness for graduate school: A survey of graduate schools. *Teaching of Psychology, 29*, 275–281.

Ilardi, S. S., Rodriguez-Hanley, A., Roberts, M. G., & Seigel, J. (2000). On the origins of clinical psychology faculty: Who is training the trainers? *Clinical Psychology: Science and Practice, 7*, 346–354.

Ingram, R. E. (1983). The GRE in the graduate admissions process: Is how it is used justified by the evidence of its validity? *Professional Psychology: Research and Practice, 14*, 711–714.

Jacob, M. C. (1987). Managing the internship application experience: Advice from an exhausted but content survivor. *The Counseling Psychologist, 15*, 146–155.

Jensen, A. R. (1998). *The g factor: The science of mental ability.* Westport, CT: Praeger.

Kaiser, J. C., Kaiser, A. J., Richardson, N. J., & Fox, E. J. (2007). Undergraduate research experiences : "Are all research experiences rated equally?" *Eye on Psi Chi, 12(2)*, 22–24.

Kalat, J. W., & Matlin, M. W. (2000). The GRE Psychology Test: A useful but poorly understood test. *Teaching of Psychology, 27*, 24–27.

Keith-Spiegel, P. (1991). *The complete guide to graduate school admission.* Hillsdale, NJ: Lawrence Erlbaum.

Keith-Spiegel, P., Tabachnick, B. G., & Spiegel, G. B. (1994). When demand exceeds supply: Second-order criteria used by graduate school selection committees. *Teaching of Psychology, 21*, 79–81.

Keith-Spiegel, P., & Wiederman, M. W. (2000). *The complete guide to graduate school admission* (2nd ed.). Mahwah, NJ: Lawrence Erlbaum.

Keller, J. W., Beam, K. J., Maier, K. A., & Pietrowski, C. (1995, April). *Research or clinical experience: What doctoral applicants need to know.* Paper presented at the annual meeting of the Southeastern Psychological Association, Savannah, GA.

Kellogg, R. T. (2003). *GRE Psychology with CD-ROM—The best test prep for the GRE.* Piscataway, NJ: Research & Education Association.

Khubchandani, A. (2002). To disclose or not to disclose: That is the question. *The APAGS Newsletter, 14*(4), 24–26.

King, D. W., Beehr, T. A., & King, L. A. (1986). Doctoral student selection in one professional psychology program. *Journal of Clinical Psychology, 42,* 399–407.

Kluger, J. (2002, June 10). Pumping up your past. *Time,* p. 45.

Kohout, J. L., & Wicherski, M. M. (1992). *1991 salaries in psychology.* Washington, DC: American Psychological Association.

Kohout, J., & Wicherski, M. (1993). *1991–1992 characteristics of graduate departments of psychology.* Washington, DC: American Psychological Association.

Kohout, J. & Wicherski, M. (1999). *1997 doctorate employment survey.* Washington, DC: American Psychological Association Research Office.

Kohout, J., Wicherski, M., & Pion, G. (1991). *Characteristics of graduate departments of psychology: 1988–89.* Washington, DC: American Psychological Association.

Kopala, M., Keitel, M. A., Suzuki, L. A., Alexander, C. M., Ponterotto, J. G., Reynolds, A. L., & Hennessy, J. J. (1995). Doctoral admissions in counseling psychology at Fordham University. *Teaching of Psychology, 22,* 133–135.

Korn, J. H. (1984). New odds on acceptance into Ph.D. programs in psychology. *American Psychologist, 39,* 179–180.

Kuncel, N. R., Hezlett, S. A., & Ones, D. S. (2001). A comprehensive meta-analysis of the predictive validity of the graduate record examinations: Implications for graduate student selection and performance. *Psychological Bulletin, 127,* 162–181.

Kupfersmid, J., & Fiola, M. (1991). Comparison of EPPP scores among graduates of varying psychology programs. *American Psychologist, 46,* 534–535.

Kyle, T. M. (2000, July/August). Investigating and choosing: The decision-making process among first-year graduate students. *APA Monitor,* p. 19.

Landrum, R. E. (2003). Graduate admissions in psychology: Transcripts and the effect of withdrawals. *Teaching of Psychology, 30,* 323–325.

Landrum, R. E., & Nelson, L. R. (2002). The undergraduate research assistantship: An analysis of benefits. *Teaching of Psychology, 29,* 15–19.

Lark, J. S., & Croteau, J. M. (1998). Lesbian, gay, and bisexual doctoral students' mentoring relationships with faculty in counseling psychology: A qualitative study. *The Counseling Psychologist, 26,* 754–776.

Lovitts, B. E., & Nelson, C. (2000, November–December). Attrition from Ph.D. programs. *Academe,* pp. 44–50.

Lubin, B. (1993, Winter). Message of the president. *Psi Chi Newsletter, 19,* 1.

Maher, B. A. (1999). Changing trends in doctoral training programs in psychology: A comparative analysis of research-oriented versus professional-applied programs. *Psychological Sciences, 10,* 475–481.

Mayne, T. J., Norcross, J. C., & Sayette, M. A. (1994). Admission requirements, acceptance rates, and financial assistance in clinical psychology programs: Diversity across the practice–research continuum. *American Psychologist, 49,* 605–611.

McWade, P. (1996). *Financing graduate school.* Princeton, NJ: Peterson's Guides.

Megargee, E. I. (1990). *A guide to obtaining a psychology internship.* Muncie, IN: Accelerated Development.

Megargee, E. I. (2001). *Megargee's guide to obtaining a psychology internship* (4th ed.). New York: Taylor & Francis.

Minke, K. M., & Brown, D. T. (1996). Preparing psychologists to work with children: A comparison of curricula in child-clinical and school psychology programs. *Professional Psychology: Research and Practice, 27,* 631–634.

Mitchell, S. L. (1996). Getting a foot in the door: The written internship application. *Professional Psychology: Research and Practice, 27,* 90–92.

Morgan, R. D., & Cohen, L. M. (2003, August). *Counseling and clinical psychology: Are we training students differently?* Poster presented at the annual convention of the American Psychological Association, Toronto.

Morrison, T., & Morrison, M. (1995). A meta-analytic assessment of the predictive validity of the quantitative and verbal components of the Graduate Record Examination with graduate grade point average representing the criterion of graduate success. *Educational and Psychological Measurement, 55,* 309–316.

Munoz-Dunbar, R., & Stanton, A. L. (1999). Ethnic diversity in clinical psychology: Recruitment and admission practices among doctoral programs. *Teaching of Psychology, 26,* 259–263.

Murray, B. (1996). Psychology remains top college major. *APA Monitor, 27,* 1, 42.

Murray, T. M., & Williams, S. (1999). *Analyses of data from graduate study in psychology: 1997–98.* Washington, DC: American Psychological Association Research Office.

National Association of Colleges and Employers. (2007). *Career Services Benchmark Survey.* Retrieved July 26, 2007 from www.naceweb.org/press/current asp.

Nauta, M. M. (2000). Assessing the accuracy of psychology undergraduates' perceptions of graduate admissions criteria. *Teaching of Psychology, 27,* 277–280.

Nevid, J. S., & Gildea, T. J. (1984). The admissions process in clinical training: The role of the personal interview. *Professional Psychology: Research and Practice, 15,* 18–25.

Norcross, J. C., Castle, P. H., Sayette, M. A. & Mayne, T. J. (2004). The Psy.D.: Heterogeneity in practitioner training. *Professional Psychology: Research and Practice, 35,* 412–419.

Norcross, J. C., Gallagher, K. M., & Prochaska, J. O. (1989). The Boulder and/or the Vail model: Training preferences of clinical psychologists. *Journal of Clinical Psychology, 45,* 822–828.

Norcross, J. C., & Goldfried, M. R. (Eds.). (2005). *Handbook of psychotherapy integration.* New York: Oxford University Press.

Norcross, J. C., Hanych, J. M., & Terranova, R. D. (1996). Graduate study in psychology: 1992–1993. *American Psychologist, 51,* 631–643.

Norcross, J. C., Hedges, M., & Prochaska, J. O. (2002). The face of 2010: A Delphi poll on the future of psychotherapy. *Professional Psychology: Research and Practice, 33,* 316–322.

Norcross, J. C., & Kaplan, K. J. (1995). Training in psychotherapy integration. Integrative/eclectic programs. *Journal of Psychotherapy Integration, 5*(3).

Norcross, J. C., Karg, R. S., & Prochaska, J. O. (1997a). Clinical psychologists in the 1990s; Part I. *The Clinical Psychologist, 50*(2), 4–9.

Norcross, J. C., Karg, R. S., & Prochaska, J. O. (1997b). Clinical psychologists in the 1990s: Part II. *The Clinical Psychologist, 50*(3), 4–11.

Norcross, J. C., Karpiak, C. P., & Santoro, S. O. (2005). Clinical psychologists across the years: The Division of Clinical Psychology from 1960 to 2003. *Journal of Clinical Psychology, 61,* 1467–1483.

Norcross, J. C., Kohout, J. L., & Wicherski, M. (2005). Graduate study in psychology, 1971–2004. *American Psychologist, 60,* 840–850.

Norcross, J. C., & Oliver, J. M. (2005, March). *An update on PsyD programs: Acceptance rates, financial assistance, and selected outcomes by program setting.* Poster presented at the 76th annual meeting of the Eastern Psychological Association, Boston, MA.

Norcross, J. C., Sayette, M. A., Mayne, T. J., Karg, R. S., & Turkson, M. A. (1998). Selecting a doctoral program in professional psychology: Some comparisons among Ph.D. counseling, Ph.D. clinical, and Psy.D. clinical psychology programs. *Professional Psychology: Research and Practice, 29,* 609–614.

O'Donohue, W., Plaud, J. J., Mowatt, A. M., & Fearon, J. R. (1989). Current status of curricula of doctoral training programs in clinical psychology. *Professional Psychology: Research and Practice, 20,* 196–197.

Oliver, J. M., Norcross, J. C., Sayette, M. A., Griffin, K., & Mayne, T. J. (2005, March). *Doctoral study in clinical, counseling, and combined psychology: Admission requirements and student characteristics.* Poster presented at the 76th annual meeting of the Eastern Psychological Association, Boston, MA.

O'Neill, J. V. (2001, September). Image seen as key to social work's future. *NASW News,* p. 3.

Osborne, R. E. (1996, Fall). The "personal" side of graduate school personal statements. *Eye on Psi Chi, 1,* 14–15.

Otto, R. K., & Heilbrun, K. (2002). The practice of forensic psychology: A look toward the future in light of the past. *American Psychologist, 57,* 5–18.

Pate, W. E. II. (2001). *Analyses of data from Graduate Study in Psychology: 1999–2000.* Washington, DC: American Psychological Association Research Office.

Peterson, D. R. (1976). Need for the doctor of psychology degree in professional psychology. *American Psychologist, 31,* 792–798.

Peterson, D. R. (1982). Origins and development of the Doctor of Psychology concept. In G. R. Caddy, D. C. Rimm, H. Watson, & J. H. Johnson (Eds.), *Educating professional psychologists* (pp. 19–38). New Brunswick, NJ: Transaction Books.

Peterson, D. R., Eaton, M. M., Levine, A. R., & Snepp, F. P. (1982). Career experiences of doctors of psychology. *Professional Psychology, 13,* 268–277.

Peterson's grants for graduate and postdoctoral study (5th ed.). (1998). Princeton, NJ: Peterson's.

Piotrowski, C., & Keller, J. W. (1996). Research or clinical experience: What doctoral applicants need to know. *Journal of Instructional Psychology, 23,* 126–127.

Prevoznak, M. A., & Bubka, A. (1999, April). *Word-a-day method in preparation for the GRE.* Poster presented at the annual meeting of the Eastern Psychological Association, Providence, RI.

Princeton Review. (2005). *Paying for graduate school without going broke* (2005 edition). Princeton: Author.

Princeton Review. (2005). *Cracking the GRE Psychology.* Princeton: Author.

Psychological Corporation. (1994). *Miller Analogies Test: Technical manual.* San Antonio, TX: Author.

Purdy, J. E., Reinehr, R. C., & Swartz, J. D. (1989). Graduate admissions criteria of leading psychology departments. *American Psychologist, 44,* 960–961.

Rader, J. (2000). Disclosing a lesbian, gay, or bisexual identity in graduate psychology programs: Risk and rewards. *APAGS, 12*(2).

Raphael, S., & Halpert, L. H. (1999). *Graduate Record Examination—Psychology* (3rd ed.). New York: Prentice Hall.

Rem, R., Oren, E. M., & Childrey, G. (1987). Selection of graduate students in clinical psychology: Use of cutoff scores and interviews. *Professional Psychology: Research and Practice, 18,* 485–488.

Resnick, J. H. (1991). Finally, a definition of clinical psychology: A message from the President, Division 12. *The Clinical Psychologist, 44*(1), 3–4.

Rheingold, H. L. (1994). *The psychologist's guide to an academic career.* Washington, DC: American Psychological Association.

Robyak, J. E., & Goodyear, R. K. (1984). Graduate school origins of diplomates and fellows in professional psychology. *Professional Psychology: Research and Practice, 15,* 379–387.

Rogers, M. R., & Molina, L. E. (2006). Exemplary efforts in psychology to recruit and retain graduate students of color. *American Psychologist, 61,* 143–156.

Sachs, M. L., Burke, K. L., & Loughren, E. A. (2006). *Directory of graduate programs in applied sport psychology* (8th ed.). Morgantown, WV: Fitness Information Technology.

Salzinger, K. (Chair). (1998, August). *Combined professional-scientific psychology: Greater than the sum of its parts?* Symposium presented at the 106th annual convention of the American Psychological Association, San Francisco, CA.

Sayette, M. A., & Mayne, T. J. (1990). Survey of current clinical and research trends in clinical psychology. *American Psychologist, 45,* 1263–1267.

Sayette, M. A., Mayne, T. J., Norcross, J. C., & Giuffre, D. E. (1999, June). *Letting a hundred flowers bloom? Ph.D. clinical psychology training in the 1990s.* Paper presented at annual meeting of the Academy of Psychological Clinical Science, Denver, CO.

Schaefer, S. E. (1995). Stigmatization of psychology doctoral program applicants who have a history of psychological counseling. *Dissertation Abstracts, 57*(02B), 1427.

Scott, W. C., & Silka, L. D. (1974). Applying to graduate school in psychology: A perspective and guide. *Journal Supplement Abstract Service,* MS. 597.

Shaffer, D. R., & Tomarelli, M. (1981). Bias in the ivory tower: An unintended consequence of the Buckley Amendment for graduate admissions. *Journal of Applied Psychology, 66,* 7–11.

Shealy, C. N. (Ed.). (2004). Special issues: The Consensus Conference and combined-integrated model of doctoral training in professional psychology. *Journal of Clinical Psychology, 60,* issues 9 and 10.

Smith, R. A. (1985). Advising beginning psychology majors for graduate school. *Teaching of Psychology, 12,* 194–198.

Snepp, F. P., & Peterson, D. R. (1988). Evaluative comparison of Psy.D. and Ph.D. students by clinical internship supervisors. *Professional Psychology: Research and Practice, 19,* 180–183.

Society for Industrial and Organizational Psychology. (2006). *Graduate training in industrial/organizational psychology and related fields.* Bowling Green, OH: Author.

Stapp, J., Tucker, A. M., & VandenBos, G. R. (1985). Census of psychological personnel: 1983. *American Psychologist, 40,* 1317–1351.

Steinpreis, R., Queen, L., & Tennen, H. (1992). The education of clinical psychologists: A survey of training directors. *The Clinical Psychologist, 45,* 87–94.

Sternberg, R. J. (Ed.). (2006). *Career paths in psychology: Where your degree can take you* (2nd ed.). Washington, DC: American Psychological Association.

Sternberg, R. J., & Williams, W. M. (1997). Does the graduate record examination predict meaningful success in the graduate training of psychologists? *American Psychologist, 52,* 630–641.

Stewart, A. E., & Stewart, E. A. (1996). A decision-making technique for choosing a psychology internship. *Professional Psychology: Research and Practice, 27,* 521–526.

Stewart, D. W., & Spille, H. A. (1988). *Diploma mills: Degrees of fraud.* New York: Macmillan.

Strickland, B. R. (1985). Over the Boulder(s) and through the Vail. *The Clinical Psychologist, 38,* 52–56.

Terry, R. L. (1996, December). Characteristics of psychology departments at primarily undergraduate institutions. *Council on Undergraduate Research Quarterly,* pp. 86–90.

Tibbits-Kleber, A. L., & Howell, R. J. (1987). Doctoral training in clinical psychology: A students' perspective. *Professional Psychology: Research and Practice, 18,* 634–639.

Tipton, R. M. (1983). Clinical and counseling psychology: A study of roles and functions. *Professional Psychology: Research and Practice, 14,* 837–846.

Titus, J. B., & Buxman, N. J. (1999, Spring). Is Psi Chi meeting its mission statement? *Eye on Psi Chi, 3,* 16–18.

Todd, D. M., & Farinato, D. (1992). A local resource for advising applicants to clinical psychology graduate programs. *Teaching of Psychology, 19,* 52–54.

Toia, A., Herron, W. G., Primavera, L. H., & Javier, R. A. (1997). Ethnic diversification in clinical psychology training. *Cultural Diversity and Mental Health, 3,* 193–206.

Toma, J. D., & Cross, M. E. (1998). Intercollegiate athletics and student college choice: Exploring the impact of championship seasons on undergraduate applications. *Research in Higher Education, 39,* 633–661.

Tryon, G. S. (1985). What can our students learn from regional psychology conventions? *Teaching of Psychology, 12,* 227–228.

Tryon, G. S. (2000). Doctoral training issues in school and clinical child psychology. *Professional Psychology: Research and Practice, 31,* 85–87.

Turkington, C. (1986). Practitioner training. *APA Monitor, 17*(1), 14, 17.

Turkson, M. A., & Norcross, J. C. (1996, March). *Doctoral training in counseling psychology: Admission statistics, student characteristics, and financial assistance.* Paper presented at the annual conference of the Eastern Psychological Association, Philadelphia, PA.

VandeCreek, L., & Fleisher, M. (1984). The role of practicum in the undergraduate psychology curriculum. *Teaching of Psychology, 11,* 9–14.

VandenBos, G. E., Stapp, J., & Kilburg, R. R. (1981). Health service providers in psychology. *American Psychologist, 36,* 1395–1418.

Walfish, S. (2004). An eye-opening experience: Taking an online practice Graduate Record Examination. *Eye on Psi Chi, Winter 2004,* 18, 19, 69.

Walfish, S., Stenmark, D. E., Shealy, J. S., & Shealy, S. E. (1989). Reasons why applicants select clinical psychology graduate programs. *Professional Psychology: Research and Practice, 20,* 350–354.

Walfish, S., & Sumprer, G. F. (1984). Employment opportunities for graduates of APA-approved and non-APA-approved training programs. *American Psychologist, 39,* 1199–1200.

Waters, J., Drew, B., & Ayers, J. (1988). Integrating conflicting needs in curriculum planning: Advice to faculty. In P. J. Woods (Ed.), *Is psychology for them?* Washington, DC: American Psychological Association.

Watkins, C. E., Lopez, F. G., Campbell, V. L., & Himmell, C. D. (1986a). Contemporary counseling psychology: Results of a national survey. *Journal of Counseling Psychology, 33,* 301–309.

Watkins, C. E., Lopez, F. G., Campbell, V. L., & Himmell, C. D. (1986b). Counseling psychology and clinical psychology: Some preliminary comparative data. *American Psychologist, 41,* 581–582.

Whitbourne, S. K. (1999, April). *A guide to personal statements.* Paper presented at the 70th annual meeting of the Eastern Psychological Association, Boston, MA.

Wicherski, M., & Kohout, J. (1992). *Characteristics of graduate departments of psychology: 1990–1991*. Washington, DC: American Psychological Association.

Wicherski, M., & Kohout, J. (2005). *2003 Doctorate Employment Survey*. Retrieved on July 27, 2007 from research .apa.org/des03.html#salaries.

Wittenberg, R. (2003). *Opportunities in social work careers*. Lincolnwood, IL: McGraw-Hill.

Young, K. S., & VandeCreek, L. (1996, March). *Ethnic minority selection procedures in clinical training graduate admissions*. Paper presented at the 67th annual meeting of the Eastern Psychological Association, Philadelphia, PA.

Zebala, J. A., Jones, D. B., & Jones, S. B. (1999). *Medical school admissions: The insider's guide*. New Haven, CT: Mustang.